THE ROY ADAPTATION
MODEL

THIRD EDITION

THE ROY ADAPTATION MODEL

Sister Callista Roy, PhD, RN, FAAN

Professor and Nurse Theorist
Connell School of Nursing
Boston College
Chestnut Hill, Massachusetts

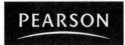

PEARSON

Upper Saddle River, New Jersey 07458

Library of Congress Cataloging-in-Publication Data
Roy, Callista.
    The Roy adaptation model / by Callista Roy.— 3rd ed.
        p.; cm.
    Includes bibliographical references and index.
    ISBN-13: 978-0-13-038497-3 (alk. paper)
    ISBN-10: 0-13-038497-6 (alk. paper)
    1. Roy adaptation model.   2. Nursing—Psychological aspects.   3. Nurse and patient.   I. Title.
    [DNLM: 1. Adaptation, Psychological.   2. Nursing Process.   3. Models, Nursing.
    WY 100 R888r 2008]
    RT84.5.R66 2008
    610.7301'9—dc22   2008027314

Publisher: Julie Levin Alexander
Publisher's Assistant: Regina Bruno
Editor-in-Chief: Maura Connor
Senior Acquisitions Editor: Pamela Fuller
Editorial Assistant: Jennifer Aranda
Managing Production Editor: Patrick Walsh
Production Liaison: Cathy O'Connell
Production Editor: Kavitha Kuttikan, Elm Street
                Publishing Services
Manufacturing Manager: Ilene Sanford

Art Director: Maria Guglielmo
Cover Designer: Bruce Kenselaar
Director of Marketing: Karen Allman
Senior Marketing Manager: Francisco Del Castillo
Marketing Specialist: Michael Sirinides
Composition: Integra Software Services, Pvt. Ltd

Cover Printer: Bind-Rite Graphics
Cover photo: Getty Images, Inc.

Notice: Care has been taken to confirm the accuracy of information presented in this book. The authors, editors, and the publisher, however, cannot accept any responsibility for errors or omissions or for consequences from application of the information in this book and make no warranty, express or implied, with respect to its contents.

The authors and publisher have exerted every effort to ensure that drug selections and dosages set forth in this text are in accord with current recommendations and practice at time of publication. However, in view of ongoing research, changes in government regulations, and the constant flow of information relating to drug therapy and drug reactions, the reader is urged to check the package inserts of all drugs for any change in indications of dosage and for added warnings and precautions. This is particularly important when the recommended agent is a new and/or infrequently employed drug.

Pearson Education LTD., London
Pearson Education Singapore, Pte. Ltd.
Pearson Education, Canada, Inc.
Pearson Education–Japan

Pearson Education Australia PTY, Limited
Pearson Education North Asia, Ltd., Hong Kong
Pearson Educación de Mexico, S.A. de C.V.
Pearson Education Malaysia, Pte. Ltd.
Pearson Education, Upper Saddle River, New Jersey

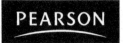

21 2021

ISBN-13:   978-0-13-038497-3
ISBN-10:   0-13-038497-6

PREFACE

This book is an introduction to the Roy Adaptation Model, developed by Sister Callista Roy, for nursing education, clinical practice, and research. The third edition of this primary source text provides an update that (1) maintains the essential concepts of the model while explaining new developments; (2) places the model developments in the context of contemporary issues of health care delivery with social and cultural sensitivity; (3) expands and clarifies the theoretical basis of each adaptive mode; (4) describes adaptive processes for each mode as integrated (effective), compensatory, and compromised (ineffective); (5) provides separate chapters for each adaptive mode at the group level; and (6) expands applications to practice for individuals and groups using clinical practice and case study examples at each step of the nursing process.

Many textbooks discuss nursing models as significant for professional nursing practice, particularly in guiding the nursing process and nurses' relationships with patients. Some texts assess the philosophical, theoretical, and conceptual bases for the views of particular nurse theorists. Other textbooks review the work of nurse theorists and provide analysis and application to practice, education, research, or administration. No other text on a nursing model has the vantage point of unifying and presenting model-based knowledge derived from more than 40 years of conceptual development and implementation in practice, education, and research.

The model was implemented as the basis of the nursing curriculum at Mount St. Mary's College in Los Angeles in March 1970. The program became the laboratory for the development of the model, with faculty, students, and graduates working with Dr. Roy to develop and publish the elements of the model. Today, the faculty and campus at Mount St. Mary's College provide the flagship implementation of the model in nursing education that is recognized throughout the world. Faculty at Mount St. Mary's continue to be friends and colleagues who provided significant input for this revision.

This book builds on the first two editions and on four previous books on the Roy Adaptation Model authored by Roy, with contributions by colleagues at Mount St. Mary's. A significant development for the Roy model publications was Roy's collaboration with Dr. Heather Andrews in 1986, 1991, and 1999. Dr. Andrews brought a wealth of knowledge and experience as an educator using the Roy Adaptation Model and also the perspective of a nursing administrator in complex health care systems in Canada. Her contribution to this edition included the original planning and authoring of the new content on the interdependence mode of relating persons at the group level.

CHANGES IN CONTENT AND ORGANIZATION

The essentials of the model were used to organize this edition, and much of the basic content from the second edition has been included. However, this edition incorporates significant changes in both content and organization.

- Each chapter on the adaptive modes has been reorganized to include the components and integrated life processes as the theoretical basis. Illustrations for self-concept, role function, and interdependence relate mode components to the life processes.
- The other two levels of adaptive processes, compensatory processes and compromised processes, are described with updated references. New content is added to provide relevant examples of adaptation at each level.

- The material on adaptive processes of groups has been moved to a separate part of the book dealing only with groups. These new chapters expand this content significantly to include group adaptive modes that parallel the development of the adaptive modes at the individual level and their use in nursing practice.
- The nursing process within each chapter is based on the theoretical content of each adaptive mode. Identifying relevant behaviors and stimuli leads to making nursing judgments about nursing diagnoses, goals, interventions, and evaluation. The tables that relate Roy's typology of positive indicators of adaptation and adaptation problems to the work of the North American Nursing Diagnosis Association have been significantly updated. Key definitions, figures, and tables have been retained, and new ones have been added as they relate to the expanded content. Presentation of nursing care planning provides case applications within each chapter; three of the chapters include a single family case study.
- A particular feature of this edition is further explanation of Roy's philosophical and scientific assumptions for the 21st century and the addition of cultural assumptions. The assumptions are discussed as they derive from a synthesis of Roy's earlier work with her thinking about cosmic knowledge in the new millennium. The aim is to update content but also to look to the future of nursing knowledge development based on the model and to the global use of the model.

ORGANIZATION

This edition of the text is divided into four parts. Part One provides the foundation for more detailed exploration of the Roy Adaptation Model. Chapter 1 introduces the reader to the profession of nursing and the developing knowledge base for practice. The role of models in nursing knowledge is described. Chapter 2 focuses specifically on the Roy Adaptation Model and describes the elements of the model using the major concepts associated with nursing in general. Chapter 3 provides the reader with an overview of the nursing process according to the model. In Chapter 4, a broad perspective of the four adaptive modes for both individuals and groups, including the theories used in their development, is presented.

Part Two addresses the adaptive modes on the individual level and how knowledge of the mode provides the basis for planning nursing care. The four adaptive modes for individuals are named the physiologic, self-concept, role function, and interdependence adaptive modes. An understanding of each mode and application in planning nursing care is the focus. Chapters 5 to 13 cover the physiologic mode for the individual. The physiologic mode chapters are organized by the five needs and four complex processes of the physiologic mode of the individual. Chapters 14, 15, and 16 present the self-concept, role function, and interdependence modes, respectively. Each of these chapters describes the process of nursing care for individuals.

Part Three includes new chapters that develop content for each adaptive mode at the group level. Chapter 17 focuses on the physical mode of the group, Chapter 18 discusses group identity, and Chapters 19 and 20 deal with the role function mode and the interdependence mode on the group level. The examples for practice use different types of groups. Although a nurse may not work with groups, the nurse is a member of many groups and can identify with the content and examples given.

Part Four consists of one chapter, Chapter 21, which focuses on the application of the model in three important areas. First, applications to nursing practice show the variety and scope of projects that apply the model in health care agencies at the unit or organizational levels. The major project reported in the second edition, the process and outcomes of implementing the Roy Adaptation Model as a basis for nursing practice at St. Joseph Regional Medical Center in Lewiston, Idaho, has been abstracted for this edition to provide some detail of practice applications. Based on the dramatic impact of technology developments in health care, the second major section of the chapter focuses on the electronic healthcare record (EHR) as a significant contemporary application in nursing practice. The final section of this chapter deals with research based on the Roy Adaptation Model. We describe a review, critique, and synthesis of 30 years of research based on the Roy Adaptation Model that includes 218 studies published in the English language. We then use the review to propose a redefinition of evidence-based-practice.

This text is intended primarily for use in educational institutions and agencies that use the Roy Adaptation Model as the basis for nursing practice and education. It provides essential content for entry-level nursing students, new nursing service personnel, and faculty. Nurses in practice with individuals, families, communities, and organizations with interest in the global society will find useful content. Master's level students will find the clarity of presentation and the updated content an efficient method to become acquainted with the essentials and recent developments of the model. Doctoral students and other nurse scholars can find within the elements of the model the basis for significant research questions and for adding to basic and clinical knowledge development. Derivations of new applications to all nursing specialties, including independent practice, are implied from the essentials described here and from the references cited.

This text provides a clear articulation of the essence of nursing to the profession, to other health care disciplines, and to the public. Every effort has been made to focus on the essential nature of nursing, its unique perspective, role, and the implications of what that role means as the systems of health care are shifting. This clarity can help facilitate the transition to effective systems that meet the needs of individuals and societal groups of the early 21st century.

ACKNOWLEDGMENTS

I am indebted to all those who have enhanced the development of this text, in particular those listed as contributors, past and present. I appreciate greatly those who have stimulated the development of the model through many years at home and around the globe. Nurses in practice, faculty colleagues, and students at all levels provide insightful observations and questions that stimulate this ongoing work.

Editorial and staff assistance has been provided by a grant from the Sisters of St. Joseph of Carondelet. Those working with me under this grant included Kate Meyers, Barbara Bellesi, and Emily Caskey. In particular, Emily's quick learning of all the details involved and commitment to the project made it possible to finally meet the final deadlines.

I appreciate the staff at Pearson Health Science, particularly Executive Acquisitions Editor Pamela Fuller; Jennifer Aranda, Editorial Assistant; and Cathy O'Connell, Production Editor, who have been patient with my efforts to update the content and organization of the text, while moving forward with production.

Sister Callista Roy

CONTRIBUTORS

I would like to acknowledge in a special way the authors of previous versions of the text (1976, 1984, 1991, and 1999) who contributed to the development of many of the basic concepts of the Roy Adaptation Model and provided the basis for the flagship implementation of the model in nursing education at Mount St. Mary's College, Los Angeles, California.

- Faculty from Mount St. Mary's College, Los Angeles, California:

Sue Ann Brown
Marjorie Buck
Zona Chalifoux
Joan Seo Cho
Edda Coughran
Marjorie Clowry Dobratz
Marie Driever
Sheila Driscoll
Jeannine R. Dunn
Janet Dunning
Edythe Ellison
Barbara Gruendemann
Joan Hansen
C. Margaret Henderson
Mary Hicks
Mary Howard
Karen Jensen

Sonja Liggett
Sister Theresa Marie McIntier
Nancy Malaznik
Kathleen Anschutz Nuwayhid
Nancy Zewen Perley
Brooke Randell
Marsha Milton Roberson
Marsha Keiko Sato
Ann Macaluso Schofield
Jane Servonsky
Mary Sloper
Nancy Taylor
Mary Poush Tedrow
Catherine Rivera Thompson
Sharon Vairo
Joyce Van Landingham

- Graduates of Mount St. Mary's College:

Lorraine Ann Marshall
Cecilia Martinez
Sally Valentine

- Colleagues of Sister Callista Roy:

Joanne Gray
Donna Romyn

- Colleague, co-author of three text books on the Roy Adaptation Model, and Honorary Lifetime member of the Roy Adaptation Association:

Heather Andrews

- Research Fellows and Assistants to the Theorist for Third Edition:

Ruthann Looper
Marguarite Tierney, CSJ

CONTRIBUTORS TO THIRD EDITION

Chapters 6 and 7:
>Heather Vallent, MS, RN
>Nursing Clinical Instructor
>Connell School of Nursing
>Boston College
>Chestnut Hill, Massachusetts

Chapters 9 and 13:
>Patti Underwood, MS, RN
>PhD Student
>Connell School of Nursing
>Boston College
>Chestnut Hill, Massachusetts

Chapter 15:
>Barbara Bellesi, MFA
>Formerly Editorial Assistant
>Boston College
>Chestnut Hill, Massachusetts

Chapter 17:
>Mary Margaret Segraves, PhD, APRN
>School Health Nurse
>Cambridge Department of Public Health
>Cambridge, Massachusetts

Chapter 20:
>Heather Andrews, PhD
>Hearing Chair and Commissioner, Appeals Commission for Alberta Workers'
>Compensation
>Edmonton, Alberta, Canada

Chapter 21:
>Pamela Senesac, PhD, RN
>Assistant Professor and Associate Director, Graduate Programs in Nursing
>Massachusetts General Hospital Institute of Health Professions
>Boston, Massachusetts

>Carolyn Padovano, PhD, RN
>Director, SNOMED Terminology Solutions

>Kathleen Connerly, MS, RN
>Vice President Patient Care Services
>St. Joseph Regional Medical Center
>Lewiston, Idaho

Susanna Ristau, RN
Program Director, Patient Care Services
St. Joseph Regional Medical Center
Lewiston, Idaho

Coralee Lindberg, RN, BSN
Director Medical/Surgical Departments
St. Joseph Regional Medical Center
Lewiston, Idaho

Mary McFarland, PhD, RN
Dean and Professor of Professional Studies
Gonzaga University
Spokane, Washington

REVIEWERS

Mary Baumberger-Henry, RN, DNSc
Associate Professor
Widener University
Chester, Pennsylvania

Mary Bliesmer, DNSc, APRN, BC
Professor and Chair
School of Nursing
Minnesota State University
Mankato, Minnesota

Diane Breckenridge, PhD, RN
Associate Professor
School of Nursing and Health Sciences
La Salle University
Philadelphia, Pennsylvania

Catherine Dearman, RN, PhD
Professor and Chair Maternal Child Health
College of Nursing
Springhill Campus
University of South Alabama
Mobile, Alabama

Pauline M. Green PhD, CNE, RN
Professor
Howard University Division of Nursing
Washington, DC

Joyce Knestrick, PhD, RN, CRNP , FAANP
Associate Professor
Wheeling Jesuit University
Wheeling, West Virginia

Hernani L. Ledesma Jr., PTA, RN, MHA, MSN
Instructor
Mount St. Mary's College
Los Angeles, California

Rebecca Otten, EdD, RN
Assistant Professor
California State University
Fullerton, California

Barbara Ponder, MS, RN, APNP, CCNS
Assistant Professor
Marian College of Fond du Lac
Fond du Lac, Wisconsin

Pamela R. Santarlasci RN, MSN, CRNP, PhD (c)
Assistant Professor of Nursing
Delaware County Community College
Media, Pennsylvania

Marsha Sato, EdD, MN, RN
Associate Professor and Director of Master of Science in Nursing Program
Mount St. Mary's College
Los Angeles, California

Kim Webb, RN, MN
Nursing Chair
Northern Oklahoma College
Tonkawa, Oklahoma

CONTENTS

PART ONE

Introduction to the Roy Adaptation Model

The Roy Adaptation Model has been considered one of the most highly developed and widely used conceptual descriptions of nursing. The model development began in the late 1960s and since that time nurses in the United States and around the world have helped Roy to clarify, refine, and extend the concepts. The presentation of the model in this text takes advantage of this ongoing work and the challenges of the 21st-century global community. The major concepts associated with nursing models—recipient of care, the environment, health, the goal of nursing, and nursing activities—are introduced in this section and discussed in further detail throughout the text.

Part 1 of this text provides the groundwork for more detailed exploration of the Roy Adaptation Model. In Chapter 1, the reader is introduced to the profession of nursing and the developing knowledge base for practice. In addition the role of models in nursing knowledge is described. Chapter 2 focuses specifically on the Roy Adaptation Model and describes the elements of the model using the major concepts associated with nursing in general. Chapter 3 provides the reader with an overview of the nursing process according to the model. Chapter 4 describes a broad perspective of the four adaptive modes for both individuals and groups. This introductory section leads to Part 2 which addresses the adaptive modes on the individual level and how knowledge of the mode provides the basis for planning nursing care.

CHAPTER 1

Nursing as a Knowledge-Based Profession

Nursing is a profession that meets health care needs in society. All professions have two characteristics. First, professions contribute to the good of society. Second, professionals are educated to use specialized knowledge to meet specific needs of society. Health and well-being are important needs for individuals, families, nations, and the global community. This chapter focuses on the nature of nursing as a knowledge-based health care profession. The kind of knowledge that is the foundation for professional nursing practice is identified. Ways of developing knowledge are described. Conceptual models for nursing practice are one approach to developing nursing knowledge. Several nursing models are described. This chapter provides background for study of the Roy Adaptation Model.

OBJECTIVES

After studying this chapter, the reader will be able to do the following:

1. Identify two characteristics of professions.
2. Describe the contributions that nursing makes to society.
3. Name two characteristics of 21st-century nursing.
4. Describe one philosophical assumption about people held by nurses.
5. List three approaches to knowledge development for the science of nursing.
6. Identify the essential elements of a conceptual model for nursing.
7. Associate specified elements of a conceptual model with the model's author.

KEY CONCEPTS DEFINED

Conceptual model for nursing: A set of concepts or images that identify and relate the essential elements of nursing, including individual, environment, health, goal of nursing, and nursing activities.

Environment: In nursing, all that influences people and their health including physical surroundings, other people, and the earth and its life-giving, but limited, resources.

Health: In general, the individual's total well-being; refers to the regular patterns of people and their environments that result in maintaining wholeness and human integrity.

Holistic: The philosophic assumption about people that refers to the physical, thinking, and feeling processes functioning together in human behavioral patterns.

Model: A description or analogy used to help visualize something that cannot be observed directly.

Knowledge: In nursing, involves philosophic and scientific principles related to people, environment, and health, particularly of human processes and patterns that can enhance health.

Nursing: A health care profession that focuses on the life processes and patterns of people with a commitment to promote health and full life-potential for individuals, families, groups, and the global society.

Philosophic assumptions: The values and beliefs that are the foundation of nursing knowledge and practice.

Profession: A group that contributes to the good of society by using specialized knowledge.

NATURE OF NURSING

Nursing is a health care profession. Nurses use specialized knowledge to contribute to the needs of society for health and well-being. Professions have developed to meet the many needs in society. Law professionals aim to maintain justice and civil order. Clergy are expected to meet spiritual needs and to interpret religious doctrine and practice. Among the needs of society, health and well-being are basic. Without health and well-being, the individual cannot live a satisfying and productive life. Human potential can be limited without health and if health care needs are not met. When people in a society are not using their full human capabilities, the society itself is threatened.

Several professions have developed to contribute to health and well-being. Medicine came about to heal illness and injury. Pharmacy developed to prepare and dispense medicinal preparations. Physical therapy uses heat, massage, and muscle training to treat illness and injury. What is the particular need for which nursing is accountable? Nursing has developed knowledge of the life patterns and processes of people and their interactions with the environment to promote health and full life-potential for individuals, families, groups, and society as a whole. The special need is for understanding people to help them manage their health. This focus is expanded upon in this chapter.

Let us begin with an example. Assume that a young mother takes her child to see a physician because the child has an earache. The physician writes a prescription for medication that can be filled by the pharmacist at the local drugstore. However, the mother does not fill the prescription. A much broader understanding of what is going on with the mother and child and in their environment is needed to promote their health and perhaps that of their community. Likely you can think of at least three areas that the nurse with a broad knowledge base might explore in this situation.

Throughout history, there have been individuals, both men and women, who tended to the sick, injured, and children. This was particularly the case in times of threats such as plague, famine, or war. As nursing evolved, the profession included both art and science. Knowledge and skill and sensitivity in using knowledge are required to meet the complex needs in contemporary society. To meet health needs in the 21st century in particular requires a broad education and understanding of people, their environments, and health.

We need to understand the place of people on our earth and how health is affected by our changing world. In one history of nursing, it was said that as professions developed it never occurred to thinkers that "it would be safer for the public welfare if nurses were educated instead of lawyers" (Robinson, 1946, ix). Modern nursing was inspired by the efforts of Florence Nightingale. Nightingale's work as a nurse during the Crimean War and in Britain provided the general principles to identify nursing's place in society.

Characteristics of 21st-Century Nursing

To describe nursing in a new century, we look to our roots. Florence Nightingale was committed to accomplishing good for those who suffered. In Victorian England she was touched by the needs she saw around her, particularly of poor children who were ill. Nightingale was determined to do more than live a life of security and comfort, supported by her family, as women of her class did in the 19th century. When her country went to war in Eastern Europe, she organized women to go with her to provide nursing care to injured and ill soldiers. Other courageous people have similarly provided nursing care in difficult situations. In civil wars in both the United States and France, women, particularly those who were in religious groups, went to the battlefields to provide care and comfort. However, in addition to her extensive health care work, Nightingale also left a legacy of writings about the nature of nursing and of her actions to improve health in her society.

In her influential writings, Nightingale emphasized that nursing was more than administering medications and applying bandages. Rather, nursing aims to promote health by using the environment to aid the natural processes of the body to heal itself. The essentials of nursing, according to Nightingale, include fresh air, light, warmth, cleanliness, quiet, and the proper selection and administration of diet. She strongly advocated that mothers, teachers, and nurses be educated in the laws of life, that is, understanding what makes for "healthy existences" (Nightingale, 1859, p. 7). Nightingale declared that nursing was a significant way to improve the health of the British nation. In the schools of nursing she established, nurses were educated to understand health and how to use the environment, both to promote health and to provide energy for the individual's natural healing processes. The Nightingale approach to nursing education came to North America in the founding of three schools in 1873: Bellevue Training School in New York City, the Connecticut Training School in New Haven, and Boston Training School (Donahue, 1996).

Writings of nurses in the last decades of the 20th century expanded richly on the characteristics of nursing that Nightingale articulated. Also during these decades great challenges were created by changes in health care. Some changes came from new developments in science and technology. Other changes were based on economics and politics. Technology makes it possible to diagnose and treat more illnesses than in the past. Still, in the United States society has not found a way to pay for health care for all. Ethical and social developments have not kept up with science. The needs of society related to health include a complex environment.

Nursing knowledge development in the 21st century builds on the advances in understanding people and their health needs. It also takes into account the unresolved concerns with health care delivery. Further, knowledge moves forward by expanding ways to develop knowledge for practice. Nurses need technical knowledge and skills related to health and recovery of health. But they need to know more than procedures and the functions of medical assistants. Nurses also need to know how to help people promote their health and deal with episodes of illness in a changing environment.

Focus of Knowledge for Nursing

As a health care profession, nursing uses specialized knowledge. For some time nurses have recognized the need to focus clinical knowledge on holism of people, processes, environment, and health (Allan & Hall, 1988). Nursing today has a strong knowledge base including each of these. This focus is noted in the nursing models used as illustrations in this chapter and in the discussion of the Roy Adaptation Model.

The goal of nursing's social commitment is to contribute to health by focusing on life processes of individuals in their environments. This goal directed the development of specialized nursing knowledge and was reflected in an influential article by Donaldson and Crowley (1978) three decades ago. These authors identified the commonalities of nursing as the following:

1. Concern with principles and laws that govern life processes, well-being, and optimum functioning of human beings, sick or well.
2. Concern with the pattern of human behavior in interaction with the environment in critical life situations.
3. Concern with the processes by which positive changes in health status are effected.

In outlining knowledge needed in the nursing practice, it has been useful to focus on understanding people (or recipients of nursing care), environment, and health. The role of nurses is to use this knowledge in promoting health.

The individual is the main focus of nursing. Nurses are involved in the health of people as individuals and in groups such as families and the communities that form society. Knowledge includes values and beliefs as well as scientific facts and principles. The values and beliefs of nursing are referred to as philosophic assumptions. Major philosophic assumptions about the individual include

1. The individual is of value, and therefore possesses dignity and is worthy of respect and care.
2. People are responsible for making decisions that influence their lives.
3. People are holistic, that is, their physical, thinking, and feeling processes function together in a unified expression of human behavioral patterns.
4. People function interdependently with other individuals in environments of the earth to create societies.

To understand the person, the nurse begins with a strong commitment to values about the individual. These beliefs are not enough, however. The nurse will also have knowledge about the science of holistic individuals. This knowledge will be biobehavioral and will include the understanding of the individual as a living system made up of cells and physiologic body systems. Nursing knowledge of individuals will also focus on how people behave holistically to influence their health. Nursing conceptual models further enhance the understanding and knowledge about individuals as a main focus of nursing knowledge. Recent developments of the Roy Adaptation Model in particular have focused on philosophical assumptions of individuals and on the description of life processes within each adaptive mode.

To know people in their life situations, the nurse learns to relate to the patient. One aspect of this relationship has been described in the literature as caring. Leininger and McFarland (2002) and Watson (2005) described caring as central to the nature of nursing. Transcultural nursing studies over many years led Leininger to identify both the commonalities of caring in all cultures and the diversities in expressions. Watson developed 10 carative factors related to what she calls the caring and sacred science of nursing. In the Scandinavian countries, caring has been a strong basis for nursing.

Since nursing's concern is with individuals in interaction with the environment, the second area of nursing knowledge is environment. Nurses in occupational health have noted that Nightingale's "broad conceptualization of the environment included recognition of the effect of social, economic, and political forces on the health of British soldiers during the Crimean War" (Salazar & Primoto, 1994, p. 317). Environment from a nursing perspective has been described as all that influences people and their health. In particular, environment refers to the individual's physical surroundings, warm or cold, comfortable or plain, and the people in one's life, whether they are supportive or indifferent. A contemporary view of environment includes the earth and its resources that are both life-giving and limited. Increasingly health providers are noting the relationship between the ecology of the earth and health as well as the future of humans and other life on the earth. Box 1–1 presents a vivid image of environment and concern for the earth.

BOX 1–1

Example of Relating Ecology and Health

Case Report

The patient is an elderly woman, beloved in her community, who comes to your office with a list of serious problems. She has night sweats and fevers that have been getting worse for the last few years. She has difficulty breathing and on examination seems to have suffered from aspiration pneumonia. She has alopecia, having lost her hair in a patchy distribution. Her normal gastrointestinal flora has been invaded by a few noxious species, and she has persistent diarrhea. Her skin is marked by an extensive dermatitis: it is fissured, inflamed, gouged, scraped, denuded, and cracking in many places. These excoriations are caused by a small but extremely industrious organism whose numbers have grown exponentially during the last few years, displacing and even eliminating other organisms that used to be widely distributed on the skin of our patient.

Interpretation: The patient is the Earth; Symptoms Night Sweats and Fevers = Global Warming; Respiratory Disease = Poor Air Quality; Alopecia = Deforestation; Diarrhea = Loss of Biodiversity; Dermatitis = Overpopulation

Differential Diagnosis: Global Environmental Change

Rosenblatt, Roger A. "*Ecological change and the future of the human species: Can physicians make a difference? (REFLECTIONS)*." *Annals of Family Medicine* 3.2 (March-April 2005): 173. Adapted with permission.

As Nightingale noted in her basic ideas about nursing, it is important for the nurse to know the laws of health or what makes for "healthy existence." In general, the concept of health refers to the individual's total well-being. The laws of health that are part of nursing knowledge refer to the regular patterns noted in people and their environments, which result in the individual's maintaining wholeness and integrity. The integrity of the individual is defined by what nurses believe about people, that is, that they are valued; are in charge of their lives; have consistency of thinking, feeling, and being; and are in balanced relationships with their world and others in it. Knowledge for nursing, then, includes understanding health.

Nursing knowledge focuses on people and how they interact with their environments to enhance well-being and human flourishing, whether sick or well. For example, nurses are concerned with how a mother of a young child can manage her child's earache, how a developmentally challenged adolescent can reach the highest level of functioning, and how the patient with Alzheimer's disease can maintain the right to make decisions as long as possible. Nursing knowledge also looks at patterns of human behavior within particular environments, and at various critical periods of life. In each lifetime, there are times that are more significant for the individual. There are expected gradual changes, such as adolescence, or more abrupt or unexpected changes, such as sudden injury or illness. Nurses deal with developing families when a baby is born. They observe how family members prepare themselves and their home when a loved one is returning to them after suffering a disabling illness, such as a stroke.

Finally, nursing knowledge deals with ways in which people can bring about positive changes in their interactions with the environment to promote health. Nurses go beyond simply learning about how certain factors threaten an individual's health. For example, we know that a high-fat diet increases the risk for heart disease. Nursing knowledge is also concerned with all aspects of the processes for promoting health. In the example of diet related to heart disease, nursing knowledge broadens to understand individual life processes. These include processes of developing eating habits and changing underlying needs and attitudes, as well as the learning processes that are most effective for a given individual. In addition, nursing knowledge considers social processes such as regional economic pressures and marketing strategies of the fast food industry. There are also political issues to look at such as debates about government regulation of foods sold in public places and individual freedom to choose what to eat.

To help people promote their health, nursing knowledge includes clinical reasoning. Nightingale (1859) alluded to this nursing thought process in her persuasive discussion about the importance of observation. She noted that the nurse "must be a sound, and close, and quick observer; and she must be a woman of delicate and decent feeling" (Nightingale, 1859, p. 71). Authors have derived models of nursing clinical judgment. The model by Gordon, Murphy, Candee, and Hiltunen (1994) distinguishes three types of clinical reasoning: diagnostic, ethical, and therapeutic. Other authors have described how intuition and analytical reasoning are both used in clinical judgments (Lamond & Thompson, 2000).

Being active in changing standards of health care and in addressing what affects health is another way that nurses promote health. Aiken (1992) noted that nurses in the United States during the 1980s gained a foothold in national, state, and local public policy arenas. In the 1990s nurses were more optimistic about using public policy to improve health care. Lynaugh (1992) assessed nursing's history in relation to society and noted that the profession is more pragmatic and confrontational, and less deferential and altruistic, than it used to be. In this sense, it is more integrated and less isolated from the larger society.

One example of nursing action to promote health was nurses as leaders from 1991 to 2004 in the privately funded national program All Kids Count Childhood Immunization Initiative. The purpose of the program was to establish immunization monitoring and follow-up systems. When combined with other local, state, and federal immunization efforts, this system helped increase immunization rates among preschool children and reduced rates of illness, disability, and death from vaccine-preventable diseases. The initiative took a simple idea and dealt with the complexities of the intersecting public and private sector responsibilities for child health care. It played a role in setting national policy for the development of an immunization registry and follow-up systems (Isaacs & Knickman, 1997).

Nurse authors are envisioning and studying health promotion at both the population-based and global levels. Butterfield (2002) encouraged nurses to consider the social, economic, and environmental origins of health problems that manifest at the population level. For example, she and her colleagues (Hill, Butterfield, & Larsson, 2006) have studied rural parents' perception of risks associated with exposure of their children to radon. Perry and Gregory (2007) focused on an ethical framework to support transcultural understanding and global social justice as well as concern for the global ecosystem. Perry (2005) researched the influence of nursing testimony on environmental justice legislation.

Thus, the characteristics of 21st-century nursing can be summarized based on the rich heritage of nursing and on the scholarly work and clinical practice of contemporary nurses. Nursing is a health care profession that focuses on the life processes and patterns of individuals. Caring is a key aspect of the nursing commitment within relationships with patients. The emphasis is on health and how mutual interactions of the individual and environment promote health. Clinical reasoning skills are needed in the practice of professional nursing. As a profession, nursing has a commitment to promote health and full life-potential for individuals, families, groups, and the global society.

Knowledge Development in Nursing

As, noted nursing is a knowledge-based profession that uses its knowledge for the good of society. With the demands of the 21st century, nurses are expanding their ways to develop knowledge. Knowledge in nursing involves philosophic assumptions and scientific principles related to individuals, environment, and health. Philosophic assumptions and scientific principles are developed by a community of scholars who also practice nursing. Florence Nightingale (1859) initially developed the profession of nursing by writing down her convictions and observations in caring for soldiers affected by war and the environment of war. The consensus of nurses, reflected in their writings, has led to the commonly held values and beliefs about people. One example of a value-based paper was developed by participants at a nursing knowledge conference designed to reach consensus about people, nursing, nursing theory, and the links to nursing practice (Roy & Jones, 2007).

The science of nursing is also developed by the community of scholars and practitioners of nursing. The development of scientific principles, however, also involves a scientific approach and evidence beyond common consensus. Nurses today are promoting the use of research in practice in a movement called evidence-based practice (Melnyk & Fineout-Overholt, 2005). Evidence may be based on empirical knowledge, but also on other ways of knowing such as personal, ethical, aesthetic, and social political (Chinn & Kramer, 2004). The purpose of science is to observe, classify, and investigate relationships. These relationships lead to understanding and the ability to deal with natural phenomena. Phenomena are the objects of study in science.

A scientific approach observes and classifies phenomena, or objects, according to a particular viewpoint. The relationships between the phenomena, or the parts of any one object, are then identified and the general theories or principles of their interaction are stated and tested. Thus, in biology, living organisms, from the smallest ones, such as invisible viruses, to the complex human being, are arranged in a hierarchy according to their various characteristics. As biologists studied living beings, they identified patterns of the activities of various species, for example, ingestion and reproduction. In this way, general theories or statements of relationships that are believed to hold true under given conditions are established. Thus, the field of biology proposes certain principles about the replication and duplication of genetic material in all living beings.

In the development of scientific knowledge for nursing, nurses observe and classify the processes of the individual interacting with the environment to promote health. The relationships among the concepts and the processes are identified and the general theories of their interactions and how nurses can affect them are stated and tested. With their growing knowledge about people's holistic processes for promoting their own well-being, nurses can have a significant impact on levels of health status.

The methods that nurses use for developing knowledge for the science of nursing include three approaches: nursing conceptual model development, theory construction, and research to test and develop new theories. Theories can be broad and are called grand theories. Theories can also be middle range when they explain specific processes, but are ones that can be applied in many clinical situations such as a theory of role transitions. In this text, discussion focuses on the first level, and specifically, the Roy Adaptation Model. From the concepts of the model many theories can be developed. Each conceptual model for nursing provides a particular focus for the study of life processes and how they can affect health status.

NURSING MODELS

A model is defined most simply as a description or analogy used to help visualize something that cannot be observed directly. When scientists work with problems of travel in space, they use models of the galaxies and models of spacecraft. The pieces of the models represent the features of the actual galaxies and spacecraft that are involved. However, these representations are in an abstract form. They can be built with Styrofoam and glue to some miniature scale of what they stand for, or they can be further abstracted to mathematical formulas and appear as dots and lines in motion on a computer screen or words in sentences that denote concepts and their relationships.

The scientific body of knowledge associated with the nursing models supports the provision of a professional service to society, namely, contributing to health by focusing on life processes of people in their environments. Just as any model is made up of the essential parts of what it represents, so a nursing model is made up of essential parts, or elements, of nursing. We define a conceptual model for nursing as a set of concepts or images that identify and relate the essential elements of nursing. The essential elements of a model for nursing practice, or concepts to be included, are as follows:

1. A description of the individual or group receiving nursing care.
2. A specified meaning for environment.
3. A definition of health.
4. A statement of the broad goal of nursing.
5. A delineation of approaches to reach the goal of nursing.

A model describes each of these concepts and shows in a general way how the concepts are related to one another. From the time of Florence Nightingale (1820–1910) to the present, the writings of nurses can be analyzed to show various ways of addressing the major concepts of nursing. Some authors identify as many as 30 different nursing models, many from the United States, but also from the United Kingdom and Scandinavian countries (Marriner Tomey & Alligood, 2006; Pearson, Vaughan, & FitzGerald, 2005). Models are sometimes referred to as grand theories or conceptual frameworks. Current textbooks describe a number of middle range theories that are derived from the nursing models or from clinical research (Peterson & Bedrow, 2004; Smith & Liehr, 2003).

For illustration, seven models are selected to describe in this chapter. This discussion can prepare the reader to pursue the expanding literature in the field. A brief description of the selected authors' views of individual, environment, health, and nursing goals and approaches are summarized in Table 1–1 and discussed in the following section.

Selected Examples

HILDEGARD PEPLAU   Hildegard Peplau had a significant influence on model development in nursing. With a background in psychiatric nursing, Peplau presented the elements of her model in a 1952 book, *Interpersonal Relations in Nursing*. Peplau's work had an impact, not only on the teaching of psychiatric nursing, but also on the shift in models of nursing from a major focus on the needs of the individual to a focus that included the nurse–patient relationship. Peplau was influential in defining nursing and served on the task force of the Congress for Nursing Practice of the American Nurses Association, which issued a landmark policy statement on the nature and scope of nursing practice (American Nurses Association, 1982).

Peplau focused attention on the individual receiving nursing care as a developing personality. Careful observations and thoughtful insights from clinical work provided the basis for the concepts of this nursing model. In addition, a study of the work of psychoanalytic theorist Harry Stack Sullivan (1953) added background for understanding the individual, and for describing the dynamic interaction that occurs during development in early infancy and childhood. The individual seeks satisfaction of physiologic demands, interpersonal security, and interpersonal contact. In this process, tensions of need, anxiety, and loneliness are created. The energy of these tensions, according to Peplau, can be transformed in positive directions.

Peplau did not define or describe the concept of environment. However, her writing reflected the general notion of environment as including the cultural and social context. Particularly, it is the cultural forces, together with the infant's biological constitution, that determine personality.

For Peplau, health is a word symbol that implies forward movement of personality and other ongoing human processes in the direction of creative, productive personal and community living. Her writing emphasized personality development and nursing as an approach to people rather than describing health or environment in detail.

Given Peplau's view of the individual, the specific goal of nursing can be stated most simply as: to foster forward movement of the personality and other ongoing human processes in the direction of creative, constructive, and productive personal and community living. Peplau noted that nurses facilitate natural ongoing tendencies in people. The nurse is an educating instrument and a maturing force, aiming at forward movement. Peplau's greatest contribution to the development of nursing science was the delineation of the interpersonal

TABLE 1–1 Examples of Nursing Models

Person	Environment	Health	Nursing Goal and Approaches
Peplau			
A developing being pursuing satisfaction and interpersonal security and contact.	Cultural and social context.	A word symbol that implies the forward movement of the personality and other ongoing human processes in the direction of constructive, productive, personal and community living.	Development of personality and other human processes through significant, therapeutic interpersonal relationships, with four phases.
Orem			
An individual with universal, developmental, and health deviation types of self-care requisites who may vary in power to engage in self-care.	Physical, chemical, biologic, and social conditions relevant to self-care requisites and basic conditioning factors.	A state of the person characterized by soundness or wholeness of developed human structures and of bodily and mental functioning that requires continuous self-care of therapeutic quality.	To help people maintain their own and dependent others' self-care demands by helping the patient accomplish therapeutic self-care and move toward independent self-care as well as become competent in providing and managing care requisites.
Rogers			
A unitary, pandimensional, negentrophic energy field identified by pattern, organization, and manifestation of characteristics and behaviors that are specific to the whole, which cannot be predicted from knowledge of the parts.	An irreducible pandimensional energy field identified by pattern and organization and integral with the human field.	A rhythmic pattern of energy exchange which is mutually enhancing and expresses full life-potential.	To strengthen the integrity of the human-environment energy field by directing and redirecting patterning, primarily by noninvasive modalities.

(continued)

TABLE 1–1 *(continued)*

Person	Environment	Health	Nursing Goal and Approaches
Roy			
An adaptive system with cognator and regulator subsystems acting to maintain adaptation in the four adaptive modes: physiologic-physical, self-concept–group identity, role function, and interdependence.	All conditions, circumstances, and influences surrounding and affecting the development and behavior of persons and groups, with particular consideration of mutuality of person and earth resources.	A state and a process of being and becoming integrated and whole that reflects person and environment mutually.	To promote adaptation for individuals and groups in the four adaptive modes, thus contributing to health, quality of life, and dying with dignity by assessing behavior and factors that influence adaptive abilities and to enhance environmental interactions.
Newman			
Pattern of consciousness that is expanding and moving through varying degrees of organization and disorganization as one unitary process.	Implicate order, or unseen multidimensional pattern, as ground or basis for all things and the explicate order, or tangibles, that periodically arise as temporary manifestations of the total pattern.	Expanding consciousness, pattern of the whole, encompassing disease and nondisease, regarded as the explication of the underlying pattern of the person and environment.	Pattern identification and expanding consciousness through personal transformations and forming shared consciousness.
Leininger			
Individual in a given cultural context that has learned, shared, and transmitted values, beliefs, norms, and lifeways that guide individual thinking, decisions, and actions in patterned ways.	The context of the totality of an event, situation, or particular experience that give meaning to human expressions, interpretations, and social interactions in particular physical, ecological, sociopolitical, and cultural settings.	A state of well-being that is culturally defined, valued, and practiced, and which reflects the ability of individuals, or groups, to perform their daily role activities in culturally expressed, beneficial, and patterned lifeways.	To focus on human care phenomena and activities in order to assist, support, facilitate, or enable individuals and groups to maintain, or regain, their well-being by using cultural care preservation and maintenance, accommodation and negotiation, and repatterning or restructuring.

TABLE 1–1 (*continued*)

Person	Environment	Health	Nursing Goal and Approaches
		Boykin and Schoenhofer	
Human mode of being is living caring and growing caring; individual is complete and whole in any given moment.	Social context of nurturing relationships, relational responsibilities and possibilities.	Living out who we are, demonstrating congruence between beliefs and behaviors, and living out the meaning of our lives.	Caring is both the goal and activity of nursing; nursing situation is lived experience of caring between the nurse and one nursed in which both enhanced; involves direct invitation, call for nursing, caring between and nursing response.

process as the approach used in nursing. The nurse improves the individual's social context by therapeutic interaction with the individual. Peplau described this process as a series of phases involving different roles for the nurse and the individual.

The orientation phase involves learning about the individual's difficulty and the extent of the need for help. The identification phase is the time that the individual is responding to the nurse and feeling a sense of belonging and identification. The exploitation phase occurs when the individual identifies with the nurse and makes full use of the services offered, including the nurse's interpersonal skills. The resolution phase generally completes the process as old ties and dependencies are relinquished and the individual prepares to resume independence. Peplau's emphasis is that the phases, and roles of nurse and patient within the phases, are fluid and tend to flow together or move backward or forward as the person moves forward or regresses. During the changing phases, the nurse can fulfill a variety of roles, including teacher, resource person, counselor, and surrogate. Within the interpersonal relationship, Peplau emphasized the specific skills of observing, communicating, and recording.

DOROTHEA OREM   Also in the late 1950s, Dorothea Orem developed another major model of nursing. Orem's initial formulations of a self-care framework stemmed from nursing practice. As a consultant at the U.S. Department of Health, Education, and Welfare, Orem (1959) developed a curriculum guideline for practical nurses. This project was the immediate stimulus for Orem to describe the subject matter of nursing. Orem worked with several work groups of nurse-scholars to further describe the basic concepts of this nursing model. The major text on the self-care model, *Nursing: Concepts of Practice,* was published in 1971 and updated five more times, as recently as 2001. Orem made significant contributions to nursing knowledge by identifying a unique focus and the boundaries of nursing as a science and an art. Orem's model is used extensively in nursing education, practice, and research. A self-care institute has been established in the United States. An International Orem Society for Nursing Science and Scholarship was founded in 1991.

Orem referred to the individual as a self-care agency. Self-care agency is the power of the individual to engage in self-care. This power is a complex acquired ability to meet one's continuing requirements for care. It regulates life processes; maintains or promotes integrity of human structure, functioning, and human development; and promotes well-being. Self-care requisites, or requirements, include the following:

1. Universal requisites: Those that apply for all people during all stages of the life cycle and are associated with life processes and the integrity of human structure and functioning.
2. Developmental requisites: Those associated with human development processes and with conditions and events occurring during various stages of the life cycle.
3. Health-deviation requisites: Those associated with people who are ill or injured, including defects or disabilities, and those under medical diagnosis and treatment.

The definition of environment used in Orem's conceptual model is the physical, chemical, biologic, and social conditions relevant to self-care requisites and basic conditioning factors. Social conditions include the family, culture, and community. Orem's definition of health stems from her concept of the individual. In this framework, health refers to the state of the individual being structurally and functionally whole or sound. Health is a state of the individual and the group and includes the ability to reflect on self, to use symbols for one's experiences, and communicate with others. Health requires self-care of therapeutic quality.

A major concept of the Orem model is the theory of the nursing system. This theory provides a specific goal and approach for nursing. It includes series and sequences of deliberate practical actions of nurses, sometimes coordinated with patient actions. The goal is to know and meet components of the patients' therapeutic self-care demands and to protect and regulate the exercise or development of the patients' self-care agency. Nursing action, according to Orem, uses concepts of intentionality and diagnosis, prescription and regulation. There are three types of nursing systems, based on the individual's self-care agency, that is, the ability to meet self-care demands.

The wholly compensatory nursing system handles the patient's therapeutic self-care, compensates for the patient's inability to engage in self-care, and supports and protects the patient. In the partly compensatory system the nurse performs some self-care measures and the patient performs some. The nurse assists the patient as required and the patient accepts care and assistance from the nurse. The third type of nursing action is the supportive-educative system, in which the patient accomplishes self-care and the nurse regulates the exercise and development of self-care agency. The eventual outcome of patient care, based on the Orem model, is that the individual is independent and able to manage universal, developmental, and therapeutic self-care requisites.

MARTHA ROGERS   Martha Rogers was involved in the scholarly discussions focused on the need to clarify the nature of nursing that were common in the late 1950s and early 1960s. In her book *Educational Revolution in Nursing,* Rogers (1961) presented the goal of nursing as the movement of the individual toward maximum health. In 1970, she described evolving views on the nature of nursing in a book entitled *An Introduction to the Theoretical Basis of Nursing.* Later, Rogers (1980) presented the basics of nursing as the science of unitary human beings. In the last decades of her life, she expanded on earlier themes in both writing (Rogers, 1990a, 1992) and speaking (Rogers, 1987, 1990b) and left the legacy of a solid conceptual system and a vision of nursing for the future (Rogers, 1994).

The major contribution of Rogers' work was a revolutionary concept of the human person. Given today's assumption of the holism of the individual, it is not easy to recognize the extent of the shift in thinking that Rogers called for in describing the individual as a unitary, four-dimensional, negentropic energy field. According to Rogers, nursing is the only learned profession that truly deals with a unitary view of the total person, since other sciences study various parts of the individual or an addition of parts. She recognized that, for nurses who have been taught other basic sciences, it is difficult to think in terms of unitary patterns rather than parts of the individual. However, Rogers energetically insisted on the unitary view of the person and of identifying concepts of holism that were not truly reflecting unitary patterns. Within Rogers' conceptual scheme, there are descriptions of the characteristics of the unitary, four-dimensional individual. The human energy field evolves rhythmically along life's non-linear, spiraling axis. This image led to representing Rogers' conceptual system by the popular child's coiled toy known as "Slinky."

Rogers was specific in the discussion of environment, which is a major concept in her theoretical formulations. Just as the individual is unitary, Rogers viewed environment as irreducible and as a pandimensional energy field. This field is also identified by pattern and organization, and most particularly is integral with the human field. Rogers' emphasis on the lack of boundaries between the individual and environment was a turning point in conceptual thinking in nursing (Newman, 1994). For Rogers, the individual–environment field is coextensive with the universe.

Rogers described health as an expression of the life process. Rogers maintained that there are no absolute norms for health. Manifestations of human and environmental field patterns deemed to have high value are labeled "wellness" by society, and those deemed to have low value are labeled "illness." However, in the glossary of terms that Rogers frequently used in public presentations of her work, she did not have a specific definition of health. When Rogers was a member of the Nurse Theorist Group of the National Conference on Nursing Diagnosis that met in the late 1970s and early 1980s, the group submitted the following definition of health that is reflective of Rogers' science of unitary human beings: Health is a rhythmic pattern of energy exchange which is mutually enhancing and expresses full life potential (Kim & Moritz, 1982, p. 246). It is important to note that Rogers' concept of unitary human–environmental fields calls for replacing the dichotomy between health and disease with a new synthesis. This idea was later expanded by another theorist, Margaret Newman (1994).

The goal of nursing, according to Rogers, is to promote health, or more specifically, to strengthen the integral human–environment energy field. She noted that the human–environment energy fields have diverse manifestations. Nursing approaches begin with pattern manifestation appraisal (Barrett, 1988), that is, the nurse becomes aware of relevant pattern information through sensations, thoughts, feelings, awareness, imagination, memory, introspective insights, intuitive apprehensions, and recurring themes and issues. In using the unitary framework, Cowling (1998) described handling the features of a case as an ensemble. The data are considered in the context of their inherent interconnectedness of field manifestations reflecting the wholeness of humans.

In later discussions, Rogers noted that this science requires new interventions and that many of these new approaches are noninvasive. Examples of such noninvasive nursing approaches include therapeutic touch, imagery, meditation, relaxation, unconditional love, attitudes of hope and humor, and the use of sound, color, and motion (Rogers, Doyle, Racolin, & Walsh, 1990). The Society of Rogerian Scholars was founded in 1986 to foster the development of the science of unitary human beings.

SISTER CALLISTA ROY   Sister Callista Roy began her work on a nursing model while she was a graduate student studying with Dorothy E. Johnson from 1963 to 1966. The first published

work on the model was an article in 1970 (Roy, 1970). The same year, the model was implemented as the basis of the baccalaureate curriculum at Mount St. Mary's College in Los
Angeles. The major concepts of the model will be discussed in greater detail in the remaining
chapters. For the purpose of this chapter, the basic elements are summarized so that they can be
compared with other nursing models selected as illustrations.

Roy described the individual as an adaptive system. As with any type of system, the
individual has internal processes that act to maintain the integrity of the individual. These
processes have been broadly categorized as a regulator subsystem and a cognator subsystem.
The regulator involves physiologic processes such as chemical, neurologic, and endocrine
responses that allow the body to cope with the changing environment. For example, when an
individual sees a sudden threat, such as an oncoming car approaching just after stepping off
the curb, a rush of energy is available from an increase of adrenal hormones.

The cognator subsystem involves the cognitive and emotional processes of interacting
with the environment. In the example of the individual who runs from an oncoming car, the
cognator acts to process the emotion of fear. The perceptions of the situation are also processed.
The individual can come to a new judgement about where and how to cross the street safely.
Both cognator and regulator activity is manifested in four ways in each individual and in groups
of people: in behaviors indicating physiologic–physical function, self-concept and group identity, role function, and interdependence. These four ways of categorizing the effects of cognator
and regulator activity are called adaptive modes. Adaptive modes and coping processes for individuals and for groups of individuals are described by the Roy model.

The Roy model defines environment as all the conditions, circumstances, and influences surrounding and affecting the development and behavior of individuals and groups.
From the perspective of the individual's place in the evolving universe, environment is a biophysical community of beings with complex patterns of interaction, feedback, growth, and
decline constituting periodic and long-term rhythms. Environment interactions are input for
the individual and for groups as adaptive systems. This input involves both internal and external factors. Roy used the work of Helson (1964), a physiologic psychologist, to categorize
these factors as focal, contextual, and residual stimuli. A specific consideration as a stimulus
is adaptation level, which represents the individuals' coping capacities. This changing level of
ability has an internal affect on adaptive behaviors.

Roy's concept of health is related to the concept of adaptation. Individuals are viewed as
adaptive systems that interact with the environment and grow, develop, and flourish. Health is
the reflection of person and environment interactions that are adaptive. Adaptive responses promote integrity. According to this model, health is defined as a process and a state of being, and
becoming whole and integrated in a way that reflects individual and environment mutuality.

Roy's view of the goal of nursing was the first major concept of her nursing model to
be described. Roy began her theoretical work by attempting to identify the unique function
of nursing in promoting health. Since a number of health care workers have the goal of promoting health, it seemed important for nursing to identify a unique goal. As a staff nurse in
pediatric settings, Roy noted the great resiliency of children in responding to major physiologic and psychologic changes. Yet nursing intervention was needed to support and promote
this positive coping. It seemed then that the concept of adaptation, or positive coping, might
be used to describe the goal or function of nursing. From this initial notion, Roy developed a
description of the goal of nursing as the promotion of adaptation for individuals and groups
in each of the four adaptive modes, thus contributing to health, quality of life, and dying
with dignity.

Nursing approaches, according to the Roy Adaptation Model, involve assessment of behavior and the factors affecting adaptation, and intervention to promote adaptive abilities and enhance environment interactions. Roy's view of adaptation, together with the other major concepts of the model, will be described in greater detail in Chapter 2.

MARGARET NEWMAN   Margaret Newman noted that her view of health as expanding consciousness is grounded in personal experience, but was stimulated by Rogers' insistence on the unitary nature of a human being in interaction with the environment (Newman, 1994). Newman first presented these concepts of nursing at a nursing theory conference in New York in 1978. Newman's clinical research, doctoral teaching, and collaboration in practice have been integral to the developing ideas explored in major publications over 3 decades.

Since the concept of health is the major focus of Newman's theoretical work, the definitions of the individual, environment, and the goal and approaches of nursing have been extrapolated from her discussions of health. The individual is viewed as a pattern of consciousness. Consciousness is defined as the information of the system that provides the capacity to interact with the environment. Newman (1994) noted that in the human system, the capacity for information processing includes not only thinking and feeling, but also all the information embedded in the nervous system, endocrine system, immune system, and genetic code. The human pattern is expanding and life is evolving in the direction of higher levels of consciousness. At the same time, there are complementary forces of order and disorder that maintain a fluctuating field. These fluctuations are what make possible the periodic transformations that shift the individual into a higher order of functioning. Organization and disorganization are one unitary process. Newman included family and community in her definition of the individual.

Newman cited Bohm's (1980) analogies of the implicate and explicate order as useful in understanding the theory underlying expanding consciousness. These terms can represent the meaning of environment in this conceptualization of nursing. The implicate order is described as the multidimensional pattern that is the ground or basis for all things. The explicate order, on the other hand, is the tangibles that periodically arise as temporary manifestations of the total pattern present in the implicate order. Environment is the patterned basis of all being. As in Rogers' work, it is not possible to separate the individual from environment since the individual's pattern is also rooted in the implicate order. Newman (1994) assumed that consciousness is coextensive in the universe and is the essence of all matter.

Newman defined health as expanding consciousness. The theorist emphasized seeing health as the pattern of the whole. By whole, she is referring to the pattern of interaction of an individual with the environment. Newman noted that disease is not a separate entity that invades the body, but rather a manifestation of the evolving pattern of individual–environment interaction. From this perspective, health is the pattern of the whole individual–environment and encompasses disease and nondisease. Disease is a manifestation of the underlying pattern and, in fact, is one way to envision a general pattern of energy flow of the individual. People also are not separate with separate diseases, but are open energy systems constantly interacting and evolving with others. Health includes the greater whole of the individual–environment pattern interacting with the family and the community.

Newman questioned the assumption that interventions are aimed at producing a particular result. To intervene with a particular solution in mind assumes that the nurse knows what form the pattern of expanding consciousness will take. Specific goal setting and approaches are not the issue. Rather, Newman (1994) directed the professional "to enter into partnership with the client, often at a time of chaos, with the mutual goal of participating in an authentic relationship, trusting that in the process of its unfolding, both will emerge at a higher level of consciousness" (p. 97). The time or event of disorganization represents an opportunity for pattern recognition, that is, the turning point in the evolution of consciousness. People have the capacity for understanding that which enables them to gain insight into their patterns. Insights lead to evolving consciousness with an accompanying gain in freedom of action. Many applications of Newman's approach to interventions have been described (Picard & Jones, 2005).

Newman (1999) discussed the importance of relating to the rhythm of another individual's interactive pattern. Recognizing irregular patterns is integral to helping people move through illness and disruptive events. In times of chaos the rhythm may be difficult to sense and the nurse will develop a tolerance for ambiguity and uncertainty as a new rhythm emerges. Nurses are reflective of their own patterns and go through personal transformations that make it possible to be partners with others in this process.

MADELEINE LEININGER   Madeleine Leininger is a nurse-anthropologist who placed human care at the center of the discipline and profession of nursing. In the mid-1950s, while working in child psychiatric nursing, Leininger observed concerns about cultural factors with which both the staff and contemporary psychodynamic theories were not prepared to deal. Leininger discussed these concerns with Margaret Mead and pursued them in intensive doctoral studies and field research in cultural and social anthropology. During the 1950s and 1960s, Leininger wrote of the common areas of knowledge in nursing and anthropology. From her insights and scholarly pursuits, she developed the field of transcultural nursing, with a national society established in 1974 and the first textbook published in 1978. Leininger was a leader in graduate education and in developing research methods and resources in many academic institutions in the United States.

Leininger published these ideas as a formal nursing theory in journal articles in 1985 and 1988. In the opening of her 1991 text, *Culture, Care, Diversity and Universality: A Theory of Nursing,* Leininger provided quotations from writing and public addresses from 1950 to 1991 to demonstrate that during these four decades, she had challenged nurses worldwide to reflect on care as the essence and central focus of nursing. Later works included *Transcultural Nursing: Concepts, Research, Theory and Practice* in 2002 and *Culture Care Diversity & Universality: A Worldwide Theory of Nursing* in 2005, both with McFarland. Although a number of nurse-theorists focus on care as the central concept of nursing, the early beginnings of Leininger's work and the depth of its development make this theory a good illustration to use.

The person, for Leininger, is the individual in a given cultural context that has learned, shared, and transmitted values, beliefs, norms, and lifeways. These experiences guide individual thinking, decisions, and actions in patterned ways. The lifeways patterns by which individuals and groups assist, support, facilitate, or enable another individual or group to maintain their well-being and health, to improve their human condition and lifeway, or to deal with illness, handicaps, or death, are called cultural care. Human care is a universal phenomenon; caring acts and processes are necessary for human birth, development, growth, survival, and peaceful death. Cultural care involves both diversity and universality. Diversity is the variability and differences in meanings, patterns, values, lifeways, or symbols of care within and among social groups. Universality is the common, similar, or dominant uniform care lifeways or symbols that are manifest among many cultures.

In Leininger's cultural care theory of nursing, environment is the context of the entire event, situation, or particular experience. The environment gives meaning to human expressions, interpretations, and social interactions in particular physical, ecological, sociopolitical, and cultural settings. Leininger uses a sunrise model to visualize different dimensions of the theory. In the top half of the rising sun, cultural and social structural dimensions are portrayed. These include technological, religious and philosophic, kinship and social, political and legal, economic, and educational factors, with cultural values and lifeways in the center.

The related definition of health used by Leininger is as follows: Health refers to a state of well-being or restorative state that is culturally constituted, defined, valued, and practiced by individuals or groups that enable them to function in their daily lives. Both generic, folk, or lay care systems and professional care systems are used to improve health conditions or to deal with handicap and death situations.

The goal of nursing, according to Leininger, is to focus on human care phenomena and activities in order to assist, support, facilitate, or enable individuals or groups to maintain or regain their well-being or health in culturally meaningful and beneficial ways, or to help people face handicaps or death. Three approaches are applied by nurses using this model to serve people: cultural care preservation and maintenance, cultural care accommodation and negotiation, and cultural care repatterning or restructuring. Nursing care decisions and actions are based on both generic care knowledge learned from the cultural group and professional knowledge obtained from research. Using the cultural care diversity and the universality theory of nursing, according to the elements of the sunrise model, the nurse keeps in mind the total picture of diverse influences to describe and explain care, with health and well-being as outcomes.

BOYKIN AND SCHOENHOFER Later work on caring by Anne Boykin and Savina Schoenhofer began while the theorists were revising a caring curriculum. The authors had the insight to focus on caring as an end rather than a means and as an intention of nursing rather than an instrument. They published *Nursing as Caring: A Model for Transforming Practice* in 1993. Boykin and Schoenhofer were influenced by the existential phenomenological theory of humanistic nursing developed by Patterson and Zderad (1988). This is reflected in their ideas of person and of nursing actions. Some of the language of their model is based on Roach's 6 "Cs"—commitment, confidence, conscience, competence, compassion, and comportment (Roach, 1987, 2002). Mayeroff's (1971) ingredients of caring were essential for the thinking of Boykin and Schoenhofer. They include knowing, alternating rhythms, patience, honesty, trust, humility, hope, and courage. The theorists have been members of a community of scholars whose studies focus on caring, and the thinkers mutually influence each other. The demonstration of use of the model in nursing administration has been a major contribution of the model. Several ongoing studies in the Florida area are examining reframing of the values and outcomes of caring within this model.

In this model the individual's human mode of being is caring. The individual is one who is living caring and growing in caring. To be an individual means to be living caring and through this process being and possibilities are fully known. Boykin and Schoenhofer consider the person complete and whole in any given moment. They do not refer to deficits, deficiency, insufficiency, or brokenness. If the nurse does not encounter the individual as whole, then he or she has not encountered the individual. Not each act of an individual is caring, but the theorists propose that nurses accept the belief that potentially and actually each individual is caring. The nurse is committed to know self and others as caring individuals. The nurse values and celebrates human wholeness as the individual living and growing in caring and active in interpersonal engagement. Caring is viewed as a lifetime process that is lived moment to moment and unfolding constantly.

As with some other models, model concepts of environment and health can be derived from the beliefs about the individual. Boykin and Schoenhofer did not define environment, but noted the importance of participating in nurturing relationships to enhance personhood; the social environment then seems most relevant. Further they note that caring is living within the context of relational responsibilities and possibilities. Similarly the theorists do not discuss health, but note that personhood is living out who we are, demonstrating congruence between beliefs and behaviors, and living out the meaning of our lives.

From this perspective of nursing as caring, both the goal and activities of nursing are nurturing the individual living and growing in caring. Boykin and Schoenhofer view the outcomes of care from values experienced in the nursing relationship. Predictable and evidence-based outcomes are not compatible with the values experienced in caring nursing.

The theorists provide richness to the concept of nursing by describing the nursing situation. The nursing situation is the lived experience of caring between the nurse and the one nursed in which both are enhanced. It involves the expression of values, intentions, and actions of two or more people choosing to live a nursing relationship. Some key parts of the nursing situation involve the direct invitation, the call for nursing, caring between, and nursing response.

In the direct invitation the nurse opens the relationship and invites the one nursed to share what matters most in this moment. The direct invitation is powerful in uniting and guiding the intention of the nurse and the one nursed. The call for nursing is a call for nurturance. The nurse is open to the call for nursing by being intentional and by having an authentic presence. The call originates within a unique individual who is living caring and has hopes of growing in caring. Thus they cannot be predicted.

The phrase "caring between" relates to the nurse entering the world of the other with the intention of knowing the other as a caring individual. The encountering of two persons brings about the phenomenon of caring between and the personhood of each is nurtured. The nurse knows the other through presence and intentionality as living and growing in caring. Nursing does not occur if the action is only in one direction. Finally, knowing the other individual as caring clarifies the call for nursing and shapes the response. The response, if mutually created in the knowing, is what really matters in the moment. The actions are specific expressions of caring nurturance to sustain and enhance the other in living and growing in caring. Storytelling is both an activity for practice and a unit of knowledge in this model.

Summary

Nursing is a health care profession that focuses on human life processes and patterns and emphasizes promotion of health for individuals, families, groups, and society as a whole. Nursing knowledge is based on a strong commitment to values about the individual and strives to understand how people interact with the environment and behave holistically to influence their health. Nurse authors since the time of Florence Nightingale have been developing concepts and knowledge related to areas of social responsibility for nursing, that is, individual, environment, health, and the goals and approaches of nursing.

This chapter included illustrations of nursing models reflected in the writings of Peplau, Orem, Rogers, Roy, Newman, Leininger, and Boykin and Schoenhofer. Nursing conceptual models are one way of developing nursing knowledge. This knowledge is then tested in research, taught in nursing education, and used to guide nursing practice. The remainder of this text will focus on the Roy Adaptation Model of nursing and on knowledge based on the model and its use in practice.

Exercises for Application

1. What does the concept "health" mean to you personally? Write down phrases that capture your understanding of and beliefs about health and then compare your definition to that provided by one of the theorists discussed in this chapter.
2. Prepare a table comparing the practice of four health care professions with which you are familiar. Are there any overlapping areas of responsibility or duplication of roles? How would you describe the contribution of nursing to health care?
3. This chapter described "the individual," or the recipient of nursing care, from the perspectives of seven nurse-theorists. Choose the one viewpoint that appears to be the closest to your perception of "the individual." What aspect(s) of the theorist's description are related to your values and beliefs?

Assessment of Understanding

QUESTIONS

1. What are the two characteristics of professions?
   (a) ____
   (b) ____
2. Which one of the following statements best describes the nursing profession's responsibility in society?
   ____ (a) care of individuals experiencing illness
   ____ (b) understanding life processes and patterns of individuals to promote health
   ____ (c) psychosocial health of individuals and families
   ____ (d) health promotion and disease prevention
3. Name two characteristics of 21st-century nursing.
   (a) ____
   (b) ____
4. Describe one philosophical assumption about people held by nurses.
   (a) ____
5. List three approaches to knowledge development for nursing.
   (a) ____
   (b) ____
   (c) ____
6. Which of the following are the five essential elements of a conceptual model for nursing?
   (a) health
   (b) pathophysiology
   (c) environment
   (d) nursing approaches
   (e) nursing's goals
   (f) health promotion
   (g) individual

7. Associate the specified element of a nursing model with the name of the nurse-author(s) who developed it.

Element
____ (a) individuals as unitary human beings
____ (b) health as adaptation
____ (c) nursing process with orientation phase
____ (d) self-care agency of individual
____ (e) living caring and growing caring
____ (f) health as expanding consciousness
____ (g) nursing as cultural care

Author(s)
1. Newman
2. Boykin & Schoenhofer
3. Rogers
4. Leininger
5. Orem
6. Roy
7. Peplau

FEEDBACK

1. (a) developed to contribute to the good of society
   (b) use specialized knowledge to meet specific social needs
2. b
3. (a) focuses on the life processes and patterns of individuals
   (b) commitment to promote health and full life-potential for individuals, families, groups, and the global society

4. Any of the following:
  (a) The individual is of value, and therefore possesses dignity and is worthy of respect and care.
  (b) Individuals are responsible for making decisions that influence their lives.
  (c) People are holistic, that is, their physical, thinking, and feeling processes function together in a unified expression of human behavioral patterns.
  (d) People function interdependently with other individuals in environments of the earth to create societies.

5. (a) nursing model development
  (b) theory construction
  (c) research to develop and test theories
6. a, c, d, e, g
7. (a) 3
  (b) 6
  (c) 7
  (d) 5
  (e) 2
  (f) 1
  (g) 4

References

Aiken, L. (1992). Charting nursing's future. In L. Aiken & C. Fagin (Eds.), *Charting nursing's future: Agenda for the 1990s* (pp. 3–12). Philadelphia: Lippincott.

Allan, J., & Hall, B. (1988). Challenging the focus on technology: A critique of the medical model in a changing health care system. *Advances in Nursing Science, 10*(3), 22–34.

American Nurses Association, (1982). *Nursing: A social policy statement.* Kansas city, MO: American Nurses Association.

Barrett, E. A. (1988). Using Rogers' science of unitary human beings in nursing practice. *Nursing Science Quarterly, 1,* 50–51.

Bohm, D. (1980). *Wholeness and the implicate order.* London: Routledge & Kegan Paul.

Boykin, A., & Schoenhofer, S. (1993). *Nursing as caring: A model for transforming practice.* New York: National League for Nursing Press.

Butterfield, P. G. (2002). Upstream reflections on environmental health: An abbreviated history and framework for action. *Advances in Nursing Science 25*(1), 32–49.

Chinn, P. L., & Kramer M. (2004). *Integrated knowledge development in nursing* (6th ed.). St. Louis, MO: Mosby.

Cowling, W. R. (1998). Unitary case inquiry. *Nursing Science Quarterly, 11,* 139–141.

Donahue, M. P. (1996). *Nursing, the finest art: An illustrated history* (2nd ed.). St. Louis, MO: Mosby.

Donaldson, S. K., & Crowley, D. (1978). The discipline of nursing. *Nursing Outlook, 26,* 113–120.

Gordon, M., Murphy, C., Candee, D., & Hiltunen, E. (1994). Clinical judgement: An integrated model. *Advances in Nursing Science, 16*(4), 55–70.

Helson, H. (1964). *Adaptation level theory.* New York: Harper & Row.

Hill, W. G., Butterfield, P., & Larsson, L. S. (2006). Rural parents' perceptions of risks associated with their children's exposure to radon. *Public Health Nursing, 23*(5), 392–399.

Isaacs, S. L., & Knickman, J. R. (Eds.). (1997). *To improve health and health care 1997: The Robert Wood Johnson Foundation anthology.* San Francisco: Jossey-Bass.

Kim, M., & Moritz, D. (1982). *Classification of nursing diagnosis: Proceedings of the third and fourth national conferences.* New York: McGraw-Hill.

Lamond, D., & Thompson, C. (2000). Intuition and analysis in decision making and choice. *Journal of Clinical Scholarship, 32*(4), 411–414.

Leininger, M. (1978). *Transcultural nursing: Concepts, theory, and practices.* New York: Wiley.

Leininger, M. (1985). Transcultural care diversity and universality: A theory of nursing. *Nursing and Health Care, 6,* 209–212.

Leininger, M. (1988). Leininger's theory of nursing: Cultural care diversity and universality. *Nursing Science Quarterly, 1*(4), 152–160.

Leininger, M. (1991). *Culture, care, diversity and universality: A theory of nursing.* New York: National League for Nursing.

Leininger, M., & McFarland, M. (2002). *Transcultural nursing: Concepts, research, theory and practice.* New York: McGraw Hill.

Leininger, M., & McFarland, M. (2005). *Culture care diversity & universality: A worldwide theory of nursing.* Sudbury, MA: Jones and Bartlett.

Lynaugh, J. (1992). Nursing's history: Looking backward and seeing forward. In L. Aiken & C. Fagin (Eds.), *Charting nursing's future: Agenda for the 1990s* (pp. 435–447). Philadelphia: Lippincott.

Marriner Tomey, A., & Alligood, M. (2006). *Nursing theorists and their work* (6th ed.). St. Louis, MO: Mosby.

Mayeroff, M. (1971). *On caring.* New York: Harper Collins.

Melnyk, B., & Fineout-Overholt, E. (2005). *Evidence-based practice in nursing & healthcare: A guide to best practice.* Philadelphia: Lippincott Williams & Wilkins.

Newman, M. (1994). *Health as expanding consciousness* (2nd ed.). New York: National League for Nursing.

Newman, M. (1999). The rhythm of relating in a paradigm of wholeness. Image: *Journal of Nursing Scholarship, 31*(3), 227–230.

Nightingale, F. (1859). *Notes on nursing: What it is and what it is not* (facsimile edition). Philadelphia: Lippincott.

Orem, D. E. (1959). *Guides for developing curricula for the education of practical nurses.* Washington, DC: U.S. Dept of Health, Education and Welfare, Office of Education, U.S. Govt. Printing Office.

Orem, D. E. (1971). *Nursing: Concepts of practice.* New York: McGraw-Hill.

Orem, D. E. (1980). *Nursing: Concepts of practice* (2nd ed.). New York: McGraw-Hill.

Orem, D. E. (1985). *Nursing: Concepts of practice* (3rd ed.). New York: McGraw-Hill.

Orem, D. E. (1991). *Nursing: Concepts of practice* (4th ed.). St. Louis, MO: Mosby Yearbook.

Orem, D. E. (1995). *Nursing: Concepts of practice* (5th ed.). St. Louis, MO: Mosby Yearbook.

Patterson, J. G., & Zderad, L. T. (1988). *Humanistic nursing.* New York: National League for Nursing Press.

Pearson, A., Vaughan, B., & FitzGerald, M. (2005). *Nursing models for practice.* Edinburgh, Scotland: Butterworth-Heinemann.

Peplau, H. (1952). *Interpersonal relations in nursing.* New York: Putnam.

Perry, D. (2005). Transcendent pluralism and the influence of nursing testimony on environmental justice legislation. *Policy, Politics & Nursing Practice, 6*(1), 60–71.

Perry, D., & Gregory, K. (2007). Global application of the cosmic imperative for nursing knowledge development. In C. Roy & D. Jones (Eds.), *Nursing knowledge development and clinical practice.* New York: Springer.

Peterson, S. J., & Bedrow, T. S. (Eds.). (2004). *Middle range theories: Application to nursing research.* Philadelphia: Lippincott Williams & Wilkins.

Roach, M. S. (1987). *Caring, the human mode of being.* Ottawa, Ontario, Canada: CHA Press.

Roach, M. S. (2002). *Caring, the human mode of being* (2nd revised ed.). Ottawa, Ontario, Canada: CHA Press.

Robinson, V. (1946). *White caps: The story of nursing.* Philadelphia: J. B. Lippincott.

Rogers, M. (1961). *Educational revolution in nursing.* New York: Macmillan.

Rogers, M. (1970). *An introduction to the theoretical basis of nursing.* Philadelphia: Davis.

Rogers, M. (1980). Nursing: A science of unitary man. In J. Riehl & C. Roy (Eds.), *Conceptual models for nursing practice* (pp. 329–337). New York: Appleton-Century-Crofts.

Rogers, M. (1987). *Rogers' framework.* Paper presented at Nurse Theorist conference, Pittsburgh, PA.

Rogers, M. (1990a). Nursing: Science of unitary, irreducible, human beings: Update 1990. In E. A. Barrett (Ed.), *Visions of Rogers' science-based nursing* (pp. 105–113). New York: National League for Nursing.

Rogers, M. (1990b). Space-age paradigm for new frontiers in nursing. In M. E. Parker (Ed.), *Nursing theories in practice* (pp. 105–113). New York: National League for Nursing.

Rogers, M. (1992). Nursing science and the space age. *Nursing Science Quarterly, 5,* 27–34.

Rogers, M. (1994). The science of unitary human beings: Current perspectives. *Nursing Science Quarterly, 7,* 33–35.

Rogers, M., Doyle, M., Racolin, A., & Walsh, P. (1990). A conversation with Martha Rogers on nursing in space. In E. A. Barrett (Ed.), *Visions of Rogers' science-based nursing* (pp. 375–386). New York: National League for Nursing.

Rosenblatt, R. A. (2005). Ecological change and the future of the human species: Can physicians make a difference? (REFLECTIONS). *Annals of Family Medicine 3*(2), 173.

Roy, C. (1970). Adaptation: A conceptual framework for nursing. *Nursing Outlook, 18,* 42–45.

Roy, C. (1997). *Knowledge as universal cosmic imperative. Proceedings of nursing knowledge impact conference 1996* (pp. 95–118). Chestnut Hill, MA: Boston College Press.

Roy, C., & Jones, D. (Eds.). (2007). *Nursing knowledge development and clinical practice.* New York: Springer.

Smith, M. J., & Liehr, P. (2003). *Middle range theory for nursing.* New York: Springer.

Sullivan, H. (1953). *The independent theory of psychiatry.* New York: Norton.

Watson, J. (1985). *Nursing: Human science and human care: A theory of nursing.* Norwalk, CT: Appleton-Century-Crofts.

Watson, J. (2005). *Caring science as sacred science.* Philadelphia: Davis.

CHAPTER 2

Elements of the Roy Adaptation Model

The first formal description of the Roy Adaptation Model was made by Sister Callista Roy while a graduate student at the School of Nursing of the University of California at Los Angeles. The roots of the model lie in Roy's personal and professional background. Roy is committed to philosophic and cultural assumptions characterized by the general principles of humanism, and by veritivity and cosmic unity, two terms given special meaning by Roy. The scientific foundation for the model is based on assumptions from systems theory, adaptation-level theory, and the challenges of the 21st century. A redefinition of adaptation for the future was used to extend the scientific assumptions.

Under the mentorship of Dorothy E. Johnson, Roy became convinced of the importance of defining nursing. She was also influenced by studies in the liberal arts and the natural and social sciences. It was her clinical practice in pediatric nursing that provided experience with the resilience of the human body and spirit. Roy began to seek ways to express these beliefs about nursing and to explore them further in her studies. The first publication on the Roy Adaptation Model appeared in 1970 (Roy, 1970). At that time Roy was on the faculty of the baccalaureate nursing program of a small liberal arts college. There, she had the opportunity to lead the implementation of this model of nursing as the basis of the nursing curriculum. During the next decade, more than 1,500 faculty and students at Mount St. Mary's College helped to clarify, refine, and develop the basic concepts of the Roy Adaptation Model for nursing. In the 1980s, Roy was influenced by postdoctoral work in neuroscience nursing. During the 1990s, as faculty member and nurse-theorist at Boston College, Roy focused on contemporary movements in nursing knowledge and the continued integration of spirituality with an understanding of nursing's role in promoting adaptation. The first decade of the 21st century included a greater focus on philosophy, knowledge for practice, and global concerns.

This chapter provides an overview of the major concepts of the Roy Adaptation Model of nursing. The model describes people in terms of holistic adaptive systems. These elements are described along with the associated philosophic, scientific, and cultural assumptions as they developed over time.

OBJECTIVES

After studying this chapter, the reader will be able to do the following:

1. Identify the philosophic, scientific, and cultural assumptions underlying the Roy Adaptation Model.
2. Identify the key terms in Roy's description of humans as adaptive systems.
3. State the difference between adaptive and ineffective responses.
4. Differentiate the three classes of stimuli.
5. Define adaptation level and identify three levels described by the Roy Adaptation Model.
6. In a situation involving an individual, identify specific behaviors as indicative of cognator or regulator activity.
7. In a group situation, label identified behaviors as indicative of stabilizer or innovator activity.
8. Define health in terms of the Roy Adaptation Model.
9. Describe the goal of nursing in terms of the Roy Adaptation Model.

KEY CONCEPTS DEFINED

Adaptation: The process and outcome whereby thinking and feeling people, as individuals or in groups, use conscious awareness and choice to create human and environmental integration.

Adaptation level: Adaptation level represents the condition of the life processes described on three levels as integrated, compensatory, and compromised.

Adaptive responses: Responses that promote integrity in terms of the goals of human systems.

Assumptions: The beliefs, values, and knowledge that are assumed to be true and on which theorists base their work to develop conceptual models for nursing.

Behavior: Internal or external actions and reactions under specified circumstances.

Cognator subsystem: For individuals, a major coping process involving four cognitive-emotive channels: perceptual and information processing, learning, judgment, and emotion.

Compensatory process: Adaptation level at which the cognator and regulator have been activated by a challenge to the integrated life processes.

Compromised process: Adaptation level resulting from inadequate integrated and compensatory life processes; an adaptation problem.

Contextual stimuli: All other stimuli present in the situation that contribute to the affect of the focal stimulus.

Coping processes: Innate or acquired ways of responding to the changing environment.

Cosmic unity: A philosophic view of reality which stresses the principle that people and the earth have common patterns and integral relationships.

Environment: All conditions, circumstances, and influences that surround and affect the development and behavior of humans as adaptive systems, with particular consideration of human and earth resources.

Focal stimulus: The internal or external stimulus most immediately confronting the human system.

Goal of nursing: Promotion of adaptation in each of the four modes.

Health: A state and process of being and becoming integrated and whole.

Human adaptive system: As an adaptive system, the human system is described as a whole with parts that function as a unity for some purpose. Human systems include people as individuals or in groups including families, organizations, communities, and society as a whole.

Humanism: The broad movement in philosophy and psychology that recognizes the individual and subjective dimensions of the human experience as central to knowing and valuing (Roy, 1988).

Ineffective responses: Responses that do not contribute to integrity in terms of the goals of the human system.

Innovator subsystem: Related to people in a group, the internal subsystem that involves structures and processes for change and growth.

Integrated life process: Adaptation level at which the structures and functions of a life process are working as a whole to meet human needs.

Regulator subsystem: For individuals, a major coping process involving the neural, chemical, and endocrine systems.

Residual stimulus: An environmental factor within or outside the human system with affects in the current situation that are unclear.

Stabilizer subsystem: For groups, the subsystem associated with system maintenance and involving established structures, values, and daily activities whereby participants accomplish the purpose of the social system.

Stimulus: That which provokes a response, or more generally, the point of interaction of the human system and environment.

System: A set of parts connected to function as a whole for some purpose and that does so by virtue of the interdependence of its parts.

Veritivity: A principle of human nature that affirms a common purposefulness of human existence (Roy, 1988).

ASSUMPTIONS OF THE ROY ADAPTATION MODEL

Nursing models, as descriptions of nursing in concepts, are based on both philosophic assumptions and scientific principles. Knowledge development for any field reflects and moves forward the philosophic and scientific thinking of the day. Nurse-theorists identify the beliefs, values, and knowledge on which they base their work and contribute to developing those ideas. For the Roy Adaptation Model, the concept of adaptation rests on scientific and philosophic assumptions which Roy has developed over time.

The scientific assumptions initially reflected von Bertalanffy's (1968) general systems theory and Helson's (1964) adaptation-level theory and later included the unity and meaningfulness of the created universe (Young, 1986). The philosophic assumptions on which the model is based were identified early as humanism and veritivity. The further development of the philosophic assumptions focuses on people's mutuality with others, the world, and a god-figure. The manner in which the major concepts of the model have been developed and expanded shows the influence of the theorist's scientific and philosophic background and global experiences. Specific assumptions underlying the development of the Roy Adaptation Model for the first few decades were based on the early scientific and philosophic perspectives. These assumptions are outlined in Table 2–1.

TABLE 2–1 Early Assumptions Underlying the Roy Adaptation Model

Scientific	
Systems Theory	Adaptation-Level Theory
Holism	Behavior as adaptive
Interdependence	Adaptation as a function of stimuli and adaptation level
Control Processes	Individual, dynamic adaptation levels
Information feedback	Positive and active processes of responding
Complexity of living systems	

Philosophic	
Humanism	Veritivity
Creativity	Purposefulness of human existence
Purposefulness	Unity of purpose
Holism	Activity, creativity
Interpersonal process	Value and meaning of life

In anticipation of nursing in the 21st century, Roy (1997) provided a redefinition of adaptation and a restatement of the assumptions that are the foundation of the model. The goal of nursing according to the Roy Adaptation Model is enhancing life processes to promote adaptation. Roy defined adaptation as the process and outcome whereby thinking and feeling people, as individuals or in groups, use conscious awareness and choice to create human and environmental integration. The development of the model elements is summarized in Box 2–1. The updating of the concept of adaptation further led to describing expanded philosophic and scientific assumptions in contemporary society and to adding cultural assumptions.

Philosophic Assumptions

Philosophy means (1) finding meaning through analysis and (2) sharing beliefs, values, and goals. A philosophic perspective affects what the individual is aware of, notices, and understands. In the first book on the model, Roy (1976) was explicit about the humanistic value base of her nursing model. Humanism is defined as the broad movement in philosophy and psychology that recognizes the individual and subjective dimensions of human experiences as central to knowing and valuing. In humanism, it is believed that humans, as individuals and in groups, share in creative power; behave purposefully, not in a sequence of cause and effect; possess intrinsic holism; and strive to maintain integrity and to realize the need for relationships.

In 1988 Roy introduced the concept of veritivity. She sought an option to total relativity. Veritivity was the term coined by Roy, based on the Latin word *veritas*. For Roy the word offered the notion of the rootedness of all knowledge being one. Within the Roy Adaptation Model, veritivity is the principle of human nature that affirms a common purposefulness of human existence. In veritivity, it is believed that people in society are viewed in the context of the purposefulness of human existence, unity of purpose of humankind, activity and creativity for the common good, and value and meaning of life.

In recent work Roy takes into account the 21st century as a time of transition, transformation, and spiritual vision. Changes in philosophy that influenced Roy included contemporary empiricism, postmodernism, and increased relevance of the human need for meaning and

BOX 2–1

Development of Roy Adaptation Model Elements

Early Development	Current Use
Adaptation	
• Responding positively to environmental changes	• The process and outcome whereby the thinking and feeling person as individuals or groups use conscious awareness and choice to create human and environmental integration
Person	
• Bio-psycho-social being in constant interaction with a changing environment • Uses innate and acquired mechanisms to adapt	• An adaptive system described as a whole comprised of parts • Functions as a unity for some purpose • Includes people as individuals or in groups—families, organizations, communities, and society as a whole
Environment	
• Focal—internal or external stimuli immediately confronting the person • Contextual—all stimuli present in the situation that contribute to the affect of the focal stimulus • Residual—a factor whose affects in the current situation are unclear	• All conditions, circumstances, and influences surrounding and affecting the development and behavior of persons and groups with particular consideration of mutuality of person and earth resources, including focal, contextual, and residual stimuli
Health	
• Inevitable dimension of person's life • Represented by a health-illness continuum	• A state and a process of being and becoming integrated and whole
Goal of Nursing	
• To promote adaptation in the four adaptive modes	• To promote adaptation for individuals and groups in the four adaptive modes, thus contributing to health, quality of life, and dying with dignity by assessing behaviors and factors that influence adaptive abilities and by intervening to enhance environmental interactions

purpose. Objective science recognized the significance of context of the subject in research (Weiss, 1995). Postmodernism acknowledged the multiple effects such as social, cultural, and economic of what could be claimed as knowledge (Rodgers, 2005). Still, this movement raised questions about whether with multiple meanings of reality there could be stability of truth.

Responding to this uncertainty and relativity seemed important in a time when people consistently face increasing threats. The world has become more violent with increasing incidents such as regional conflicts and global terrorism as well as neighborhood crime and abuse within families. Roy focused on describing the unity of knowledge (Roy, 2007a), which provided a broad world view that enhanced the assumption of veritivity.

Roy (1997) drew upon the richness of diverse cultures and research into the origins of the universe to derive a philosophic view of reality. She called this stance cosmic unity, which stresses the principle that people and the earth have common patterns and integral relationships. Swimme and Berry (1992) highlighted the patterns of the earth as unity, diversity, and subjectivity. They described how to be is the state of being related and connected in unity. The authors noted "In the very first instance when the primitive particles rushed forth, every one of them was connected to every other one in the entire universe. At no time in the future existence of the universe would they ever arrive at a point of disconnection (p. 77)." The destiny of each galaxy in the universe is united to the destiny of all other galaxies. We are one with our universe and one with each other. Still, beings of the universe have evolved differently from each other. We have the natural beauty of mountains and plains, delicate flowers and gigantic trees, oceans and tadpole ponds. The diversity of the earth helps us understand the diversity of people. The self expression of each entity makes the whole universe. Roy referred to this pattern as self identity. Thus, the whole universe or community emerges into being from the unique personhood of each individual. The full potential of each individual contributes to society.

The belief in a purposeful universe is also basic to understanding the philosophic assumptions of the Roy Adaptation Model. One scientist (Young, 1986), noted the irony of mainstream scientific thought restating its denial of meaning or purpose in the cosmos, at the same time that more remarkable facts have been emerging from cosmology, geology, and the study of life that seem to point to a purposeful and ordered universe. Another author noted that the evolutionary advance of the universe suggests a cosmic aim (or purpose) toward increasingly more intense forms of ordered novelty, that is, toward heightening the beauty and value of the universe (Haught, 1993).

Many enduring religious traditions affirm that the world is orderly and good—that God is transcendent and purposeful and that the world is dependent on God. The Abrahamic traditions of Judaism, Christianity, and Islam all believe in a creator God from whom all come and to whom all will return. All people share in the purposefulness of the created universe. A belief in purposefulness does not negate, but rather emphasizes individual freedom.

Roy holds a belief that individuals stand united in a common destiny and find meaning in mutual relations with each other, the world, and a God-figure. She emphasizes commonality that includes the unity and diversity of people. The common purposefulness and a common destiny of humankind provide profound insights into the dignity of people in their individuality and sacred depth of a shared humanity. Nursing sees people as co-extensive with their physical and social environments. Nurse scholars take a value-based stance. Rooted in beliefs and hopes about the individual, they develop professional knowledge that participates in the well-being of people (Roy, 1997).

Beliefs about people in society included in the principle of veritivity are summarized in the Philosophic Assumptions listed in Table 2–2.

Scientific Assumptions

The scientific assumptions for the Roy Adaptation Model began with systems theory and adaptation-level theory. As the concepts associated with the model have evolved, so too has the understanding of the scientific assumptions upon which the model is based. The contribution of systems theory to the scientific foundation of the Roy Model is evident in the description of humans as adaptive systems. Roy views human adaptive systems as functioning with

TABLE 2–2 Assumptions of the Roy Adaptation Model for the 21st Century

Philosophic Assumptions

Persons have mutual relationships with the world and a God-figure.

Human meaning is rooted in an omega point convergence of the universe.

God is intimately revealed in the diversity of creation and is the common destiny of creation.

Persons use human creative abilities of awareness, enlightenment, and faith.

Persons are accountable for entering the process of deriving, sustaining, and transforming the universe.

Scientific Assumptions

Systems of matter and energy progress to higher levels of complex self organization.

Consciousness and meaning are constitutive of person and environment integration.

Awareness of self and environment is rooted in thinking and feeling.

Human decisions are accountable for the integration of creative processes.

Thinking and feeling mediate human action.

System relationships include acceptance, protection, and fostering interdependence.

Persons and the earth have common patterns and integral relations.

Person and environment transformations are created in human consciousness.

Integration of human and environment meanings results in adaptation.

Cultural Assumptions

Experiences within a specific culture will influence how each element of the RAM model is expressed.

Within a culture there may be a concept that is central to the culture and will influence some or all of the elements of the RAM to a greater or lesser extent.

Cultural expressions of the elements of the RAM may lead to changes in practice activities such as nursing assessment.

As RAM elements evolve within a cultural perspective, implications for education and research may differ from experience in the original culture.

---

interdependent parts acting in unity for some purpose. Control mechanisms are central to the functioning of human systems. The systems theory concepts related to inputs (stimuli) and outputs (behaviors) also contribute important concepts to the model. Living systems, however, are regarded as nonlinear, multifaceted, and complex phenomena. The process is never viewed as a single stimulus initiating a given response. Rather, living systems, particularly human adaptive systems, involve complex processes of interaction.

Adaptation-level theory (Helson, 1964) forms the parent theory for the origin of the Roy adaptation concept and the description of humans as adaptive systems having the capacity to adapt and to create changes in the environment. The ability to respond positively to these changes is a function of the human system's adaptation level, a changing point influenced by the demands of the situation and internal resources. Three levels of adaptation described in this book are integrated, compensatory, and compromised. Roy (1997) combined expanded notions of systems theory and adaptation theory in the light of her worldview into the set of scientific assumptions listed in Table 2–2. The ideas and language of systems theory is compatible with views of the universe as progressing in structure, organization, and complexity. Rather than a system acting to maintain itself, the emphasis shifts to the purposefulness of human existence in a universe that is creative. Roy further emphasizes that science does not negate a creator or the meaningfulness of human existence. Rather there is an increasing literature on the integration of faith and science (Smith-Moran, 2001).

Cultural Assumptions

Roy began her global travels in 1980 and eventually visited about 30 countries on five continents. She was always inspired by the dedicated nurses who eagerly sought new knowledge and ways to improve nursing practice. Roy also felt enriched by the people of many cultural backgrounds who shared their homes and lives with her. Roy continued to give the message that the ideas of the Roy Adaptation Model could be adjusted to their cultural needs. However, no particular guidelines for many such adjustments existed.

Two members of the Roy Adaptation Association executive board met with Roy in 2007 to discuss the issue of cultural adjustments. Martha Velasco-Whetsell and Keville Frederickson also had extensive experience with nurses from other countries, particularly in Central and South America. They were concerned that nurses in other countries were frustrated that some concepts of the model did not fit with their experience. Their discussion was based on their cross-cultural research on the culture-bound process of analyzing concepts such as anxiety (Frederickson, Acuna, Whetsell, & Tallier, 2005). Roy wrote the Cultural Assumptions listed in Table 2–2. The purpose of making these assumptions explicit is to encourage the growth of the Roy Adaptation Model in ways that are culturally relevant in each country.

The three sets of underlying assumptions are the basis for and are evident in the specific description of the major concepts of the Roy Adaptation Model—humans as adaptive systems as both individuals and groups, the environment, health, and the goal of nursing.

PEOPLE AS ADAPTIVE SYSTEMS

From the perspective of the discipline of nursing, people are the focus of nursing activities. The view of people as adaptive systems provides a paradigm for the way nurses relate to and interact with individuals; their families; and the groups, organizations, communities, and societies of which they are a part.

Roy describes people in terms of holistic adaptive systems. The term holistic stems from the philosophic assumptions underlying the model and relates to the idea that people function as wholes in one unified expression of meaningful human behavior. They are, then, more than the sum of their parts. People represent unity in diversity. Similarly, there is diversity among people and their earth, yet all are united in a common destiny. The term adaptive is an integral concept in the scientific assumptions underlying the model. Human adaptive systems have thinking and feeling capacities, rooted in consciousness and meaning, by which they adjust effectively to changes in the environment and, in turn, affect the environment. People and the earth have common patterns and mutuality of relations and meaning.

To begin understanding people as adaptive systems, it is important to understand the concept of a system. Broadly defined, a system is a set of parts connected to function as a whole for some purpose and this functioning requires the interdependence of its parts. In

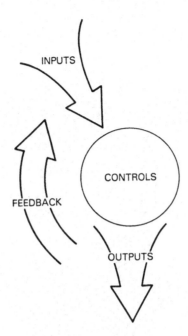

FIGURE 2–1 Diagrammatic representation of a simple system.

addition to having wholeness and related parts, systems can be viewed as experiencing inputs, outputs, and control and feedback processes. This dynamic and multifaceted interaction is simplified and shown in Figure 2–1.

Roy has applied this general systems theory in the description of people as adaptive systems. As illustrated in Figure 2–2, input for people has been termed stimulus. A stimulus has been defined as that which provokes a response. It is the point of interaction of the human system and environment. Stimuli can come externally from the environment (external stimuli) or may originate in the internal environment (internal stimuli). Certain stimuli pool to make up a specific internal input, the adaptation level.

Adaptation level represents the condition of the life processes. Three levels are described: integrated, compensatory, and compromised life processes. Adaptation level affects the individual's ability to respond positively in a situation. The behavior (output) of the individual(s) is a function of the input stimuli and the individual or group adaptation level. This changing level is significant as people and their environment are constantly in the process of change. An integrated life process may change to a compensatory process, which evokes attempts to reestablish adaptation. If the compensatory processes are not adequate, compromised processes result.

In this model, the major processes for coping are termed the regulator and the cognator subsystems as they apply to individuals, and the stabilizer and innovator subsystems as applied to groups. The cognator–regulator and stabilizer–innovator act to maintain integrated life processes for the individual or group. The life processes—integrated, compensatory, or compromised—are manifested in behavior. Over time, the behavior of the basic life processes reoccur in patterns that can be recognized as indicative of a given individual or group.

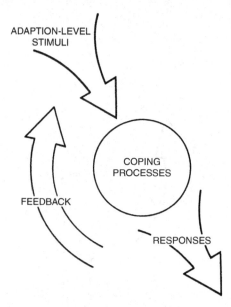

ADAPTION-LEVEL
STIMULI

COPING
PROCESSES

FEEDBACK

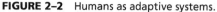

RESPONSES

FIGURE 2–2   Humans as adaptive systems.

Behavior as the output of human systems takes the form of adaptive responses and in-effective responses. These responses act as feedback or further input to the system, allowing people to decide whether to increase or decrease efforts to cope with the stimuli. As will be evident, when people as adaptive systems are explored further, all the various aspects of human systems are interrelated. Anything happening in one aspect of the system affects the whole system and all its parts. Similarly, viewing adaptive systems from different perspectives will allow emphasis on different aspects of the individual or group. The image of the kaleidoscope is used to understand how elements change places and reflect different patterns with each turn of the device. Another image that provides a similar insight is that of the changing patterns of a computer-generated laser light show. Images are larger or smaller, stand up straight or turn in circles, while colors are changing and lights appear in different places and perspectives. The individual is always a unified whole; however, at any given time, one perspective or another may be more apparent to the viewer.

It has been noted that human systems are affected by and, in turn, affect the world around and within. In the broadest sense, this world is called the environment (external and internal). According to the Roy Adaptation Model, the environment is more specifically classified as stimuli: focal, contextual, and residual. At any point in time, adaptation level is a significant internal stimulus. For purposes of developing knowledge to understand adaptive people and groups, adaptation levels are described as integrated, compensatory, or compromised. The varying adaptation levels significantly affect the ability to cope with the changing environment. Based on the environment and the current adaptation level, people make a response. Responses are observed as behavior and can be adaptive or ineffective.

The nurse soon learns that people never act in isolation, but are influenced by the environment and, in turn, affect the environment. Environment is both physical and social. Understanding this ongoing interaction of people with their world and with others in it is important to nursing practice.

Stimuli

The Roy Adaptation Model describes three classes of stimuli that form the environment. The names of these stimuli and their original descriptions are based on the work of a physiologic psychologist, Harry Helson (1964). The use of these categories by thousands of nurses has clarified their meaning within the nursing framework.

The focal stimulus is the internal or external stimulus most immediately in the awareness of the individual or group—the object or event most present in consciousness. For example, an individual may turn around quickly when a loud noise comes from behind or be annoyed by head noise of an internal buzzing sound. The individual focuses on the stimulus and spends energy dealing with it. In this example of internal or external noise, the individual tries to find its source to decide how to handle it. For a family, a violent act against a member can be an event that commands the attention of the others and elicits energy and action to deal with it. The 2001 terrorist attacks on sites in the United States became a focal stimulus for the country as people from throughout the United States were aware strongly of these events and united to assist those victimized by the events.

With the environment constantly changing, many stimuli never become focal, that is, they never command the attention of the individual(s). We generally are not conscious of the weather unless it is particularly pleasant, unpleasant, or changing. Similarly, positive or negative changes in the environment can become focal. When individuals or groups encounter a focal change, they are required to respond.

As the nurse using the Roy Adaptation Model views the patient, many stimuli that may be focal will be noted. For the surgical patient, pain may be a focal stimulus, the one on which the patient focuses attention and energy. For the pediatric patient, being away from home may be the focal change. When the nurse is working in the home with an elderly patient who is recovering from a stroke, it may be apparent that the individual focuses conscious awareness mainly on the fear of another stroke.

Similarly, in a community setting, a polluted water supply may not command the attention of members of the community until several people become severely ill as a result of consuming contaminating substances in the water. An outbreak of tuberculosis becomes a focal stimulus for the entire community.

Contextual stimuli are all other stimuli present in the situation that contribute to the affect of the focal stimulus. That is, contextual stimuli are all the environmental factors that present to the human adaptive system from within or outside but which are not the center of attention or energy. These factors will influence how the people can deal with the focal stimulus.

In our common experience with the weather, it is not the temperature alone that makes us react to the heat or cold. When high humidity is added to high temperatures, the heat is less tolerable, and when a wind chill is added to cold temperature, one is more affected by the cold. While more attention is devoted to the focal stimulus, the contextual stimuli are those that also can be identified as affecting the situation.

As noted a patient may have many environmental changes that can be focal. Each of these situations can have many contextual stimuli. The individual in pain may be more distressed by pain when the cause of it is unknown. Similarly, pain may be better tolerated when the individual knows that it is expected and that it is temporary. A little girl may handle being away from her family more easily when she can have her own toys with her and expects her parents to return. The man who fears another stroke may find that this fear is intensified by memories of his own stroke and of the death of a brother from a stroke. A community with significant economic resources may find it easier to deal with a disastrous situation than a community with few economic advantages. In these examples, it can be seen that the contextual stimuli are also within or outside human systems and that they can be positive or negative factors.

Residual stimuli are environmental factors within or outside human systems, the effects of which are unclear in the current situation. There may not be an awareness of the influence of these factors, or it may not be clear to the observer that they are having an effect. For example, an individual who is frightened in a storm may have forgotten being lost once in a storm as a child. A friend who observes that the individual is very frightened may have a hunch that there has been a bad experience in the past. However, in describing what is causing the fright, the observer can only consider this as a possibility since the individual has never mentioned such an experience.

Understanding of communities and their development such as that described by Kretzmann and McKnight (1993) suggest that the manner in which society approaches assistance to disadvantaged groups may be one factor (stimulus) that actually exacerbates the problems of the community. The traditional "needs-based approach" may be a residual stimulus that ignores capabilities and strengths within the community, thus actually contributing to failure of programs intended to help. This possibility constitutes a residual stimulus with an affect on the community that is yet to be understood.

In looking at what is affecting people in a given nursing situation, it is useful for the nurse to consider possible influencing stimuli and, in this way, further describe the situation. For example, a nurse may observe the child's reaction to being away from home and consider that this might be the child's first separation from her family. The nurse frequently uses the category of residual stimuli to place general knowledge about what influences the type of behavior observed. The nurse then gets to know the situation and those involved well enough to decide whether that stimulus is focal, contextual, or perhaps not applicable to the patient. By using the category of residual stimuli, one has a place to include even uncertain influencing stimuli and the nurse's intuitive impressions.

The nurse recognizes that focal, contextual, and residual stimuli change rapidly. The person and environment interaction is constantly changing and the significance of any one stimulus is changing. What is focal at one time soon becomes contextual and what is contextual may slip far enough into the background to become residual, that is, just a possible influence. For example, an individual watching a national weather report may be vaguely aware of the weather patterns in another part of the country. However, if that individual will be traveling to that area soon, attention is focused on what is said about that location. The relevance of the stimulus draws the individual's attention to it. Again, the image of the changing patterns of a kaleidoscope or laser light show is brought to mind in recognizing changing stimuli affecting human experiences.

The adaptation model emphasizes the individual or group's coping capacity as an important stimulus. Understanding of this stimulus is being furthered by development of a middle range theory of coping and adaptation processing. Several research studies have been based on this developing theory. The hope is that this approach can inform exploration of the concept of "capacity-focused development" on both the individual and community level. By moving away from focusing on "needs, deficits, and problems" we may use the positive stimulus of coping capacity to enhance adaptation. Throughout this text, there are examples of the three types of stimuli and their importance in providing nursing care according to the Roy Adaptation Model.

Adaptation Level

Among the focal, contextual, and residual stimuli is a significant internal input, the adaptation level. Adaptation level is the name given to three possible conditions of the life processes of the human adaptive system: integrated, compensatory, and compromised. The Roy Adaptation Model has always identified adaptation level as a stimulus. However, the concept was defined and described only briefly until the 1999 edition of this text (Roy & Andrews, 1999). In developing knowledge related to basic life processes of each component of the adaptive modes (demonstrated in the chapters in Parts 2 and 3), the model now specifies that these processes will vary at three levels: integrated, compensatory, and compromised. The first adaptation level is termed integrated. The term *integrated* describes the structures and functions of the life process working as a whole to meet human needs. For example, intact skin acts as a nonspecific defense to protect against infection. Integrated adaptation level thus constitutes a stimulus for the individual or group. It is assessed by observing integrated processes described within each of the adaptive mode components.

The second adaptation level is the compensatory level at which the cognator and regulator (or stabilizer and innovator for groups) have been activated by a challenge to the integrated processes. An example of a compensatory adaptation level is fever, which inhibits the multiplication of bacteria and increases metabolic rate to enhance repair. The discussion of each adaptive mode provides examples of compensatory processes that the nurse assesses.

The third adaptation level is the compromised level. When both integrated and compensatory processes are inadequate, an adaptation problem can result. Such problems become part of the nurse's consideration of the individual or group as having a compromised adaptation level. Disrupted skin integrity and infection are two examples of compromised processes of the basic life process of protection. Again, the examples of compromised processes and how the nurse identifies them are provided in each chapter on an adaptive mode for both individuals and groups.

As noted, life processes are discussed further in relation to each adaptive mode. Adaptation level is described by identifying whether the life process is integrated, compensatory, or compromised. As a stimulus, the changing condition of adaptation level affects the individual or group ability to respond positively in a situation. Assessment of adaptation level is part of the assessment of stimuli. However, when the nursing process is described in Chapter 3, it will be noted that what is a compromised process affecting the individual as a whole may also be the outcome of the assessment and described as a given nursing diagnosis. This shows the characteristic of the model that requires a nurse to look at a human experience from different perspectives, similar to changing patterns of the kaleidoscope or laser lights.

Helson (1964) first used the term adaptation level in a technical sense. The human system's ability to deal with an event comes from two conditions: the demands of the event and the current internal situation. An example from Helson's work relates to an individual lifting a series of varying lead weights and judging their heaviness. The individual's response to each weight is influenced by the actual weight of the object and other factors in the event, such as the weight of the object lifted just prior or physical fitness relative to weight lifting. Thus, ability to respond positively depends on all three types of stimuli and the current situation of relevant life processes of the individual. The focal stimulus is judged to have the greatest effect because it will determine which life processes are relevant in describing the current adaptation level. There may also be many related contextual stimuli and any number of residual stimuli that can be considered. The condition of the internal capacities, described by adaptation level, will be a key factor in the given environment.

Beyond the description given by Helson, the concept of adaptation level has been developed further to identify knowledge for nursing. The notion of adaptation level conveys that the human adaptive system is not passive in relation to the environment. People and the environment are in constant interaction with each other. A given individual or group, on most days, maintains integrated life processes. According to the Roy Adaptation Model, the regulator and cognator of the individual, and innovator and stabilizer for the group, are the internal subsystems for changing adaptation levels from one condition to another. If the ability to deal with a new experience is limited, information and learning about the new situation may be actively sought. For example, in setting up a new household, a young person may choose to take a short course on finances. In this way, individuals change their own adaptation level. Learning creates a compensatory process to reach a new adaptation level. Without such learning, the individual's adaptation level could have been compromised, resulting in debt and eventual bankruptcy.

Similarly, people also change the external environment. For example, if a group of employees finds that a focal concern for them is the unrealistic demands of their employer, they may take positive action together to change the employer's expectations. In this way, people are active participants in the dynamic process of interacting purposefully with the environment and adjusting adaptation levels.

When thinking of adaptation level in clinical terms, it is important to note that nurses meet people who have varying levels of capacity to cope with changing circumstances. Some life processes are integrated, others may be at a compensatory level, and others may be compromised. These varying levels reflect both the challenges and strengths of the internal and external environment. At any given time, people will respond on the basis of the combined effect of the internal and external environment. Adaptation level identifies a key factor of the internal environment. As has been noted, the current internal state includes the affects of the individual and group's past experiences, even those of which one has little or no awareness. The nurse is impressed often by the extent to which people can cope with potentially overwhelming situations. Many parents and families of children with birth defects respond with love, concern, and appropriate planning. This response is related to the pooled effect of all that these people bring to this demanding situation and to the new levels of adaptation they attain.

Adaptation level, then, describes the condition of the life processes as a significant focal, contextual, or residual stimulus in a situation. The adaptation level and all other stimuli present determine a range of coping for the human system. Many positive life experiences provide a broad range of capacities to deal with life's changes. A changing situation can limit that range. For example, a single parent may have worked very hard to maintain a family and home using a broad range of coping skills that is an example to friends and colleagues. However, recognizing that he or she is the sole support and parent of that family, the parent may find it unusually difficult to handle an illness that requires even a short hospitalization. Nurses can play an important role in supporting life processes and helping people to use cognator and regulator processes, or stabilizer and innovator processes, to develop integrated and compensatory adaptation levels.

Nurses are aware of both the strengths and limitations of the people with whom they deal, whether they are individual patients, families, groups, communities, or coworkers. Nurses also recognize minor fluctuations in their own changing adaptation levels in situations such as fatigue and anxiety. Furthermore, they know that, at times, working with cases of high demand, they must call on all their resources, and sometimes those outside themselves, to deal with the physical and emotional demands of the situation. Nurses do not avoid these experiences, but can see them as new opportunities for growth. They can help further extension of inner resources, and expand coping capacity that can result in a higher level of adaptation levels.

Behavior

As has just been described, stimuli and adaptation level serve as input to human adaptive systems. Simply speaking, processing of this input through control processes results in behavioral responses. As noted in Chapter 1 nursing knowledge focuses on human experiences related to health in a broad way rather than on specific needs or pathology. The Roy

Adaptation Model suggests a particular way of viewing human experiences and responses. Within the model, responses are not limited to problems, needs, and deficiencies. Rather, the model reflects all responses of the human adaptive system including capacities, assets, knowledge, skills, abilities, and commitments. These responses are called behavior.

Behavior is defined in the broadest sense as internal or external actions and reactions under specified circumstances. An individual who responds to a loud noise by walking toward the noise is making an external response. At the same time, the individual's increased heart rate is an internal response.

Human systems such as organizations also demonstrate behavior. In response to fiscal constraints and other environmental factors such as too many hospital beds for the population base, many hospitals responded with downsizing and mergers with other organizations. In response to such change, anxiety, conflict, and confusion tend to be behaviors that permeate the organization.

Behaviors, whether individual or in groups, can be observed, sometimes measured, or subjectively reported. The ANA's Social Policy Statement (2003) noted that nurses integrate objective data with knowledge gained from an understanding of the patient or group's subjective experience. For example, one can see the individual walk across the room, a monitor can measure heart rate, or the individual can share feelings of being frightened. The "mood" of the organization can be observed in the interaction with the employees, measured through employee satisfaction surveys, or is evident in the quality of services provided.

As the nurse views a human adaptive system, the output behavior shows how well the system is adapting in interaction with the environment. This observation is key to nursing assessment and intervention. The nurse's assessment of behaviors is discussed in detail in Chapter 3. The reader is also referred to the *Nursing Manual: Assessment Tool According to the Roy Adaptation Model* (Cho, 1998).

An important concern is whether the behavior is adaptive or ineffective. In general, understanding the effectiveness of behaviors can take place only in collaboration with those involved, the individual or those in a group. The understanding is specific to that human system and the inherent conditions and circumstances. However, the Roy Adaptation Model provides broad guidelines for nursing judgments about adaptive behaviors.

Adaptive responses are those that promote the integrity of the human system in terms of the goals of adaptation: survival, growth, reproduction, mastery, and human and environment transformations. To drink water when one's body fluids are depleted is an adaptive response contributing directly to survival. Similarly, to seek out new educational experiences contributes to growth, mastery, and higher levels of adaptation. Reproduction includes the continuation of the human species by having children, but it also involves the many ways that people extend themselves in time and space by creative works and moral presence.

From a societal perspective, the Native American grandfather lives on in the life of his grandchild by instilling the values of the tribe in the child. One's personal contributions are propagated both through individuals and to the whole society. The cultural heritage left by poets and artists can be viewed as their own adaptive responses related to reproduction.

Human systems, as individuals, families, groups, organizations, communities, or the global society must sense changes in the environment and make adaptations in the way they function to accommodate new environmental requirements. In some situations and at some developmental stages, the appropriate response may be discontinuation of the system. Death is a reality that each individual faces.

Adaptive responses, then, promote the goals of adaptation and promote the integrity of the human system. In turn, the human system's adaptation has an effect on the broader society. Based on Roy's definition of adaptation for the 21st century (Roy, 1997), new knowledge can be developed related to higher levels of complex self-organization; consciousness and meaning; integration of creative processes; common human and earth patterns; diversity and destiny; convergence and transformation of the universe; and human creative abilities of awareness, enlightenment, and faith.

Ineffective responses, on the other hand, are those that neither promote integrity nor contribute to the goals of adaptation and the integration of people with the earth. That is, they can, in the immediate situation or if continued over a long time, threaten the human system's survival, growth, reproduction, mastery, or people and environment transformations. To refuse to eat for one day may not be a serious threat to survival, but to continue such a fast over many weeks may be a serious threat and is ineffective for survival. Inability of an organization such as a hospital to respond to environmental changes may result in its closure or reconstitution into a different entity.

In judging effectiveness, then, one looks at the effect of the behavior on the general goals of adaptation and a broad understanding of the term as it pertains to human systems. At the same time, the system's individual goals are a major consideration. On the personal level, for example, there has been much discussion of the right to die. In certain stages of illness, sheer survival may not be the individual's highest goal. Rather, the individual may choose to be free from medical intervention to enter the final developmental stage of life, that is, preparation for death. One author (Dobratz, 1984, 2004, 2005) has described this developmental stage according to the Roy model as life closure. Goals of reproduction, in the sense of legacy of self, and mastery are more prominent at this time. The total integrity of the individual may be at its highest point as all the experiences of life are brought together in this closure. Using the words of the philosophic assumptions for the 21st century, the individual strives for an omega point and God as the common destiny of creation. Ineffective responses in this situation would be those that do not contribute to the individual's own adaptive goals.

Another example is a family situation. At a certain stage in the life of a dysfunctional family, it may be appropriate for the members to consider pursuing different directions, particularly if that response promotes adaptation for other family members. Such may be the case in the situation of an abusive parent who is threatening the integrity of the children.

In addition to these broad guidelines for determining adaptive and ineffective responses, the nurse's knowledge of the coping processes—regulator and cognator coping capacities for the individual and stabilizer and innovator subsystems for the group—can offer further guidelines. In general, indications of adaptive difficulty for an individual can be observed in pronounced regulator activity and cognator ineffectiveness. For example, an individual can have a rapid pulse and tense muscles, but deny any concern. The nurse recognizes that the body is automatically responding to some threat, but the individual is not effectively using cognitive and emotional processes to deal with the situation. The response that there is no concern is ineffective in handling the threat. Other people may identify the threat, but be ineffective in having strategies to cope.

Indication of adaptive difficulty in groups can be observed in situations of pronounced stabilizer activity with innovator ineffectiveness. Malphurs (1993) described this phenomenon in declining churches. He suggested that many churches become stagnant because their members are intent on preserving the status quo and refuse to respond to environmental factors that necessitate adaptation and change. Attempts at revitalization are strongly resisted. The group is exhibiting pronounced stabilizer activity with innovator ineffectiveness.

Chapter 3 includes further discussion of the nurse's assessment of adaptive and ineffective behavior and how the basic concepts of the Roy Adaptation Model are used in conjunction with established norms.

COPING PROCESSES AND CAPACITY

In applying the notion of a simplified system's control processes to human adaptive systems, the Roy model conceptualizes the complex dynamics within the individual as the coping processes. Broadly categorized, these processes are the regulator subsystem and the cognator processes for individuals, and the stabilizer and innovator subsystems for groups.

Coping processes are defined as innate or acquired ways of interacting with, that is, responding to and influencing the changing environment. Innate coping processes are genetically determined or common to the species and are generally viewed as automatic processes; people do not have to think about them. An example of an innate coping process is the ability to concentrate hemoglobin. When an individual moves to a high altitude where the oxygen saturation of the air is less, hemoglobin concentration in the blood gradually increases. The blood cells can then carry sufficient oxygen to the organs of the body. This response is automatic, unconscious, and innate.

Acquired coping processes are developed through strategies such as learning. The experiences encountered throughout life contribute to customary responses to particular stimuli. A child soon learns an appropriate response to a mother's call to get up for school. The mother's voice (stimulus) activates acquired coping processes that result in a series of actions to get out of bed and start getting ready for school (response). The response is deliberate, conscious, and acquired.

Cognator and Regulator Coping Subsystems

In consideration of the individual as an adaptive system, the Roy model further categorizes these innate and acquired coping processes into two major subsystems, the regulator and the cognator. A basic type of adaptive process, termed the regulator subsystem, responds through neural, chemical, and endocrine coping channels. Stimuli from the internal and external environment act as inputs through the senses to the nervous system and affect the fluid, electrolyte, and acid–base balance, and the endocrine system. The information is channeled automatically in the appropriate manner and an automatic, unconscious response is produced. At the same time, inputs to the regulator subsystem have a role in forming perceptions.

A mother in labor provides an example of regulator subsystem activity. During the birth process, internal stimuli, both chemical and neural, initiate endocrine and central nervous system activity to produce physiologic responses of labor such as uterine contractions and the opening of the cervix to permit birth of the baby. External stimuli, such as medications administered during labor, for example, a drug with an action that intensifies uterine contractions, also affect regulator subsystem activity and, subsequently, body response.

All aspects of the regulator subsystem are so interrelated that one cannot isolate any one system as being the only active system in a particular process. As in the example of the labor of childbirth, both chemical and neural processes are involved. These complex interrelationships are further evidence of the holistic and integrated nature of the individual.

The second major coping process of the individual is termed the cognator subsystem. This subsystem responds through four cognitive-emotional channels: perceptual and information processing, learning, judgment, and emotion. Perceptual and information processing includes the activities of selective attention, coding, and memory. This component of the cognator is discussed further in Chapter 12. Learning involves imitation, reinforcement, and insight whereas the judgment process encompasses such activities as problem solving and decision making. Through the individual's emotions, defenses are used to seek relief from anxiety and to make affective appraisal and attachments.

An example that illustrates all four cognitive-emotional channels is that of an individual driving a car. Learning (imitation, reinforcement, and insight) is involved in mastering the skills needed to operate the vehicle. When gear shifting is required, insight as to the position and function of the various gear ratios and correct positioning of the gearshift are essential. The "rules of the road" and their application are handled by perceptual and information processing, and the judgment process is continuously active, although at some times it may be more effective than at others. Even the emotions are called into action, especially when another driver has suddenly cut into the line of traffic.

As with the regulator subsystem, internal and external stimuli including social, physical, and physiologic factors act as inputs to the cognator subsystem. This information is processed through the four channels mentioned previously and responses made.

Thinking again of the driver, the traffic light ahead has just turned yellow. The driver is already 10 minutes late for an appointment (external and internal stimuli). Through the judgment process, the driver decides to go through the yellow light instead of stopping. The response would probably be to step a little harder on the accelerator.

Coping Capacity

Based on the grand theory concepts of cognator and four adaptive modes, Roy has developed a middle-range theory of coping and adaptation processing. The theory development process involved thinking of coping as multidimensional with all four adaptive modes and hierarchical with levels of information processing. Inductive and deductive research was used to identify coping strategies. Patients facing diagnostic tests and those recently hospitalized were interviewed to describe how they were coping in each adaptive mode and using regulator and cognator processes. Patients with neurologic difficulties were observed for input, central, and output information processing strategies. An instrument to measure coping and adaptation processing was developed and tested (Roy, 2007b). Key factors for positive coping capacity were using self and others to be resourceful while focusing on the issue. Those with less coping capacity were more fixed in their responses and had more physical responses. One researcher used the tool to measure how coping capacity could be changed by nursing interventions with patients who had cardiac conditions (Gonzalez, 2007).

Stabilizer and Innovator Control Processes

Just as control processes are central to the functioning of individuals, so control processes are inherent in the functioning of human social systems. With respect to groups, Roy and Anway (1989) categorized the control mechanisms as the stabilizer and the innovator subsystems to coincide with the regulator and cognator subsystems associated with the individual.

Groups, in this perspective, have two major goals, one related to stability, the other to change. Thus, the term stabilizer is used to refer to the structures and processes aimed at system maintenance. Just as the adaptive individual has neural-chemical-endocrine activities and engages in processes that act to maintain homeostasis, equilibrium, and growth potential, so the group, as an adaptive system, has strategies and engages in processes that act to stabilize. The stabilizer subsystem involves the established structures, values, and daily activities whereby participants accomplish the primary purpose of the group and contribute to common purposes of society. For example, within a family unit, specified members fulfill wage-earning activities; others may be primarily responsible for nurturance and education of children. The family members possess values that influence how they respond to their environment and fulfill their daily responsibilities to each other and society. The same can be said for other social clusters such as community groups, organizations, and society as a whole.

The second control process described by Roy relative to people in groups is the innovator subsystem. This subsystem involves the structures and processes for change and growth in human social systems. Just as the cognator for the individual involves cognitive and emotional channels for responding to a changing environment, groups have parallel information and human processes for innovation and change. The innovator dynamism involves cognitive and emotional strategies for change to higher levels of potential. Both established long-term and short-term strategies are included. For example, in organizations, strategic planning activities, think tanks, team-building sessions, and social functions constitute innovator strategies. When the innovator subsystem of a group is intact and operating well, new goals emerge and new growth and mastery are achieved, as well as individual and environment transformation. Senesac (2004) used these concepts to work with nurses to create organizational change in practice.

The examples of coping processes and strategies have been simplified for the purposes of illustration. Roy and Roberts (1981) described possible ways to conceptualize the interrelationships of the regulator and cognator subsystems. The complex relationships within and between the two dimensions of the individual system and a group system further illustrate the holistic nature of humans as adaptive systems.

THE ADAPTIVE MODES

Although it has been possible to identify specific processes inherent in the regulator–cognator and stabilizer–innovator subsystems, it is not possible to observe directly the functioning of these systems. Only the responses that are created can be observed. The behaviors that result from the control processes can be observed in four categories or adaptive modes for individuals developed by Roy to serve as a framework for assessment. These four modes, initially developed for human systems as individuals, were expanded to encompass groups. These are termed the physiologic–physical, self-concept–group identity, role function, and interdependence modes. It is through these four major categories that responses to and interaction with the environment are carried out and adaptation can be observed. The four adaptive modes are discussed in greater detail in the chapters of Parts 2 and 3; a description of each is provided here.

The category of behavior pertaining to physical aspects of human systems is termed the physiologic–physical mode for individuals and groups. The physiologic part of the mode in the Roy Adaptation Model is associated with the way people as individuals interact as physical beings with the environment. Behavior in this mode is the manifestation of the physiologic activities of all the cells, tissues, organs, and systems comprising the human body. For the individual, the physiologic mode has nine components. There are five basic needs: oxygenation, nutrition, elimination, activity and rest, and protection. In addition, four complex processes are involved in physiologic adaptation. These are the senses; fluid, electrolyte, and acid–base balance; neurologic function; and endocrine function. The underlying need for the physiologic mode is physiologic integrity.

For humans in groups it is more appropriate to use the term physical in referring to the first adaptive mode. At the group level, this mode relates to the way the human adaptive system of the group manifests adaptation relative to basic operating resources, that is, participants, physical facilities, and fiscal resources. The basic need associated with the physical mode for the group is resource adequacy, or wholeness achieved by adapting to change in physical resource needs.

Some fluctuations in the quality and strength of any one or more physiologic or physical factors over time are expected; however, prolonged ineffectiveness or compromised state of functioning can have dramatic and negative consequences for the individual or group as a whole. For example, if a community continues to permit pollution of its rivers from industries in its environment, the physical health of the community members will be affected. The individual may not show the effects of pollutants immediately, but gradually will show vague symptoms, then a more defined pattern of illness.

The category of behavior related to the personal aspects of human systems is termed the self-concept–group identity mode. The basic need underlying the self-concept mode for the individual has been identified as psychic and spiritual integrity, the need to know who one is so that one can be or exist with a sense of unity. Self-concept is defined as the composite of beliefs and feelings that an individual holds about him- or herself at a given time. Formed from internal perceptions and perceptions of others, self-concept directs one's behavior. Components of the self-concept mode are the physical self, including body sensation and body image; and the personal self, including self-consistency, self-ideal, and moral-ethical-spiritual self.

Group identity is the relevant term used for the second mode related to groups. Identity integrity is the need underlying this group adaptive mode. The mode is comprised of interpersonal relationships, group self-image, social milieu, culture, and shared responsibility of the group.

A nurse can have a self-concept seeing self as physically capable of the work involved. In addition, the nurse feels comfortable meeting self expectations of being a caring professional. In a social system, such as a nursing care unit, an associated culture can be described. There is a social environment experienced by the nurses, administrators, and other staff that is reflected by those who are part of the nursing care group. The group feels shared values and counts on each other. As such, the self-concept–group identity mode can reflect adaptive or ineffective behaviors associated with an individual nurse or the nursing care unit as an adaptive system.

The category of behavior pertaining to roles in human systems is termed the role function mode for both the individual and the group. From the perspective of the individual, the role function mode focuses on the roles that the individual occupies in society. A role, as the functioning unit of society, is defined as a set of expectations about how an individual occupying one position behaves toward an individual occupying another position. The basic need underlying the role function mode has been identified as social integrity, the need to know who one is in relation to others so that one can act.

Roles within a group are the vehicle through which the goals of the social system are actually accomplished. They are the action components associated with group infrastructure. Roles are designed to contribute to the accomplishment of the group's mission, or the tasks or functions associated with the group. The role function mode includes the functions of administrators and staff, the management of information, and systems for decision making and maintaining order. The basic need associated with the group role function mode is termed role clarity, the need to understand and commit to fulfill expected tasks, so that the group can achieve common goals.

The category of behavior related to interdependent relationships of individuals and groups is the interdependence mode, the final adaptive mode Roy describes. For the individual, the mode focuses on interactions related to the giving and receiving of love, respect, and value. The basic need of this mode is termed relational integrity, the feeling of security in nurturing relationships. For groups, the interdependence mode pertains to the social context in which the group operates. Integrity of the mode for the group includes relational, developmental, and resource adequacy. Two specific relationships are the focus within the interdependence mode for the individual: significant others, people who are the most important to the individual, and support systems, others contributing to meeting interdependence needs. For the group, the components include context, infrastructure, and member capability.

Individual and group behavior is viewed in relation to the four adaptive modes. The modes provide a particular form or manifestation of cognator–regulator and stabilizer–innovator activity within human adaptive systems. In the chapters that follow, the adaptive modes are described separately, including their theoretical basis and guidelines for assessment and the other steps of the nursing processes. However, as has been noted several times, the nurse is aware that the individual or group is to be viewed as a whole and cannot be separated into parts. The four modes are depicted as four overlapping circles in Figure 2–3. At the center of the figure is a circle representing the coping processes. An illustration of the interrelationship of the modes is noted by the intersection of the physiologic–physical mode in the diagram by each of the other three modes. Behavior in the physiologic–physical mode can have an effect on or act as a stimulus for one or all of the other modes. For example, if one loses the use of an arm, it challenges adjustments in self concept and role function. In addition, a given stimulus can affect more than one mode, or a particular behavior can be indicative of adaptation in more than one mode. Such complex relationships among modes further demonstrate the holistic nature of humans as adaptive systems.

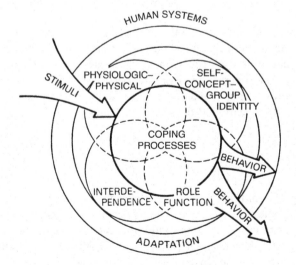

FIGURE 2–3 Diagrammatic representation of human adaptive systems.

ENVIRONMENT

Environment is the second major concept of a nursing model. It is understood as the world within and around humans as adaptive systems. According to the Roy Adaptation Model, human systems interact with the changing environment and make adaptive responses. For people, life is never the same. It is constantly changing and presenting new challenges. The human system has the ability to make new responses to these changing conditions. As the environment changes, people have the continued opportunity to grow, develop, and transform the meaning of life for everyone. One example of a positive response to changing circumstances is the patient who reorders life's priorities after suffering a near-fatal heart attack. Altering a style of living can provide a more satisfying life for the individual and the family. For example, the individual may make a decision to spend more time with a spouse and children and less time at work.

Another example illustrates the group perspective. The Institute of Medicine (2003) published a report entitled "Unequal Treatment: Confronting Racial and Ethnic Disparities in Healthcare." Many questions were raised about the environment in which health care is provided ranging from location of services to the possibility of racial bias. The result has been an increase in research to study the issue and to make recommendations for improvement. One positive outcome reported is that counseling about health risks and the quality of health providers' communication skills improved in the black non-Hispanic population by the Midcourse Review of Healthy People 2010 (2007, p. 22).

In describing the environment, Roy has drawn upon the work of Helson (1964). This physiologic psychologist described adaptation as a function of the degree of change taking place and the human system's adaptation level. The three types of stimuli described previously pool to make up the adaptation level. Adaptation level has been described as part of the internal environment of integrated, compensatory, or compromised life processes. Stimuli immediately confronting the human system are termed focal stimuli. All other stimuli present that can be identified as influencing the situation are called contextual stimuli. The residual stimuli are those that may influence the adaptation level, but whose affect has not been confirmed.

Thus, environment includes all conditions, circumstances, and influences that surround and affect the development and behavior of humans as adaptive systems, with particular consideration of human and earth resources. Another definition compatible with broad notions of individual and environment interactions from the perspective of an evolving universe is the description of the environment as a biophysical community of beings with complex patterns of interaction, feedback, growth, and decline, constituting periodic and long-term rhythms (Swimme & Berry, 1992).

HEALTH

As an understanding of health has been sought over the past decades by both professionals and the public, the complexity of the concept has become increasingly apparent. No consistent view of health exists in the literature and only recently has published research dealing with perceptions of health been available. It is generally agreed that an understanding of the complex nature of health continues to evolve.

Traditionally, health was viewed as a concept anchoring one end of a health–illness continuum. This view of health is now seen as simplistic and unrealistic since it does not accommodate the coexistence of wellness and illness and excludes individuals with chronic disabilities or terminal illness who, in spite of their condition, are dealing effectively with life's challenges.

Health, defined as the absence of disease, is a Western biomedical perspective with a biologic focus. Thus, the diagnosis and treatment of disease have become widely synonymous with health care. This perspective, however, excludes consideration of cultural, social, and psychological constructs of health as perceived by individuals and their families and friends. It does not emphasize health promotion as an important approach to improving health or the use of complementary therapies as effective health treatments.

Some views of health have come to be accepted by both the lay public and health care professionals. One of the more common perspectives on health is that published by the World Health Organization (WHO). Health is "a state of complete physical, mental and social well-being and not merely the absence of disease or infirmity" (World Health Organization et al., 1986). Fitzgerald (1994, p. 197) expressed concern about the widespread acceptance of this definition by stating, "We now act as if we really believe that disease, aging, and death are unnatural acts and all things are remediable. All we have to do, we think, is know enough (or spend enough), and disease and death can be prevented or fixed." Fitzgerald endorsed the notion of health as presented by Illich (1974). Illich maintained that health is not freedom from the inevitability of death, disease, unhappiness, and stress, but the ability to cope with them in a competent way.

Health was defined by Pender (1987, p. 27) as "the actualization of inherent and acquired human potential through goal-directed behavior, competent self-care, and satisfying relationships with others while adjustments are made as needed to maintain structural integrity and harmony with the environment." Pender and colleagues developed a nursing theory for health promotion (Pender et al., 2002). The American Nurses Association noted in Nursing's Social Policy Statement (2003) that health and illness are human experiences, but that the presence of illness does not preclude health nor does optimal health preclude illness.

Many authors have emphasized the contextual nature of health. For example, Watson (1985, 2005) viewed health as an individually defined phenomenon. Sorrell and Smith (1993) portrayed the Navajo view of health as "a holistic state, where harmony and balance between individual's physical, social, and spiritual state and the physical, social, and spiritual environment are achieved" (p. 336). Fryback (1993) provided a perspective on health in terms of terminal and chronic disease. Each of these presentations emphasizes the importance of contextual factors when defining health.

Healthy People 2010 is a major initiative that provides a vision for achieving improved health for all Americans. Through a national process of input from scientists, health providers, and the public, the project identified two overarching goals—to increase quality and years of health life and to eliminate health disparities. The U.S. Department of Health and Human Services set out specific objectives in 28 focus areas. Focus areas include access to quality health services; arthritis, osteoporosis, and chronic back conditions; cancer; chronic kidney disease; disability and secondary conditions; educational and community-based programs; environmental health; family planning; and food safety. The status of the national objectives were assessed midway through the decade by reviewing data trends and considering new science that was available in January 2005.

While acknowledging limitations of the data, the review found progress toward the target for 70 percent of the 507 objectives and sub-objectives when tracking data in Healthy

People 2010. In relation to the overall goal of helping individuals of all ages to increase quality and years of health life, reviewers using one measure found that life expectancy continues to increase. However, significant gender and racial and ethnic differences remain. For example, men's years of health life lag behind women; black men and women currently do not live as long as white men and women. Similarly, the second goal calling for eliminating health disparities shows mixed results. While there are improvements in rates for most populations, there is little evidence of systematic reductions in disparity. The decreases noted for some objectives, for example, were offset by increases in disparity between racial and ethnic populations for 14 objectives and between men and women for 15 objectives.

An understanding of the description of health as presented in the Roy Adaptation Model depends on understanding the concepts of the human adaptive system and the environment as presented earlier in this chapter. This understanding of health is also deeply rooted in the scientific, philosophic, and cultural assumptions that are the foundation of the model. It is recognized that, with further consideration of the model from the theoretical perspective and its increasing use in practice globally, the clarity with which this concept can be described will be enhanced.

Earlier in the chapter, people were described as adaptive systems constantly growing and developing within changing environments. Health for human adaptive systems can be described as a reflection of this interaction or adaptation.

In earlier discussion, adaptation was viewed as a positive response of human systems that promotes survival, growth, reproduction, mastery, and human and environment transformations. Adaptive responses were said to promote integrity or wholeness relative to these goals, with the use of integrity to mean soundness or an unimpaired condition leading to wholeness. Health is viewed in light of human goals and the purposefulness of human existence. The fulfillment of purpose in life is reflected in becoming integrated and whole. Thus, in the Roy Adaptation Model, health is defined as a state and a process of being and becoming an integrated and whole human being. Lack of integration represents lack of health.

Consider the following two situations. In the first case, a 29-year-old woman, as a result of an accident, is quadriplegic. Although confined to a wheelchair and assisted by mechanical devices, she has developed a fruitful and meaningful life as a wife, author, and painter. Her perspective on life is an encouragement to all those with whom she comes in contact.

In the second case, a 20-year-old male college student is becoming increasingly dependent on drugs to see him through his academic year. Where initially he was using them during stressful periods of examinations, now he is finding that he cannot function on a day-to-day basis without their assistance. His grades are falling and he is considering withdrawing from school.

In considering health as a reflection of adaptation with a goal of becoming integrated and whole, it is the first situation that exemplifies health. The woman is demonstrating the integration indicative of successful adaptation while the young man is responding ineffectively to his changing environment. The need for intervention is apparent.

GOAL OF NURSING

Generally speaking, nursing's goal is to contribute to the overall goal of health care, that is, to promote the health of individuals and society. The goal of nursing according to the American Nurses Association is reflected in the revised definition of professional nursing.

Nursing is the protection, promotion, and optimization of health and abilities, prevention of illness and injury, alleviation of suffering through the diagnosis and treatment of human response, and advocacy in the care of individuals, families, communities and populations. (p. 6)

The document goes on to note that the knowledge base for nursing practice is concerned with human experiences and responses across the life span. Nurses address a number of issues in partnering with individuals, families, communities, and populations. Some of these issues include promotion of health and safety; care and self-care processes; physical, emotional, and spiritual comfort, discomfort, and pain; adaptation to physiologic and pathophysiologic processes; and emotions related to experiences of birth, growth and development, health, illness, disease, and death. Nursing practice, then, is based on understanding the human condition across the life span and the relationship of the individual within the environment.

According to the Roy Adaptation Model, the profession of nursing focuses on human and environment interactions that promote maximum human development and well-being. As discussed in depth in Chapter 3, nursing activities in terms of the Roy Adaptation Model involve assessment of behavior and the stimuli that influence adaptation. Nursing judgments are based on this assessment and interventions are planned to manage these stimuli. The goal of nursing is to promote adaptation. Consider the situation of a first-time mother hospitalized for the birth of her child. Following the birth, nursing care for the mother would be directed toward helping her adapt to her new role. In addition to physiologic concerns such as nutrition, elimination, and protection from infection, goals would relate to the mother's ability to care for the child, the support systems that she may have in place when help is required, and the integrity of her self-concept throughout the adjustment period. In this case, the goal of nursing care is to assist the new mother in all aspects of adaptation. The nurse will identify the mother's adaptation level and coping capacity, identify difficulties, and intervene where necessary to promote the mother's adaptation. In this manner, the integrity of the mother and the newborn child as well is maintained.

In nursing situations involving advanced practice, nurses are involved in providing care to people in groups, whether they are families, organizations, communities, or society as a whole. Again, nursing activities involve the assessment of group behaviors and the stimuli that influence adaptation of the group. Nursing judgments are based on this assessment and interventions are planned to manage these stimuli. The goal of nursing for groups also is to promote adaptation.

Another example of this goal is a nurse who is involved as an occupational health nurse for employees in a hospital. When the incidence of needle-stick injuries is observed to be increasing, that nurse will work with employees to determine what factors appear to be influencing this trend. The interventions in this instance are focused on addressing the matters that are contributing to the problem.

Thus, Roy defines the goal of nursing as the promotion of adaptation in each of the four modes, thereby contributing to health, quality of life, or dying with dignity. It must be recognized that complete physical, mental, and social well-being, the common understanding of optimal health, is not possible for every human system. It is the nurse's role to promote adaptation in situations of health and illness and to enhance the interaction of human systems with the environment, thereby promoting health. In keeping with the assumptions of the model, nurses aim to enhance system relationships through acceptance, protection, and fostering of interdependence and to promote personal and environmental transformations.

Summary

In summary, the Roy Adaptation Model defines people, both individually and in groups, as human adaptive systems, with coping processes acting to maintain adaptation with respect to four adaptive modes. The concept of humans as adaptive systems was depicted in Figure 2–3. Stimuli from the internal and external environment activate the coping processes—the regulator and cognator subsystems of individuals, and the stabilizer and innovator subsystems of groups—which in turn produce behavioral responses relative to the physiologic–physical, self-concept–group identity, role function, and interdependence modes for individuals and groups. These responses can be either adaptive, and thus promote the integrity or wholeness of the human system (as depicted by the arrow remaining within the adaptation circle), or ineffective, and not contributing to the goals of the human system (as shown by arrows extending beyond the adaptation circle). Although, for descriptive purposes, it has been necessary to present each aspect of the human adaptive system as a separate entity, the model is based on the belief that human systems function in a holistic manner with each aspect related to and affected by the others.

Health, according to the Roy Adaptation Model, is a state and a process of being and becoming integrated and whole. It is a reflection of adaptation, that is, the interaction of the human adaptive system and the environment. Nurses act to promote this adaptation. The goal of nursing is stated as the promotion of adaptation in each of the four modes. In promoting adaptation, the nurse contributes to the health of the human adaptive system, the quality of life, and dying with dignity.

The scientific, philosophic, and cultural assumptions that form the basis for these ideas are systems theory, adaptation-level theory, humanism, veritivity, and cosmic unity and diversity. As the major concepts of the model are explored in more depth, the influence of these foundational assumptions will become increasingly evident.

Exercises for Application

1. Review the assumptions of the Roy Adaptation Model and identify the ones that you find closest to your thinking and the ones that you would need to know more about before you could form an opinion of whether or not they are like your own thinking.

2. Imagine yourself in rush-hour traffic approaching an intersection at which the light for your direction of traffic has just turned to yellow. Suggest focal, contextual, and residual stimuli that might have an effect on your judgment as to what action to take.

3. From your personal experience of taking an important examination such as your initial licensure exam, suggest focal, contextual, and residual stimuli that serve (a) to broaden your adaptation level or range of coping capabilities, and (b) to limit that range.

4. In considering your own behavioral responses during the last minute, suggest two responses that can be (a) observed, (b) measured, and (c) subjectively reported.

5. Suggest two behavioral responses that would be considered adaptive in promoting your mastery of the content presented in this chapter and two that would be considered ineffective. An example of an adaptive response would be underlining important concepts; an ineffective response would be daydreaming.

6. Jot down phrases that are descriptive of your personal perception of health. Compare them to the definition of health identified in the Roy Adaptation Model.

7. Identify several examples of nursing situations in which health care is provided for groups. An example would be an occupational health nurse in an industrial situation.

Assessment of Understanding

QUESTIONS

1. Associate the specific assumptions in Column A with the appropriate major philosophic, scientific, and cultural perspectives in Column B (note all that apply).

Column A

_____ (a) human systems possess intrinsic holism

_____ (b) control processes are central to human functioning

_____ (c) human systems behave purposefully

_____ (d) there is unity of purpose of humankind

_____ (e) concepts central to a culture

_____ (f) persons and the earth have common patterns and integral relationships

Column B

1. systems theory
2. cultural expressions
3. veritivity
4. cosmic unity

2. Fill in the missing words.
   In human systems, inputs have been termed _____ and _____ _____. The controls, or _____ _____, are central to function and their activity is manifest by _____, which act as feedback and further input to the system.

3. Label each of the following descriptions according to whether it indicates an adaptive (A) or ineffective (I) response.
   (a) _____ disrupts integrity
   (b) _____ does not contribute to survival, growth, reproduction, mastery, or transformations
   (c) _____ promotes integrity
   (d) _____ contributes to the goals of the human system

4. Situation: A four-year-old child is having a plaster cast changed. He has been wearing casts on his left ankle since he was 6 months old to correct a congenital problem. The instant the plaster saw comes into view, he begins to scream, calling for his mother. On previous occasions, the staff had to restrain him and proceed as quickly as possible with their task.
   Label the following stimuli as focal (F), contextual (C), or residual (R).
   (a) _____ past experience with cast removal
   (b) _____ the sight of the plaster saw
   (c) _____ previous cut due to saw blade

5. Which of the following statements apply to adaptation level?
   (a) It represents the condition of the life processes.
   (b) It is an individual's state of health.
   (c) It affects human system's ability to respond positively.
   (d) It can be described as integrated, compensated, or compromised.

6. Classify the underlined behaviors in the following situation as being indicative of regulator or cognator activity.
   As a young woman was <u>driving calmly down the street</u>, smelling fresh spring air, a small child suddenly ran out in front of her car. She <u>slammed on the brakes</u> and <u>swerved to the left</u> to avoid hitting him. As the child ran off, oblivious to the near accident, she was left in silence with <u>fierce pounding of her heart</u> in her chest and her <u>body shaking</u> with fright.

7. Classify the underlined behaviors in the following group situation as indicative of stabilizer or innovator activity.
   The staff of the Pregnancy Crisis Center has recently had a change in leadership. In an effort to <u>develop new direction</u> for the agency, the new leaders are <u>holding a daylong retreat</u> for all staff. Karen, a long-time employee, has been appointed to arrive early to save seats at a table so that <u>"the gang" can sit together</u>. She and her friends are <u>critical of the decision to devote an entire day to planning activities</u>. The Center has been <u>working well in the same way for years</u>. "This business of <u>strategic planning</u> is a waste of time."

8. Insert the appropriate words in the following description of health according to the Roy Adaptation Model.

Health is a _____ and a _____ of being and becoming _____ and _____.

9. Which of the following statements relate to the goal of nursing as described in the Roy Adaptation Model?
   (a) to achieve the health of individuals and groups in society
   (b) to enhance the interaction of human systems and the environment
   (c) to promote adaptation
   (d) to promote complete physical, mental, and social well-being for every person

FEEDBACK

1. (a) 1
   (b) 1
   (c) 1 and 3
   (d) 3 and 4
   (e) 2
   (f) 4
2. stimuli, adaptation level, coping processes, responses or behaviors
3. (a) I
   (b) I
   (c) A
   (d) A
4. (a) C
   (b) F
   (c) R
5. a, c, d
6. Behaviors indicative of regulator activities: pounding of her heart, body shaking. Behaviors indicative of cognator activity: driving calmly down the street, slammed on the brakes, swerved to the left.
7. Behaviors indicative of stabilizer activity: "the gang" can sit together, critical of the decision to devote an entire day to planning activities, working well in the same fashion for years. Behaviors indicative of innovator activity: change in leadership, develop new direction, holding a daylong retreat, strategic planning.
8. state, process, integrated, whole
9. b, c

References

American Nurses Association. (1995). *Nursing's social policy statement.* Kansas City, MO: American Nurses Association.

American Nurses Association. (2003). *Nursing's social policy statement.* Washington, DC: American Nurses Association.

Cho, J. (1998). *Nursing manual: Assessment tool according to the Roy Adaptation Model.* Glendale, CA: Polaris Publishing.

Dobratz, M. C. (1984). Life closure. In C. Roy (Ed.), *Introduction to nursing: An adaptation model* (2nd ed., pp. 497–518). Englewood Cliffs, NJ: Prentice Hall.

Dobratz, M. C. (2004). Life closing spirituality and the philosophic assumptions of the Roy adaptation model. *Nursing Science Quarterly, 17*(4), 335–338.

Dobratz, M. C. (2005). A comparative study of life-closing spirituality in home hospice patients. *Research and Theory for Nursing Practice, 19*(3), 243–256.

Fitzgerald, F. T. (1994). The tyranny of health. *New England Journal of Medicine, 331,* 196–198.

Frederickson, K., Acuna, V. R., Whetsell, M., & Tallier, P. (2005). Cross-cultural analysis for conceptual understanding: English and Spanish perspectives. *Nursing Science Quarterly, 18*(4), 286–292.

Fryback, P. B. (1993). Health for people with a terminal diagnosis. *Nursing Science Quarterly, 6*(3), 147–159.

Gonzalez, Y. M. (2007). *Efficacy of two interventions based on the theory of coping and adaptation processing.* Paper presented at 8th Annual Roy Adaptation Association Conference, Los Angeles.

Haught, J. F. (1993). *The promise of nature: Ecology and cosmic purpose.* New York: Paulist Press.

Helson, H. (1964). *Adaptation level theory.* New York: Harper & Row.

Illich, I. (1974). Medical nemesis. *Lancet, 1*(7863), 918–921.

Institute of Medicine, Committee on Understanding and Eliminating Racial and Ethnic Disparities in Health Care. Washington, DC: National Academies Press, 2003.

Johnson, M., Mass, M., & Moorhead, S. (2000). *Nursing outcome classification* (NOC; 2nd ed.). St. Louis, MO: Mosby.

Kretzmann, J. P., & McKnight, J. L. (1993). *Building communities from the inside out.* Evanston, IL: Center for Urban Affairs and Policy Research, Northwestern University.

Malphurs, A. (1993). *Pouring new wine into old wineskins: How to change a church without destroying it.* Grand Rapids, MI: Baker Books.

McCloskey, J. C., & Bulechek, G. M. (Eds.). (1992). *Nursing Interventions Classification* (NIC). St. Louis, MO: Mosby Year Book.

Pender, N. (1987). *Health promotion in nursing practice* (2nd ed.). Norwalk, CT: Appleton & Lange.

Pender, N. J., Murdaugh, C. L., & Parsons, M. A. (2002). *Health promotion in nursing practice* (4th ed.). Upper Saddle River, NJ: Prentice-Hall.

Rodgers, B. L. (2005). *Developing nursing knowledge: Philosophical traditions and influences.* Philadelphia: Lippincott Williams & Wilkins.

Roy, C. (1970). Adaptation: A conceptual framework for nursing. *Nursing Outlook, 18,* 42–45.

Roy, C. (1976). *Introduction to nursing: An adaptation model.* Englewood Cliffs, NJ: Prentice Hall.

Roy, C. (1984). *Introduction to nursing: An adaptation model* (2nd ed.). Englewood Cliffs, NJ: Prentice Hall.

Roy, C. (1988). An explication of the philosophical assumptions of the Roy Adaptation Model. *Nursing Science Quarterly, 1*(1), 26–34.

Roy, C. (1990). Theorist's response to "Strengthening the Roy Adaptation Model through conceptual clarification." *Nursing Science Quarterly, 3*(2), 64–66.

Roy, C. (1997). Future of the Roy model: Challenge to redefine adaptation. *Nursing Science Quarterly, 10*(1), 42–48.

Roy, C. (2007a). Knowledge as universal cosmic imperative. In C. Roy & D. A. Jones (Eds.), *Nursing Knowledge Development and Clinical Practice* (pp. 145–161). New York: Springer.

Roy, C. (2007b). *Coping and Adaptation Processing Scale* (CAPS). Boston: Boston College.

Roy, C., & Andrews, H. A. (1999). *The Roy Adaptation Model* (2nd ed.). Stamford, CT: Appleton & Lange.

Roy, C., & Anway, J. (1989). Roy's Adaptation Model: Theories and propositions for administration. In B. Henry, C. Arndt, M. DeVincenti, & A. Marriner-Tomey (Eds.), *Dimensions and issues of nursing administration.* St. Louis, MO: Mosby.

Roy, C., & Roberts, S. (1981). *Theory construction in nursing: An adaptation model.* Englewood Cliffs, NJ: Prentice Hall.

Smith-Moran, B. (Ed.). (2001). *The Journal of Faith and Science Exchange* (Vol. 5). Newton Centre, MA: The Boston Theological Institute.

Sorrell, M. S., & Smith, B. A. (1993). Navajo beliefs: Implications for health professionals. *Journal of Health Education, 24*(6), 336–338.

Swimme, B., & Berry, T. (1992). *The universe story.* San Francisco: Harper.

U.S. Department of Health and Human Services (HHS). *Healthy People 2010: Midcourse Review, Section 1. Health of the nation.* More information available at: http://www.healthypeople.gov/data/midcourse/default.htm; accessed May 21, 2008.

von Bertalanffy, L. (1968). *General systems theory.* New York: Braziller.

Watson, J. (1985). *The philosophy and science of caring.* Boulder: Colorado Associated University Press.

Watson, J. (2005). *Caring science as sacred science.* Philadelphia: Davis.

Weiss, S. (1995). Contemporary empiricism. In A. Omery, C. E. Kasper, & G. G. Page (Eds.). *In Search of Nursing Science* (pp. 13–26). Thousand Oaks, CA: Sage.

Wilkinson, J. (2000). *Nursing Diagnosis Handbook with NIC interventions and NOC outcomes* (7th ed.). Upper Saddle River, NJ: Prentice-Hall.

World Health Organization, Health and Welfare Canada, Canadian Public Health Association. (1986). *Ottawa charter for health promotion.* Ottawa, Canada: WHO, HWC, CPHA.

Young, L. B. (1986). *The unfinished universe.* New York: Simon & Schuster.

Additional References

Roy, C. (1983). Roy Adaptation Model and application to the expectant family and the family in primary care. In J. Clements & F. Roberts (Eds.), *Family health: A theoretical approach to nursing care* (pp. 255–278, 298–303, 375–378). New York: Wiley.

Roy, C. (1984). *The Roy Adaptation Model in nursing: Applications in community health nursing.* Paper presented at the eighth annual Community Nursing Conference, Chapel Hill, NC.

Roy, Sr. C., & Corliss, C. (1993). The Roy Adaptation Model: Theoretical update and knowledge for practice. In Parker, M. Parker (Ed.), *Patterns of nursing theories in practice* (pp. 215–229). New York: National League for Nursing.

Senesac, P. (2004). *The Roy Adaptation Model: An Action Research Approach to a Pain Management Organizational Change Project.* PhD Dissertation, Boston College, Chestnut Hill, MA.

The Nursing Process According to the Roy Adaptation Model

The goal of nursing is to contribute to the overall aim of health care, that is, to promote the health of individuals and society. To achieve this goal, nurses involve the full and active participation of the individual (American Nurses Association [ANA], 2003) and collaborate with other health care professionals to develop a plan of health care. Each health care discipline has an area of independent practice but also functions in overlapping and interdependent areas. In a rapidly changing health care environment, nurses recognize that nursing's scope of practice is dynamic and continually evolving. It has a flexible boundary that is responsive to the changing needs of society and the expanding knowledge base of its theoretical and scientific domains (ANA, 2003, p. 8). It is knowledge about people from the view of nurses and the nursing process related to the social concern of the profession that distinguishes nursing from other health-related disciplines.

A number of discussions of the definition of nursing were based on an earlier statement that referred to nursing as the diagnosis and treatment of human responses to health and illness (quoted in ANA, 1995, p. 6). However, current definitions place more emphasis on human experiences and responses to health and illness without restriction to a problem-focused orientation (ANA, 2003). As noted, the document by the ANA described the knowledge base for nursing practice as concerned with human experiences and responses across the life span in which nurses address a number of issues in partnering with individuals, families, communities, and populations, including promotion of health and safety and finding meaning in health and illness.

The Roy Adaptation Model suggests a particular way of viewing human experiences and responses. Within the model, responses are not limited to problems, needs, and deficiencies. Rather, the model reflects all responses of the human adaptive system including capacities, assets, knowledge, skills, abilities, and commitments. These responses are called behavior.

The recipients of nursing care are people as individuals and as collectives of people such as families, groups, organizations, communities, society as a whole, and the global community. Nursing practice is carried out by using the nursing process, a problem-solving approach for gathering data, identifying capacities and needs, establishing goals, selecting and implementing approaches for nursing care, and evaluating the outcomes of care provided.

Each model of nursing presents nursing knowledge and nursing goals and activities as rooted in the beliefs, values, and concepts that are foundational to the nursing model. For the Roy Adaptation Model, this foundation rests on the philosophic, scientific, and cultural assumptions and the description of human beings as adaptive systems with life processes.

The nursing process described by Roy relates directly to the view of human beings as adaptive systems. The process assumes that the values and beliefs about people, environment, and culture are primary. Six steps have been identified in the nursing process according to the Roy Adaptation Model.

1. Assessment of behavior
2. Assessment of stimuli
3. Nursing diagnosis
4. Goal setting
5. Intervention
6. Evaluation

This chapter explores each of these steps and relates it to Roy's view of human adaptive systems and the goal of nursing to promote adaptation.

OBJECTIVES

After studying this chapter, the reader will be able to do the following:

1. Given a situation, identify the behaviors demonstrated by an individual or group.
2. Apply criteria to evaluate specified behaviors as adaptive or ineffective.
3. In a given situation, identify stimuli influencing designated behaviors.
4. Classify designated stimuli as being focal, contextual, or residual.
5. Identify the specific stimulus of adaptation level as integrated, compensated, or compromised in a given situation.
6. In a given situation, make a nursing diagnosis.
7. Derive complete goal statements when provided with assessment data and nursing diagnoses.
8. In a given situation identify actions that could serve to alter a specific stimulus.
9. Propose approaches to strengthen regulator and cognator processes as nursing interventions for given nursing diagnoses.
10. Given goal statements, describe the evidence that would indicate that nursing interventions were effective.

KEY CONCEPTS DEFINED

Adaptation problems: Broad areas of concern related to adaptation. These describe deviations from the indicators of positive adaptation.

Adaptive behavior: Responses that promote the integrity of the human adaptive system in terms of the goals of survival, growth, reproduction, mastery, and human and environment transformations.

Behavior: Actions or reactions under specified circumstances.

Contextual stimuli: All other stimuli, internal or external, affecting the situation; contribute to the behavior triggered by the focal stimulus.

Evaluation: Judging the effectiveness of nursing interventions in relation to the behavior of the individual or group.

Focal stimulus: The stimulus, internal or external, most immediately confronting the adaptive system of the individual or group.

Goal setting: The establishment of clear statements of the behavioral outcomes of nursing care.

Ineffective behavior: Responses that disrupt or do not contribute to integrity of the human adaptive system in terms of the goals of survival, growth, reproduction, mastery, and individual and environment transformations.

Intervention: Nursing approaches selected to promote adaptation by changing stimuli or strengthening adaptive processes.

Intuition: The process of immediately knowing something without seeming to use conscious thinking.

Norms: Generally accepted guidelines and expectations used to guide judgment about the effectiveness of behavior.

Nursing diagnosis: A judgment process resulting in statements conveying the adaptation status of the individual or group.

Nursing process: A problem-solving approach for gathering data, identifying the capacities and needs of people or groups as adaptive systems, selecting and implementing approaches for nursing care, and evaluating the outcome of care provided.

Residual stimuli: Those stimuli having an indeterminate affect on the behavior of the individual or group; their affect cannot be, or has not been, validated.

THE NURSING PROCESS

The last chapter focused on the description of people and groups as adaptive systems. This chapter highlights the nursing process as it is described within the Roy Adaptation Model. In outlining the steps of the process it is important to recognize three underlying characteristics of the nursing process: the holistic nature of the process, the importance of intuitive and subjective processes, and the autonomy of the individual.

First, although the steps of the nursing process have been named and discussed separately for clarity, the process is ongoing and simultaneous. For example, the nurse could be assessing behaviors in one adaptive mode while implementing an intervention in another. This approach is similar to the manner in which Roy's conceptualization of the human adaptive system is presented. It is necessary to focus on different parts of the adaptive system separately, however, one keeps in mind the belief that human systems function as a whole. Each part is related to, and affected by, the others. The image of the kaleidoscope or laser light show, again, exemplifies the whole individual or the whole nursing process, both of which can be viewed from different perspectives at different points in time.

The second underlying characteristic of the nursing process is that it uses intuitive processes and insights as well as objective clinical reasoning. Intuition refers to the process of immediately knowing something without seeming to use conscious thinking. Knowing the patient is an outcome of the nurse's relating to the patient. These relationships often occur in critical life situations or over time in planning for health promotion. The melding of objective and subjective processes is reflected in the quote from Florence Nightingale noted earlier that the nurse "must be a sound, and close, and quick observer; and she must be a woman of delicate and decent feeling" (Nightingale, 1859, p. 71). Nurses demonstrate compassion, caring, and interpersonal skills in addition to highly developed cognitive, behavioral, and technical competencies.

The third characteristic underlying the nursing process is the right of people to manage their own lives and to make choices they feel are best. Nurses are aware of the value of autonomy, that is, the belief that individuals have the right to be involved in making informed choices about themselves and their future. In carrying out the nursing process, nurses hold a profound respect for human consciousness, meaning, and common destiny. These beliefs are held for individuals and groups receiving care, other care givers, and nurses themselves. Nurses promote the right of individuals to define their own health-related goals and seek out health care that reflects their values. Some nursing research has focused on ways to help people develop what is called their own voice in planning their care (Demarco, et al., 1998). Similarly, professional advocacy requires that nurses be aware of the accountability to look at how the larger health care system is meeting the needs of society (Grace, 2001).

STEP 1: ASSESSMENT OF BEHAVIOR

The first step of the nursing process as described in the Roy Adaptation Model is the assessment of behavior. The indicator of how a human adaptive system manages to cope with, or adapt to, changes in health status is behavior. Thus, the first step in the nursing process involves gathering data about the behavior of the human adaptive system and the current state of adaptation. In Figure 3–1, each step of the nursing process as it relates to Roy's description of the human adaptive system is shown.

The Roy Adaptation Model views people individually and collectively as holistic, adaptive systems. Input, in the form of stimuli from the internal and external environment, activates coping processes that act to maintain adaptation with respect to the four adaptive modes. The result is behavioral responses, which are identified as either adaptive or ineffective. Adaptive behavior promotes the integrity of the human adaptive system in terms of the goals of survival, growth, reproduction, mastery, and human and environment transformation. Ineffective behavior disrupts or does not contribute to this integrity.

The responses of the human adaptive system are the focus of the first step of the nursing process, assessment of behavior. Behavior is defined as actions or reactions under specified circumstances. It can be observable or nonobservable. Nonobservable behavior can occur when an individual feels anxious, as in the phenomenon commonly described as "butterflies in the stomach." Nonobservable behavior must be reported by the individual or be otherwise demonstrated. On the other hand, observable behavior can be seen by another. The crying of a frightened child would be an observable behavior.

Under usual circumstances, most human adaptive systems cope effectively with changes that occur in their environments, internal and external. However, there may be times, during an illness or life transitions, for example, when stress is placed on an individual's coping capacities. The stimuli or changes encountered may call for more than the individual's usual adaptive strategies. Adaptation levels become vulnerable and integrated life processes may become compensatory or compromised. It is often at these times that the nurse encounters the individual or the group.

In a nursing situation, the primary concern is a certain type of behavior, behavior that requires further adaptive responses as a result of environmental changes straining the coping processes of the human adaptive system. It is important for the nurse to know how to assess these behaviors, compare them to specific criteria in order to evaluate their contribution to the maintenance of integrity, and identify the strengths of the coping processes and the demands faced. Throughout each step of the nursing process, nurses rely on highly developed technical, interpersonal, and intuitive skills as they assess and initiate interventions involving approaches such as physical care, anticipatory guidance, health teaching, and counseling.

Gathering Behavioral Data

In assessing behavior, the nurse systematically considers responses in each adaptive mode of the individual or group. As noted in Chapter 2, the four adaptive modes for the individual and the group system are a classification of ways of coping that manifest coping processes. The adaptive modes include physiologic–physical, self-concept–group identity, role function, and interdependence. It is in relation to these four major categories that responses are carried out and that observable and nonobservable behaviors occur.

All behavior is not directly obvious to another individual. Nonobservable behavior must either be reported by the individual or group or be demonstrated in some other way. Observable behaviors typically can be seen, heard, or measured. Thus, in assessing behavior in each adaptive mode, the nurse uses the skills of observation and insight, measurement and interviewing to identify behavioral data. The scope of this text permits only a brief look at each of these methods of behavioral assessment. Expertise in their use is achieved through knowledge and practice of the principles involved.

The nurse, when applying observational skills, uses the senses to obtain data about the behavior of the individual or group. In the case of the individual, the nurse may see cyanotic skin color, feel a weakened pulse, smell body odor, or hear unusual breath sounds. Observation is used together with insight and intuition. There may be a sense of the patient's discomfort, even though the individual denies it and does not look uncomfortable. In a situation with a family, the nurse may observe physical indications such as bruising on a child's arm (an observable behavior) and uses insight beyond the observation to consider whether one should suspect child abuse.

Behavioral responses can be measured and the measurements compared to preestablished criteria. The nurse may take a blood pressure reading, test a urine specimen, or have an individual read an eye chart. In a family situation, special assessment tools can be administered to provide indication of possible abusive behavior toward the child. The scoring of the tool becomes the behavioral data.

The nurse uses interviewing skills to listen and purposefully question to obtain behavioral data. For example, an individual's expression of pain alerts the nurse to ask questions regarding the nature of the pain (as discussed further in Chapter 10). The individual's verbal response becomes the behavioral data that the nurse identifies and records. When a nurse performs a community assessment, interviewing can be the vehicle for understanding the capacities and needs of that particular human adaptive system. These are behavioral data for the community as an adaptive system.

Effective communication among the nurse, patients, families, and the other members of the health care team is important in assessing behavior, and throughout the nursing process. A number of nursing textbooks provide learning exercises for therapeutic communication and the strengthening of partnerships (Antai-Otong, 2007). Consideration is always given to cultural meanings beyond possible differences in language. A caring approach may take priority over a problem-solving approach; however, generally caring and problem solving go together. A sensitive nurse will know when to slow down formal data collection to focus on immediate patient feelings and concerns. The emphasis on communication and caring strategies contributes to the effectiveness of all nursing actions (Boykin & Schoenhofer, 1993; Leininger & McFarland, 2002; and Watson, 2005).

The process of data collection related to behavior is systematic. In later chapters, specific behavioral data for each of the adaptive modes are identified. In addition, the reader is referred to the *Nursing Manual: Assessment Tool According to the Roy Adaptation Model* (Cho, 1998). In initial assessment, the specific data are gathered by means of skillful observation and intuitive sensitivity, accurate measurement, and purposeful interview within the nurse-patient relationship. An initial nursing judgment is made as to whether the behavior is adaptive or ineffective. Criteria have been established to assist in this decision.

Tentative Judgment of Behavior

As presented in Chapter 2, adaptive responses are those that promote the integrity or wholeness of the human adaptive system in terms of the goals of survival, growth, reproduction, mastery, and individual and environment transformation. Ineffective responses are those that do not contribute to these goals and disrupt integrity.

The individualized adaptive goals of the individual or group are a major consideration. Chapter 2 provided an example of the individual in the final developmental stage, preparing for death. At this point, the individual's highest goal may not be survival; rather, integrity of the self and interdependent relationships becomes the priority.

Although the range for what are considered adaptive responses is wide, in some areas, normal values are available to guide judgments about the effectiveness of behavior. For example, based on data from large numbers of people, charts have been developed to identify average weights and heights for specific age groups, and we know normal ranges for values of pulse, blood pressure, and temperature. In other areas, norms, that is, expectations or generally accepted guidelines, are evident. When behavior does not match these generally accepted norms, guidelines, or expectations, there is reason to suggest that it may be ineffective. For example, there are some general expectations as to how a new mother behaves toward her baby. These are based on common cultural norms and nursing research. In some cultural groups, babies represent a responsibility for the entire community. In Hutterite communities in Canada, a baby is regarded as the colony's child. The baby's grandmother has a significant role in providing instruction for the new mother. All members of the colony bear some responsibility for the child's nurturing and education. In dominant North American cultures, the baby's mother often assumes the primary role of providing physical care and affection for the child.

In situations where norms are not available, Roy has hypothesized general indications of difficulty in adaptation. For individuals, these indications are described as pronounced regulator activity with cognator ineffectiveness. Some signs of pronounced regulator activity are as follows:

1. Increase in heart rate or blood pressure
2. Tension

3. Excitement
4. Loss of appetite
5. Increase in serum cortisol

Signs of cognator ineffectiveness include:

1. Faulty perception and information processing
2. Ineffective learning
3. Poor judgment
4. Inappropriate affect

Similar indications of difficulty with adaptation are demonstrated in systems involving groups of individuals. This is pronounced stabilizer activity with innovator ineffectiveness. In some situations, the loss of a family member could prompt such behavior. Pronounced stabilizer activity would be demonstrated by increased levels of unproductive activity, refusal to acknowledge and accept the death of the family member, and inability to initiate the necessary changes. Signs of innovator ineffectiveness include faulty assessment of environmental factors such as the cause of death, poor judgment regarding changing roles in the family, and inappropriate responses such as delaying burial arrangements. Such behaviors require energy that could be used more effectively to respond to other stimuli. Furthermore, they limit the full potential of the human adaptive system and can ultimately affect integrity.

In making the initial judgment as to whether behavior is adaptive or ineffective, it is important that nurses continually involve those for whom they are caring. Included in the understanding of human adaptive systems is an appreciation of the immense capacities and responsibilities associated with each individual. Nurses include in their practice acceptance, protection, and fostering of human and environment integral relationships. The coping capacities of people are used for personal well-being and for creating and enhancing the well-being of the earth and of all creation. In all steps of the nursing process, the nurse holds a deep conviction about the importance of involving the recipients of care as partners in observations and plans related to their health care.

The patient's perceptions associated with the effectiveness of behavior is essential in determining if behavior is adaptive or ineffective. For example, a nurse may observe, after checking a number of times during the night, that a patient slept soundly for 8 hours during the night. The nurse judges that this behavior was adaptive in meeting the patient's need for rest. However, when asked about the night's sleep, the patient responded, "I only slept about 2 hours. I couldn't get to sleep." By validating an observation with the individual, the nurse changes the judgment of behavior from adaptive to ineffective. Through a tentative assessment of behaviors as adaptive or ineffective, the nurse has a basis on which to set priorities of concern. The primary concern would be the behaviors that are disrupting the integrity of the human system and not promoting adaptation. However, the importance of identifying, maintaining, and enhancing adaptive behaviors is acknowledged, as well.

Consider the following example. In a community called Riverside, frequent minor interpersonal disputes are becoming major issues and are increasingly requiring intervention by law enforcement personnel. The behavior from the perspective of the community as an entity would be the increasing number of interpersonal disputes. This behavior is assessed as being ineffective and interfering with the identity integrity of the community. The group members are not able to relate effectively and efficiently to maintain and enhance the identity of the group and move it toward its goal achievement.

The nurse identifies indications of whether the individual or group is coping effectively with changes in the environment, internal and external. The nurse sets priorities with respect to the next step of the nursing process, assessment of stimuli.

STEP 2: ASSESSMENT OF STIMULI

As discussed in Chapter 2, change in the stimuli, internal and external, places stress on the coping capacities of the individual or group. The behavior of the system shows whether or not coping activity is effective in dealing with changes. The first level of assessment in the nursing process involves the assessment of behavior and a tentative judgment as to whether it is adaptive or ineffective. The second step of the nursing process is based on the first and involves the identification of internal and external stimuli that are influencing the behaviors.

The skills used in assessing stimuli are the same as those used in assessing behaviors, namely, astute observation, sensitive intuition, accurate measurement, and perceptive interview. Behavior manifesting a threat to integrity is a primary concern. To assist in setting priorities for the behavior of concern, the nurse, in collaboration with patients and others relevant in the situation, identifies the focal, contextual, and residual stimuli influencing these responses. In addition, the nurse identifies the particular stimulus of the adaptation level, that is, integrated, compensatory, and compromised life processes that contribute to adaptive or ineffective behavior. Examples of integrated, compensatory, and compromised life processes are provided in chapters on the adaptive modes. Additional specific stimuli have been suggested by Roy and colleagues as having an affect on behavior in each adaptive mode. These common stimuli can be focal, contextual, or residual, depending on the situation. They are identified in Box 3–1.

Identifying Focal, Contextual, and Residual Stimuli

A stimulus is defined as that which provokes a response. Stimuli can be internal or external and include all conditions, circumstances, and influences surrounding or affecting the development and behavior of the human adaptive system. A term for all internal and external stimuli is environment. Stimuli are assessed in relation to the behaviors identified in the first level of assessment. Behaviors of disrupted integrity, or the ineffective responses, would be a primary concern. Ineffective behaviors are of concern since it is the goal of nursing to promote

---

BOX 3–1

Common Stimuli Affecting Adaptation

- Culture. Socioeconomic status, ethnicity, belief system.
- Family/aggregate participants. Structure and tasks.
- Developmental stage. Age, sex, tasks, heredity, genetic factors, longevity of aggregate, vision.
- Integrity of adaptive modes. Physiologic (including disease pathology); physical (including basic operating resources); self-concept–group identity; role function; interdependence modes.
- Adaptation levels. Integrated, compensatory, or compromised life processes.
- Cognator–innovator effectiveness. Perception, knowledge, skill.
- Environmental considerations. Changes in internal or external environment; medical management; use of drugs, alcohol, tobacco; political or economic stability.

adaptation. The nurse assists in changing ineffective behaviors to adaptive ones. Adaptive behaviors are also important. They are to be maintained and enhanced. The stimuli are a key to accomplishing this goal. Changes in stimuli challenge the coping capacities of the individual or group's adaptive system. In many situations stimuli can be altered, thereby enabling more effecting coping. This idea will be discussed further in subsequent steps of the nursing process. In other situations, the nurse uses knowledge of regulator–cognator and stabilizer–innovator activity so that the coping processes can be dealt with more directly to promote adaptation.

In assessing stimuli, the nurse uses skills of perceptive observation, measurement, and interview. As the stimuli affecting each priority behavior or set of behaviors are identified, they are classified as focal, contextual, and residual. As with step 1, and with each step of the nursing process, collaboration with those involved in the situation and validation of observations are important. The focal stimulus is defined as stimulus, internal or external, most immediately confronting the adaptive system of the individual or group. In assessing the focal stimulus, the nurse is looking for the most immediate trigger of the identified behavior. Consider the example of an individual asking for suggestions about beginning an exercise program. The focal stimulus in this situation is recently receiving information about an evaluation for risk for cardiac disease. The information that data showed a high risk is the stimulus or change in environment with which the individual is coping. Possible focal stimuli have been identified for given behaviors relative to each adaptive mode. These common stimuli are identified in the chapters discussing each adaptive mode. They are summarized in the *Nursing Manual: Assessment Tool According to the Roy Adaptation Model* (Cho, 1998). It is important to note that behavior in one adaptive mode or system can act as a focal stimulus in another. For example, as a manifestation of anxiety regarding final exams, a teenage girl begins eating while she is studying and subsequently gains weight. This weight gain, a physiologic behavior, may become a stimulus to the self-concept mode causing low self-esteem when she does not meet her own and others' expectations that she remain slim. From the organizational point of view, consider an organization that is experiencing a threat to its existence. In an effort to resist the threat, the organization launches litigation proceedings over petty issues. This interdependence behavior becomes a stimulus to the physical mode by placing significant pressure on the organization's fiscal resources and actually adding another pressure that further compromises the organization's continued existence.

Also reflective of the holism of adaptive systems, one focal stimulus can affect more than one adaptive mode. The loss of a limb not only affects an individual's physiologic mode but it may disrupt the self-concept, role function, and interdependence modes. Not only is the individual's mobility affected, self-image, ability to perform roles, and interrelationships with others may be disrupted, as well. In the situation of a collective group, legislation affecting an organization's role will have significant impact on the physical mode, that is, operating resource requirements such as capacities of participants, physical facilities, fiscal adequacy, and capital resources. The group identity mode, including group self-image, social milieu, and culture will be affected. The group's interdependence mode, for example, interorganizational relations and the group's infrastructure, may also change.

Contextual stimuli are defined as all other internal or external stimuli affecting the situation. They contribute to the behavior triggered by the focal stimulus. Consider, again, the individual receiving information about cardiac risk. One contextual stimulus may be that the individual has noted a decreasing physical energy since beginning a new job that requires mostly work at a desk. This recognition contributes to the information about being at high risk for cardiac disease. Contextual stimuli are important because they often are tied to the meaning ascribed to the situation. An individual with concerns about high risk for cardiac disease who has a family member who has had a heart attack may react entirely differently from one who does not.

Residual stimuli are the next category of stimuli influencing behavior to be assessed. These stimuli are defined as those having an indeterminate effect on the behavior of the individual or group adaptive system. Their effect has not, or cannot, be validated. Roy identifies two ways in which validation of a stimulus can occur. First, there can be confirmation by those involved that the stimulus is having an effect. Second, the nurse may have theoretical or experiential knowledge to establish confirmation. Residual stimuli become contextual or focal once they have been validated. The rationale for this change in naming the stimuli is that they are now confirmed present in the situation just as are the focal and contextual stimuli. When residual stimuli are identified as affecting the situation, they are no longer possible influencing stimuli; their effect on the behavior of the human adaptive system has been confirmed. Residual stimuli affecting the individual dealing with concerns of being at high risk for cardiac disease could be lifelong health habits that are also related to cardiac risk. If one is able to confirm that good habits of diet and exercise are not part of the individual's routine self care, the stimulus then becomes contextual. Probable influencing factors can be identified through research and understanding of people. Still, based on philosophic and cultural assumptions, Roy maintains that parts of people as individuals and as groups remain a mystery.

It is important to note that changing circumstances can alter the significance of the stimuli, as has been noted in using the image of the kaleidoscope or laser lights. What is contextual at one point in time might be focal at another. For example, at the point in time when the individual learned of being at high risk for a heart attack, the most immediate cause of concern was the new information. This focal stimulus later becomes a contextual factor when the individual focuses on increasing energy levels by exercise. In the previous example relating to the community of Riverside, it was determined that many of the community members were not skilled at resolving conflict when disputes were minor in nature. As a result, many problems that were readily resolvable early on became major issues when left unattended. Thus, the stimulus in this situation involves the level of capability or skill of the community participants, a factor that is related to resource adequacy in the physical system.

Common Influencing Stimuli

As discussed in Chapter 2 the environment is considered to be all the internal and external stimuli affecting the development and behavior of human adaptive systems. Because of their common influence in the environment, certain stimuli are identified as having an affect on behavior in all of the adaptive modes. Box 3–1 presents an overview of these common influencing stimuli. Sato (1984) discussed culture, family, and developmental stage as primary considerations for stimuli affecting human adaptation. Culture is described as involving socioeconomic status, ethnicity, and belief systems. Socioeconomic status provides an indication of the style of living and the material resources upon which the human adaptive system has to draw. Different stimuli are evident in situations of different socioeconomic status. For example, an impoverished community with many inhabitants suffering from malnutrition is affected by entirely different stimuli than those affecting a situation involving a malnourished teenager from an upper-middle-class family. Ethnicity is viewed as including language, practices, philosophies, and associated values. Ethnic background may influence health practices and responses to illness. Sorrel and Smith (1993) addressed Navajo beliefs and their influence on health practices. For example, consent for a medical procedure or treatment must involve consultation with the family members. It is recognized that ethnicity is a stimulus in an individual's response to pain. Generally the experience of pain is believed to be universal. However, perception and behavior in response to pain are influenced by cultural beliefs and practices. Behavior related to pain is taught and socialized within a culture, thus allowing more or less expression of the pain experience by people of different cultural groups. Belief systems, as a component of culture, involve spiritual beliefs, practices, and philosophies and may influence all aspects of life for people as adaptive systems. As well as being a major support system, belief systems can have a specific influence on health practices and adaptation. For example, attitudes toward death are affected to a great extent by belief systems and the extent to which the beliefs are carried into practice. Religion and spirituality will affect one's deepest beliefs. Often it is important for a Catholic, even one who has not been an active church member, to see a priest when death is imminent.

Another common influencing stimulus relates to the family or group and its associated structure and tasks. Consider the different stimuli associated with a single-parent family as opposed to a nuclear or extended family. A family in the beginning stages of child-rearing has different duties and responsibilities from a family with children who are grown and have left home. There is increasing knowledge about the genetic factors that are part of the individual's family history. Genetic information is inherited from both parents. The term for the total genetic information for an individual is the phenotype. Genetic factors are considered stimuli because they are influencing factors that often require given environments, sometimes of other genetic entities, before any effect is realized. Nurses have developed specialized roles as genetic counselors to help people understand and process the information they receive about human genetics. They support patients, families, or prospective parents in dealing with the effects of inherited genes on health conditions. Factors related to developmental stage are important in assessment of contextual stimuli affecting adaptation. Based primarily on the classic developmental stages and tasks identified by Erikson (1963), it is known that factors such as age and gender influence individual behavior, especially relating to the role function mode. For people in groups, longevity of the group is important to consider. Families and groups proceed through transitional phases much as individuals do, and often the challenges encountered are associated with their particular stage of development.

The interrelationships among the parts of the human adaptive system cannot be overemphasized. As described earlier, it is important to recognize that a stimulus being assessed may be a behavior in another adaptive mode or system, just as a laser light image may be viewed as a light seen by the individual or as a light generated by a computer program operator. Thus, lack of integrity in any area of functioning will, in turn, act as a stimulus for another area. Since the nurse often encounters individuals during treatment for illness, an important consideration relative to adaptation in the physiologic mode is the presence of disease pathology. This lack of integrity in the physiologic mode will act as a stimulus for behavior in each of the other modes and, likewise, lack of integrity of the physical mode will affect the group. In Chapter 2 it was noted that, at any point in time, adaptation level is a significant internal stimulus. Adaptation levels in individuals and in groups can be described as integrated life processes, or compensatory or compromised life processes. The Roy Adaptation Model has always identified adaptation level as a stimulus. However, in early publications the concept was only briefly defined and described. Knowledge related to the basic life processes of each component of the adaptive modes is developed in the following chapters. Understanding the processes made it possible to see how they will vary at the three levels of integrated, compensatory, and compromised. Another stimulus demonstrating the interrelated aspects of human adaptive systems relates directly to acquired coping capacities, the cognator of the individual and innovator of the group. Coping processes involve the effectiveness with which the particular subsystem is functioning. Inherent in the stimulus of coping processes are the knowledge, perception, and skill to assist in coping with environmental stimuli. Consider an example of a malnourished individual. If the individual does not recognize what nutrients constitute a balanced diet, the knowledge necessary to provide for adaptive behavior related to nutritional health is not present. Therefore, the cognator subsystem cannot perform effectively. Lack of knowledge is a stimulus affecting adaptation level. The previous example with the community illustrates this notion with respect to the innovator coping processes. The last stimulus to be mentioned relates to the environment. Changes in environment can have a profound effect on the system's state of adaptation. These changes tend to affect the senses and include such stimuli as temperature changes, different noise levels, or unusual diet. The presence of unfamiliar people or absence of familiar ones may be part of an environmental change. Also related to the environment are drugs, alcohol, and tobacco. The use of each of these has a distinct effect on the individual's internal environment. For the collective adaptive system, political and economic stability are important environmental considerations affecting adaptation.

The effect on adaptation of each of the common stimuli identified is a study in itself, as is the reciprocal effect of the individual and groups on the environment. The discussion in this chapter is an attempt to identify common stimuli affecting adaptation for individuals and groups as adaptive systems. It is not meant to be exhaustive. Many other stimuli will be evident as each situation is assessed. The stimuli that have been described, however, include those that have been found to be important in the assessment of the stimuli affecting the behavior of human systems relative to each adaptive mode. Such assessment also contributes to the nurse's general understanding of the context and meaningfulness of the world for the human adaptive system.

STEP 3: NURSING DIAGNOSIS

Since the nursing process is described as a problem-solving process, behavioral data must be gathered and interpreted. Data collected thus far in the nursing process take the form of statements about the behavior of the human adaptive system that have been observed, intuited, measured, or subjectively reported. Also, data include statements about the focal, contextual, and residual stimuli that are, or may be, influencing these behaviors. The third step of the nursing process involves making statements that interpret these data. Such a statement is the nursing diagnosis and is depicted in the diagrammatic representation of the Roy Adaptation Model in Figure 3–1. The nursing diagnosis is an interpretive statement about the human adaptive system. This interpretation is made by considering the behaviors, as assessed in the first level of assessment, with the stimuli affecting those behaviors, as assessed in the second level of assessment.

Nursing diagnosis is defined in the Roy Adaptation Model as a judgment process resulting in statements conveying the adaptation status of the individual or group. In setting up nursing diagnoses within the framework provided by the model, Roy suggests the development of statements that identify behaviors together with the most relevant influencing stimuli. Consider the assessment data associated with the following physiologic adaptation problem. An individual's pulse is rapid and thready, breathing is rapid and shallow, blood pressure tends to rise at first and then fall. The individual feels clammy, looks pale, and seems agitated and confused. All these behaviors are indicative of inadequate circulation

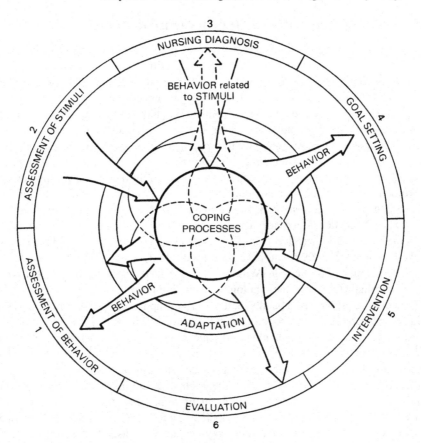

FIGURE 3–1   The nursing process as it relates to Roy's description of the human adaptive system.

and, thus, insufficient oxygenation of body tissue. They can result from a variety of factors, or stimuli, such as loss of blood volume, an infectious process in the body, or a stressful physical or emotional event. Formulating these data into a nursing diagnosis, the nurse may determine, "blood pressure of 90/60 due to hemorrhage from incision." This would represent one nursing diagnosis related to the problem described. Stated as such, the nursing diagnosis provides specific indication for nursing intervention since, as will be seen later in this chapter, nursing interventions often relate directly to stimuli.

The concept of nursing diagnosis is similarly applicable in situations where the nurse is providing nursing care for humans in groups. Consider the example of a single-parent family with a newborn. The mother is a young girl who has not had access to prenatal care. She has little understanding of the requirements of a newborn and has few material resources. From the perspective of the family, many of the deficiencies are indicative of physical mode difficulties. A nursing diagnosis relevant in this situation might be "lack of knowledge about baby's requirements due to inadequate prenatal care." The wording of the nursing diagnosis in this way becomes important to facilitate the step of goal setting in the nursing process according to the Roy Adaptation Model.

Relating Nursing Diagnosis to Clinical Classifications

Nursing diagnosis is primarily a process of critical thinking or judgment by the nurse. The process results in a statement about the patient status. During the past 35 years there has been an effort to develop diagnostic categories to describe the health status of the individual, family, or community from a nursing perspective. The categories are not meant to take the place of the nurse's process of reasoning and coming to a clinical judgment about the patient status observed in the assessment phase of the nursing process. Rather, the various classification systems and taxonomies that have been developed have the specific purpose of aiding the process of nursing diagnosis by providing a common language to communicate the nurse's clinical judgment. The effort has been to provide names for concerns that are within the domain of nursing practice. Many textbooks and clinical agencies currently use the North American Nursing Diagnosis Association (NANDA) Diagnostic Classification System (NANDA-International, 2007). Other typologies have been developed for nursing interventions and nursing outcomes. Nursing Interventions Classifications (NIC) were first published by scholars at the University of Iowa (McCloskey & Bulechek, 1992) and have been regularly updated. A second group worked on the Nursing Outcomes Classification (Wilkinson, 2000). NANDA, NIC, and NOC have worked together to coordinate the use of the typologies in nursing practice.

One author has developed a handbook that links the approved NANDA diagnosis to current NOC and NIC research-based outcomes and interventions (Wilkinson, 2000). The goal is to help nurses and students to develop individualized patient care plans. To facilitate a unified nursing language and computerized health care records, each diagnosis is listed. Then the suggested outcomes follow. These are the outcomes that nurses can influence. Nursing interventions given for each diagnosis are from the NIC project. Other nursing activities are listed and are written in NIC language. The linkages are based on an extensive process used by a research team. The process included the judgments of experts in practice and research. One example from an author's work is as follows: The definition of anxiety is given, then she lists the defining characteristics, related factors, and suggestions for use along with suggested alternative diagnoses. The suggested NOC Outcomes include aggression control, anxiety control, impulse control, self-mutilation restraint, and social interaction skills. Each of these is briefly defined. Examples of goals and evaluation criteria are provided. The NIC priority intervention is listed as anxiety reduction, which is described as minimizing apprehension, dread, foreboding, or uneasiness related to an unidentified source of anticipated danger. The author listed nursing activities under these headings: assessment, patient/family teaching, and collaborative activities. A final section, called "other," lists helpful suggestions such as encourage patient to verbalize thoughts and feelings, to externalize anxiety, and suggest alternative therapies for reducing anxiety that are acceptable to the patient.

The participants in the development of the NANDA, NIC, and NOC systems have been involved in national efforts in the United States to use nursing language in electronic health care records (discussed further in Chapter 21). Since the NANDA taxonomy is a widely used classification system, and because Roy was involved in its development from 1973 through 1983, this classification system will be related throughout this text to the clinical classifications based on the Roy Adaptation Model.

Considering the goal of nursing described in the model, namely, to enhance positive life processes and to promote adaptation, Roy has identified the utility of a typology of indicators of positive adaptation associated with each of the four adaptive modes. Table 3–1 presents the typology for individuals and Table 3–2 for groups. Adaptation problems, defined as broad areas of concern related to adaptation, also have been derived to describe deviations

TABLE 3–1 Typology of Indicators of Positive Adaptation for the Individual

Physiologic Mode

Oxygenation

- Stable processes of ventilation
- Stable pattern of gas exchange
- Adequate transport of gases
- Adequate processes of compensation

Nutrition

- Stable digestive processes
- Adequate nutritional pattern for body requirements
- Metabolic and other nutritive needs met during altered means of ingestion

Elimination

- Effective homeo static bowel process
- Stable pattern of bowel elimination
- Effective processes of urine formation
- Stable pattern of urine elimination
- Effective coping strategies for altered elimination

Activity and Rest

- Integrated processes of mobility
- Adequate recruitment of compensatory movement processes during inactivity
- Effective pattern of activity and rest
- Effective sleep pattern
- Effective environmental changes for altered sleep conditions

Protection

- Intact skin
- Effective healing response
- Adequate secondary protection for changes in skin integrity and immune status
- Effective processes of immunity
- Effective temperature regulation

Senses

- Effective processes of sensation
- Effective integration of sensory input into information
- Stable pattern of perception, i.e., interpretation and appreciation of input
- Effective coping strategies for altered sensation

Fluid, Electrolyte, and Acid–Base Balance

- Stable processes of water balance
- Stability of electrolytes in body fluids

(continued)

TABLE 3–1 *(continued)*

- Balance of acid–base status
- Effective chemical buffer regulation

Neurologic Function

- Effective processes of arousal and attention; sensation and perception; coding; concept formation, memory, language; planning, and motor response
- Integrated thinking and feeling processes
- Plasticity and functional effectiveness of developing, aging, and altered nervous system

Endocrine Function

- Effective hormonal regulation of metabolic and body processes
- Effective hormonal regulation of reproductive development
- Stable patterns of closed-loop negative feedback hormone system
- Stable patterns of cyclical hormone rhythms
- Effective coping strategies for stress

Self-Concept Mode

- Positive body image
- Effective sexual function
- Psychic integrity with physical growth
- Adequate compensation for bodily changes
- Effective coping strategies for loss
- Effective process of life closure
- Stable pattern of self-consistency
- Effective integration of self-ideal
- Effective processes of moral-ethical-spiritual growth
- Functional self-esteem
- Effective coping strategies for threats to self

Role-Function Mode

- Role Clarity
- Effective processes of role transition
- Integration of instrumental and expressive role behaviors
- Integration of primary, secondary, and tertiary roles
- Effective pattern of role performance
- Effective processes for coping with role change
- Role performance accountability
- Effective role integration
- Stable pattern of role mastery

TABLE 3–1 (*continued*)

Interdependence Mode

- Affectional adequacy
- Stable pattern of giving and receiving love, respect, and value
- Effective pattern of dependency and independency
- Effective coping strategies for separation and loneliness
- Developmental adequacy of learning and maturing in relationships
- Effective relations and communication
- Nurturing ability to provide growth-producing care and attention
- Security in relationships
- Adequate significant others and support systems to achieve affectional and developmental adequacy

TABLE 3–2 Typology of Indicators of Positive Adaptation for Groups

Physical Mode

- Adequate fiscal resources
- Member capability
- Availability of physical facilities
- Adequate number of participants
- Adequate knowledge and skills of participants
- Stable membership
- Satisfactory physical facilities
- Effective structure and processes to meet changing physical needs
- Effective planning for future adequacy of participants, physical facilities, and fiscal resources

Group Identity Mode

- Effective interpersonal relationships
- Supportive milieu and culture
- Shared goals and values
- Shared expectations
- Expressing self in the context of others
- Values in action
- Understanding and support
- Shared leadership
- Positive morale
- Flexibility in functions
- Unity in crisis

(*continued*)

TABLE 3–2 *(continued)*

Role-Function Mode

- Role clarity
- Effective processes of socialization for role expectations
- Structuring of expectations to accomplish goals of the group
- Effective processes for reciprocating roles
- High mutual dependence in division of labor
- Effective processes for integrating roles
- Regulating responsibilities and expectations between individuals in complementary and relating roles
- Flexibility in carrying out all roles to meet group demands
- Sufficient mentoring for role development

Interdependence Mode

- Relational adequacy
- Developmental adequacy
- Resource adequacy

from the indicators of positive adaptation. These are presented in Table 3–3 for individuals and Table 3–4 for groups. In this way, the capacities, capabilities, and skills of the people and groups as adaptive systems are considered in addition to circumstances that may result in a need or problem. From the typology of commonly recurring adaptation problems listed in Table 3–3, the behavioral assessment information in the postoperative patient example can be

TABLE 3–3 Typology of Commonly Recurring Adaptation Problems for the Individual

Physiologic Mode

Oxygenation

- Hypoxia
- Shock
- Ventilatory impairment
- Inadequate gas exchange
- Inadequate gas transport
- Altered tissue perfusion
- Poor recruitment of compensatory processes for changing oxygen need

Nutrition

- Nausea and vomiting
- Nutrition more or less than body requirements
- Weight 20% to 25% above or below average
- Anorexia
- Ineffective coping strategies for altered means of ingestion

TABLE 3–3 *(continued)*

Elimination

- Diarrhea
- Flatulence
- Bowel incontinence
- Constipation
- Urinary incontinence
- Urinary retention
- Ineffective coping strategies for altered elimination

Activity and Rest

- Immobility
- Activity intolerance
- Restricted mobility, gait, and/or coordination
- Disuse syndrome
- Inadequate pattern of activity and rest
- Sleep deprivation
- Potential for sleep pattern disturbance

Protection

- Disrupted skin integrity
- Pressure ulcer
- Itching
- Delayed wound healing
- Infection
- Potential for ineffective coping with allergic reaction
- Ineffective coping with changes in immune status
- Ineffective temperature regulation
- Fever
- Hypothermia

Senses

- Impairment of a primary sense
- Potential for injury
- Loss of self-care abilities
- Stigma
- Sensory overload and deprivation
- Sensory monotony or distortion
- Potential for distorted communication
- Pain
- Acute pain

(continued)

TABLE 3–3 *(continued)*

- Chronic pain
- Perceptual impairment
- Ineffective coping strategies for sensory impairment

Fluid, Electrolyte, and Acid–Base Balance

- Dehydration
- Edema
- Intracellular water retention
- Shock
- Hyper- or hypocalcemia, -kalemia, or -natremia
- Acid–base imbalance
- Ineffective buffer regulation for changing pH

Neurologic Function

- Decreased level of consciousness
- Defective cognitive processing
- Memory deficits
- Instability of behavior and mood
- Ineffective compensation for cognitive deficit
- Potential for secondary brain damage

Endocrine Function

- Ineffective hormone regulation
- Ineffective reproductive development
- Instability of hormone system loops
- Instability of internal cyclical rhythms
- Stress

Self-Concept Mode

- Body image disturbance
- Sexual ineffectiveness
- Rape trauma syndrome
- Unresolved loss
- Anxiety
- Powerlessness
- Guilt
- Low self-esteem

Role-Function Mode

- Ineffective role transition
- Prolonged role distance
- Role conflict–intrarole and interrole

TABLE 3–3 (*continued*)

- Role failure
- Role ambiguity

Interdependence Mode

- Ineffective pattern of giving and receiving
- Ineffective pattern of dependency and independency
- Ineffective communication
- Lack of security in relationships
- Insufficient significant others and support systems for affection and relationship needs
- Separation anxiety
- Alienation
- Loneliness
- Ineffective development of relationships

TABLE 3–4 Typology of Commonly Recurring Adaptation Problems for Groups

Physical Mode

- Inadequate fiscal resources
- Capability deficits
- Inadequate physical facilities
- Shortage of personnel
- Debt for family, organization, community, nation
- Homelessness
- Health disparities
- Global hunger
- Inadequate potable water
- Ineffective response to disaster

Group Identity Mode

- Ineffective interpersonal relationships
- Values conflict
- Oppressive culture
- Low morale
- Outgroup stereotyping
- Abusive relationships

(*continued*)

TABLE 3–4 *(continued)*

Role-Function Mode

- Role confusion
- Inadequate socialization for role expectations
- Failure of some roles in group
- Ineffective give and take in role responsibilities
- Uneven distribution of responsibilities to detriment of goals of the group
- Interrole conflict
- Caregiver or other role strain
- Inadequate role development to meet growing needs of group

Interdependence Mode

- Isolation
- Ineffective development
- Inadequate resources
- Pollution
- Aggression

clustered and labeled "shock." Shock is a common adaptation problem of the physiologic mode, specifically, the individual's need for oxygenation. A nursing diagnosis using this example from the typology of commonly recurring adaptation problems could be "shock due to incisional hemorrhage." The related categories from the NANDA classification are "fluid volume deficit" and "altered tissue perfusion." This method of stating nursing diagnoses from established classifications is useful in the complex situations encountered in nursing practice. It is important to be aware that the label stands for a multifaceted clinical situation and points to an established set of cues, signs and symptoms, possible causes, or etiologies (Carpenito-Moyet, 2004). The label represents scientific nursing knowledge that can be used in planning nursing interventions. Diagnostic classifications are useful shorthand ways of communicating with other nurses and with other health care providers, including the federal agencies and private insurance companies that finance health care.

In using the nursing process based on the Roy Adaptation Model, the nurse concludes the first three steps with a clear understanding of patient behavior, the stimuli affecting the behavior, and a diagnostic statement. This statement reflects a nursing judgment about the adaptation status of the individual or group.

STEP 4: GOAL SETTING

Goals are established once the nurse has assessed the behavior of the individual or group and the stimuli influencing the behavior and has identified a nursing diagnosis from the assessment information. Goal setting is defined as the establishment of clear statements of the behavioral outcomes of nursing care. The general goal of nursing intervention, as defined earlier, is to maintain and enhance adaptive behavior and to change ineffective behavior to adaptive. The behavior of the individual or group is the focus of this general statement, and similarly, when establishing specific goals, the behavior of the individual or group is the focus. Throughout the first and second levels of assessment, the behavior and the stimuli influencing it have been identified and recorded. This information was put together into nursing diagnoses. Step 4 of the nursing process, goal setting, involves the statement of behavioral outcomes of nursing care that will promote adaptation. Figure 3–1 illustrates goal setting as it relates to the other steps of the nursing process.

Recall from previous discussion the individual who, following surgery, was demonstrating a progressive drop in blood pressure caused by hemorrhage from the incision. A nursing diagnosis could be expressed as "blood pressure 90/40 related to hemorrhage." A goal for this individual could be stated as follows: "The patient's blood pressure measurement will stabilize in a range of 100/70 to 130/80 within 30 minutes." This is a short-term goal that identifies a behavioral outcome promoting adaptation. Goals can also be long term. A long-term goal pertaining to the example might be, "The patient will return to his job within 3 weeks." The designation of goals as long or short term is relative to the situation involved. For some problems, especially those that are life threatening, short-term goals may be formulated on a minute-to-minute basis, and long-term goals on a day-to-day basis. In other situations, related to self-concept, group identity, or role function, for example, short-term goals may involve the time frame of a week, and long-term goals, months. In situations of community nursing, goals may span much broader time frames. It may take a year or more for a community to make progress in addressing situations of ineffective adaptation.

A goal statement should designate not only the behavior to be observed but the way the behavior will change (as observed, measured, or subjectively reported) and the time frame in which the goal is to be attained. Consider the following.

1. The patient's blood pressure measurement will stabilize (behavior) within a range of 110/70 to 130/80 (change expected) within 30 minutes (time frame).
2. The patient will be able (behavior) to return to his job (change expected) within 3 weeks (time frame).
3. The new mother will demonstrate increased ability (change expected) to care for her new baby (behavior) within 2 days (time frame).
4. Within 1 year (time frame) there will be a 25% decrease (change expected) in the frequency with which law enforcement personnel will need to be involved in dispute resolution (behavior).

Notice how each of the goals demonstrates the three elements identified above. These elements are important in the evaluation of goal attainment. In these examples, the goals focus on ineffective behaviors in an attempt to change them to adaptive behaviors. However, it may be just as important to focus on adaptive behaviors in an effort to maintain and enhance them. Consider the following situation: A 5-year-old boy, admitted for same day surgery, was interacting readily with the child next to him until it was time for his mother to leave. At this time he began to cry and cling to her. In this situation, the goal might focus on the adaptive behavior of interaction with the other child. The goal might be, "Within 5 minutes of mother's departure, child distracted from the separation as evidenced by interactive talking between the children." In the previous community situation, many members are willing to be involved in learning activities and voluntary programs. This is a physical mode (human resource) adaptive behavior that could be enhanced to help address the problem associated with dispute resolution.

The individuals involved in the situation are actively involved in developing behavioral goals whenever possible. This involvement provides the nurse with the opportunity to explore the rationale behind certain goals and gives the participants, as individuals or a group, the chance to suggest goals and evaluate whether goals are realistic. Those who are actively involved in setting a goal are more likely to be committed to achieving the goal. Consider the following goal: "Within 1 hour after surgery, the patient will stand unsupported by the bed for 5 minutes." Generally, it is considered important for people undergoing surgery to be mobile as soon as possible following return from the operating room. The patient involved in the formulation of this goal who understands the underlying rationale is more likely to try to achieve it than someone awakening to, "It's time to get you out of bed," while in pain and still drowsy.

It can be noted that individual behavioral goals are aimed at the goals of adaptation, that is, survival, growth, reproduction, mastery, and human and environment transformations. Thus, the nurse helps people strive for full human potential.

STEP 5: NURSING INTERVENTION

Once the goals have been established relative to behaviors that will promote adaptation, the nurse determines how best to assist the individual or group in attaining these goals. This is the fifth step of the nursing process, intervention, as described in the Roy Adaptation Model. Intervention is described as the selection of nursing approaches to promote adaptation by changing stimuli or strengthening adaptive processes.

Intervention With Stimuli and Coping Processes

In Roy's description of human adaptive systems, stimuli from the internal and external environment activate the coping processes to produce behaviors. When ineffective behavior is identified, there is evidence that the coping processes are not able to adapt effectively to the stimuli affecting them. Interventions can then be focused on both stimuli and coping processes. The first three steps of the nursing process involved the assessment of behaviors and related stimuli and synthesis of this information into a nursing diagnosis. Subsequent goal setting is the statement of the desired behavioral outcomes of nursing care relative to the problem areas identified. Intervention focuses on the way in which these goals can be reached. Whereas the focus of goal setting is the behavior of the human system, the focus of intervention is the stimuli influencing the behavior or the ability to cope with the stimuli. Figure 3–1 illustrates this in terms of the Roy Adaptation Model.

As was identified in Chapter 2, the ability of the human system to adapt or respond positively to a change depends on the focal stimulus and adaptation level. The focal stimulus is the degree of change taking place. The adaptation level is the changing condition of the life processes. It is an internal stimulus, which affects the ability of the individual or group to respond positively in a situation. To promote adaptation, it may be possible to manage the focal or other stimuli present. Management of stimuli involves altering, increasing, decreasing, removing, or maintaining them. Altering the stimuli brings them within the capacity of the coping processes of the human system to respond positively. The result is adaptive behavior. In getting the patient out of bed for the first time, the nurse adds positive stimuli to the simple request to get out of bed. This is done in the form of providing specific instructions for each move, for example, to sit on the side of the bed before standing. At the same time, the nurse provides both physical and emotional support.

Nurses are increasing their knowledge about individuals and groups as regulatory and stabilizer systems. Likewise, they better understand how thinking and feeling people promote health for individuals and groups through cognator–innovator systems. Based on this developing knowledge, the nurse increasingly becomes able to design nursing interventions specific to the coping processes. To return to the example of getting the postoperative patient out of bed for the first time, the nurse can affect the cognator by changing perception. Without adequate explanation, the individual may perceive the request to stand at the bedside one hour after surgery only as an occasion of pain and discomfort. The nurse can provide the opportunity to change this perception by explaining the positive effects of getting out of bed after surgery and increase the perception of this action as beneficial to healing and getting well.

Identification and Analysis of Possible Approaches

The identification of possible approaches to nursing intervention involves the selection of which stimuli to change. Roy incorporates the nursing judgment method as initially presented by McDonald and Harms (1966) in a description of this fifth step of the nursing process. In this method, possible approaches are listed and the approach with the highest probability of attaining the goals is selected. In applying this method to the Roy model, the stimuli affecting specific behaviors are listed and relevant coping processes are identified. Next, the consequences of changing each stimulus, or affecting a coping process, are identified together with the probability of their occurrence. The outcome of the consequence is judged as desirable or undesirable. This is accomplished in collaboration with the individual or group involved. Consider an example of the individual who is unable to sleep in the hospital environment. The second level of assessment yielded the following stimuli as contributing to this sleeplessness.

- Noise level (focal)
- Uncomfortable bed (contextual)
- Hunger (contextual)

Application of the nursing judgment method to these factors is illustrated in Table 3–5. The first approach, altering the stimulus of noise level, has the best probability of accomplishing the desired goal with undesirable consequences having a low probability. On the other hand, the third approach has a moderate probability of achieving the desired result, but the undesirable consequence of disrupting plans for surgery is highly probable. Whenever possible, the focal stimulus should be the focus of nursing interventions. However, when this is not possible, contextual stimuli or the coping mechanisms are considered in an effort to change adaptation

TABLE 3–5 The Nursing Judgment Method as Applied to Selection of Approaches

Alternative Approach	Consequence	Probability	Value
Alter noise level	Enhance sleep	High	Desirable
	Not enhance sleep	Low	Undesirable
Alter comfort of bed	Enhance sleep	High	Desirable
	Not enhance sleep	Low	Undesirable
	Disrupt intravenous	Low	Undesirable
Alter hunger	Enhance sleep	Moderate	Desirable
	Not enhance sleep	Moderate	Undesirable
	Disrupt plans for surgery in morning	High	Undesirable

levels. It also may be appropriate to use several approaches in combination. For example, an individual can be suffering severe pain caused by the focal stimulus of a terminal disease process. In this case, it is not possible to deal with the disease itself, and efforts must be directed toward contextual factors enabling the individual to handle the pain and be more comfortable. A personal support system may be one of the stimuli that must be increased or maintained. Other factors related to pain management that include strategies for intervening with the regulator and cognator are discussed in Chapter 10.

In the earlier example related to the community with dispute resolution problems, second level assessment indicated that the following stimuli contributed to the problems:

- No resources for dispute resolution other than the law enforcement personnel (contextual).
- Community members not versed in dispute resolution methods (contextual).
- Little positive interaction among neighbors (contextual).

Application of the nursing judgment method in this situation is illustrated in Table 3–6. From this analysis, it appears as if initiating a volunteer mediation program has the highest potential of producing a desirable result, that is, one that would promote the adaptation of the community.

Implementation of Selected Approach

Once the appropriate approach to nursing intervention has been selected, the nurse works with those involved to determine and initiate the steps that will alter the stimulus and enhance coping. Having decided that altering the noise level is the best approach to the patient's sleep-lessness, the nurse must determine how to do it. Shutting the door to the individual's room might help. It may be possible to reduce the volume of discussions at the nursing station. It may be necessary to move the individual away from a disruptive roommate. To initiate a community mediation program, the nurse works with other agencies and representatives from the community to develop a plan and a strategy to engage and train volunteer mediators. It is also necessary to provide the required infrastructure to operate the program. The law enforcement agencies may offer to fulfill this role in recognition of the extent to which the volunteer mediation program will alleviate their involvement in minor disputes.

From a broad perspective, the nurse is aware of accountability for nursing interventions. The American Nurses Association statement on social policy noted that nurses are

TABLE 3–6 Application of Nursing Judgment Method to Community Situation

Alternative Approaches	Consequence	Probability	Value
Increase law-enforcement capacity	Increased resources to deal with conflict	Low	Undesirable
	Increased cost	Low	Undesirable
Initiate community mediation program	Disputes handled in early stages	High	Desirable
	Community participants develop capabilities	High	Desirable
Prioritize disputes and assist in most serious	Number of unresolved disputes escalates	High	Undesirable

"legally accountable for actions taken in the course of professional nursing practice as well as for actions assigned by the nurse to others assisting in the provision of nursing care" (ANA, 2003, p.13). Having initiated or accomplished the nursing intervention, the nurse then proceeds with the evaluation of its effectiveness.

STEP 6: EVALUATION

The last step of the nursing process as described in the Roy Adaptation Model is evaluation. Evaluation involves judging the effectiveness of the nursing intervention in relation to the behavior of the individual or group. Was the goal reached that was set in the fourth step of the nursing process? To make this judgment, the nurse assesses the behavior after the interventions have been implemented. As in the initial assessment steps, the skills of observation, intuition, measurement, and interview are used. The nursing intervention would be judged effective if the behavior of the individual or group matches that of the goal set.

Evaluation as a Reflection of Goals

Understanding the nursing process according to the Roy Adaptation Model thus far, the reader knows that behavior shows how effective the coping processes are in adapting to the stimuli affecting the human adaptive system. Nursing interventions are directed toward altering stimuli in an effort to enhance the ability of the coping processes to respond effectively, or are directed to the coping processes. When goals are established in step 4 of the nursing process, they are set in terms of the behavior and they aim to maintain and enhance the adaptive behavior and to change ineffective behavior to adaptive. To evaluate the effectiveness of nursing interventions in terms of these goals, the nurse in collaboration with the individual(s) involved looks again at the behavior. Have the behavioral goals been achieved? This evaluation is the sixth and final step of the nursing process. The relations of evaluation to the previous steps and to Roy's description of the human adaptive system are illustrated in Figure 3–1.

Skills Used in Evaluation

As in the first assessment steps of the nursing process, the nurse uses the skills of observation, intuition, measurement, and interview to evaluate the effectiveness of nursing interventions. Consider the earlier example of the individual who was hemorrhaging following surgery. Some of the ineffective behaviors identified were falling blood pressure (measured), a large amount of blood on the dressing (observed), and a decreasing level of consciousness (observed through purposeful questioning). Goals relative to these behaviors relate to stabilizing blood pressure, cessation of bleeding, and regaining of consciousness, respectively. To evaluate the effectiveness of nursing interventions related to the goals, the nurse measures the individual's blood pressure, observes the amount of blood on a fresh dressing, and uses an established format for determining the level of consciousness (see Chapter 12). These are all skills used in making the initial assessment. In the example of the community with dispute resolution problems, the goal addressed the extent to which law enforcement officers were required to intervene in interpersonal disputes. Evaluation of attaining this goal involves noting the frequency with which officers became involved and determining the change 1 year after the initiation of the program. There would most likely be other qualitative measures that could also be employed to measure effectiveness. A survey of those who had used the volunteer mediators to assist with their dispute resolution would constitute a good measure of the effectiveness of the program in increasing the ability of group members to relate to each other.

Continuity of the Nursing Process

For the nursing intervention to be judged effective, the behavior of the individual or group will reflect the mutually set goals. If the goals are not achieved, the nurse proceeds to discover why the behavior did not change as anticipated. The goals may have been unrealistic or unacceptable to the individual or group involved, the assessment data may have been inaccurate or incomplete, or the selected interventions may need to be approached in a different way. The nurse returns to the first step of the nursing process to look closely at behaviors that continue to be ineffective and to work with the individuals involved to further understand the situation. In the postoperative example, the nurse may evaluate that the individual's blood pressure has stabilized and that bleeding has stopped, but there may not be a change in the level of consciousness. Although it is still important to ensure that the stable blood pressure and cessation of bleeding are maintained, the nurse would begin to focus on the individual's level of consciousness and proceed through the steps of the nursing process again to identify any other stimuli that might point to the use of an alternative approach to address the ineffective behavior of a decreasing level of consciousness.

The steps of the nursing process have been identified and discussed separately for the purpose of clarity. It is important, however, to recognize that the nursing process is ongoing. In fact, many of the steps occur simultaneously. The nurse may be assessing behavior in one adaptive mode while proceeding with a nursing intervention in another. She may be assessing behavior and stimuli at the same time and discussing goals in another area.

Summary

The six-step nursing process described in the Roy Adaptation Model has been presented in this chapter. The nurse assesses the behavior of the individual or group and the stimuli influencing that behavior and proceeds to state nursing diagnoses. Goals establishing behavioral outcomes are formulated, and interventions designed to manage stimuli and enhance coping are planned and implemented. Evaluation involves judging the effectiveness of the nursing interventions in relation to the adaptive system's behavior.

Each step of the nursing process is informed by the assumptions and concepts that describe persons according to the Roy Adaptation Model. The importance of collaboration with the individuals involved throughout the steps of the nursing process has been emphasized. The effectiveness of the nurse in assisting the people in promoting adaptation depends on the nurse's understanding of the situation and related knowledge as well as effectiveness of collaboration with those involved.

Exercises for Application

1. Suggest a behavioral goal that could apply to you, as the reader of this text, on your completion of this chapter. It should apply to the knowledge gained from reading this chapter.
2. Imagine yourself as a student who has just received a failing grade on an examination. Suggest several stimuli (focal, contextual) that may have influenced the poor performance. Identify and analyze possible approaches to the problem related to the stimuli or your coping strategies. Use the following table as a guideline. Select the approach with the highest possibility of success.

Alternative Approach	Consequence	Probability	Value

3. Describe a situation in which you think you used intuition rather than, or with, conscious thinking in assessing a patient.

4. Assume that, as of last week, you have applied the nursing process to yourself relative to your daily diet and have set the goal that you will begin immediately to eat a nutritionally balanced diet containing all the recommended daily allowances for nutrients. In light of this goal, evaluate your intake of food in the past 24 hours and suggest whether your observations match the preset goal or are ineffective in moving toward the goal. Proceed through all the steps of the nursing process related to your own situation.

Assessment of Understanding

QUESTIONS

1. Underline the behaviors demonstrated by the child in the following situation.

    A mother noticed that her 5-year-old son was not actively participating in play with other children. When she questioned him, he stated that he did not feel well and had a sore throat. The mother noticed that he appeared flushed and felt warm to her touch. Looking down his throat, she noticed that it was reddened and two rather large masses of tissue were protruding from either side.

2. Using the criteria presented in this chapter, label the following behaviors as adaptive (A) or ineffective (I) and provide rationales for your decision.

    (a) _____ A woman is 5 feet tall and weighs 80 pounds.

    (b) _____ The nurse measured the patient's blood pressure at 125/75.

    (c) _____ The patient asked the nurse three times to explain a simple procedure.

    (d) _____ In assessing the family's eating habits, the nurse noted that they never planned meals, they all ate at different times, and that their diet virtually excluded fruits and vegetables.

    (e) _____ Almost 50% of children in the elementary school were home from school with flu-like symptoms.

3. In the following situation, suggest stimuli that might be influencing the individual's behavior of refusing to taste the food.

    An 80-year-old patient who had been placed on a salt-restricted diet received her first salt-free meal. She announced to her nurse that she would rather go hungry than eat such tasteless food. The entire meal was left untouched.

4. In the following situation identify the stimuli that contributed to the student's performance and classify them as being focal, contextual, and residual.

    In preparation for an important exam, an anxious student who was having persistent problems in a course studied all night before the day of the test. During the writing of the exam she found that she was having trouble concentrating on the questions and remembering what she had studied. Handing in her paper, she commented to the instructor, "That exam was really hard; I know I didn't make it." Later she found out that her evaluation of her performance was correct.

5. State a nursing diagnosis statement related to the behaviors and stimuli underlined in the situation below. Your statement need not include all behaviors and stimuli.

    A 55-year-old woman has lost the use of the right side of her body as a result of a stroke. She is presently in a program of rehabilitation, which is aimed at helping her achieve a degree of independence relative to her activities of daily living. She appears to lack enthusiasm for the program and states that she can see no reason to make an effort to become active again as she has lost her position as an executive secretary. Since she lives alone, she feels she could not manage on her own anyway.

6. Formulate several goal statements for each of the following segments of assessment information and nursing diagnoses.

Behavior	Stimuli	Nursing Diagnosis

a.16-year-old girl.
   Weight 85 pounds.
   Height 5 feet 7 inches.
   States she does not eat
   breakfast and only has
   candy bars for lunch.
   Feels tired.
   Appears drawn and pale.
	Inadequate caloric and
	nutritive intake.
	Always short of time.
	Peer group does not eat lunch.
	Parents work; must prepare
	meals herself.
	Does not understand principles
	of good nutrition.
		Malnutrition due to inadequate
		intake of food and lack of
		knowledge.

b.Elderly male patient.
   Withdrawn and
   uncommunicative.
   Refuses to do anything for
   himself.
   States "No one cares
   whether I'm dead or alive."
   States "I'll never leave this
   place."
	Long-term hospitalization.
	Hospital is long distance from
	home and family.
	Has one close relative (a son)
	who can visit only
	occasionally.
		Loneliness due to absence of
		support systems.

7. The school nurse in an urban high school has been consulted by the administrative staff and a group of parents to help address a problem of teenage pregnancy among students. The following table represents a segment of information from steps 1 to 4 of the nursing process obtained when the nurse began discussions with a number of girls in the school. Continue with step 5 of the nursing process and identify interventions that could assist in the achievement of the specified goals.

Behavior	Stimuli	Nursing Diagnosis	Goals
Increasing pregnancy rate among high school girls.	Lack of knowledge about consequences and complications associated with teenage pregnancy.	Unwanted pregnancy related to lack of knowledge about sexual activity and lack of evaluative thought prior to decision making.	Within 6 months, the pregnancy rate among students will have decreased.
All state that they had not intended to become pregnant. Many girls state that they acted on impulse and without consideration of long-term outcomes. Girls stated that their peers expected sexual activity. Parents of girls are concerned about sexual activity.	Lack of information on which to base decision about sexual activity. Lack of information about birth control. Lack of parental involvement in sex education.	Inadequate knowledge about sexual behavior and potential outcomes.	Within 1 month, all the students at the school will state confidence in the adequacy of their knowledge related to sexual activity and its ramifications.

8. For the following goal statements, identify what one would look for in the behavior of the individuals or groups that would indicate that nursing interventions had been effective.
   (a) Within 1 week, the patient will have regained full use of his hand as evidenced by his ability to perform a full range of motion.
   (b) Within 6 months, 80% of the staff of the hospital will have received an immunization for hepatitis B.
   (c) Within 1 month, the family will document 1 week's nutritional intake that reflects all the recommended daily requirements.

FEEDBACK

1. Five-year-old, not actively participating in play, stated that he did not feel well and had a sore throat, appeared flushed, felt warm, (throat) reddened, large masses of tissue were protruding.
2. (a) I: Normally people of 5 feet weigh much more.
   (b) A: A blood pressure reading of 125/75 is within normal limits.
   (c) I: The patient appears to be demonstrating ineffective learning.
   (d) I: The family is not eating a balanced diet and their nutritional requirements are not being met.
   (e) I: The health status of the school participants indicates that there is a problem affecting half of the school population.
3. Stimuli contributing to the individual's refusal to eat: tastelessness of food, inadequate explanation of reason for salt-free diet, diminished acuity of taste sensation associated with aging.
4. Had trouble concentrating and remembering (focal). Studied all night (contextual). Had persistent problems (contextual). Was anxious (contextual). The exam was important (contextual).
5. Examples of nursing diagnosis statements:
   "Appears to lack enthusiasm for rehabilitation and states she sees no reason to make an effort since she has lost her job and feels she will be dependent." This is a statement of behavior connected to the relevant stimuli.

"Loss of body function due to stroke." The woman has lost the use of the right side of her body as a result of a stroke. She can no longer physically perform her job or care for herself. "Loss" is a common problem associated with the physical self-concept.

6. Examples of goal statements:
   (a) Patient will begin to gain weight as evidenced by a measured gain of 5 pounds in 1 month.
   Patient will eat regular nutritious meals within 1 week as evidenced by a daily diary of food intake that contains all the recommended daily allowances of nutrients.
   Patient's appearance will improve within 6 months as evidenced by weight gain and improved coloring.
   Patient will have more energy within 1 week as evidenced by her statements that she feels less tired and has more energy.
   (b) The patient will begin to interact with other patients and staff by becoming involved actively in an occupational therapy session on a daily basis beginning tomorrow.
   Within 2 days, the patient will begin to assume responsibility for several self-care tasks as demonstrated by shaving himself and cleaning his own teeth.
   Within 2 weeks, the patient will begin to demonstrate optimism about the future by inquiring about potential for discharge to alternative care agency.
7. Examples of interventions:
   In consultation with the students, develop an informational program to address their lack of knowledge.
   Work with the students to enhance their decision-making process by developing several scenarios that illustrate the ramifications and responsibilities of sexual activity.
8. In each case, nursing interventions would be judged effective if the behavior of the human system as identified in the goal statement was attained within the time frame specified.

References

American Nurses Association. (1995). *Nursing's social policy statement.* Kansas City, MO: American Nurses Association.

American Nurses Association. (2003). *Nursing's social policy statement.* Washington, DC: American Nurses Association.

Antai-Otong, D. (2007). *Nurse-client communication: A life span approach.* Sudbury, MA: Jones and Bartlett Publishers.

Boykin, A., & Schoenhofer, S. (1993). *Nursing as caring: A model for transformation practice.* New York: National League for Nursing Press.

Carpenito-Moyet, L. J. (2004). *Nursing diagnosis: Application to clinical practice.* Philadelphia: Lippincott Williams & Wilkins.

Cho, J. (1998). *Nursing manual: Assessment tool according to the Roy Adaptation Model.* Glendale, CA: Polaris Publishing.

DeMarco, R. F., Miller, K., Patsdaughter, C., Grindel, C., & Chisholm, M. (1998). From silencing the self to action: Experiences of women living with HIV/AIDS. *Women's Health Care International, 19*(6), 539–552.

Erikson, E. H. (1963). *Childhood and society* (2nd ed.). New York: Norton.

Grace, P. J. (2001). Professional Advocacy: Widening the scope of accountability. *Nursing Philosophy, 2*(2), 151–162.

Johnson, M., Mass, M., & Moorhead, S. (2000). *Nursing outcome classification* (NOC; 2nd ed.). St. Louis, MO: Mosby.

Leininger, M., & McFarland, M. (2002). *Transcultural nursing: Concepts, research, theory and practice.* New York: McGraw Hill.

McCloskey, J. C., & Bulechek, G. M. (Eds.). (1992). *Nursing Interventions Classification* (NIC). St. Louis, MO: Mosby Year Book.

McDonald, F. J., & Harms, M. (1966). Theoretical model for an experimental curriculum. *Nursing Outlook, 14*(8), 48–51.

NANDA-International. (2007). *Nursing diagnoses: Definitions and classifications, 2007–2008.* Philadelphia: NANDA-I.

Nightingale, F. (1859). *Notes on nursing: What it is and what it is not* (facsimile edition). Philadelphia: Lippincott.

Sato, M. K. (1984). Major factors influencing adaptation. In C. Roy, (Ed.), *Introduction to nursing: An adaptation model* (2nd ed., pp. 64–87). Englewood Cliffs, NJ: Prentice Hall.

Sorrel M. S., & Smith, B. A. (1993). Navajo beliefs: Implications for health professionals. *Journal of Health Education, 24*(6), 336–338.

Watson, J. (2005). *Caring science as sacred science.* Philadelphia: Davis.

Wilkinson, J. (2000). *Nursing diagnosis handbook with NIC interventions and NOC outcomes* (7th ed.). Upper Saddle River, NJ: Prentice-Hall.

CHAPTER 4

Overview of Adaptive Modes

Roy's description of persons, individuals, and groups as adaptive systems includes four major categories in which coping processes can be observed. These categories are named the four adaptive modes: the physiologic–physical mode, the self-concept–group identity mode, the role function mode, and the interdependence mode. One way to observe human behavior is in these four major categories. Understanding the adaptive modes also helps to identify adaptation levels. Part 2 of this text explores these four adaptive modes for individuals. Part 3 considers the adaptive modes for groups. Each mode for both individuals and groups identifies integrated processes, compensatory processes, and compromised processes. Knowledge of the processes provides a basis for assessment and planning of nursing care. The physiologic needs and processes are presented first, followed by the other modes, on the individual level then the group level. The intent is to move from simple to complex and from concrete to abstract. The understanding gained about one adaptive mode is helpful in understanding the other modes. Similarly knowledge of the processes, behavior, and influencing stimuli for individuals in each mode provides the basis for understanding groups. These concepts are applied to using the adaptation model in nursing practice situations. In this chapter the authors provide an overview of each of the four adaptive modes on the individual and group levels.

OBJECTIVES

After studying this chapter, the reader will be able to do the following:

1. Identify the basic need underlying each of the four adaptive modes for both individuals and groups.
2. Provide examples of the theoretical basis of each adaptive mode.
3. Identify the five basic needs and their associated life processes inherent in physiologic integrity.

4. Describe the four complex physiologic processes that serve to mediate regulator activity and integrate physiologic functioning.

5. Demonstrate beginning application of the concepts associated with the physical mode as it applies to groups or collective human systems.

KEY CONCEPTS DEFINED

Biobehavioral knowledge: Focus of nursing knowledge that balances understanding of people as both physiologic beings in a physical world and as thinking and feeling beings with human experience in a cosmic world.

Capacities: The assets that participants in group adaptive systems bring to the situation including knowledge, skills, abilities, commitments, and associations with others.

Fiscal resources: The component of the physical mode related to the monetary capacity of the group adaptive system.

Identity integrity: The basic need of the group identity mode; implies the honesty, soundness, and completeness of identification with the group; involves the process of shared identity and goals.

Operating integrity: The underlying need of the physical adaptive mode; wholeness achieved by adapting to changes in operating resource requirements; encompasses participants, physical facilities, and fiscal resources.

Participants: The component of the physical mode related to those involved in, or members of, the group adaptive system.

Personal self: The individual's appraisal of personal characteristics, expectations, values, and worth.

Physical facilities: The component of the physical mode related to capital and material capacities required for ongoing operation and effective adaptation of the group adaptive system.

Physical mode: The way the group adaptive system manifests adaptation relative to needs associated with basic operating resources.

Physical self: An individual's appraisal of personal physical being including physical attributes, functioning, sexuality, health-illness states, and appearance.

Physiologic integrity: The underlying need of the physiologic mode; physiologic wholeness achieved by adapting to changes in physiologic needs.

Physiologic mode: One of the four adaptive modes in which an individual manifests the physical and chemical processes involved in the functions and activities of a living organism.

Physiology: A science dealing with knowledge about the physical and chemical phenomena involved in the function and activities of a living organism.

Process: A series of activities or changes that proceed from one to the next.

Psychic and spiritual integrity: The basic need of the self-concept mode on the individual level; the need to know who one is so that one can be or exist with a sense of unity, meaning, and purposefulness in the universe.

Relational integrity: The underlying need of the interdependence mode; wholeness achieved in terms of the needs for affection, development, and resources.

Role: The functioning unit of society; each role exists in relation to another.

Role clarity: Basic need associated with the role function mode for groups; the need to understand and commit to fulfill expected tasks, so that the group can achieve common goals.

Self-concept: The composite of beliefs and feelings that is held about oneself at a given time, formed from internal perception and perceptions of others' reactions.

Significant others: Persons who are most important to the individual.

Social integrity: The basic need of the role function mode for individuals; the need to know who one is in relation to others so that one can act.

Support systems: Other people contributing to meeting interdependence needs.

THE FOUR ADAPTIVE MODES

The adaptive modes, as described in the Roy Adaptation Model, are related to the way human systems respond to stimuli from the environment. Adaptive systems are studied on both the individual and group levels. The behaviors of both individuals and groups that result from coping activity can be observed in four categories, or adaptive modes. Roy has developed an understanding of each mode from a broad knowledge base to serve as a framework for assessment and planning of nursing care. These four modes are as follows:

1. The physiologic for individuals and the physical for groups
2. The self-concept for individuals and group identity for groups
3. Role function for both individuals and groups
4. Interdependence for both individuals and groups

In the following section an overview of each of the four modes is provided. The use of the adaptive modes to plan nursing care is provided in a case study that begins in this chapter and is continued in other chapters as examples of the adaptive modes of individuals in the family and of the family as a group.

PHYSIOLOGIC–PHYSICAL MODE

The behavior related to the material aspects of adaptive systems is termed the physiologic mode for individuals and the physical mode for groups. Each of these has been developed to guide the assessment of the effectiveness of adaptation from the material perspective of individuals and groups. The components of the physiologic mode of people are addressed in Chapters 5 to 13 and the physical mode of the group is discussed in Chapter 17.

Physiologic Mode

The physiologic mode includes the physical and chemical processes involved in the function and activities of living organisms. An understanding of physiologic behavior uses knowledge of anatomy and physiology of the human body as well as of the pathophysiology underlying disease processes. The nurse will be knowledgeable about normal body processes to recognize compensatory processes and compromised processes of physiologic adaptation. The underlying need of the physiologic mode is physiologic integrity. Integrity has been defined as the degree of wholeness achieved by adapting to changes in needs. When a person's physiologic needs are met, physiologic integrity is achieved.

Behavior in this mode is the expression of the physiologic activities of all the cells, tissues, organs, and systems of the human body. As with each of the adaptive modes, stimuli activate the coping processes, creating adaptive and ineffective behavior. In this case, the coping processes are those associated with physiologic functioning and the resulting responses are physiologic behaviors. It is the person's physiologic behavior that indicates whether the coping processes are able to adapt to the stimuli affecting them. Five needs are identified in the physiologic mode relative to physiologic integrity: oxygenation, nutrition, elimination, activity and rest, and protection. Each of the physiologic needs involves integrated processes. These needs and associated processes are briefly described here and addressed individually in following chapters.

1. Oxygenation. This need involves the body's requirements for oxygen and the basic life processes of ventilation, exchange of gases, and transport of gases.
2. Nutrition. This need involves a series of integrated processes associated with digestion; that is, the ingestion and assimilation of food and metabolism, provision of energy, building of tissue, and regulation of metabolic processes.
3. Elimination. The need for elimination includes the physiologic processes involved in the excretion of metabolic wastes, primarily through the intestines and kidneys.
4. Activity and rest. The need for balance in the basic life processes of mobility and sleep provides optimal physiologic functioning of all body components and periods of restoration and repair.
5. Protection. The need for protection includes two basic life processes: nonspecific defense processes and specific defense processes, or immunity.

A discussion of physiologic adaptation includes complex processes involving senses; fluid, electrolyte, and acid–base balance; neurologic function; and endocrine function.

1. Senses. The sensory processes of sight, hearing, touch, taste, and smell enable people to interact with their environment. The sensation of pain is a particular focus in this mode component.
2. Fluid, electrolyte, and acid–base balance. Complex processes associated with fluid, electrolyte, and acid–base balance are required for cellular, extracellular, and systemic function.
3. Neurologic function. Neurologic channels function to control and coordinate body movements, consciousness, and cognitive-emotional processes, as well as to regulate activity of body organs.
4. Endocrine function. Endocrine processes through hormone secretion serve, along with neurologic function, to integrate and coordinate body functioning. Endocrine activity plays a significant role in the stress response.

These four complex processes are viewed as mediators of regulatory activity, and they include many physiologic functions of the person. The nine components listed are described within the model as a basis for nursing assessment of the physiologic mode of an individual. The theoretical understanding of each component is used with the assessment of behaviors and stimuli to plan nursing care.

Theoretical Basis for the Physiologic Mode

The theoretical background of the physiologic mode for the individual human system lies in basic life sciences, particularly anatomy, physiology, pathophysiology, and chemistry. In addition, meeting human needs is influenced by psychologic processes such as motivation and concepts from sociology, anthropology, religious studies, and other disciplines within the humanities. For example, literature can provide understanding of how fictional characters are developed to deal with basic themes of life. The relevant theoretical fields can be described briefly as follows.

Anatomy. The study of the structure of the human body, human anatomy provides the structural basis for the physiologic mode.

Physiology. Physiology provides the nurse with knowledge of the processes involved in the functioning and activities of the human body. This knowledge is the basis for the judgment of adaptive and ineffective physiologic behavior.

Pathophysiology. The study of the abnormal physiologic changes accompanying illness, pathophysiology provides the nurse with a rationale for the identification of ineffective behavioral responses and the stimuli influencing them.

Chemistry. Knowledge from chemistry, dealing with the composition, properties, and reactions of substances, provides the basis for an understanding of body processes such as those involved in fluid, electrolyte, and acid–base balance activity.

Psychology. The study of the mind and behavior provides a basis for the understanding of psychosocial processes related to self, role, and interdependence, and how the processes relate to dealing with illness.

Sociology. The study of the development, structure, interaction, and behavior of organized groups of people provides a foundation for the nurse's assessment of the self, role, and interdependence modes and their influence on physiologic function in situations of effective and ineffective adaptation.

Anthropology. The study of people in relation to their distribution, origin, classification, and the relationship of ethnic groups including physical character, environmental and social relationships, and culture. This knowledge contributes to the nurse's ability to identify the impact of these factors on the manifestation of physical needs and the integrity of the adaptive modes.

Religious studies and spirituality. The study of specific religions and approaches to spirituality provides insight into the beliefs and values of people. It enables consideration of factors that may influence how one meets given needs and the responses to particular environmental influences. This diversity is significant in providing nursing care.

Humanities. Knowledge from other disciplines focusing on the attributes or qualities of the human person enables the nurse more effectively to consider the experiences of people and to intervene appropriately in situations of need.

Physical Mode

The physical mode for people interacting in groups corresponds with the physiologic mode for the individual. It has been described as the way in which the group adaptive system manifests adaptation concerning basic resources for operating. These basic resources include participants of the group, physical facilities, and fiscal resources. The basic need associated with the physical mode is operating integrity, or the wholeness of having what is needed for system survival and for adapting to changes in participants, facilities, or resources.

The component of the physical mode called participants relates to the people who are involved in the group adaptive system. In the case of a family, this includes the relevant family members. Some terminology to describe family members includes the nuclear family (two parents and child or children), single-parent family (one parent and child or children), and the extended family (including relatives beyond parent(s) and children). Some families include adults, with or without children, living together, who are bound by legal, kinship, or other relations. For other groups, the participants would consist of members of the group, both formal and informal. In organizations, the participants are those who are involved in or employed by the organization or have some other role to fulfill as part of the organization. Community participants tend to be those who reside in a particular community; however, geographic location may not be a determinant for community membership. In the case of some ethnic communities the participants can reside in several locations. Participants in the society as a whole typically are located within the societal boundaries. Whatever the collective of people in a group, the participants are those who would name themselves as part of the group.

Just as the goals of the individual human adaptive system are identified in the Roy Adaptation Model, so are the goals of adaptation for systems that are groups of people. Effective responses of groups such as families, organizations, communities, or society relate to goals. The basic goals of groups are ongoing existence of the group and its continuing growth. Within these goals are the ability of the group to transmit beliefs, values, and cultural heritage. Adaptation includes confidence and success in fulfilling the group's vision and objectives. The capacities of participants are a major resource for the human adaptive system. Included in the notion of capacities are the knowledge, skills, capabilities, commitments, and health of the individuals within the group system. The basic need of the physical adaptive mode, operating integrity, cannot be fulfilled unless the participants possess the capacities required to support the collective entity. Identifying, refining, and enhancing the capacities of participants of the group can enable meeting the goals of adaptation.

Physical facilities are an important component for group adaptive systems. This aspect of the physical system includes a physical plant such as shelter for the family, a meeting place for a group, offices for organizations, or territorial integrity for a nation. Also included in this component are the operational resources required to fulfill the purpose of the group. In a family situation, food and clothing are examples of operational resources. In an organization, supplies and equipment constitute physical resources, for example, books and computers in schools and bedsheets and exercise equipment in a rehabilitation facility. Some group systems have need for technologic resources as well. A community requires communication systems, road maintenance equipment, and trash disposal. All these physical commodities contribute to meeting the need for resource adequacy in the physical system.

Many resources are dependent on fiscal adequacy. Inadequate levels of funding compromise the ability of the system to maintain the integrity of the particular group. In a family situation, if there is not enough food for the members, health of the adults or children can be compromised. If an organization is unable to purchase operating supplies, it will experience difficulty remaining in business. Capital resources are also an important aspect of fiscal adequacy for most collective human adaptive systems. Capital resources relate to the significant and infrequent purchases that may be required to support the ongoing integrity of the collective system. In a family situation, this can be a major health care expenditure on behalf of a member or the purchase of a house for the family. For a baseball team, it may be the purchase of uniforms so that the team can play in an organized league. Organizations, communities, and societal groups often have major requirements for capital resources to support their ongoing and orderly operation. For example, as a hospital or a university expands it may purchase land to construct additional buildings for its services. If inadequate funding persists over time, the integrity of the entire system is compromised; ineffective behaviors result. This notion will be explored further as the nursing process is applied to the physical mode.

Theoretical Basis for the Physical Mode

Understanding the physical mode draws upon some of the theoretical basis identified for the physiologic mode. The psychologic understanding of human behavior helps to recognize how people act in groups. Sociology and anthropology, described briefly above, contribute theories to understand group behavior. Similarly, just as religious studies and spirituality explain effects on individuals, these studies add to appreciating behaviors of groups. In addition, the theoretical basis for the physical mode includes family studies, organizational behavior, economics, community studies, and ecology and cosmology. These additional fields of study with application to group adaptive systems are described briefly as follows.

Family studies. The study of family interactions includes the stages of the family life cycle and consideration of contemporary issues, for example, changing family structures and family violence.

Organizational behavior. The study of organizations and their environment, strategies, and structures is basic to understanding groups as adaptive systems.

Economics. The study of the principles of economics provides insight into the effects of employment, inflation, monetary policy, and fiscal policy on health and the provision of health care. The knowledge also leads to understanding of major stimuli affecting individuals and groups.

Community studies. The study of community dynamics includes the development, structure, interaction, and collective behavior of community members and is useful to understanding groups as adaptive systems.

Ecology and cosmology. The study of the earth and universe, developmental stages and future, helps nurses understand decisions made by people concerning the environment and the integrity of earth resources.

These disciplines provide some of the knowledge needed to support understanding of all four modes and the study of nursing as a knowledge-based profession. The view of nursing based on the Roy Adaptation Model indicates what knowledge is relevant and what knowledge needs to be developed. From their experience with people who are in all stages of health, nurses can determine what knowledge is relevant for nursing care. As with each of the modes, consideration of the physiologic–physical mode involves knowledge from a variety of related disciplines. This knowledge is viewed in the light of nursing's concept of the person as an individual or group system and of the goal of promoting adaptation. Nursing knowledge is biobehavioral. Such knowledge balances understanding of persons as both physiologic beings in a physical world and as thinking and feeling beings with human experience in a cosmic world.

An understanding of the physiologic and physical modes is the basis for the nursing process according to the Roy Adaptation Model. Application of the nursing process to the adaptive modes was illustrated in general in the diagrammatic conceptualization of the model in Figure 3–1.

An example of assessment related to a family facing major health concerns is provided in Box 4–1. The health concerns affect all adaptive modes; however, the physical mode is the focus of this example. Nursing assessment according to the Roy Adaptation Model

---

BOX 4–1

Case Study of Robles Family: Part I Assessment in Physical Mode

---

The Robles family, as a result of a motor vehicle accident, is adjusting to a 2-year-old child who is totally paralyzed and ventilator dependent. After a lengthy hospitalization, the child is now stable and plans are being made to move her out of the acute care setting.

Behaviors	Stimuli
Capacities of family members	Culture
• Mother learned knowledge and skills to care for an individual on a ventilator; is committed to assuming care for 8 hours a day, 5 days a week • Father expressed willingness to learn, has not yet demonstrated competence • Two young siblings cannot yet be involved in care	• Family ethnic origin generally noted to have very strong commitments to fellow members; high sense of responsibility regarding family tasks • Extended family highly supportive and involved; willing to assist with the child in home care
Physical facilities	Socioeconomic status
• Plans to renovate home • Special room close to family activity altered to accommodate the mobile bed and equipment • Entrance altered to provide wheelchair access	• Family is considered in upper quartile in income; believes they can bear additional financial expenses
	Environmental considerations
	• Family lives in a spacious house with flexibility for renovation to accommodate the particular needs of handicapped child

---

involves two considerations: the assessment of behavior and the assessment of relevant influencing stimuli. Although these steps are separated in the example, the nurse will identify behaviors and stimuli simultaneously while interacting with the family for the purposes of nursing assessment.

Based on assessment of behaviors and stimuli, the nurse plans care as illustrated in Box 4–2. Diagnoses, goals, interventions, and evaluations are listed for selected issues of the physical mode of the family. The method of stating a nursing diagnosis according to the Roy Adaptation Model was presented in Chapter 3. This involves relating the observed behavior to the most relevant stimuli. The goal of nursing, when applied to behavior in the adaptive modes, is to maintain and enhance adaptive behavior and to change ineffective behavior to adaptive. Thus, the focus of goal setting is the behavior of the adaptive system. The goal statement consists of the three entities identified in Chapter 3, the behavior to be observed, the change expected, and the time frame for achievement of the goal. Interventions to promote adaptation manage the stimuli influencing the behavior under consideration. The nurse may change the stimuli or broaden the adaptation level by supporting cognator and regulator or stabilizer and innovator activity. In selecting approaches, the nurse considers possible alternatives and then selects the approach with the highest probability of achieving the agreed-upon goal. The final step of the nursing process, evaluation, involves assessment of

---

BOX 4–2

Case Study of Robles Family: Planning Nursing Care

Nursing Diagnosis	Goal
• Planning to accommodate handicapped child in home supported by family commitment and capabilities and adequate fiscal resources • Inadequately trained personnel to care for child on a 24-hour basis since the mother is the only on-site caregiver at this point in time	• One week prior to discharge (time frame), physical accommodations for handicapped child in home (change expected) completed (behavior) • Two weeks prior to discharge (time frame), plans will be in place (change expected) for 24-hour nursing care coverage (behavior)

Intervention	Evaluation
• Collaborate with staff of other agencies to develop a workable plan for sufficient nursing care coverage • Pursue support above current provision of health insurance plan in exceptional circumstance; family willing to take on the care, otherwise requiring institutional care • Explore with family the possibility of involvement of members from the extended family	• 24-hour nursing care planned for the child at discharge from hospital • If goal not accomplished, the nurse and the family would proceed with further assessment and reconsideration of the goal; perhaps caring for the child in the home is not realistic; perhaps there are other sources of funding such as voluntary organizations to approach for assistance • Success in achieving goal leads to further detailed planning for the child's imminent discharge and the support and achievement of the integrity of the family unit

---

the behavioral response in relation to the established behavioral goal. If the goal has been achieved, the intervention was effective; if not, further assessment and reconsideration of goals and intervention is required.

SELF-CONCEPT–GROUP IDENTITY MODE

The adaptive mode related to the personal aspect of human systems is termed the self-concept mode for the individual and the group identity mode for groups. Knowledge of self for persons and groups has been developed to guide assessment of the effectiveness of adaptation of the self-concept and group identity mode. Chapter 14 expands on the self-concept adaptive mode of persons and Chapter 18 discusses the group identity adaptive mode.

Self Concept Mode

Self concept is defined as the composite of beliefs and feelings held about oneself at a given time. Self concept is formed from internal perceptions and perceptions of others' reactions. The fused sense of self is used to direct one's behavior. The self-concept mode is viewed as having two components. The physical self includes body sensation and body image. The personal self is composed of self-consistency, self-ideal, and a moral-ethical-spiritual self. Some examples of these components include the statement, "I look like I haven't slept in a week!" a behavioral statement related to body image. The statement, "I know I can figure out how to add photos to my PowerPoint presentation," illustrates self-ideal behavior. In the self-concept mode, the underlying basic need is psychic and spiritual integrity, or the need to know who one is so that one can be or exist with a sense of unity, meaning, and purposefulness in the universe. Psychic and spiritual integrity is basic to health. Adaptation problems in integrity of self can interfere with the person's ability to recover or to do what is necessary to maintain health. It is important for the nurse to have knowledge about the self-concept mode to assess behaviors and stimuli influencing the person's self-concept.

Theoretical Basis for the Self Concept Mode

The description of the self-concept mode is based on a number of specific psychologic, biologic, and social theories and principles, synthesized by Driever (1976) and expanded by Roy. These provide direction for the assessment of behavior and stimuli of the self concept of the individual and for each of the other steps of the nursing process. The following is an identification of the theoretical bases of the self-concept mode described in the Roy Adaptation Model. The works of the identified theorists can enhance knowledge in application of the Roy Adaptation Model.

Freud (1949), Piaget (1954), Erikson (1963), Bowlby (1969), Neugarten (1969, 1979), Kolberg (1981), and Gilligan (1982). Developmental theories based on physical, social, cognitive, and moral maturational.

Markus (1977). Self schemas describing cognitive generalizations that guide processing of self-related information.

Mead (1934), Sullivan (1953), Cooley (1964), and Goffman (1959, 1967). Symbolic interaction theories focusing on social interaction as a basis for developing and maintaining a sense of self.

Luft (1984). A theoretical framework for describing levels of self-awareness as expressed in relating to others; uses a two-way matrix to form a graphic metaphor of a window to awareness.

Lecky (1969), Rogers (1951, 1961), Elliott (1986), and Antonovsky (1986). Theories based on self-consistency, self-organization, and coherence.

McMahon (1993). Focusing as a term to include being in touch with self in a way that surfaces hope, energy, continuity, meaning, purpose, and pride to be an individual self within the whole human community.

Campsey (1985), Johnson (1983), Montagu (1986), Johnson and Levanthal (1974), and Amman-Gainotti (1986). Focused on body sensation, sexuality, and coping relevant for nursing assessment and intervention.

Festinger (1962) and Andrews (1990). Theory of cognitive dissonance in which the individual's behavior reflects an endeavor to minimize perceived discrepancies between the self concept and other aspects of experience.

Rosenberg (1965, 1979), Driever (1976), and Crocker and Park, (2003). Self-esteem described as stemming from values of self-attributions and as a pervasive aspect of self.

Kübler-Ross (1969) and Dobratz (1984, 2004, 2005). Described five stages of death and dying, and the process of life closure. Understanding is commonly used in promoting resolution of the issue of the meaning of one's life and accepting the reality of death. In addition, the nurse helps people grow through grieving.

Group Identity Mode

The group identity mode is analogous to the self-concept mode. It reflects how people in groups perceive themselves based on environmental feedback. The group identity mode is comprised of interpersonal relationships, group self-image, social milieu, and culture. The basic need underlying the group identity mode is termed identity integrity, the ability of group members to relate to each other with the honesty, soundness, and completeness of identification with the group. Identity integrity involves the process of shared identity and goals. In a social system such as a school, one can describe an associated culture. There is a social environment experienced by the teachers and students, and a group identity that is reflected by those who are part of the school group. As such, the group identity mode can reflect adaptive or ineffective behaviors associated with the school as a social organization.

Theoretical Basis for the Group Identity Mode

Lewin (1948). Theory of small group interaction.

Kimberly (1997). Described processes and structures of groups and the bases of cohesiveness as the relationships among liking or attraction, norms and values, and effective pursuit of goals and good working relations.

Rabbie and Lodewijks (1996). Goal-directed behavior of groups are a function of the perceived external environment and shared cognitive, emotional, motivational, and normative understandings of social systems; behavioral interaction model for studying groups that includes demands and distance, external social environment, and leadership and responsibility.

Zohar (1990) and Swimme and Berry (1992). The creative self and the human capacity for unity of consciousness and relational wholes. Transaction adds that as persons interact with environment, both are changed and integration and mutual transformations are possible.

Singer (2002). Begin to consider ourselves members of community of the world.

Hanna (2004, 2005). Provided a revised definition of moral distress based on study of the Roy Adaptation Model and its philosophic assumptions.

Chinn (2008). Presented a process of transformation based on experiences of women's groups and represented by the five words: praxis, empowerment, awareness, consensus, and evolvement (PEACE).

Perry (2004, 2005). Developed the framework of transcendent pluralism to support evolution of social consciousness that is grounded in human dignity, leading to understanding and justice.

Stanger and Lange (1994). Social identity theory resulting in ingroup and outgroup awareness.

Satir (1991). Patterns of behavior are transmitted through family generations.

This text introduces the theoretical basis for self concept and group identity. Understanding of people and groups as adaptive systems that strive for psychic and spiritual integrity and identity integrity is described. Nurses will find that continued study and experience can expand upon this knowledge. In this way, they are enabled to practice nursing with the Roy Adaptation Model at the increasing level of complexity required in contemporary health care.

ROLE FUNCTION MODE

The category of behavior that relates to roles of people is termed the role function mode for both the individual and the group. Knowledge of this adaptive mode has been developed in further detail to guide assessment of the effectiveness of adaptation as it relates to the roles that people occupy relative to each other.

Individual

From the perspective of the individual, the role function mode focuses on the roles that the individual occupies in society. A role, as the functioning unit of society, is defined as a set of expectations about how a person occupying one position behaves toward a person occupying another position. The basic need underlying the role function mode has been identified as social integrity. Social integrity is the need to know who one is in relation to others so that one can act. The role set is the complex of positions that an individual holds. A classification of role sets as involving primary, secondary, and tertiary roles has been used in the Roy Adaptation Model. Associated with each role are instrumental behaviors and expressive behaviors. Instrumental behaviors are goal oriented and expressive behaviors relate to feelings. Each type of behavior can be illustrated with the role of a mother. Caring for a baby's physical needs involves instrumental behaviors; holding and cuddling the baby are expressive behaviors. The manner in which the individual fulfills role expectations is an indication of adequacy of role mastery. Assessment of behaviors provides an indication of social adaptation related to role function.

Group

Roles within a group are how the goals of the group are actually accomplished. They are the action components associated with the group or collective infrastructure. Roles are designed to contribute to the accomplishment of the group's mission or the tasks and functions associated with the group. The role function mode includes the functions of officers and workers, the management of information, and systems for decision making and maintaining order. The basic need associated with the role function mode at the group level is termed role clarity, the need to understand and commit to fulfill expected tasks so that the group can achieve common goals. In a business, the management function constitutes a role subsystem as do decision-making processes and performance assessment systems. In a family, roles relate to such functions as earning a living, maintaining a place to live, and child rearing. Interrelated roles are the aggregated role sets of all members and constitute the role function mode for the group.

Theoretical Basis for the Role Function Mode

The description of the role function mode is based on a number of specific theories and principles from sociology, psychology, management, globalization, social justice, and nursing. These provide direction for the assessment of behaviors and stimuli relative to the role function mode and for each of the other steps of the nursing process. The following is an identification of major theorists and a statement of their important theoretical concepts that are the basis of the role function mode for individuals and groups as described in the Roy Adaptation Model.

Parsons and Shils (1951) and Patterson (1996). Classic structural approach to roles. Identification of role requirements and instrumental and expressive behaviors associated with roles; structural and functional considered.

Mead (1934) and Blumer (1969). Interaction approach to roles. One defines the situation as one "sees it" and acts on the perception.

Banton (1965) and Erikson (1963). Described roles as primary, secondary, and tertiary; age-related developmental stages and social expectations.

Turner (1979). Role-taking by three standpoints. Described internal and external validation of roles.

Merton (1957). Identified six processes for integrating role sets.

Eagly (1987). View of social role theory that deals with how gender affects roles in society, particularly occupations.

Brehm and Kassin (1996). Described social perception as involving observations of raw data, analyzing behavior, and attributing characteristics to the other. Stereotyping involves beliefs that associate certain groups of people with certain types of characteristics and then these beliefs influence judgments of individuals.

Meleis (1975) and Meleis et al. (2000). Role transitions require incorporation of new knowledge, altering one's behavior, and changing one's definition of self. Role modeling described as a nursing intervention; middle-range theory regarding the complexities of the transition experience.

Roy (1967) and Clarke and Strauss (1992). Role cues described and tested as intervention in role transition; role supplementation involves clarification, role-taking, role modeling, and role rehearsal.

Marquis and Huston (2006). Clarified role expectations by role models, preceptors, and mentors.

Lambert and Lambert (2001). Working with preceptor allows student to observe and acquire knowledge about the role; work in the environment and be in climate that fosters motivation to meet role demands.

Vance (1977, 1982) and Prestholdt (1990). A mentor serves many roles including model, guide, teacher, tutor, coach, confidant, and visionary-idealist; mentoring is viewed as a long-term adult developmental process with active involvement in a close personal relationship.

Gray (2003). Described series of reciprocating roles taken on in any new position.

Worchel (1996). Described six stages of development from observing ongoing groups that are useful in group-based analysis, including nursing assessment.

Chinn (2008). Chinn recommended that groups rotate leadership and responsibility. In this approach the formal structures are minimized while all group members are given the equal opportunity to participate regardless of any informal structures that develop. The purpose is to reverse the familiar structure with a linear chain of command. In the old structure a single individual or elite group manages the group and assumes leadership and control. The author describes instead a group convener who facilitates announcements, focuses the discussion, and provides leadership for the process. However, whoever is speaking is the leader.

Zohar and Marshall (1994) and Derber (2003). Described a global society where community draws on common culture and collective patterns of thinking, feeling, and acting. The search for meaningful social norms goes beyond individualism or collectivism to creative use of both freedom and ambiguity; new movement to explicitly organize a challenge to how globalization is emerging; an alternative to a corporate-dominated world system; people think globally about markets, democracy, and social justice; organized by networks to sustain cooperation among thousands of different groups and communities both in the United States and around the globe.

Vision Points of the Global Cooperation for a Better World (2004). Group-developed vision of a process of change based on an ethic of cooperation to stimulate and strengthen the appropriate social, human, moral, and spiritual values; based on belief that human progress requires a collective will.

The theoretical basis for understanding the goals of the role function mode, that is, social integrity and role clarity, includes structural, interaction, and collective pattern approaches. These approaches are congruent with the assumptions outlined in the Roy Adaptation Model. The melding of diverse theories provides a rich perspective of the role function adaptive mode. Again, the reader will find it useful to continue professional development as it relates to theories of roles in society.

INTERDEPENDENCE MODE

Behavior relating to interdependent relationships of individuals and groups is termed the interdependence mode. Theoretical development of the mode guides the assessment of the effectiveness of interdependence adaptation of individuals and groups. The interdependence mode focuses on the close relationships of people, one to one and in groups. For any given relationship, the interdependence mode helps describe the purpose, structure, and development. Each interdependent relationship exists for some purpose and it is through such relationships that people continue to grow as individuals and as contributing members of society. Interdependent relationships involve the willingness and ability to give to others and accept from them all that one has to offer such as love, respect, value, nurturing, knowledge, skills, commitments, material possessions, time, and talents. People who have a comfortable balance in interdependent relationships feel valued and supported by others, and can express the same for others. These people have learned to live successfully in a world of others including people, animals, objects, and the environment. The basic need of this mode, for both individuals and groups, is termed relational integrity or the feeling of security in relationships. This basic need consists of three components: affectional adequacy, developmental adequacy, and resource adequacy.

Individual

Two specific relationships are the focus of the interdependence mode as it applies to individuals. The first relationship is with significant others, persons who are the most important to the individual. The second is with support systems, that is, others contributing to meeting interdependence needs. Specific to these relationships, two major areas of interdependence behavior have been identified (Randell, Tedrow, & VanLandingham,

1982): receptive behavior and contributive behavior. These behaviors apply respectively to the receiving and giving of love, respect, and value in interdependent relationships. For example, a significant other for a child would be the mother. In this interdependent relationship, receptive behavior on the child's part would be allowing the mother to give comfort when the child is hurt. Contributive behavior would be the child's giving the mother a hug and a kiss on leaving for school. The assessment of receptive and contributive behaviors, or giving and receiving, provides an indication of social adaptation relative to the interdependence mode.

Group

The interdependence mode as it applies to relating people, groups, and collectives has been described in terms of three interrelated components.

1. The context of internal and external influences in which the group operates.
2. The infrastructure such as procedures, processes, and systems of the group.
3. The people who are participants.

Subcomponents of the context of the interdependence mode include governing and political systems, laws, availability of resources, judicial and legal processes, government regulations, ecological concerns, the general economic climate, interorganizational relations, and customer and supplier relationships. The internal context encompasses such aspects as the group's mission, vision, values, and plans.

The infrastructure consists of the procedures, processes, and systems within and by which the collective human system operates. This includes the way members relate to each other, how they communicate, and how they meet the needs for group functioning. The third component, the people, encompasses the knowledge, skills, attitudes, and commitments of all those involved. For the group to be successful in goal attainment, all three components must be in alignment and compatible. Otherwise, dissonance occurs that is disruptive and adaptation problems are evident. Many hospitals in the 1990s and the early part of this century experienced merger and consolidation with other health care agencies. For the health care organization, the three components of context, infrastructure, and people become important considerations associated with their interdependent relationships. Of course, economic factors and other external context variables also play significant roles in such relationships.

Theoretical Basis for the Interdependence Mode

The description of the interdependence mode is based on a number of sociologic, psychologic, management, nursing, and behavioral theories and principles. These provide direction for the assessment of behaviors and stimuli relative to the interdependence mode and for each of the other steps of the nursing process. The following is an identification of the theorists and a statement of their important theoretical concepts that are the basis of the interdependence mode described in the Roy Adaptation Model.

Andrews, Cook, Davidson, Schurman, Taylor, and Wensel (1994). Interdependence mode consisting of three components: context, infrastructure, and people.

Berkman (1978). Development of the social contact index.

Cobb (1976). Described individuals as involved in networks of mutual obligation.

Ellison (1976) and Koch and Haugk (1992). Described different types of aggression, including physical, nonverbal, verbal, and passive.

Erikson (1963) and Selman (1980). Eight stages of development and their implication for interdependent relationship; stages of friendship related to affectional needs.

Havighurst (1953). Developmental tasks for the infant to the mature adult.

Ainsworth (1964) and Mead (1971). Studied children in other cultures.

House, Landis, and Umberson (1988), Cohen (1985), and Gottlieb (1981). Relationship between interdependence and health.

Kane (1988) and Caplan (1974). Conceptual model of family social support with three interaction factors: reciprocity, advice and feedback, and emotional involvement.

Klaus and Kennel (1981), Bowlby (1969), Mahler (1979), and Spitz (1945). Theories related to emotional bonding and attachment and the effects of separation.

Maslow (1999). Hierarchy of needs of the individual as physiologic needs, safety needs, need for belongingness, and love-esteem needs.

Randell, Tedrow, and VanLandingham (1982). Identification and description of receiving and giving behaviors.

Tuckman and Jensen (1977). Stages of groups as they become effective in accomplishing goals.

Stanford (1977). Described group behaviors during the process of termination and closure.

Selman and Andrews (1994). Described successful coordination in relationships as the coordination of commitments.

Benner (1984). Described development of nursing practice from novice to expert.

Dunn (2003). Explores horizontal violence.

Individual and group behavior is viewed in relation to the four adaptive modes. They provide a particular form or manifestation of cognator–regulator and stabilizer–innovator activity within the human adaptive process. Although these modes are frequently viewed separately for teaching and assessment purposes, the nurse remembers that they are interrelated.

In Figure 4–1, the four modes are depicted as four overlapping circles, central to which is a circle representing the coping processes as introduced in Chapter 2. As an illustration of interrelationships, we note that the physiologic–physical mode in the diagram is intersected by each of the other three modes. Behavior in the physiologic–physical mode can have an affect on, or act as a stimulus for, one or all of the other modes. In addition, a given stimulus can affect more than one mode, or a particular behavior can be indicative of adaptation in more than one mode. Such complex relationships among modes further demonstrate the holistic nature of people as individuals or group adaptive systems. The kaleidoscope image or laser light show example illustrates these multifaceted interrelations and how changing the position of one's perspectives changes the patterns perceived.

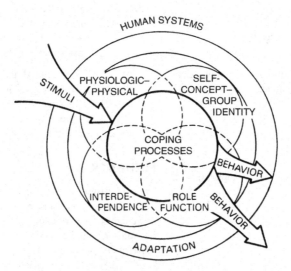

FIGURE 4-1 Diagrammatic representation of human adaptive systems.

Summary

Understanding the four adaptive modes for both individuals and groups is significant knowledge according to the Roy Adaptation Model. The theoretical basis for, and the behaviors to be assessed in each adaptive mode provides the background for applying the Roy Adaptation Model in nursing practice, education, and research. The chapters that follow will build on the general overview of the four adaptive modes to enhance understanding of the modes in both theory and application.

Exercises for Application

1. Select one of the adaptive modes and suggest behaviors that would be important to consider. Check your list with those suggested in the relevant following chapters.
2. Compare the head-to-toe assessment framework for physical assessment of an individual to assessment suggested by the physiologic mode in the Roy Adaptation Model. Look particularly for commonalities.
3. Select a group (family, organization, community) of which you are a part. Identify behaviors and stimuli that are part of the physical, self identity, role function, and interdependence modes.

Assessment of Understanding

QUESTIONS

1. Match the basic need in Column A to the associated adaptive mode in Column B.

Column A Basic Needs	Column B Adaptive Mode
(a) social integrity	**1.** _____ physical mode
(b) relational adequacy	**2.** _____ group identity mode

(continued)

(c) physiologic integrity
(d) identity integrity
(e) psychic and spiritual integrity
(f) resource adequacy

2. Name five disciplines that form the theoretical basis for the physiologic mode.
   (a) _____
   (b) _____
   (c) _____
   (d) _____
   (e) _____

3. Identify the basic life processes associated with the five basic needs.
   (a) oxygenation (3)
   (b) nutrition (2)
   (c) elimination (2)
   (d) activity and rest (2)
   (e) protection (2)

4. Name the four complex physiologic processes that mediate regulator activity and integrate physiologic functioning.
   (a) _____
   (b) _____
   (c) _____
   (d) _____

5. Label the following factors as related to one of the three components of the physical mode: participants (P), facilities (F), resources (R).
   (a) _____ knowledge
   (b) _____ physical plant

3. _____ self-concept mode
4. _____ interdependence mode
5. _____ role function mode
6. _____ physiologic mode

   (c) _____ operational resources
   (d) _____ monetary resources
   (e) _____ physical commodities
   (f) _____ commitments
   (g) _____ health

FEEDBACK

1. (a) 5, (b) 4, (c) 6, (d) 2, (e) 3, (f) 1
2. Any five of: anatomy, physiology, pathophysiology, chemistry, psychology, sociology, anthropology, religious studies and spirituality, and humanities.
3. (a) Oxygenation: (1) ventilation (2) exchange of gases, (3) transport of gases.
   (b) Nutrition: (1) digestion, (2) metabolism.
   (c) Elimination: (1) intestinal elimination, (2) elimination from kidneys.
   (d) Activity and rest: (1) mobility, (2) sleep.
   (e) Protection: (1) nonspecific defense processes, (2) specific defense processes.
4. (a) senses
   (b) fluid, electrolyte, and acid–base balance
   (c) neurologic function
   (d) endocrine function
5. (a) P, (b) F, (c) F, (d) R, (e) F, (f) P, (g) P

References

Ainsworth, M. D. (1964). Patterns of attachment shown by the infant in interaction with his mother. *Merrill Palmer Quarterly, 10*(1), 51–58.

Amman-Gainotti, M. (1986). Sexual socialization during early adolescence: The menarche. *Adolescence, 21*, 703–710.

Andrews, H. A., Cook, L. M., Davidson, J. M., Schurman, D. P., Taylor, E. W., & Wensel, R. H. (Eds.). (1994). *Organizational transformation in health care: A work in progress.* San Francisco: Jossey-Bass.

Andrews, J. D. W. (1990). Interpersonal self-confirmation and challenge in psychotherapy. *Psychotherapy, 27*(4), 485–504.

Antonovsky, A. (1986). The development of a sense of coherence and its impact to stress situations. *The Journal of Social Psychology, 26*(2), 213–225.

Banton, M. (1965). *Roles: An introduction to the study of social relations.* New York: Basic Books.

Benner, P. (1984). *From novice to expert: Excellence and power in clinical nursing practice.* Menlo Park, CA: Addison-Wesley.

Berkman, B. (1978). Mental health and the aging: A review of the literature for clinical social workers. *Clinical Social Work Journal, 6*, 230–245.

Blumer, H. (1969). *Symbolic interactionism: Perspective and method.* Englewood Cliffs, NJ: Prentice Hall.

Bowlby, J. (1969). *Attachment and loss: Attachment* (Vol. 1). New York: Basic Books.

Brehm, S. S., & Kassin, S. M. (1996). *Social psychology* (3rd ed.). Boston: Houghton Mifflin.

Campsey, J. (1985). The sexual dimension of patient care. *Nursing Forum, 22*(2), 69–71.

Caplan, G. (Ed.). (1974). *Support systems and community mental health*. New York: Behavioral Publications.

Chinn, P. L. (2008). *Peace and power: Creative leadership for building community* (7th ed.). Sudbury, MA: Jones and Bartlett.

Clarke, B. A., & Strauss, S. S. (1992). Nursing role supplementation for adolescent parents: Prescriptive nursing practice. *Journal of Pediatric Nursing, 7*(5), 312–318.

Cobb, S. (1976). Social support as a moderator of life stress. *Psychosomatic Medicine, 38,* 300–312.

Cohen, S. S. L. (1985). *Social support and health*. New York: Academic Press.

Cooley, C. H. (1964). *Human nature and the social order*. New York: Schocken.

Crocker, J., & Park, L. E. (2003). Seeking self-esteem: Construction, maintenance, and protection of self-worth. In M. R. Leary & J. P. Tangney (Eds.), *Handbook of self identity* (pp. 291–313). New York: The Guilford Press.

Derber, C. (2003). *People before profit: The new globalisation in an age of terror, big money, and economic crisis*. London: Souvenir Press.

Dobratz, M. C. (1984). Life closure. In C. Roy (Ed.), *Introduction to nursing: An adaptation model* (2nd ed., pp. 497–518). Englewood Cliffs, NJ: Prentice Hall.

Dobratz, M. C. (2004). Life closing spirituality and the philosophic assumptions of the Roy Adaptation Model. *Nursing Science Quarterly, 17*(4), 335–338.

Dobratz, M. C. (2005). A comparative study of life-closing spirituality in home hospice patients. *Research and theory for nursing practice, 19*(3), 243–256.

Driever, M. J. (1976). Theory of self-concept. In C. Roy (Ed.), *Introduction to Nursing: An adaptation model* (pp. 255–283). Englewood Cliffs, NJ: Prentice Hall.

Dunn, H. (2003). Horizontal violence among nurses in the operating room. *AORN Journal, 78*(6), 977–980, 982, 984–988.

Eagly, A. H. (1987). *Sex differences in social behavior: A social-role interpretation*. Hillsdale, NJ: Erlbaum.

Elliot, G. (1986). Self-esteem and self-consistency: A theoretical and empirical link between two primary motivations. *Social Psychology Quarterly, 49*(3), 207–218.

Ellison, E. (1976). Problem of interdependence: Aggression. In C. Roy (Ed.), *Introduction to nursing: An adaptation model* (pp. 330–341). Englewood Cliffs, NJ: Prentice Hall.

Erikson, E. H. (1963). *Childhood and society* (2nd ed.). New York: Norton.

Festinger, L. (1962). *A theory of cognitive dissonance*. Palo Alto, CA: Stanford University Press.

Freud, S. (1949). *An outline of psychoanalysis* (James Strachey, Trans.). New York: W. W. Norton.

Gilligan, C. (1982). *In a different voice: Psychological theory and women's development*. Cambridge, MA: Harvard University Press.

Goffman, E. (1959). *The presentation of self in everyday life*. New York: Anchor.

Goffman, E. (1967). *Interactional ritual*. New York: Anchor.

Gottlieb, B. H. (Ed.). (1981). *Social networks and social support*. Beverly Hills, CA: Sage.

Gray, J. J. (2003). Role transition. In P. S. Yoder-Wise (Ed.), *Leading and Managing in Nursing* (3rd ed.). St. Louis, MO: Mosby.

Hanna, D. (2004). Moral distress: The state of science. *Research and Theory for Nursing Practice, 18*(1), 73–94.

Hanna, D. (2005). The lived experience of moral distress: Nurses who assisted with elective abortions. *Research and Theory for Nursing Practice 19*(1), 95–124.

Havighurst, R. J. (1953). *Human development and education*. New York: Longman.

House, J., Landis, K., & Umberson, D. (1988). Social relationship and health. *Science, 241,* 540–545.

Johnson, D. (1983). *Body*. Boston: Beacon Press.

Johnson, J. E., & Levanthal, H. (1974). Effects of accurate expectations and behavioral instructions on reactions during a noxious medical examination. *Journal of Personality and Social Psychology, 2,* 55–64.

Kane, C. F. (1988). Family social support: Toward a conceptual model. *Advances in Nursing Science, 10*(2), 188–225.

Kimberly, J. C. (1997). *Group processes and structures: A theoretical integration*. Lanham, MD: University Press of America.

Klaus, M. H., & Kennel, J. H. (1981). *Parent-infant bonding* (2nd ed.). St. Louis, MO: Mosby.

Koch, R. N., & Haugk, K. C. (1992). *Speaking the truth in love*. St. Louis: Stephen Ministries.

Kohlberg, L. (1981). *The philosophy of moral development* (Vol. 1). San Francisco: Harper & Row.

Kübler-Ross, E. (1969). *On death and dying*. New York: Macmillan.

Lambert, C. E., & Lambert, V. A. (2001). Preceptorial experience. In A. J. Lowenstein & M. J. Bradshaw (Eds.). (2001). *Fuszard's innovative teaching strategies in nursing* (3rd ed.). Gaithersburg, MD: Aspen Publishers, Inc.

Lecky, P. (1969). *Self-consistency: A theory of personality*. New York: Doubleday.

Lewin, K. (1948). *Resolving social conflicts*. New York: Harper & Row.

Luft, J. (1984). *Group Processes: An introduction to group dynamics*. San Francisco: Mayfield Publishing Co.

Luft, J., & Ingram, H. (1963). The Johari window: A graphic model of awareness in interpersonal interactions. In J. Luft (Ed.), *Group Processes* (pp. 50–125). Palo Alto, CA: National Press Books.

Mahler, M. S. (1979). *The selected papers of Margaret Mahler: Separation-individuation* (Vol. 2). New York: Jason Aronson.

Markus, H. (1977). Self-schemata and processing information about the self. *Journal of Personality and Social Psychology, 35*(2), 63–78.

Marquis, B. L., & Huston, C. J. (2006). *Leadership roles and management functions in nursing: Theory and application* (5th ed.). Philadelphia: Lippincott Williams & Wilkins.

Maslow, A. H. (1999). *Toward a psychology of being* (3rd ed.). New York: John Wiley & Sons.

McMahon, E. M. (1993). *Beyond the myth of dominance: An alternative to a violent society*. Kansas City, MO: Sheed & Ward.

Mead, G. (1934). *Mind, self, and society*. Chicago: University of Chicago Press.

Mead, M. (1971). *Coming of age in Samoa*. New York: Morrow.

Meleis, A. I. (1975). Role insufficiency and role supplementation: A conceptual framework. *Nursing Research, 24*(4), 264–271.

Meleis, A. I., Sawyer, L. M., Im, E., Hilfinger Messias, D. K., & Schumacher, K (2000). Experiencing transitions: An emerging middle-range theory. *Advances in Nursing Science, 23*(1), 12–28.

Merton, R. K. (1957). *Social theory and social structure*. New York: Free Press.

Montagu, A. (1986). *Touching: The human significance of the skin* (3rd ed.). New York: Harper & Row.

Neugarten, B. (1969). Continuities and discontinuities of psychological issues in adult life. *Human Development, 12*, 121–130.

Neugarten, B. L. (1979). Time, age, and the life cycle. *The American Journal of Psychiatry, 136*(7), 887–894.

Parsons, T., & Shils, E. (Eds.). (1951). *Toward a general theory of action*. Cambridge, MA: Harvard University Press.

Patterson, M. L. (1996). Social behavior and social cognition: A parallel process approach. In J. I. Nye & A. M. Brower (Eds.), *What's social about social cognition? Research on socially shared cognition in small groups* (pp. 87–105). Thousand Oaks, CA: Sage Publications.

Perry, D. (2004). Self-transcendence: Lonergan's key to integration of nursing theory, research, and practice. *Nursing Philosophy, 5*(1), 67–74.

Perry, D. (2005). Transcendent pluralism and the influence of nursing testimony on environmental justice legislation. *Policy, Politics & Nursing Practice, 6*(1), 60–71.

Piaget, J. (1954). *The construction of reality in the child* (M. Cook, Trans.). New York: Basic Books.

Prestholdt, C. O. (1990). Modern mentoring: Strategies for developing contemporary nursing leadership. *Nursing Administration Quarterly, 15*(1), 20–27.

Rabbie, J. M., & Lodewijks, H. F. M. (1996). A behavioral interactional model: Toward an integrative theoretical framework for studying intra- and intergroup dynamics. In E. Witte & J. H. Davis (Eds.), *Understanding group behavior: Small group processes and interpersonal relations* (Vol. 2, pp. 255–294). Mahwah, NJ: Erlbaum.

Randell, B., Tedrow, M., & VanLandingham, J. (1982). *Adaptation nursing: The Roy conceptual model made practical*. St. Louis, MO: Mosby.

Rogers, C. (1951). *Client centered therapy*. Boston: Houghton Mifflin.

Rogers, C. (1961). *On becoming a person*. Boston: Houghton Mifflin.

Rosenberg, M. (1965). *Society and adolescent self-image*. Princeton, NJ: Princeton University Press.

Rosenberg, M. (1979). *Conceiving the self*. New York: Basic Books.

Roy, C. (1967). Role cues and mothers of hospitalized children. *Nursing Research, 16*, 178–182.

Satir, V. (1991). *The Satir model: Family therapy and beyond.* Palo Alto, CA: Science and Behavior Books.

Selman, J. C., & Andrews, H. A. (1994). Effective relationships: Rethinking the fundamentals. In H. A. Andrews, L. M. Cook, J. M. Davidson, D. P. Schurman, E. W. Taylor, & R. T. Wensel (Eds.), *Organizational transformation in health care: A work in progress* (pp. 53–69). San Francisco: Jossey-Bass.

Selman R. L. 1980. *The Growth of Interpersonal Understanding.* Academic Press, Inc: New York.

Singer, P. (2002). *One world: the ethics of globalization* (2nd ed.). New Haven, CT: Yale University.

Spitz, R. A. (1945). Hospitalism: An inquiry into the genesis of psychiatric conditions in early childhood. In O. Fenechel, P. Greenacre, H. Hartmann, E. B. Jackson, E. Kris, L. S. Kubie, B. D. Lewin, M. C. Putnam, & R. A. Spitz (Eds.), *The psychoanalytic study of the child* (pp. 53–74). New York: International Universities Press.

Stanford, G. (1977). *Developing effective classroom groups.* New York: Hart.

Stangor, C., & Lange, J. (1994). Mental representations of social groups: Advances in understanding stereotypes and stereotyping. *Advances in Experimental Social Psychology, 26*, 357–416.

Sullivan, H. S. (1953). *The interpersonal theory of psychiatry.* New York: Norton.

Swimme, B., & Berry, T. (1992). *The universe story.* San Francisco: Harper.

Tuckman, B. W., & Jensen, M. A. (1977). Stages of small group revisited. *Group and Organization Studies, 2*(4), 419–427.

Turner, R. H. (1979). Role-taking, role standpoint and reference group behavior. In B. J. Biddle & E. J. Thomas (Eds.), *Role theory: Concepts and research* (pp. 151–159). New York: Krieger Publishing.

Vance, C. N. (1982). The mentor connection. *The Journal of Nursing Administration, 12*(4), 7–13.

Vision Points of the Global Cooperation for a Better World. (2004). Retrieved May 22, 2008, from http://www.bkun.org/socdev/wit7.html

Worchel, S. (1996). Emphasizing the social nature of groups in a developmental framework. In J. L. Nye & A. M. Brower (Eds.), *What's social about social cognition? Research on socially shared cognition in small groups* (pp. 261–281). Thousand Oaks, CA: Sage Publishing.

Zohar, D. (1990). *The quantum self: Human nature and consciousness defined by the new physics.* New York: Quill/Morrow.

Zohar, D., & Marshall, I. (1994). *The quantum society: Mind, physics, and a new social vision.* New York: Quill/Morrow.

PART TWO

The Adaptive Modes for the Individual

Roy describes the person as an adaptive system. Adaptation can be observed in four major categories for the individual. These categories are termed the four modes or ways in which people adapt. The modes are named the physiologic, self concept, role function, and interdependence adaptive modes. It is in relation to these four major categories that responses are carried out and that adaptation levels can be observed. Part 2 of this text focuses on understanding the basic concepts and processes of the modes and how this understanding helps to plan nursing care. The description of each mode includes their integrated processes, compensatory processes, and compromised processes. The knowledge of the processes provides the basis for an overview of assessment and planning of nursing care.

The focus of Chapters 5 to 13 is the physiologic mode for the individual. The physiologic mode chapters are organized by the five needs and four complex processes for the individual. Chapters 14, 15, and 16 present the self-concept, role function mode, and interdependence mode, respectively. Each of these chapters describes and provides examples of the nursing care for individuals. The intent of presenting the physiologic needs and processes first and then following with a presentation of the other modes is to move from simple to complex, concrete to abstract. Complete discussion of the four adaptive modes on the individual level provides the basis for understanding the application of the adaptation model to more complex nursing practice situations with groups, discussed in Part 3.

CHAPTER 5

Oxygenation

Oxygenation is identified in the Roy Adaptation Model as one of five physiologic needs. The three basic life processes that provide oxygenation are ventilation, gas exchange, and transport of gases. Understanding the physiology of these processes provides the framework for determining adaptation in relation to oxygenation. Concepts from pathophysiology are helpful in identifying ineffective behaviors. In this chapter the three basic life processes of oxygenation are addressed. Illustrations of innate and learned adaptive responses to compensate for ineffective processes related to oxygenation are described. Examples of compromised processes are discussed. Finally, guidelines for planning nursing care related to the need for oxygenation by assessing behaviors and stimuli, formulating diagnoses, establishing goals, selecting interventions, and evaluating nursing care are described.

OBJECTIVES

After studying this chapter, the reader will be able to do the following:

1. Describe the three basic life processes associated with the need for oxygenation.
2. Describe one compensatory process for each of the basic life processes associated with oxygenation.
3. Name and describe two situations of compromised processes of oxygenation.
4. Identify important first-level assessment factors for each of the basic life processes associated with the need for oxygenation.
5. List common stimuli affecting oxygenation.
6. Develop a nursing diagnosis, given an adaptation problem related to oxygenation.
7. Derive goals for an individual with ineffective oxygenation in a given situation.
8. Describe nursing interventions commonly implemented in situations of ineffective oxygenation.
9. Propose approaches to determine the effectiveness of nursing interventions to meet needs for oxygenation.

KEY CONCEPTS DEFINED

Apnea: The periodic absence of respiration.

Arrhythmia: Irregular pulse rhythm.

Barrel chest: An abnormal condition where the anterior chest diameter is increased and the ribs are more horizontal rather than the normal downward slant.

Bradycardia: A pulse rate below 60 beats per minute.

Bradypnea: Respiratory rate below 10 breaths per minute.

Cheyne-Stokes Respiration: A pattern of periods of deep breathing alternating with periods of not breathing.

Dyspnea: The subjective distressing sensation of difficulty breathing.

Gas exchange: At the alveolar level the movement of oxygen and carbon dioxide across the alveolocapillary membranes by diffusion.

Gas transport: Movement of oxygen from the alveolocapillary membrane to the mitochondria within the cells and the movement of carbon dioxide from tissue capillaries to the alveolocapillary membrane.

Kussmaul's respirations: Abnormal increase in rate and depth of respirations.

Oxygenation: The processes of ventilation, gas exchange, and transport of gases by which cellular oxygen supply is maintained in the body.

Pulse rhythm: The time intervals between heartbeats.

Respiratory arrest: Prolonged period of apnea.

Shortness of breath: Observable difficulty with respirations.

Tachycardia: A pulse rate above 100 beats per minute.

Tachypnea: Respiratory rate above 24 breaths per minute.

Tidal volume: The amount of air moved into and out of the lungs during normal respiration.

Ventilation: The complex process of respiration that exchanges air between the lungs and the atmosphere.

BASIC LIFE PROCESSES OF OXYGENATION

Oxygenation refers to the processes by which cellular oxygen supply is maintained in the body. The basic life processes responsible for oxygenation are ventilation, alveolar and capillary gas exchange, and transport of gases to and from the tissues. If these processes are functioning effectively and the environmental oxygen is sufficient, then there is adequate oxygenation of the body tissues. The life of all body tissues depends on maintaining oxygenation; thus, this need is a high priority in the clinical situation.

Process of Ventilation

Ventilation is the complex process of breathing that exchanges air between the lungs and the atmosphere. This process involves both neural control and muscle activity. The neural control is based in a group of neurons referred to as the respiratory center located in the medulla oblongata and lower pons of the brain stem. Afferent and efferent neural pathways transmit signals to the respiratory center to regulate breathing. Further, the peripheral chemoreceptor system, including carotid and aortic bodies, is responsive to changes in oxygen, carbon dioxide, and hydrogen ion concentrations and transmits signals to the main center. This control system operates to maintain an adequate oxygen supply, a fundamental need of all cells.

Process of Exchange of Gases

In ventilation, atmospheric air reaches the alveoli, where the process of exchange of gases begins. Oxygen and carbon dioxide are exchanged across the alveolocapillary membranes. This transfer of gases at the alveolar level is a result of diffusion. Diffusion is determined by the partial pressures of the gases on both sides of the alveolocapillary membrane. There is a larger amount of oxygen and a smaller amount of carbon dioxide in the alveoli than in the blood. Thus, oxygen diffuses across the membrane and enters the hemoglobin molecules in the blood. Blood circulation carries oxygen to the body's cells. Carbon dioxide diffuses in a reverse direction across the membrane into the alveoli to be exhaled out of the body. Normal gas exchange depends on the concentration gradients of the gases, on the intact alveolar membrane, and on adequate perfusion of the alveoli.

Process of Transport of Gases

After diffusion across the alveolocapillary membranes, oxygen is transported to the tissues for uptake. Gas transport includes the processes involved in the movement of oxygen from the alveolocapillary membrane to the mitochondria within the cells and the movement of carbon dioxide from tissue capillaries to the alveolocapillary membrane. Blood transports oxygen in two ways. First, approximately 98% of the oxygen is carried in chemical combination with hemoglobin. Second, the remaining 2% is carried in physical solution as dissolved oxygen in the plasma. Under normal conditions, hemoglobin has a high affinity for oxygen, which means it readily absorbs the oxygen transported from the lungs and releases it at the tissue level. The oxygen is carried by the hemoglobin to the capillaries where it moves out of the red blood cell into the plasma, crossing the capillary wall, and goes into the interstitial fluid. By this transport process the oxygen becomes available to the cells.

At the tissue level, carbon dioxide is picked up and returned to the lungs for disposal. The blood transports carbon dioxide in three forms: bicarbonate ions; dissolved carbon dioxide in the plasma; and as a compound with other proteins, mainly hemoglobin. Carbon dioxide diffuses 20 times more rapidly than oxygen; however, only 7% reaches the lungs dissolved in plasma (P_{CO2}). More importantly, hemoglobin plays a major role in converting carbon dioxide to bicarbonate. Once formed, bicarbonate diffuses out of the red blood cells into the plasma, where it combines with sodium to form sodium bicarbonate. Thus, 70% of the carbon dioxide is carried back to the lungs in the form of sodium bicarbonate. The remaining 23% returns in the form of compounds, mainly attached to hemoglobin proteins.

COMPENSATORY ADAPTIVE PROCESSES OF OXYGENATION

Viewed as an adaptive system (see Chapter 2) the individual has innate and acquired ways of responding to the changing environment. Roy conceptualizes these complex adaptive dynamics as the coping processes of the regulator and cognator subsystems. This chapter identifies that the need for oxygenation is met through processes of ventilation, gas exchange, and gas transport. However, when the processes of oxygenation are not stable or adequate, the regulator and cognator activate processes of compensation. Canon (1932), an early physiologist, used the term *the wisdom of the body* to describe the automatic self-regulation of physiologic processes. This phrase is useful when studying Roy's concept of the regulator subsystem. Likewise, the thinking and feeling individual, by way of cognator activity, can do much to affect any need of the physiologic mode, oxygenation in particular. Regulator and cognator abilities, then, are important internal stimuli for the individual. These subsystems provide compensatory adaptive responses that extend the effectiveness of behavior in reaching the goals of adaptation.

Compensatory abilities that respond to oxygenation requirements include both automatic homeostatic functions of the regulator and voluntary or behavioral activities of the cognator. The nurse will understand as fully as possible the wisdom of the body to identify and interpret changes in the patient's condition. Important to this understanding is the study of physiology and pathophysiology. One particular illustration of a regulator compensatory activity is given to illustrate compensatory adaptation related to oxygenation.

A protective mechanism that helps maintain an open airway is mucociliary clearance. The layer of mucus that covers the upper and lower airway traps particles from the inspired air. Cilia then propel the mucus, with entrapped foreign material, toward the pharynx, where it can be swallowed or expectorated. An automatic compensatory response that assists mucociliary clearance is the cough reflex. A cough is caused by stimulation of irritant receptors in the airway. In particular, these receptors respond to chemical and mechanical stimulation from substances such as dust in the air, noxious fumes, aspiration of foreign material, and mucus accumulation. The complex act of coughing generally involves one deep inspiration, followed by several forced expirations that expel large volumes of air from the lungs. The function of the cough is to clear the upper airways of the irritant. Thus, a cough is a compensatory adaptive response to the need for oxygenation.

An illustration of a compensatory response to oxygen need by way of the cognator is the conscious recruitment of accessory muscles of respiration. Likewise, adequate ventilation depends on respiratory muscles pumping air into and out of the lungs. When oxygen need is challenged, such as in chronic obstructive lung disease, the patient can be taught to recruit additional muscles for ventilation. The individual learns to use sternomastoid, intercostal, and abdominal muscles to assist with breathing. Even mandibular, facial, and gluteal muscles can be used (Breslin, Roy, & Robinson, 1992). Similarly, through the cognator, the individual can be taught to increase the effectiveness of an automatic regulatory compensating response, such as a cough. Some environmental changes related to oxygen need, particularly in a state of illness, can have an overwhelming effect on the individual's ability to adapt. When the demands are greater than the compensatory processes can handle, this may lead to compromised processes of oxygenation.

COMPROMISED PROCESSES OF OXYGENATION

Adaptation problems can be caused by difficulties in any or all of the processes of oxygenation since ventilation, gas exchange, and gas transport are all interdependent. Two specific examples of compromised processes of oxygenation will be discussed here. Hypoxia is the most pressing concern that reflects a compromised process of oxygenation. Shock is a generalized syndrome that can have many causes; however, a common feature is inadequate tissue perfusion.

Hypoxia

Hypoxia has been classified into four main types: hypoxic, anemic, circulatory, and histo-toxic (Berne, 1998). Hypoxic hypoxia is caused by a decrease in oxygen pressure in the inspired air or in the lungs, or by conditions that prevent or interfere with the diffusion of oxygen across the alveolar membrane. Examples of causes are exposure to high altitudes, obstruction of the airway, asthma, pneumonia, and congenital cardiovascular disease. Anemic hypoxia results from a compromised ability of the blood to carry enough oxygen due to a decrease in hemoglobin. Examples of this are anemia and carbon monoxide poisoning. Circulatory hypoxia occurs when there is inadequate circulation of the blood to the tissue cells, even though the oxygen-carrying capacity of the blood may be normal. Examples of causes include congestive heart failure or other forms of reduced cardiac output; shock; and arterial spasm or other local obstruction to arterial blood flow. Histotoxic hypoxia occurs when there is interference with the ability of the cells to utilize oxygen. Causative examples are alcohol, narcotics, and poisons such as cyanide.

Although it is possible to compensate for moderate hypoxia over a period of time, this is not true of acute hypoxia. People have essentially no oxygen reserve. When exposed to an acute inter-ruption of oxygen, symptoms of hypoxia appear quickly. Symptoms vary widely with individuals and differing abilities to adjust physiologically. However, in general, the higher levels of the brain will show the effects of oxygen deficit very early. Cognitive function is impaired. The individual is confused and usually unaware of what is happening. Early signs also include changes in vital signs resulting from the cardiovascular response to hypoxia. Tachycardia may occur and respira-tions increase in depth and rate. The systolic blood pressure rises slightly as cardiac output increases. As hypoxia increases, a wide variety of central nervous system symptoms may appear including headache, agitation, irritability, drowsiness, apathy, dizziness, decreased concentration, impaired judgment, diminished visual acuity, emotional disturbances, euphoria, poor muscular coordination, fatigue, stupor, and unconsciousness. When the hypoxic state becomes more advanced and the body's compensatory efforts fail, both blood pressure and pulse rate fall precipi-tously. Hypoxia is also accompanied by changes in the gastrointestinal and renal systems. These changes can occur as a direct result of the hypoxia on the involved tissues or indirectly through the effects of hypoxia on the nervous system. The individual can experience anorexia, nausea, and vomiting, as well as oliguria. Since the kidney is very sensitive to hypoxia, frequent measurement of urine output is an important part of the nursing assessment of the patient with acute hypoxia.

The emotional responses of individuals who are unable to breathe are evident. An indi-vidual may be apprehensive and anxious and compound the problem by hyperventilating. People who are having difficulty breathing will try to sit upright if possible. If an oxygen mask is being used, they may try to push it away because of the sensation that it is stifling them. Respirations become increasingly gasping and as the individual's fears increase, the energy requirement increases. This places an even greater load on the already overburdened respiratory and cardiac systems, thus increasing the hypoxia.

The most important measure in treating hypoxia is oxygen administration. The purpose of oxygen therapy is to deliver to the patient a greater concentration of oxygen than is avail-able from the air in the room (21%). There are a wide variety of devices for delivering oxy-gen. Low-flow systems referred to as supplemental oxygen include nasal cannula, simple mask, and partial nonbreathing and nonrebreathing masks with reservoir bags. High-flow systems provide oxygen sufficient to supply the entire inspired tidal volume. Two kinds of high-flow systems are oxygen under pressure and mechanical ventilation.

Specific plans for nursing care for the individual with hypoxia are based on careful individual assessment and collaboration with the medical team. However, general interventions can be outlined here. Essential components of oxygen therapy include the following:

- Careful observation of respiratory status, vital signs, and reaction to therapy
- Use of aseptic technique to assist in preventing infections
- Thorough explanation to the individual of the procedures being used
- Understanding and correct usage of the equipment being used

Positioning for comfort and correct body alignment are also important for the patient with hypoxia. The individual can usually get maximum ventilation from an upright position, sometimes leaning slightly forward, such as on an over-bed table. A calm, confident, and supportive manner on the part of the nurse, as well as a calm physical environment, can help alleviate the stress encountered in breathing difficulties.

Shock

Shock is ordinarily associated with poor tissue perfusion and usually characterized by systemic hypotension. The decrease in blood pressure can be caused by different mechanisms. Thus, shock occurs in several forms, including hemorrhagic, septic, cardiogenic, neurogenic, hypoglycemic, traumatic, and anaphylactic. Each of these clinical situations and their treatment are described in textbooks on pathophysiology and medical science. However, a general nursing assessment and approaches to care can be outlined.

The shock syndrome can be as simple as fainting at the sight of an accident on the highway, or as complex as a medical emergency for the accident victim with internal bleeding. The common feature is inadequate perfusion and oxygenation of cells, tissues, and organs. The usual cause is a decrease in blood pressure. The circulation becomes progressively inadequate. The behaviors of the individual reflect low arterial pressure and increased activity of the sympathetic nervous system in the body's attempt to deal with the emergency. The individual in shock appears pale, and the skin is cool and moist. The pupils are dilated and the individual is visibly anxious. Early in the chain of events, an individual may be quite restless and agitated, but this progresses to apathy and confusion. Thirst is a common symptom, but usually little water can be tolerated because of nausea. Urinary output is progressively decreased. Breathing is rapid and shallow, and as shock becomes more severe, the pulmonary function progressively deteriorates. Pulse rate is rapid but thready. Arterial blood pressure, particularly systolic pressure, rises early in shock for a brief period and then falls. Further, the pulse pressure tends to be narrow. Medical therapy of shock aims to restore fluid volume, correct metabolic acidosis, and increase cardiac output. Nursing responsibilities involve careful observation of the patient's appearance, vital signs, and response to treatment, as well as supportive care.

The three stages of the shock syndrome are important in understanding this compromised process. In the initial or compensatory stage, many physiologic reactions occur in adapting to the shock state. During the decompensated or progressive stage, the shock state is continuing and the patient's condition is increasingly worse. In some people, there is a final, refractory stage that can become irreversible. At this point, neither the various compensatory mechanisms nor the treatment is effective in reversing the state of shock, and the prognosis is poor.

The patient in shock should lie flat, or in the case of neurogenic shock, horizontally with moderate elevation of the legs. The position of the head lower than the body is not used because the pressure of the abdominal viscera on the lungs impairs ventilation. Supportive care for the respiratory system can include oxygen therapy, suctioning, mechanical ventilation, and pulmonary physiotherapy. Supportive care for the cardiovascular system involves intravenous fluids, either blood or electrolyte solutions, depending on the patient's needs. Cardiac monitoring is continuous and identifying arrhythmia is essential. Renal and gastrointestinal support is provided by accurate monitoring of intake and output with hemodialysis and parenteral nutrition as needed. The nursing challenge is to anticipate the development of shock and intervene before the serious progressive changes occur. This challenge involves careful monitoring for early recognition of any changes in the patient's condition (Burrell, Gerlach, & Pless, 1997).

NURSING PROCESS RELATED TO OXYGENATION

Oxygenation of body tissues is a priority need for the individual's physiologic adaptation. In using the nursing process, the nurse will make a careful assessment of behaviors and stimuli related to the basic life processes of ventilation, gas exchange, and gas transport. To assess factors influencing oxygenation need, structural and functional influences are considered along with regulator and cognator effectiveness in initiating compensatory processes. Based on thorough first- and second-level assessment, the nurse makes a diagnosis, sets goals, selects interventions, and evaluates care.

Assessment of Behavior

In the first level of assessment of oxygenation, behaviors that the nurse observes relate to how the individual is coping with factors that affect the processes of oxygenation, ventilation, gas exchange, and gas transport.

VENTILATION   Given the importance of ventilation to the individual's physical and psychological integrity, the nurse assesses oxygenation needs based on the understanding of ventilation as a human life process. Specific assessment factors are used to determine the adequacy of ventilation and to identify any existing adverse consequences of ventilatory problems.

VENTILATORY PATTERNS   Normal respiratory rate in adults is 12 to 18 breaths per minute when awake. Rates above 24 per minute are termed tachypnea, and below 10 per minute, bradypnea. Apnea means the periodic absence of respirations. Respiratory arrest is the term used for a prolonged period of apnea, a behavior incompatible with life. Normal respiratory rhythm consists of equal intervals between respiratory cycles with the inspiratory phase shorter than the expiratory phase. Depth of respirations determines the tidal volume. This is the amount of air moved in and out of the lungs during normal respiration. Tidal volume during quiet breathing is approximately 500 mL in a 70-kg male, with lower capacities in women. Tidal volume is estimated by observing chest movements during inspiration and expiration. The measurement of air flow in the respiratory track examines air flow versus volume. Direct measurement of tidal volume is done using a spirometer. Spirometry can be done at the bedside or in an outpatient setting using simple equipment. At times, spirometry is done in a pulmonary function laboratory with sophisticated equipment and protocols. One important measurement that can be taken at home on a small device is peak expiratory flow (PEF), the amount of air that can be forcibly exhaled after maximal inhalation. This provides a quick measure of disease exacerbation or response to medications such as bronchodilators.

Some patterns of altered ventilatory control have specific names. Two patterns most commonly encountered are Cheyne-Stokes respiration (CSR) and Kussmaul's respiration. Cheyne-Stokes respiration is a pattern of periods of deep breathing alternating with periods of not breathing. Rate and depth gradually increase and then decrease, followed by a period of apnea, and another cycle of increasing rate and depth. This type of breathing may occur normally in the elderly during sleep, but it may also be seen in patients prior to death or in severe cases of heart failure and drug overdose. Kussmaul's respiration is a term used to describe an abnormal increase in rate and depth of respiration that is seen in cases of metabolic acidosis such as diabetic ketoacidosis. Other types of periodic breathing are described by their characteristics, such as hyperpnea alternating with apnea. Sleep apnea is a syndrome associated with altered ventilatory control. Obese individuals are at risk for losing tone in the pharyngeal muscles and consequently having an obstructed airway during sleep. The individual exhibits obstructive sleep apnea with episodes of potentially dangerous hypoxemia.

BREATH SOUNDS   Another assessment parameter is breath sounds. Breath sounds are produced by air flow through the airway and are audible through a stethoscope. Normal breath sounds vary in pitch and intensity over different parts of the lungs. The sounds heard over much of the lung fields are soft and low-pitched, with the air moving through the bronchioles and filling the alveoli. Abnormal breath sounds are commonly described as crackles, fine or coarse; wheezes, sibilant or sonorous (formerly called rhonchi); and pleural friction rub. Nurses learn to distinguish different abnormal breath sounds in studying techniques of physical assessment.

SUBJECTIVE EXPERIENCE   The patient's subjective experience of breathing should be perceived as effortless and without conscious thought. Shortness of breath is a term indicating observable difficulty with respirations. Dyspnea is the subjective distressing sensation of difficulty breathing. It is reported by the patient and often is the symptom that limits the individual's daily activities. In the case of difficult respirations caused by obstruction, respiratory sounds are audible without the use of a stethoscope. For example, obstruction of the trachea produces a harsh crowing sound (stridor) on inspiration, as seen in a child with acute croup, or laryngotracheitis. Obstruction caused by a foreign body is called aspiration. Severe constriction of the bronchioles, as in asthma, produces wheezing that is continuous, high-pitched, and whistling, as air is forced through narrowed respiratory passages. Assessment of gas exchange is not made directly since it is not possible to see, hear, or touch the diffusion of gases. However, there are a number of ways to infer the adequacy of gas exchange from noninvasive techniques and from blood samples.

OXYGEN CONCENTRATION   A variety of technologies are available to evaluate in a noninvasive way the arterial oxygen saturation (PaO_2) and partial pressure of serum oxygen and carbon dioxide (P_{CO2}) in the critically ill patient. These include pulse oximeters and transcutaneous monitoring devices. Adequate gas exchange also can be inferred from arterial blood gas levels. If there is a normal concentration of oxygen and carbon dioxide in the blood, it is assumed that there is adequate gas exchange across the alveolar and capillary membranes. Blood gas levels are determined in laboratory testing of blood samples taken from the patient. Often in the intensive care unit, the nurse obtains the arterial blood sample from an indwelling arterial catheter. The most important laboratory finding to determine if there is a problem of oxygen exchange is the level of PaO_2. This reading indicates the partial pressure of oxygen in the arterial blood and generally is about 95%, with variations as noted in the discussion of factors influencing gas exchange. The transport of gases is heavily dependent on cardiac output. For this reason, pulses, blood pressure, and heart sounds provide important behavioral indicators in assessing the transport of gases.

PULSES   The apical pulse is felt at the apex of the heart and peripheral pulses are felt in the body's periphery, for example, in the neck, wrist, or foot. In a healthy individual, the peripheral pulse is equivalent to the heartbeat. Normal adult pulse rates range from 60 to 100 beats per minute. A rate below 60 is called bradycardia and above 100 is called tachycardia. Pulse rates out of the normal range may not necessarily indicate a pathologic condition. Increased exercise, or any condition that increases the need for tissue oxygenation, will automatically increase the heart rate. When an individual is frightened or anxious, stimulation of the sympathetic nervous system will cause temporary tachycardia. Pulse rhythm is normally regular, that is, the time intervals between beats are of equal duration. Pulse rhythm is recorded as either regular or irregular. An irregular rhythm is referred to as an arrhythmia or dysrhythmia. A pulse deficit exists if the apical pulse, on auscultation, is higher than the radial pulse rate, indicating a weakness in the ventricular contractions. Peripheral pulses are assessed for their presence and strength and are important indicators of the oxygenation status of distal tissues. Patients with cardiac health problems or peripheral vascular disorders may have absent or diminished strength in the peripheral pulses.

In addition to assessing rate and rhythm, the nurse also considers the force of the pulse. The force is an indication of stroke volume and is noted by assessing the pressure exerted to feel the pulse. A full, bounding pulse is difficult to obliterate and is exemplified by the pulse after exercise. Full force of the pulse is also found in a variety of alterations in health, including fever. A weak, thready pulse is easy to obliterate. It may indicate an alteration in health such as hemorrhage. The expected force of a pulse is felt clearly with a reasonable pressure and does not disappear when pressure on the pulse site is slightly adjusted.

BLOOD PRESSURE   Blood pressure readings reflect the ebb and flow of blood in waves within the systemic arteries. The systolic pressure occurs at the height of the wave, when the left ventricle contracts, and is recorded as the upper reading. Between the contractions, the heart is at rest and reflects the diastolic pressure, which is recorded as the lower reading. Normal blood pressure readings vary widely in healthy adults. The general norm of 120/80 is used, but it is important to know the patient's blood pressure range to make a correct interpretation of adaptive or ineffective behavior relative to the reading obtained. For example, if a patient's normal range is 150/86 to 138/80, then a sudden change to 106/60 will alert the nurse to possible problems that need further assessment and medical treatment. Useful assessment information is also obtained from taking the blood pressure in several positions, such as lying down, sitting, and standing. Decreased fluid volume can be reflected in changes in blood pressure, which in turn leads to decreased transport of gases. From supine to the standing position, the systolic pressure normally should not drop more than 15 mmHg and the diastolic pressure not more than 5 mmHg. The most common abnormality seen in systolic and diastolic pressure is hypertension. Further important information about transport of gases is obtained by differentiating and interpreting heart sounds. Discussion of the procedures associated with auscultation of heart sounds can be found in physical assessment resources such as Bickley and Hoekelman (1999).

DIAGNOSTIC TESTS   Although the nurse cannot assess gas exchange and transport directly, it is possible to evaluate cellular oxygenation. When cellular impairments are identified, they reflect alterations in the homeostatic relationship between the delivery of oxygen and its cellular utilization. Delivery of oxygen depends on the structure and function of the cardiovascular system. A number of tests for this vary in levels of invasiveness and risk. A chest x-ray provides information about cardiac enlargement, pulmonary congestion, cardiac calcifications, and placement of any equipment being used internally. More invasive tests like arteriography show the arterial vessels by fluoroscopy and the use of contrast media. Coronary arteriography is done by cardiac catheterization—the most invasive, but most definitive, test. Exercise electrocardiography is known as a stress test and helps to determine the functional capacity of the heart. Nurses can broaden their understanding of expanding technologies such as myocardial nuclear perfusion imaging, magnetic resonance imaging (MRI), and electronic-beam computed tomography scan (EBCT) as well as hemodynamic monitoring.

PHYSIOLOGIC INDICATORS   In completing a first-level assessment of oxygenation, the nurse is aware that other components of the physiologic mode can be useful behavioral indicators. The skin, mucous membranes, and nail beds are often considered for their protective functions. However, pallor and cyanosis of these are seen in situations of decreased tissue perfusion. Decreased cellular oxygenation stimulates the sympathetic nervous system response, causing the skin to be cool and clammy. A decreased level of consciousness can be an early indicator of cerebral hypoxia. With respect to elimination, decreased urinary output can indicate a decrease in cardiac output. Monitoring hourly output of urine is important in some situations. If the nurse detects a production of less that 30 mL/hr, this signifies ineffective behavior. Such decreased urinary output is reported to the attending physician for immediate treatment.

Assessment of Stimuli

In the second level of assessment, assessment of stimuli, the nurse gathers data about internal and external factors that influence the behaviors identified in the first level of assessment of the adaptation nursing process. This includes stimuli related to ventilation and exchange and transport of gases. Second-level assessment of the need for oxygenation, as with other adaptive mode components, includes identifying stimuli that influence adaptive and ineffective behaviors. Changes in structure or function can compromise the basic breathing processes and affect respiratory rate, rhythm, depth, and ease as well as exchange and transport of gases. Disease and injury are particular stimuli that have significant effects on processes of oxygenation. Other environmental factors also affect the processes of oxygenation.

STRUCTURAL AND FUNCTIONAL INTEGRITY   A patent airway; musculoskeletal structure of the rib cage; and functioning muscles, neural control centers, and pathways are important for effective ventilation. Assessment of the patency of the patient's airway is a primary responsibility of the nurse. Foreign bodies in the airway; inflammatory reactions from infections, irritants, and allergens; and aspiration of fluids or emesis are all factors that can impede airway clearance. Pathologic processes can lead to deformity or atrophy of musculoskeletal structures of the rib cage and chest. Skeletal problems of the thoracic cage, such as scoliosis and rib fractures, affect ventilation by decreasing thoracic expansion. Barrel chest, as seen in emphysema, is an abnormal condition where the anterior chest diameter is increased and the ribs are more horizontal rather than the normal downward slant. This change in appearance of the chest results from trapped air due to increased bronchial resistance and the chronic over-use of expiratory muscles. Any condition that decreases the pumping ability of the heart will cause oxygenation problems because there will be a deficiency in the number of red blood cells reaching the tissues. Inflammatory conditions of the heart such as bacterial endocarditis, myocardial infarction, and congestive heart failure are disorders which can interfere with the pumping ability of the heart. Hemorrhage and dehydration are common causes of a decrease in cardiac output and circulating blood volume.

OTHER DISEASE PATHOLOGY   Pathology in the lungs can affect the blood supply to the alveoli. Specific examples are diseases that alter the expandability and elastic recoil of lung tissue such as pneumonia, tuberculosis, chronic bronchitis, and emphysema. Pulmonary emboli or thrombi are examples of situations that directly interfere with blood supply to the alveoli. Further, if the alveolar membrane is thick and fibrotic, or if the alveoli are filled with exudate or fluid, as in cystic fibrosis, there will be inadequate gas exchange.

Neuromuscular diseases restricting ventilation include skeletal muscle disorders such as muscular dystrophy; neuromuscular junction disorders such as myasthenia gravis and botulism; and spinal cord disorders such as Guillain-Barré syndrome, poliomyelitis, spinal cord injuries, and tetanus.

TRAUMA   Head injuries that cause trauma and bleeding in the central nervous system can result in increased intracranial pressure which, in turn, can affect the respiratory center in the brain. Traumatic injuries from motor vehicle accidents, shootings, or stabbings can result in tears of the diaphragm or pleura causing pneumothorax. In this critical condition, air at atmospheric pressure enters the pleural space and causes the lungs to collapse. This interferes with both ventilation and tissue perfusion because it also affects gas exchange and transport.

RESULTS OF DIAGNOSTIC STUDIES   The study of samples of blood can show factors that affect oxygenation. A decrease in the number of red blood cells or lack of hemoglobin will decrease the oxygen-carrying capabilities of the blood. Under certain circumstances, the ability of hemoglobin to carry oxygen is compromised. Acidosis and increase in body temperature are situations which decrease the uptake of oxygen at the alveolar level. On the other hand, alkalosis and decreased body temperature depress oxygen release at the tissue level. There are numerous studies used specifically to evaluate the effectiveness of the respiratory and cardiovascular systems. A detailed discussion of relevant diagnostic procedures and findings can be found in medical, surgical, or laboratory textbooks. The most common studies are hematocrit, hemoglobin, red cell count, arterial blood gases, chest x-ray, and electrocardiogram. The hematocrit, hemoglobin, and red cell count provide information about oxygen-carrying capabilities of the red blood cells. Arterial blood gas studies, and other noninvasive techniques noted before, reflect the amount of oxygen and carbon dioxide in the blood.

The chest x-ray provides information about the gross structures of the lungs and pleural cavity, indicating abnormal growth, inflammation, and fluid within the lungs. Special studies such as angiography, bronchography, lung scans, pulmonary angiography, and nuclear medicine studies, including MRI and PET scanning, can reveal information not obtained in standard chest x-rays. The electrocardiogram (EKG) is a noninvasive test that shows a graphic record of the electrical impulses that stimulate contractions of the heart. Electrodes from the chest and extremities are connected to an EKG machine or telemetry unit for the graphic recording. EKGs also can be monitored by a unit used by an ambulatory patient. EKGs reveal abnormal rhythms and other functional changes that affect cardiac output.

ENVIRONMENTAL CONDITIONS   Besides the basic structure and functional factors affecting oxygenation, noxious environmental stimuli such as tobacco smoke, allergens, and irritating fumes can be considered individually as stimuli affecting oxygenation. Environmental stimuli are often part of the pathogenesis of many of the disease conditions mentioned previously. These stimuli and other risk factors can be considered contextual stimuli. While not causing an acute oxygen deficit, they contribute to the situations resulting in compromised oxygenation. Depression of the respiratory center can occur with the use of narcotics and anesthetics.

Exercise, stress, changes in altitude, and temperature changes are all stimuli that alter the oxygen demands of the body. Concentration of oxygen in the air can be decreased in some situations. Changes of these stimuli are a normal part of the individual's external environment. The body, if healthy, adapts to these stimuli with innate regulatory responses. The individual can also use learned adaptive responses to enhance processes of oxygenation. Assessment of behaviors and stimuli are the basis for making nursing judgments of issues to be addressed in the step of the nursing process referred to as nursing diagnosis.

Nursing Diagnosis

As introduced in Chapter 3 nursing diagnosis, according to the Roy Adaptation Model, is a judgment process in which the nurse makes an interpretive statement about the individual or group as an adaptive system. The statement is formulated by considering the data of the first- and second-level assessment. The statement can include a summary of observed behaviors with the most relevant influencing stimuli. A nursing diagnosis illustrating adaptation and summarizing both behavior and stimuli is, "Adequate oxygenation of toes of left foot due to good circulation in leg with cast." Also using a summary of behavior and stimuli, the nurse states an adaptation problem as, "Ventilatory impairment related to copious secretions in the airways."

An alternate way of stating a nursing diagnosis is to use a summary label that best identifies the nurse's judgment of the clinical situation from an established classification system. The Roy model has two classification lists, one for indicators of adaptation and one for commonly recurring adaptation problems. The complete classification lists for the Roy model are included in Chapter 3. In Table 5–1, the Roy model nursing diagnostic categories for the physiologic need of oxygenation are shown in relation to nursing diagnosis labels approved by the North American Nursing Diagnosis Association (NANDA International, 2007).

An example of use of a summary diagnosis can be considered. Mrs. Jones is an 87-year-old woman who lives alone and has had emphysema for the past 20 years. For many years, she worked outside the home and was a heavy smoker until approximately 12 years ago, when she reportedly quit. The nurse from a neighborhood clinic visits Mrs. Jones and makes a nursing assessment. Mrs. Jones is sitting in a chair and leaning forward on a TV tray. Her rate of respiration is 30 and her lips have a slightly blue tinge. She says she is not really having difficulty breathing, but that she is conscious of every breath. Mrs. Jones has been trying some exercises that the nurse gave her. One is to lift her buttocks and try to use the muscles to help force air out of her lungs. Mrs. Jones says she thinks the exercises are helping but that she is afraid she will

TABLE 5–1 Nursing Diagnostic Categories for Oxygenation

Positive Indicators of Adaptation	Common Adaptation Problems	NANDA Diagnostic Labels
• Stable processes of ventilation • Stable pattern of gas exchange • Adequate transport of gases • Adequate processes of compensation	• Hypoxia • Shock • Ventilatory impairment • Inadequate gas exchange • Altered tissue perfusion • Inadequate gas transport • Poor recruitment of compensatory processes for changing oxygen need	• Impaired gas exchange • Impaired spontaneous ventilation • Ineffective breathing pattern • Risk for suffocation • Risk for aspiration • Ineffective airway clearance • Risk for peripheral neurovascular dysfunction • Risk for sudden infant death syndrome • Dysfunctional ventilatory weaning response • Ineffective tissue perfusion • Decreased cardiac output • Activity intolerance • Risk for activity intolerance

forget to do them. Mrs. Jones has asked her friend Sally to help remind her. Sally calls Mrs. Jones every day and asks how her exercises are going. The nurse uses a handheld spirometer to measure Mrs. Jones' ventilatory capacity and notes that it has improved over the last measurement 2 weeks ago. The nurse makes the diagnosis of, "Improving processes of compensation for oxygenation need resulting from respiratory exercises."

The statement of nursing diagnoses, the third step of the nursing process, provides direction for the next step. Based on the nursing diagnosis, the nurse proceeds to the fourth step of the nursing process, known as goal setting.

Goal Setting

Goal setting, according to the Roy Adaptation Model, involves the establishment of clear statements of behavioral outcomes for the individual as the result of the nursing care provided. A complete goal statement contains the behavior of focus, the change expected, and the time frame in which the goal should be achieved. Goals may be short term or long term, and these time frames are relative to the situation. Consider the example of a patient with a newly applied leg cast. Although the nursing diagnosis indicated that there was adequate oxygenation to the tissue in the toes at that time, the nurse should be aware that swelling often occurs after the application of a new cast, and should monitor the patient's leg. A short-term goal pertaining to this situation could be, "Toes will remain warm and pink within the next hour." The behavior in this goal is, "Toes will be warm and pink." The change expected is no change; that is, oxygenation will remain adequate as evidenced by the toes being warm and pink. The time frame is stated as "within the next hour."

In the case of a patient whose diagnosis is "ventilatory impairment related to copious secretions in the airways," the behavior the goal will focus on is ventilatory impairment. The goal is stated, "Within 10 minutes, the patient will be breathing effortlessly." The patient's breathing is the behavior of focus, the criterion is "effortlessly," and the time frame is "within 10 minutes." In the case of Mrs. Jones, the nurse plans to make the next visit in 1 week. For the diagnosis, "improving processes of compensation for oxygenation need," the nurse sets the goal with the patient that, "Processes of compensation for oxygenation will improve in 1 week." The processes of compensation are the focus of the goal, improvement beyond this week's level is the criterion, and "1 week" is the time frame.

Generally, the nursing goal for oxygenation is to ensure an adequate level of oxygen supply to all parts of the body. This goal is operationalized by the identification of the specific goals that address ventilation, gas exchange, transport of gases, and compensatory adaptive responses. The importance of anticipating potential problems associated with oxygenation involves monitoring the individual's condition to detect oxygenation problems before they become serious. Thus, many goals established for the patient may be preventive in nature rather than focusing on adaptation problems. In order to assist the patient in achieving the established goals, the nurse proceeds to plan nursing interventions.

Intervention

The four previous steps of the nursing process, based on an understanding of oxygenation processes, provide specific direction for the identification of nursing interventions to assist the patient. Whereas the goal focused on specified patient behaviors, the interventions address the stimuli that are affecting the behaviors. The management of stimuli involves altering, increasing, decreasing, removing, or maintaining the influencing factors. Some nursing measures used to facilitate ventilation and gas exchange focus on functioning of the associated structures of respiration, an important factor influencing oxygenation. These include deep breathing and coughing, positioning to encourage maximal breathing capacity, using lung inflation devices, providing oxygen therapy, promoting drainage and removal of tracheobronchial secretions, providing hydration, and providing adequate pulmonary resuscitation in situations of respiratory arrest. The nurse may be responsible for the care of patients on mechanical ventilation and frequently use suctioning techniques to remove respiratory secretions.

Nursing interventions to enhance gas transport include maintaining adequate circulation through proper positioning and nonrestrictive clothing, providing adequate intake of iron, and promoting effective pumping action of the heart. In the previous situation involving the patient with the new cast, the stimulus that could interfere with oxygenation of the toes is swelling within the cast and the subsequent interruption of blood flow to the toes. In considering interventions to prevent such an occurrence, the nurse would identify and analyze possible approaches and then select the approach with the highest probability of achieving the goal. Possible interventions could be splitting the cast, elevating the leg on a pillow, or packing the leg in ice to prevent swelling. The last alternative may have a detrimental effect on the plaster cast; the first is not something that would be tried as a preventive measure. Thus, the nurse would select the intervention of elevating the leg on a pillow in an attempt to minimize swelling before it becomes a problem.

Nursing intervention in situations of oxygenation disruption involves facilitating the processes of ventilation, gas exchange, and gas transport. For a patient with ventilatory impairment due to bronchial secretions, the nursing intervention focuses on clearing the secretions from the individual's airway. Possible interventions include positioning of the patient, postural drainage, encouraging the patient to cough, and suctioning of the patient's airway. The approach selected would depend on the circumstances. An individual with an altered level of consciousness may require suctioning while a patient who is aware and can follow instructions may benefit by assistance and encouragement for effective coughing. In addition to intervention, the nurse can promote improved respiratory health by encouraging the patient to make healthful adjustments to one's lifestyle. Recommendations include regular exercise; refraining from smoking or using other tobacco products; avoiding secondhand smoke; making sure that one's residence is well ventilated; and avoiding prolonged exposure to noxious fumes (Sheldon, 2001). Whatever the nursing interventions selected, their effectiveness in reaching the goals is addressed through evaluation.

Evaluation

As is evident from the initial description of behaviors related to the three basic life processes associated with oxygenation (ventilation, gas exchange, and gas transport), the key to evaluation lies generally in four important behavioral areas: respiratory status, cardiac status, renal status, and mental status. The key to evaluating the effectiveness of specific nursing interventions is determining if the behavior identified in the patient-specific goal changed within the stated time frame. Consider the goal, "Within 10 minutes, the patient will be breathing effortlessly." If it is effortless within the 10-minute time frame, the goal has been achieved. Suppose that within 1 hour, the nurse identified that the patient with the cast was demonstrating decreased circulation to his toes in that they were dusky in color and the patient was reporting numbness. This situation would necessitate immediate action on the part of the nurse to continue reassessment with further intervention. With Mrs. Jones and her goal to improve the processes of oxygenation compensation, evaluation of the success of the interventions would relate to compensatory processes and the effectiveness she is experiencing as the result of her exercising. Measurement of ventilatory capacity with the spirometer would provide an indication of this. If no improvement is observed, both the goals and the interventions will need to be reevaluated to determine whether an alternative approach is indicated.

Such situations demonstrate the simultaneous and continuous nature of the nursing process. Although the steps are addressed separately for purposes of teaching and learning, experienced nurses assess behavior and stimuli simultaneously, perhaps while setting goals with the patient and carrying out interventions. The interrelatedness of the steps of the process, based on Roy's concept of the individual human system as a whole, becomes increasingly evident as the nurse becomes more experienced in its application.

Summary

This chapter focused on applying the Roy Adaptation Model to the physiologic need of oxygenation. An overview of the basic life processes—ventilation, gas exchange, and gas transport—associated with oxygenation was provided. Illustration of innate and learned adaptive compensatory responses related to oxygenation were described and examples of two compromised processes, hypoxia and shock, were provided. The identification of parameters for assessment of behaviors and stimuli was discussed. Finally, guidelines for the formulation of nursing diagnoses, goals, and interventions were explored and an evaluation of nursing care was described.

Exercises for Application

1. Develop a tool to assist you with the assessment of oxygenation. Address in the tool important behavioral indicators and stimuli that affect ventilation, gas exchange, and gas transport.

2. Using the tool developed in exercise 1, assess a patient's status relative to oxygenation. Assess the adequacy of your assessment tool by comparing it to an oxygenation assessment guideline in a physical assessment resource.

Assessment of Understanding

QUESTIONS

1. Identify the appropriate basic life process of oxygenation in Column A with the associated descriptor(s) in Column B.

   Column A
   Basic Life Process

   Ventilation (V)
   Gas exchange (GE)
   Transport of gases (TG)

   Column B
   Descriptor

   (a) _____ depends on concentration gradient of gases
   (b) _____ inspiratory phase and expiratory phase
   (c) _____ movement of oxygen to the mitochondria within cells
   (d) _____ involves alveolocapillary membrane
   (e) _____ diffusion of gases
   (f) _____ exchanges air between lungs and atmosphere

2. Label each assessment parameter with the basic life process to which it most closely relates.
   Ventilation (V), Gas exchange (GE), Transport of gases (TG)
   (a) _____ breath sounds
   (b) _____ arterial blood gas levels
   (c) _____ tidal volume
   (d) _____ pulse rate
   (e) _____ pulse oximetry

   (f) _____ respiratory rate
   (g) _____ pulse rhythm
   (h) _____ blood pressure

3. Name two factors that influence each of the basic life processes associated with oxygenation.
   (a) Ventilation: _____ and _____.
   (b) Exchange of gases: _____ and _____.
   (c) Transport of gases: _____ and _____.

4. Provide an example of a compensatory process related to oxygenation that is illustrative of (a) regulator coping mechanism activity and (b) cognator coping mechanism activity.
   (a) _____
   (b) _____

5. Name two serious adaptation problems indicative of compromised processes of oxygenation.
   (a) _____
   (b) _____

6. Situation: A young man has been brought into the emergency department from the scene of an automobile accident. He appears very pale. His skin is cool and moist. His pupils are dilated, and he is restless and agitated. He complains of thirst and nausea. His pulse is rapid and thready, and his blood pressure is lower than normal and is falling. He is being examined for possible internal injury, and a ruptured spleen is anticipated but has not yet been confirmed.
   (a) Develop a nursing diagnosis related to the situation described.
   (b) Develop one short-term and one long-term goal relative to the behavior of the falling blood pressure. Each goal should include the behavior of concern, the change expected, and the time frame involved.

7. List five nursing interventions commonly used in situations of hypoxia.
   (a) _____
   (b) _____
   (c) _____
   (d) _____
   (e) _____

8. Which of the following evaluative methods would be appropriate for assessing the effectiveness of the nursing interventions aimed at enhancing tissue perfusion in the patient demonstrating shock?
   (a) cardiac status
   (b) renal status
   (c) respiratory status
   (d) mental status
   (e) all the above

FEEDBACK

1. (a) GE, (b) V, (c) TG, (d) GE, (e) GE, (f) V
2. (a) V, (b) GE, (c) V, (d) TG, (e) GE, (f) V, (g) TG, (h) TG
3. (a) Examples: impairment of structure or function, increased intracranial pressure, trauma to diaphragm or pleura.
   (b) Examples: oxygen concentration in air, adequacy of blood supply to alveoli, thickness and surface area of alveolar membrane.
   (c) Examples: cardiac function, circulating blood volume, hemorrhage, dehydration.
4. (a) Regulator coping mechanism activity: coughing, sneezing, yawning, increased heart rate upon exertion.
   (b) Cognator coping mechanism activity: use of additional muscles to facilitate air exchange, use of positioning with head elevated on extra pillows, mouth breathing in situations of high spinal cord injury.
5. (a) hypoxia
   (b) shock
6. (a) Example of nursing diagnosis: Altered tissue perfusion due to decrease in circulating bloodvolume; or shock due to possible internal hemorrhaging.
   (b) Example of a short-term goal: Within 5 minutes, the patient's blood pressure will have stabilized.
   Example of a long-term goal: Within 1 hour, the patient's blood pressure will demonstrate an upward trend.
7. (a) oxygen administration
   (b) comfortable and aligned positioning
   (c) calm and supportive physical environment
   (d) correct usage of oxygen equipment
   (e) thorough explanation of procedures being used
8. e

References

Berne, R. (1998). *Physiology*. St. Louis, MO: Mosby.

Bickley, L. S., & Hoekelman, R. A.(1999). *Bates' guide to physical examination and history taking* (7th ed.). Philadelphia: Lippincott.

Breslin, E., Roy, C., & Robinson, C. (1992). Physiological nursing research in dyspnea: A paradigm shift and a metaparadigm exemplar. *Scholarly Inquiry for Nursing Practice, 6*(2), 81–104.

Burrell, L. O., Gerlach, M. J. M., & Pless, B. S. (1997). *Adult nursing: Acute and community care* (2nd ed.). Stamford, CT: Appleton & Lange.

Canon, W. (1932). *The wisdom of the body.* New York: Norton.

NANDA International (2007). *Nursing diagnoses: Definitions & classification, 2007–2008.* Philadelphia: NANDA International.

Sheldon, L. K. (2001). *Oxygenation.* Thorofare, NJ: SLACK Inc.

Additional References

Grimes, J., & Burns, E. (1992). *Health assessment in nursing practice* (3rd ed.). Boston: Jones and Bartlett.

Marieb, E. N. (2007). *Human anatomy and physiology* (7th ed). San Francisco: Pearson Benjamin Cummings.

Porth, C. (2005). *Pathophysiology: Concepts of altered health states* (7th ed.). Philadelphia: Lippincott Williams & Wilkins.

Seidel, H. M., Ball, J. W., Dains, J. W., & Benedict, G. W. (1995). *Mosby's Guide to Physical Examination.* St. Louis, MO: Mosby.

Vander, A., Sherman, R., & Luciano, D. (1998). *Human physiology: The mechanisms of body function* (7th ed.). Boston: WCB McGraw-Hill.

West, J. B. (2005). *Respiratory physiology: The essentials.* Philadelphia: Lippincott Williams & Wilkins.

CHAPTER 6

Nutrition

Nutrition is identified in the Roy Adaptation Model as one of five physiologic needs. Nutrition relates to the series of processes by which the individual takes in and assimilates food necessary for maintenance of human functioning, promotion of growth, and replacement of injured tissues. Unfortunately, nutrition is often overlooked in health care. However, society today faces a number of major health concerns related to nutrition throughout the life span. We are familiar with the increasing rate of childhood obesity. With an increasingly aging population, it is significant to note some authors determined that with attention to nutritional needs, unintentional weight loss in the elderly can be prevented (Splett, Roth-Yousey, & Vogelzang, 2003). This is significant because "adequate nutritional intake is important to maintain body functions, healthy tissues, and body temperature; to promote healing; and to build resistance to infection" (Craven & Hirnle, 2007, p. 998). These observations have important implications for nurses in their goal of promoting health. Level of nutrition influences every phase of metabolism and plays a major role in each individual's overall health. Consideration of the individual's state of nutrition and promotion of an optimal nutritional level are important nursing activities in the holistic role that nurses occupy in the promotion of adaptation and health.

Basic life processes of nutrition as described within the Roy Adaptation Model include digestion and metabolism. Understanding the physiology of these processes provides the framework for determining adaptation related to nutrition. Concepts from pathophysiology and other disciplines are helpful in identifying ineffective behaviors. In this chapter, the two basic life processes of nutrition are addressed. Illustrations of compensatory and compromised processes related to nutrition are described. Finally, guidelines for planning nursing care by identifying the factors for assessment of behaviors and stimuli, formulating nursing diagnoses, establishing goals, selecting nursing interventions, and evaluating the plan are provided.

OBJECTIVES

After studying this chapter, the reader will be able to do the following:

1. Describe the two basic life processes associated with the need for nutrition.
2. Describe one compensatory process of the basic life processes associated with nutrition.
3. Name and describe two situations of compromised processes of nutrition.

4. Identify important first-level assessment parameters for the basic life processes associated with the need for nutrition.

5. List common stimuli affecting each basic life process associated with nutrition.

6. Given a situation related to nutrition, develop a nursing diagnosis.

7. In a given situation, derive goals for an individual with ineffective nutrition.

8. Describe nursing interventions commonly implemented in situations of ineffective nutrition.

9. Propose approaches to determine the effectiveness of nursing interventions.

KEY CONCEPTS DEFINED

Absorption: The movement of digested substances, plus vitamins, minerals, and water, from the GI tract through the mucosal cells into the blood or lymph for transport to body cells.

Appetite: A pleasant sensation involving the individual's desire for and anticipation of food and fluids.

Body Mass Index (BMI): A measure of obesity that is an index of weight related to height. The BMI is calculated by multiplying weight in pounds by 705 and dividing by height in inches squared.

Chemical digestion: A series of steps to break down complex food molecules into their chemical building blocks so they are small enough to be absorbed. This is accomplished by enzymes in various parts of the GI tract.

Defecation: The elimination of contents of the bowel, that is, feces.

Digestion: A series of mechanical and chemical processes by which food is taken into the body and prepared for absorption into the blood and lymph for transport to the body cells.

Hunger: A physiologically aroused sensation related to the body's need for food.

Ingestion: The process of taking food and liquids into the digestive tract.

Mechanical digestion: The breakdown of food to physically prepare it for chemical digestion. Food components are broken into smaller parts by chewing, mixing, and churning.

Nausea: An unpleasant sensation reported as a feeling of sickness with the urge to vomit.

Nutrition: The series of processes by which an individual takes in nutrients and assimilates and uses them to maintain body tissue, promote growth, and provide energy.

Propulsion: The movement of food through the gastrointestinal tract by peristalsis.

Thirst: A desire for fluid or the dry sensation resulting from a lack of or need for water.

Vomiting: The forceful ejection of stomach contents through the mouth.

BASIC LIFE PROCESS OF NUTRITION

The concept of nutrition encompasses the food people eat and how the body makes use of the food. It is defined as the series of processes by which the individual takes in nutrients and assimilates and uses them to maintain body tissue, promote growth, and provide energy. Second only to the need for oxygen, nutrition provides the foundation for life and health. For purposes of this overview of nutrition, two major processes are identified: digestion and metabolism. Although it is difficult to separate the concept of assessment related to digestion and metabolism, for purposes of discussion here, the assessment of digestion pertains to the physiologic processes associated with foods and fluids that are ingested. Assessment of metabolism, on the other hand, addresses factors associated with the adequacy of nutrient intake relative to the body's requirements.

Process of Digestion

Digestion is described as a series of mechanical and chemical processes by which food is taken into the body and prepared for absorption into the blood and lymph for transport to the body cells. The organs of the digestive system function to keep the body supplied with the nutrients required by the body tissues and organs. The structures involved in digestion are categorized into two main groups. The gastrointestinal (GI) tract, also called the alimentary canal, consists of the mouth, pharynx, esophagus, stomach, small and large intestines, and the anus, the terminal opening. Within the GI tract, food is digested, digested fragments are absorbed, and undigested substances are eliminated. The teeth, tongue, gallbladder, salivary glands, liver, and pancreas (together, sometimes referred to the accessory digestive organs) assist in the process of digestive breakdown of foods.

Marieb and Hoehn (2007, pp. 884–885) described digestion in terms of the following five major processes.

1. Ingestion: The process of taking food and liquids into the digestive tract usually by way of the mouth.
2. Propulsion: The movement of food through the GI tract by swallowing, which is voluntary, and by peristalsis, which is involuntary wavelike contractions of the smooth muscles of the digestive system that propel the contents through the tract.
3. Mechanical digestion: The breakdown of food to physically prepare it for chemical digestion. Food components are broken into smaller parts by chewing, mixing, and churning.
4. Chemical digestion: A series of steps to break down complex food molecules into their chemical building blocks so they are small enough to be absorbed. This is accomplished by enzymes in various parts of the GI tract.
5. Absorption: The movement of digested substances, plus vitamins, minerals, and water from the GI tract through the mucosal cells into the blood or lymph for transport to body cells.

Process of Metabolism

The process of metabolism can be summarized by three life sustaining tasks: breaking down complex substances into smaller ones (catabolism), building simpler substances into larger structures (anabolism), and utilizing nutrients to produce cellular energy. Through the process of metabolism, nutrients are synthesized to fulfill these tasks.

Nutrients are described as substances that provide nourishment to the body and are used by the body to promote normal growth, maintenance, and repair. Essentially, nutrients can be organized into two categories, major and minor nutrients. The major nutrients include carbohydrates, lipids, and proteins. Minor nutrients are vitamins and minerals. Water is also considered a major nutrient by some sources and is about 60% by volume of what we eat. Carbohydrates, some lipids, and some proteins are converted into chemical energy (metabolic products), electrical energy (brain and nerve activity), mechanical energy (muscle activity), and thermal energy (warmth). Proteins and other nutrients including minerals, vitamins, and fatty acids contribute to building cells, to replacing worn structures, or to synthesis of functional molecules. Other nutrients contribute to regulation and control within body systems.

COMPENSATORY ADAPTIVE PROCESSES

Viewed as an adaptive system (see Chapter 2) the individual has innate and acquired ways of responding to the changing environment. Further, Roy conceptualizes these complex adaptive dynamics for the individual as the coping processes of the regulator and cognator subsystems. As described in this chapter, the need for nutrition is met through processes of digestion and metabolism. However, when the processes of nutrition are not integrated, then the regulator activates processes of compensation. Further, the thinking and feeling individual, by way of cognator activity, can do much to affect any need of the physiologic mode, nutrition in particular. Regulator and cognator abilities, then, are important internal stimuli for the individual. Compensatory abilities that respond to nutritional needs include both automatic homeostatic functions of the regulator and voluntary, or behavioral, activities of the cognator. The nurse needs to understand as fully as possible the "wisdom of the body" to identify and interpret changes in the patient's condition. Study of physiology and pathophysiology are important to this knowledge. One particular illustration of a regulator compensatory activity is given to illustrate compensatory adaptation related to nutrition.

The hypothalamus contains the hunger and satiety centers of the body and is the principal organ involved in the physiologic regulation of eating. A functioning hypothalamus is responsible for initiating internal cues that signal the individual to eat in order to supply the body with needed energy. Hunger is the physiologically aroused sensation related to the body's need for food. The hypothalamus again signals through the satiety center to tell the individual to stop eating. A healthy individual who responds to these internal cues that regulate energy balance is able to maintain a normal weight and control appetite. At particular times of rapid, specialized growth throughout the life cycle, the body's nutritional demand is heightened. This is particularly true during pregnancy and lactation, in the first year of life, and at the onset of puberty. It is the regulator mechanisms within the body that stimulate enhanced appetite at these crucial times.

Another example of a regulator compensatory response is related to nutrition and hydration at the end of life. Although the research is limited by its very nature, there have been studies that demonstrate withholding nutrition and hydration are humane based on the body's ability to compensate for this need. A review by Winter (2000) discussed how the body accommodates this change. The body begins to utilize fats for energy instead of carbohydrates, and continues to conserve protein stores for brain metabolism. Eventually, the brain begins to utilize ketones for energy and the use of ketones triggers the body to decrease amino acid metabolism. As a result, there is a reduction in metabolism which reduces the sense of hunger. It is speculated that this compensatory response may induce a sense of euphoria or well-being (Ersek, 2003).

An illustration of a compensatory response to nutritional need by way of the cognator is an individual with a medical diagnosis of diabetes mellitus. This metabolic disorder of energy balance involves the body's production of or response to the hormone insulin. Many people with this disorder have learned to effectively manage their diabetes by balancing food intake, exercise, and insulin requirements. In some cases, this means self-administration of insulin; in other situations, dietary control is effective. The keystone of effective management is sound diet therapy. Many people with the disorder become skilled at determining dietary and insulin requirements based on self-assessment of blood sugar levels and exercise requirements. They are compensating for a physiologic problem through their cognator coping processes—perceptual and information processing, learning, judgment, and emotion. Some changes in the environment related to nutrition, particularly in a state of illness, can have an overwhelming effect on the individual's ability to adapt. The demands are greater than what compensatory processes can handle, and the result can be compromised processes of nutrition.

COMPROMISED PROCESSES OF NUTRITION

Adaptation problems can be caused by difficulties in any or all of the processes of nutrition since digestion and metabolism are interdependent. Two specific examples of compromised processes of nutrition will be discussed here. Obesity is a common nutritional problem in North American society. According to the Center for Disease Control's National Center for Health Statistics (2006), approximately 66% of United States adults and 17% of children are considered to be overweight or obese. These staggering statistics have led to many comorbidities in adults and early onset type 2 diabetes mellitus in children, as well as many other issues. Anorexia, or the loss or lack of appetite for food, is another common problem; it can be a result of such factors as medications, depression, and cancer. The eating disorder, anorexia nervosa, is a psychiatric disorder that is particularly prevalent among adolescent females.

Obesity

Obesity is a clinical term for excess body weight with an abnormally high proportion of body fat. The term obese is generally applied to those who have a BMI > 30 kg/m^2, and an individual is considered overweight if they have a BMI > 25 kg/m^2. This is one of the most common adaptation problems related to nutrition in contemporary North America. Excessive accumulation of fat in the body increases the weight beyond the recommended measures with regard to bone structure, height, and age. Although many individual differences exist in the factors contributing to obesity, the most common cause is an imbalance between the amount of food ingested and the amount of energy expended. Dudek (2006) described the increase in overweight children:

> Although multifactorial in origin, the bottom line is that overweight and obesity result from an imbalance between caloric intake and caloric expenditure. Over the last 25 years, the average caloric intake of American children has increased and portion sizes have grown. On the other side of the energy equation, physical inactivity is seen as a major contributor to weight gain in children. (p. 333)

Overweight children often develop low self-esteem and experience social isolation, as well as many physical complications.

Unfortunately, there are no easy answers to successful weight control. Although bariatric surgery has been shown to be effective even long term, the individual must subscribe to an entirely different lifestyle postoperatively, and the surgery is not without risks. All effective weight management programs must be personalized for the individual. The individual must focus on healthy lifestyle eating and exercise behaviors, and include stress management with supportive interpersonal relationships. The nurse's primary role in supporting people with a weight management problem is to teach and encourage healthy dietary patterns.

In many situations, referral to a health professional involved exclusively in dietetics and nutrition may be required. In situations where further physiologic problems are suspected, referral to a physician specializing in metabolic disorders may be required.

Anorexia Nervosa

The National Institute of Mental Health (2001) observed the large impact society has on eating disorders and noted, "Dieting to a body weight leaner than needed for health is highly promoted by current fashion trends, sales campaigns for special foods, and in some activities and professions" (p. 3). Unfortunately, many individuals develop a poor body image and subsequently are diagnosed with an eating disorder such as anorexia nervosa. Dudek (2006) vividly described the disorder in the following quote, "Clients with anorexia nervosa pursue thinness compulsively through semistarvation and compulsive exercise. They are intensely preoccupied with weight and food, and their distorted perception causes them to see themselves as fat when they are emaciated" (p. 402). In clinical terms, anorexia nervosa diagnostic criteria is defined as adults who have a BMI < 18 kg/m^2 and children who have a BMI that is less than the 5th percentile for their age and gender. The typical individual with anorexia nervosa is a teenage girl who is a high achiever and who seeks perfection. Food consumption becomes a way to feel in control. Obviously, serious problems including altered growth and development, lowered resistance to infection, poor general health, and reduced strength can result from being seriously underweight. Without help, the disorder can lead to fatality. Treatment of a serious psychological disorder such as anorexia nervosa requires the therapy of a skilled team of professionals—physicians, nurses, psychologists, and nutritionists. The nurse's role is one of teaching and supporting the individual and family with respect to healthy lifestyle, balanced diet, and support for a realistic perception of expectations and accomplishments. Ongoing monitoring and the support of treatment regimen may be required. Understanding processes related to nutrition at the three levels of adaptation provide the knowledge for the planning of nursing care.

NURSING PROCESS RELATED TO NUTRITION

Adequate nutritional status is a priority requirement of the individual's physiologic adaptation. In applying the nursing process, the nurse will make a careful assessment of the behaviors and stimuli related to the basic processes of eating, digestion, and metabolism. In assessing stimuli influencing the need for nutrition, a number of common influencing factors including regulator and cognator effectiveness in initiating compensatory processes will be considered. Based on these thorough first- and second-level assessments, the nurse makes a nursing diagnosis, sets goals, selects nursing interventions, and evaluates care.

Assessment of Behaviors

There are a number of factors to consider in assessing behaviors related to the processes of nutrition. In first level assessment the nurse observes the following categories of behavior: eating patterns, nutrient profile, sense of taste and smell, condition of the oral cavity, appetite and thirst, height and weight, food allergies, pain, altered ingestion, and any relevant laboratory indicators.

EATING PATTERNS The nurse obtains a diet history listing the quantities of all food and fluids ingested during a 24-hour period. Of particular interest with respect to digestion are types of foods ingested, times of food intake, the situations associated with mealtimes and eating, and the individual's bodily response in terms of the digestive process. Many of these factors are specified further in the following discussion.

NUTRIENT PROFILE Dudek (2006) stated that, "A healthy diet provides enough of all essential nutrients to avoid deficiencies but not excessive amounts that may increase the risk of nutrient toxicities or chronic disease…" (p. 178). Accepted standards for recommended daily allowances of nutrients have been developed over time and by multiple organizations. The optimal diet provides a caloric level that will meet the energy needs of the body. Dudek also noted that, "As the science of nutrition grew, it became clear that nutrient excesses contribute to chronic disease and that recommendations needed to expand their focus from simply preventing deficiencies to achieving optimal health and avoiding excesses" (p. 178). People should eat food that promotes health and provides a measure of prevention in protecting them from illness throughout all stages of the life cycle.

The established nutrient profile must be acceptable to the individual or family. Acceptability includes establishing a diet that includes culturally defined differences such as those noted later in this chapter. Taking into account such differences is possible since there are many kinds and combinations of foods that constitute a well-balanced diet. Finally, the diet chosen should promote a good supply of energy for optimum performance of the individual's activities of daily living and total human functioning.

Given expanded knowledge of nutrition, scientists have developed many different ways to determine appropriate nutritional intake. In 2005, the United States Department of Agriculture (USDA) augmented its original idea of a food pyramid to account for serving amounts; this guide can be reviewed at www.mypyramid.gov. This guide provides a flexible framework to help people achieve nutrient needs as outlined in the recommended daily dietary allowances. The Harvard School of Public Health developed another nutritional guide in 2001 that is currently printed on many nutritional labels. The aim of this guide is to reduce the number of chronic diseases. In planning a diet, the individual should be encouraged to choose a variety of foods that he or she likes and can afford, and that have good nutritional benefit. Refer to nutrition textbooks for further information about nutritional requirements and dietary planning.

SENSE OF TASTE AND SMELL The taste and smell of food to the individual have a significant influence on the individual's response to it. The majority of taste buds are located on the tongue. Four basic sensations are experienced: sweet, sour, bitter, and salty. The sensory receptors for taste are the glossopharyngeal nerve (cranial nerve IX) and the facial nerve (cranial nerve VII). The ability to taste relies heavily on the ability to smell. As a result, nasal passages should be patent. Testing each nostril separately, the individual should be able to identify such odors as coffee or cinnamon.

CONDITION OF THE ORAL CAVITY Appraisal of the oral cavity, that is, the lips, teeth, gums, and tongue, is useful in determining the individual's nutritional health and in identifying deficiencies. The lips of the healthy adult are smooth and free from lesions. The skin is thin with many vascular structures, which give the lips their reddish appearance. The oral mucosa is normally smooth, moist, and pink-red in color, with expected variations based on ethnic differences. The adult has 32 permanent teeth. They are examined for conditions that decrease their grinding action, such as loose or missing teeth, cavities, or wear. If dentures are used, they are removed to allow complete inspection of the mouth. Normal gums are solid in turgor and free of inflammation or bleeding. The tongue is pink in color. The dorsal surface is rough and the ventral surface is smooth.

APPETITE AND THIRST   Appetite is a pleasant sensation involving the individual's desire for and anticipation of food and fluids. Frequently, the appetite is affected by such specific stimuli as the sight, smell, and thought of food. It is psychological and is dependent on memory and associations. An example of an adaptive appetite behavior would be the statement, "I have a good appetite in the morning and eat a well-balanced breakfast," whereas an ineffective appetite behavior would be, "Although I ate a large lunch, the smell of freshly baked cinnamon rolls got to me and I ate two large rolls. I now feel very uncomfortable."

Thirst is a desire for fluid or the dry sensation resulting from a lack of or need for water. Often this sensation of dryness is felt in the mouth and the back of the throat. Thirst is usually a reliable guide to the body's need for water. The normal adult should consume a minimum of 1 and 1/2 liters of water or other liquids daily to provide a sufficient amount of water for all physiologic processes. Water is available to the body through other sources, such as beverages, solid foods, and a small amount through the oxidation of essential nutrients. The maintenance of water balance is explored further in Chapter 11.

HEIGHT AND WEIGHT   In a behavioral assessment of nutrition, the nurse measures and records the height and the weight of the individual. Height measurements are taken without shoes and the weight, preferably, is taken without clothing. A daily weight is also useful when assessing an individual's fluid balance. In this case, it is particularly important that the weight be taken at the same time of day and on the same scale. When an individual is underweight or overweight, measurements taken over a period of time are more useful than a single measurement. The official measure of obesity and body fatness is the Body Mass Index (BMI), an index of weight related to height. The BMI is calculated by multiplying weight in pounds by 705 and dividing by height in inches squared. The BMI is divided into four classifications (underweight, normal, overweight, and obese), and each classification has different risk factors associated with it. Standard and reference growth charts for infants, children, and adolescents have been established and used in practice for many years. More recently, BMI is also being used for the pediatric population, especially with the increase in overweight children.

FOOD ALLERGIES   The nurse assesses whether the individual has a known food allergy or sensitivity. An allergic reaction to a certain food or food group is the result of an antibody–antigen reaction in the body. Foods causing problems are identified. The behaviors that occur if the food is ingested are noted such as skin rash, swelling of the face or mouth, or gastrointestinal reaction. For example, the increasing occurrence of individuals with allergies to peanuts has changed the American culture from the school cafeteria to the local ice cream stand.

PAIN   The nurse assesses for any pain related to the ingestion of food or fluids. Pain can be noted as a behavior by listing the individual's statements regarding discomfort and pain following ingestion of food. For example, an individual may identify a burning sensation, or "heartburn," after the ingestion of spicy foods. Another example is odynophagia (painful swallowing) as a result of radiation therapy. All verbal and nonverbal behaviors are recorded. Pain is further specified in terms of severity; duration; onset (gradual or abrupt, before or after meals); location, spread, and radiation; precipitating factors; frequency; and quality (sharp, dull, burning, pressure, stabbing). In addition, treatment measures (diet, rest, position, and medications), aggravating factors, associated symptoms, and the patient's attitude toward the pain are explored.

ALTERED INGESTION   If the individual is unable to eat and drink normally, the altered means of nutritional intake are assessed. Dysphagia, or alteration in the ability to swallow, may require individuals to be nourished in alternative ways. For example, an individual may be nourished through a nasogastric or gastrostomy tube, therefore bypassing the need to swallow. The amount and substance ingested should be noted. If the individual is receiving intravenous fluid or a hyperalimentation solution, the solutions and rate of delivery are recorded. The knowledge and skills related to these particular altered means of ingestion are continually developing. The nurse is challenged to maintain the knowledge and skill necessary to provide nursing care in these situations through reading, clinical practice, and continuing education.

LABORATORY INDICATORS   Many laboratory tests provide indicators of the body's nutrition status. Plasma protein measures of albumin and prealbumin assist in the detection of protein and iron deficiencies. Twenty-four hour urine tests measure products of protein metabolism. Elevated levels may indicate excess body tissue breakdown. Other important laboratory indicators include lipid panel, complete blood count (CBC), and glycated hemoglobin assay (Hgb A1C). In advanced nursing practice roles, nurses may be involved in ordering such laboratory procedures as further behavioral indicators of the patient's nutrition and metabolic status.

Assessment of Stimuli

Assessment of stimuli involves the identification of the factors that appear to be influencing the individual's behavior related to nutrition. Common stimuli affecting the processes of nutrition include the physical structures and physiologic functions of digestion, nutrient requirements, availability of food, conditions of eating, cues for eating including weight consciousness, cognator effectiveness, culture, and medication.

INTEGRITY OF STRUCTURE AND FUNCTION   The digestive system consists of the GI tract and accessory digestive organs. The GI tract or gut described earlier is responsible for the digestion and absorption of nutrients. The accessory organs are the teeth, tongue, gallbladder, and glands including salivary, liver, and pancreas. When food is ingested, a series of physical and chemical changes occur by action of the GI tract and accessory organs. These processes prepare the nutrients for absorption and utilization by the cells. The GI tract is regulated by the neural, chemical, and endocrine processes that Roy describes as the regulator subsystem (see Chapter 2). Residue remaining after digestion and absorption is then excreted from the body (elimination is further discussed in Chapter 7). Through physical assessment of the structures associated with the process of digestion, the nurse identifies whether or not a condition is present that affects the normal processes of the digestive system. Such examination involves inspection of the oral cavity, abdomen (inspection, auscultation, percussion, and palpitation), and a rectal examination, in addition to inquiring about the individual's experiences surrounding ingestion and elimination. Examples of disease states influencing digestive function include such conditions as obstructive lesions of the esophagus and malabsorption. These diseases are explained in general textbooks of pathophysiology and medical science. Also, the nurse assesses for conditions that prohibit the individual from eating, such as impending or recent surgery, and for restricted or special diets, such as that for an individual with the medical diagnosis of diabetes mellitus.

NUTRIENT REQUIREMENTS Factors affecting nutrient requirements are age, gender, size, activity, temperature, diet, climate, pregnancy, and endocrine functioning. For example, an infant, because of a high rate of metabolism and relatively large body surface area, requires more calories per kilogram of body weight than an adult. An individual exposed to severely cold weather expends additional calories to maintain body temperature. In periods of rapid growth during infancy, adolescence, and pregnancy, there is an increased caloric need. Males, who usually have a greater body size and greater proportion of lean body tissue, have a greater caloric requirement than do females. As an individual ages, there is a steady decline in caloric need starting with the early adult years. In the older adult, caloric needs decrease but the other nutritional requirements remain similar to that of a middle age adult. Exercise patterns of the individual are assessed, as they will also influence caloric requirements.

AVAILABILITY OF FOOD The nurse considers the availability of food to the individual including financial and other resources. Brainstorming with the patient, the nurse can help with the affordability of nutritious foods for those experiencing financial difficulties. For example, an elderly individual may find it difficult to travel to the store and may have limited financial resources with which to purchase food. For pregnant women or families with young children, there are government-funded food assistance programs.

CONDITIONS OF EATING The nurse identifies who purchases and prepares the food the individual eats. In the family setting, the health beliefs of the food purchaser and preparer regarding nutrition will greatly influence the eating behaviors of all members. The nurse determines whether or not the family meal plan provides a well-balanced diet and notes what social and moral values are placed on eating. For example, is eating a highly social event, and is food used as a punishment or reward? The nurse further identifies the level of family or peer group influence regarding eating and considers if the individual or family sets aside a special time for mealtime. For example, are the meals taken alone, with a group, at home, at fast-food services, or in a restaurant? Another important consideration is the individual's familiarity with different types of food, and his or her understanding of the nutritional benefit of the foods chosen, as noted in the discussion of cognator effectiveness.

CUES FOR EATING When assessing factors influencing the individual's food intake and the process of digestion, it is important to identify the internal and external cues to which the individual responds. A healthy, functioning hypothalamus sends the individual internal cues that signal that enough food has been ingested. In cases of overeating, the nurse helps the individual identify what external cues they are responding to when eating. Generally, other cues are being used when the individual is failing to respond to internal cues relating to satiety and hunger control. For example, some people might overeat as a means of coping with the stresses of daily living. The nurse identifies if the individual's eating and drinking behaviors are influenced by emotions, social pressures, habits, or the good taste and palatability of food, rather than the internal cues that control appetite. Cues from the external environment, such as a pleasant environment and freedom from pain and stress, also influence ingestion. In addition, the nurse identifies the individual's desire to gain, lose, or maintain body weight. This weight consciousness is a cue that influences the individual's present and future eating patterns.

COGNATOR EFFECTIVENESS The individual's level of knowledge regarding nutrition and perception of what constitutes a healthy and nutritious diet is a major stimulus. The nurse assesses this knowledge and perception since it greatly influences what the individual is ingesting or what the individual desires to eat. The individual's knowledge can be a major factor in either adaptive or ineffective patterns of nutrition. The nurse can help an individual read the nutrition labels and determine appropriate serving sizes. Based on the patient's level of knowledge about sound nutrition, diet counseling may be required. The nurse explores the individual's beliefs regarding types of food eaten. Some people, for religious, economic, health, ethical, or ecologic reasons, are vegetarians. Such beliefs are taken into account in diet counseling.

CULTURE The nurse inquires about the individual's cultural, social, and religious patterns that influence eating and drinking. Food habits and preferences based on cultural experience begin early in life. Cultural patterns affect both the kinds of foods used and the way they are prepared. As examples, two cultural perspectives described by Purnell & Paulanka (2003) are cited here. Basic dietary laws for Jewish people are identified in the Laws of Kashrut, and the food that satisfies that requirement is considered Kosher. These apply to the slaughter, preparation, and serving of meat; the combining of meat and milk; types of fish eaten; and eggs. Some food is restricted. Pork is not used; no combining of meat and milk is allowed; and only fish with fins and scales are to be eaten. Orthodox Jewish people strictly observe these laws, and the less conservative Jewish person determines his or her own degree of restrictions. It is important for the nurse to understand and observe the individual's preference in this regard. A second example pertains to the food patterns of people subscribing to traditional Japanese heritage. Rice is considered the staple for all three meals, and to some Japanese religions it has symbolic meaning. The Japanese diet also consists of beef, poultry, pork, seafood, and many fruits and vegetables. Unfortunately, many favorites of the Japanese culture include a large amount of sweets or are high in sodium. It is thus important that culture be assessed as a factor potentially influencing meeting the need for nutrition.

MEDICATION The nurse identifies whether or not the individual takes any medication that can influence the intake of food or the digestive process. For example, drugs that can decrease the appetite may be taken if the individual is attempting to lose weight. In contrast, there are drugs that can increase appetite when an individual is trying to gain weight or has lost interest in eating. It is important to ascertain whether supplemental vitamins, herbs, or minerals are used, as well.

Nursing Diagnosis

As has been described previously in this text, the assessment information related to behaviors and stimuli are interpreted in the form of a nursing diagnosis. The diagnostic statement is made by considering the data of the first- and second-level assessment. The statement can include a summary of observed behaviors with the most relevant influencing stimuli. An example of a nursing diagnosis illustrating adaptation and summarizing behavior and stimuli is, "Eating patterns show intake of recommended nutrients related to knowledge of balanced diet for body requirements and availability of food." In situations where problems exist related to the need for adequate nutrition, it is important that the nursing diagnosis convey the essence of the problem so that direction is provided for the subsequent steps of the nursing process. This is facilitated by the recommended structure of a nursing diagnosis: a statement of observed behaviors with most relevant influencing stimuli. Consider an example of a 75-year-old man who has recently become a widower. Although he has been in good health, he has been losing weight gradually since his wife's death. When asked about his eating patterns, he states that he does not bother cooking for himself. Rather, he eats primarily cereals and bread, never cooks meat or vegetables, but occasionally enjoys baked food that his neighbor prepares. A nursing diagnosis relevant to this situation might be, "Weight loss related to inadequate intake of required nutrients."

A summary label is an alternate way of stating a nursing diagnosis. The nurse's judgment of the clinical situation may be expressed by using a statement from an established classification system. The Roy model has two classification lists, one for indicators of adaptation and one for commonly recurring adaptation problems. The complete classification lists for the Roy model are included in Chapter 3. In Table 6–1, the Roy model nursing

TABLE 6–1 Nursing Diagnostic Categories for Nutrition

Positive Indicators of Adaptation	Common Adaptation Problems	NANDA Diagnostic Labels
• Stable digestive processes • Adequate nutritional pattern for body requirements • Metabolic and other nutritive needs met during altered means of ingestion	• Nausea and vomiting • Nutrition more or less than body requirements • Weight 20% to 25% above or below average • Anorexia • Ineffective coping strategies for altered means of ingestion	• Impaired swallowing • Imbalanced nutrition: Less than body requirements • Imbalanced nutrition: More than body requirements • Risk for imbalanced nutrition: More than body requirements • Effective breast-feeding • Ineffective breast-feeding • Interrupted breast-feeding • Ineffective infant feeding pattern • Risk for impaired liver function • Risk for unstable blood glucose level • Readiness for enhanced nutrition

diagnostic categories for the physiologic need of nutrition are shown in relation to nursing diagnosis labels approved by the North American Nursing Diagnosis Association (NANDA International, 2007). Labels that summarize a behavioral pattern when more than one mode is being affected by the same stimuli are often very meaningful to experienced nurses. They convey much information in a single term. An example of such a label would be the term anorexia nervosa. As described earlier, stimuli contributing to this disorder are often very complex and are associated with modes in addition to the physiologic mode. For example, the self-concept and interdependence modes may be involved. The individual may feel attractive only at a weight of less than 100 pounds. Significant others may reinforce this belief by commenting adversely whenever additional weight becomes evident. A nursing diagnosis illustrating this could be, "Limited food intake related to peer pressure and low self-esteem."

Another nursing diagnosis related to altered nutrition is "Changing nutrient profile with increased carbohydrate and fat intake related to picking up fast foods near new work site." This diagnosis defines the state in which an individual experiences or is at risk of experiencing an intake of nutrients that exceeds metabolic needs. The behaviors and stimuli related to these diagnoses are individual and may include such assessment factors as sedentary activity level or responding inappropriately to internal and external cues for eating. It is important to consider metabolic and endocrine factors that may be contributing to the problem. If physiologically based factors do not exist, other stimuli should be explored. A diagnosis of "altered nutrition, less than body requirements related to poverty" is defined as the state in which an individual experiences an intake of nutrients insufficient to meet metabolic needs based on limited financial resources. Other stimuli that can relate to inadequate nutrition may include the individual's ability to ingest or digest food or absorb nutrients because of psychological, biologic, or economic factors. An individual is considered to have an insufficient nutrient intake to satisfy metabolic needs when his or her BMI is less than 18 kg/m^2 for gender and age. The behaviors and stimuli related to this diagnosis are varied and can include such assessment factors as lack of interest in food; decreased availability of food; or painful, inflamed condition of the mouth.

Nausea and vomiting are other common adaptation problems related to nutrition. These problems are frequently associated but can be experienced separately. Nausea is an unpleasant sensation reported as a feeling of sickness with the urge to vomit. Vomiting is the forceful ejection of stomach contents through the mouth. The vomiting reflex can be stimulated by a number of intrinsic and extrinsic factors, for example, unpleasant odors, tastes, sights; sensations such as severe pain; chemical agents used in the treatment of disease; and radiation therapy. Identification of the stimuli contributing to the problem is an important factor in its solution. Once the nursing diagnosis related to nutrition has been established, the nurse proceeds to formulate individualized goals that address each of the identified problems or support areas in which adaptation has been observed.

Goal Setting

In the fourth step of the nursing process as described in the Roy Adaptation Model, the nurse establishes goals in collaboration with the individual receiving care. Statements of clear behavioral outcomes of nursing care are planned with the individual. The goal should address the behavior, the change expected, and the time frame in which the goal is to be achieved. Goals may be short term or long term, and these time frames are relative to the situation involved.

When setting a goal for the individual experiencing an intake of nutrients exceeding metabolic needs, it is realistic and healthy to establish a goal providing for gradual weight loss of 1 to 2 pounds per week while eating a well-balanced diet. An appropriately worded goal could be, "The patient will lose 2 pounds each week for the next 4 weeks." In this objective, the individual's weight is the behavior of focus, the change expected is the loss of 2 pounds each week, and the time frame is 4 weeks. An appropriate goal for the situation described previously of the elderly man experiencing weight loss related to inadequate intake of required nutrients would be eating a well-balanced, high-caloric diet so as to initially stabilize the weight and then increase weight gradually. A short-term goal may relate to the daily intake, "Today Mr. Smith will ingest an evening meal that is balanced in nutrients and of sufficient caloric content to meet his energy requirements." A longer term goal could be related to his status in 1 month: "By this date next month, Mr. Smith will have gained 5 pounds and documented a balanced intake containing all recommended nutrients."

For the individual experiencing the adaptation problems of nausea and vomiting, the goal should directly reflect a decrease in the stated assessed behavior or an increased ability to cope with it. As has been identified before, goals pertain directly to the individual's behavior and are stated in behavioral terms from the patient's perspective.

The focus for the next step of the nursing process, nursing intervention, is the change of the stimuli identified as contributing to the observed behaviors and the strengthening of compensatory processes.

Nursing Intervention

Once the goals have been established related to behaviors that will promote adaptation, the nurse determines the nursing interventions that will assist the individual in meeting stated goals. Nursing interventions for promotion of nutrition depend on the stimuli and, particularly, the coping processes identified. The nurse manages the stimuli by either promoting or reinforcing them, or by taking action to change or eliminate them. For example, if the stimulus related to overeating is an identified response to internal cues of feeling stressed, then the nurse can assist the individual in establishing coping strategies to adapt to the stresses of daily living. Additionally, if a decreased exercise pattern is identified as a stimulus, the nurse can assist the individual with measures to increase activity level. New coping strategies may be learned, such as taking a walk to handle stress.

If an individual wants to change a situation of being overweight, it is important to establish the motivation for the desired weight-loss regimen. One reason for wanting to lose weight may include an improved health status in order to avoid the many chronic disorders linked to obesity. Other motivators may be a desire for improvement in personal appearance and peer pressures from family and friends to lose weight. A nursing intervention that has been used successfully for changing an obese individual's response pattern of eating because of external cues is behavior modification (Berkel, Poston, Reeves, & Forreyt, 2005). Behavior modification entails a variety of strategies to alter an individual's behavior and thought processes to accomplish the intended results. It is often helpful for the individual to write down specific feelings before eating to identify whether the eating is in response to emotions such as anxiety, boredom, or loneliness. Writing down observations is a self-monitoring strategy. The individual is then instructed to try to substitute other activities in place of eating at these times. This behavior is a stress management strategy. Other techniques in this approach include slowing down and making the act of eating a conscious acknowledged action, which is helpful as a problem solving strategy. Another strategy of behavior modification is to reward oneself with a nonfood item such as a new outfit when one meets goals.

In the previous situation of the elderly man, the short-term goal focused on one balanced meal. In addressing the stimuli involved in the situation, it was evident that Mr. Smith had never received instruction related to proper nutrition, or had the opportunity to do any cooking. By reviewing the dietary requirements associated with a balanced meal and discussing preparation methods with him, Mr. Smith made a commitment to make a list and go to the grocery store to buy the required supplies, and then cook himself a meal. He invited his neighbor to observe the cooking session, intervene in case of a problem, and share the meal with him. This scenario utilizes the behavior modification strategies of cognitive restructuring and social support, particularly important for the man whose wife died recently.

General nursing interventions for nausea and vomiting will focus, where possible, on the stimuli causing the problem. For example, unpleasant, strong odors in the environment should be eliminated; or the individual's environment should be kept quiet and sudden movements prevented. If pain is causing the problem, it may be that something can be done to alleviate it. Other conservative treatments for nausea and vomiting include limiting the individual's food and fluid intake until the problem subsides. Ice chips may be tolerated, and oral hygiene is refreshing for the patient. Positioning the patient with the head raised and turned to the side may assist and will be necessary if vomiting is occurring. If none of these nursing interventions is successful, it may be necessary to administer an antiemetic medication as prescribed. When the problem subsides and the diet is resumed, offering foods that are bland, such as dry toast or plain crackers, is often appropriate. If nausea and vomiting persist, the use of intravenous fluids to prevent fluid and electrolyte imbalance may be warranted. One nursing intervention by the nurse related to nutrition planning may be to provide a referral to a health professional involved exclusively in dietetics and nutrition.

Evaluation

Evaluation involves judging the effectiveness of nursing interventions in relation to the individual's behavior and in terms of the agreed upon goals. The nursing interventions are identified as effective if the individual's behavior is in accordance with the stated goal. For example, in a previous illustration, the goal was, "The patient will lose 2 pounds each week for the next 4 weeks." The goal would be achieved if the individual loses 2 pounds each week for 4 weeks. Achievement of this goal is measured by weekly assessment of weight. For Mr. Smith, evaluation would be accomplished as he reported on his success with his first meal and, eventually, his ability to continue to consume a balanced diet. Further evaluation would include observing for evidence of subsequent weight stabilization and gain. If this expected scenario did not materialize, other approaches to the problem are sought. If the goal has not been achieved, the nurse identifies alternative nursing interventions or approaches by reassessing the behavior and stimuli, particularly the use of compensating strategies, and continuing with the other steps of the nursing process.

Summary

This chapter has focused on the application of the Roy Adaptation Model to the physiologic need of nutrition. An overview of the basic life processes of digestion and metabolism that meet the need for nutrition was provided. Illustrations of innate and learned adaptive compensatory processes related to nutrition were described. Two examples of compromised processes, obesity and anorexia nervosa, were explained. Finally, guidelines for planning nursing care through identification of factors for assessment of behaviors and stimuli, the formulation of nursing diagnoses, goals, and nursing interventions were explored and evaluation of nursing care was described.

Exercises for Application

1. Assess your own eating patterns by recording a diet history for a 24-hour period. Determine if the quantity and quality of the nutrients ingested are adaptive or ineffective.
2. For your eating pattern, list the factors that you think most influence your behavior.
3. Identify an individual with good eating habits and preferences based on cultural experience that is different from your own. Determine the cultural, social, and religious patterns that influence that individual's ingestion of food and fluids.

Assessment of Understanding

QUESTIONS

1. List the five major processes associated with the basic life process of digestion.
   (a) _____
   (b) _____
   (c) _____
   (d) _____
   (e) _____
2. Label the following examples of compensatory responses as associated with regulator (R) or cognator (C) mechanisms.
   (a) _____ In situations of illness, the individual often loses his or her appetite for food.
   (b) _____ When blood glucose levels are too low, the liver breaks down stored glycogen and releases glucose into the blood.
   (c) _____ To lose weight, the individual alters intake of fats and increases his or her exercise pattern.
   (d) _____ When caloric intake is inadequate for the body's level of activity, fat and even tissue proteins begin to break down to satisfy the body's requirements.
   (e) _____ The diabetic individual calculates daily requirement for insulin and self-administers the required amount.
3. An altered means of ingestion can be the outcome of compromise related to a particular process involved in nutrition. In the situation of an individual being fed through a gastrostomy tube, identify two processes that could be compromised to warrant such an alternative.

4. List three categories of behaviors associated with the basic life processes of nutrition.
   (a) _____
   (b) _____
   (c) _____
5. The following is the list of common influencing factors that were identified in Chapter 3. Identify the factors that are of concern with respect to the need for nutrition.
   (a) Culture
   (b) Family and aggregate participants
   (c) Developmental stage
   (d) Integrity of modes and systems
   (e) Cognator and innovator effectiveness
   (f) Environmental considerations

SITUATION

Nancy James is a 40-year-old career woman who works as an executive for a publishing company. She commutes 2 hours each day, leaving early and arriving home late. She rarely has time for breakfast and does not bother preparing dinner for herself. She frequently has business luncheons and does not feel hungry until later in the evening. Whenever she does feel hungry, she snacks on soda pop, chocolate bars, and chips since the dispensing machine is located close to her office. Nancy wants to lose some weight. She is 5 feet 2 inches tall and weighs 160 pounds. She states, "I can't understand why I keep putting on weight. I usually eat only one meal a day!"

6. Formulate a nursing diagnosis for the described situation.

_____

_____

7. State a goal to address weight loss in the described situation. Identify the behavior, the change expected, and the associated time frame.

Goal: _____

Behavior: _____

Expected change: _____

Time frame: _____

8. List two nursing interventions that might assist Nancy in the achievement of the goal stated. What stimuli are being managed?

Nursing Interventions   Stimuli

_____   _____

_____   _____

9. What behavior would provide evidence that the identified goal had been achieved?

_____

FEEDBACK

1. (a) ingestion
   (b) propulsion
   (c) mechanical digestion
   (d) chemical digestion
   (e) absorption

2. (a) R, (b) R, (c) C, (d) R, (e) C
3. Ingestion: The individual may be unable to swallow. Movement of food: It may not be possible for food to move down the esophagus.
4. Any three of: eating patterns, nutrient profile, sense of taste and smell, oral cavity, appetite, height and weight, food allergies, pain, altered ingestion, laboratory indicators.
5. All of the factors are relevant to the need for nutrition.
6. Nursing diagnosis example: "High caloric eating pattern related to lack of awareness of intake in excess of body requirements and long work hours."
7. Goal example: Within 4 weeks, Nancy will have lost 10 pounds.
   Behavior: weight
   Change expected: loss of 10 pounds
   Time frame: within 4 weeks
8. Nursing Interventions and Stimuli
   Documentation of intake (nursing intervention)
   Cognator effectiveness (stimuli): Nancy's perception of how much she eats is erroneous.
   Adherence to 1,800-calorie diet (nursing intervention)
   Nutrient requirements (stimuli): Nancy's diet will be based on her required nutritional intake and her desire for weight loss.
9. Within 4 weeks, Nancy will have lost 10 pounds.

References

Berkel, L. A., Poston, W. S. C., Reeves, R. S., & Foreyt, J. P. (2005). Behavioral interventions for obesity. _Journal of the American Dietetic Association, 105_, (Supp. 1), S35–S43.

Centers for Disease Control and Prevention, National Center for Health Statistics, Fast Facts A to Z. Available at: http://www.cdc.gov/nchs/fastats/overwt.htm. Accessed May, 2008.

Craven, R. F., & Hirnle, C. J. (2007). _Fundamentals of nursing human health and function_ (5th ed.). Philadelphia: Lippincott Williams & Wilkins.

Dudek, S. G. (2006). _Nutrition essentials for nursing practice_ (5th ed.). Philadelphia: Lippincott Williams & Wilkins.

Ersek, M. (2003). Artificial nutrition and hydration: Clinical issues. _Journal of Hospice and Palliative Nursing, 5_(4), 221–230.

Kavey, R-E. W., Allada, V., Daniels, S. R., Hayman, L. L., McCrindle, B. W., Newburger, J. W., et al. (2007). Cardiovascular risk reduction in high-risk pediatric patients. _Journal of Cardiovascular Nursing, 22_(3), 218–253.

Marieb, E. N., & Hoehn, K. (2007). _Human anatomy and physiology_ (7th ed.). San Francisco: Pearson Benjamin Cummings.

McCance, K. L., & Huether, S. E. (2002). _Patho physiology: The biologic basis for disease in adults & children_ (4th ed.). St. Louis, MO: Mosby.

NANDA International (2007). _Nursing Diagnoses: Definitions and classifications, 2007–2008_. Philadelphia: NANDA-1.

National Institute of Mental Health. (2001). _Eating disorders: Facts about eating disorders and the search for solutions_ (NIH Publication No. 01–4901). Bethesda, MD: Author.

Nelms, M., Sucher, K., & Long, S. (2007). *Nutrition therapy and pathophysiology*. Australia: Thomson Brooks/Cole.

Purnell, L. D., & Paulanka, B. J. (2003). *Transcultural health care: A culturally competent approach* (2nd ed.). Philadelphia: F. A. Davis Company.

Splett, P. L., Roth-Yousey, L. L., & Vogelzang, J. L. (2003). Medical nutrition therapy for the prevention and treatment of unintentional weight loss in residential healthcare facilities. *Journal of the American Dietetic Association, 103*(3), 352–362.

Winter, S. M. (2000). Terminal nutrition: Framing the debate for the withdrawal of nutritional support in terminally ill patients. *The American Journal of Medicine, 109*, 723–726.

Additional References

Harvard School of Public Health. (2007). The Healthy Eating Pyramid. Available from: http://www.hsph.harvard.edu/nutritionsource/pyramids.html

Ignatavicius, D. D., & Workman, M. L. (2006). *Medical-surgical nursing: Critical thinking for collaborative care* (5th ed.). St. Louis, MO: Elsevier Saunders.

National Heart, Lung, and Blood Institute. (2000). *The practical guide: Identification, evaluation, and treatment of overweight and obesity in adults* (NIH Publication No. 00–4084). Bethesda, MD: National Heart, Lung, and Blood Institute.

National Institute of Diabetes and Digestive and Kidney Diseases. (2007). Weight-control Information Network: Statistics related to overweight and obesity. Available from: http://win.niddk.nih.gov/statistics/index.htm

United States Department of Agriculture. (2005). MyPyramid—Getting Started. Available from: http://www.mypyramid.gov

Women, Infants, and Children Program. Available from: http://www.fns.usda.gov/wic

CHAPTER 7

Elimination

Elimination is a basic life process essential to adaptation. Just as nutrients are provided for survival and maintenance of physiologic balance by digestion and metabolism processes, so do metabolic waste products need to be eliminated. As Smith and Watson (2005) stated, "Nutrients, water and salts are absorbed from digested food and all products that cannot be absorbed are retained in the digestive tract until they are eliminated" (p. 13). Waste materials are expelled to maintain homeostasis. In addition to excretion from the intestines, metabolic wastes are eliminated by the kidneys, the skin, and the lungs. Chapter 5 addresses excretion by the lungs through gas exchange with the environment, and Chapter 9 deals with excretion by the skin through perspiration. In this chapter, the basic life processes of intestinal elimination and urinary elimination are addressed. Illustrations of compensatory and compromised processes related to elimination are described. Guidelines for planning nursing care include identifying behaviors and stimuli for assessment, formulating diagnoses, establishing goals, selecting nursing interventions, and evaluating nursing care.

OBJECTIVES

After studying this chapter, the reader will be able to do the following:

1. Describe two basic life processes associated with the need for elimination as presented in this chapter.
2. Describe one compensatory process related to each of the basic life processes associated with elimination.
3. Name and describe two situations of compromised processes of elimination.
4. Identify important first-level assessment behaviors for the need for elimination.
5. List second-level assessment common stimuli that affect elimination.
6. Develop a nursing diagnosis, given a situation related to elimination.
7. Derive goals for an individual with ineffective elimination in a given situation.
8. Describe nursing interventions commonly implemented in situations of ineffective elimination.
9. Propose approaches to determine the effectiveness of nursing interventions.

KEY CONCEPTS DEFINED

Anuria: The complete suppression of urine formation by the kidneys.

Bowel incontinence: The involuntary passage of stool.

Constipation: A condition in which the fecal matter in the bowel is too hard to pass with ease, or a state in which the bowel movements are so infrequent that uncomfortable symptoms occur. It is clinically defined as less than three bowel movements per week.

Diarrhea: The rapid movement of the fecal material through the intestines, resulting in poor absorption of water, essential nutrients, and electrolytes, and an abnormally frequent passage of watery stool.

Flatulence: Gas or air in the gastrointestinal tract that can result in pain or feelings of abdominal fullness.

Intestinal elimination: The expulsion from the body of undigested substance via the anus in the form of feces.

Micturition: The process by which the bladder is emptied.

Oliguria: Diminished urine secretion in relation to fluid intake.

Peristalsis: Movements of the intestinal tract that both mix and propel the mixture of food and enzymes that comes from the digestive process in the stomach.

Urinary elimination: The elimination of fluid wastes and excess ions as a result of the filtering process in which the kidneys maintain the purity and constancy of internal fluids.

Urinary incontinence: The involuntary passage of urine from the bladder.

Urinary retention: The inability to void, with the resultant accumulation of urine within the bladder.

BASIC LIFE PROCESSES OF ELIMINATION

Although many life processes are involved in elimination of waste products from the body, the focus of this chapter is intestinal and urinary elimination. Intestinal elimination is the expulsion from the body of undigested substances by way of the anus in the form of feces. Urinary elimination is the elimination of fluid wastes and excess ions as a result of the filtering process of the kidneys to maintain the purity and constancy of internal fluids. As mentioned, other elimination processes are addressed in other chapters of this text.

Process of Intestinal Elimination

Maintenance of adequate intestinal elimination requires a functioning gastrointestinal tract. As noted in Chapter 6, the primary function of the gastrointestinal tract, or alimentary canal, as a whole is to provide water, electrolytes, and nutrients to sustain life. Basic structures of the upper gastrointestinal (GI) tract consist of the mouth, esophagus, and stomach. The lower gastrointestinal tract is made up of the small intestine—the duodenum, jejunum, and ileum. The large intestine includes the cecum and the ascending, transverse, descending, and sigmoid colon and the rectum and the anus. The GI tract carries out three functions: the movement of food through the tract; secretion of digestive juices; and absorption of the digested nutrients, water, and electrolytes. The upper GI tract deals with ingestion and digestion of food. The small intestine involves both digestion and absorption of nutrients. The function of the large intestine is primarily the absorption of water and electrolytes, and the elimination of the waste products of digestion through the anus. Movements of both the small and large intestine are key to the process of elimination. Peristalsis is the term used to describe the smooth muscle movement of contraction and relaxation in the stomach. This movement allows for both mixing and propelling of the mixture of food and enzymes that comes from the digestive process in the stomach, called chyme. The peristaltic waves are set by multiple valves and pacemaker cells within the stomach. In the small intestine, rapid segmental contractions chop the solid food particles to promote mixing with digestive secretions from the liver and pancreas. "The process of food digestion is accelerated during the chyme's tortuous journey of three to six hours through the small intestine…" (Marieb & Hoehn, 2007, p. 919).

The proximal half of the colon is concerned primarily with absorption, and the distal half with storage. Less intense mixing movements are required for these functions. Thus, in the colon, the fecal material is gradually turned over and exposed to the surface of the large intestine, where fluid is progressively absorbed. In this way, about 500 mL of chyme enters the large intestine each day but only approximately 150 mL are excreted as feces (Marieb & Hoehn, 2007). The propulsive movements of small and large intestines also differ. Instead of segmentation, primarily mass movements occur in the large intestine. The movements involve slow but powerful contractile waves initiated by a reflex in the colon. This reflex is stimulated by the presence of food in the stomach. The action forces the fecal material as a mass down the colon. These movements usually occur only a few times a day, most frequently for about 15 minutes during the first hour or so after eating. On the other hand, segmentation movements of the small intestine occur throughout the day, but are greatly increased after a meal, similar to the peristaltic waves of the stomach.

Defecation is the action whereby feces are emptied from the rectum. A weak sphincter approximately 20 cm from the anus, at the juncture between the sigmoid colon and the rectum, keeps the rectum empty of feces most of the time. Normally, when a mass movement forces feces into the rectum, the process of defecation is initiated. This process includes the defecation reflex mediated by the spinal cord and voluntary sphincter control. Control of fecal evacuation involves two sphincters working in tandem. The internal sphincter is a circular mass of smooth muscle that involuntarily constricts immediately inside the anus. The external anal sphincter is composed of striated voluntary skeletal muscle and surrounds the internal sphincter, slightly distal to it. Stretching of the rectal wall by feces initiates the defecation reflex, ordinarily resulting in defecation. Sensory nerve fibers in the rectum carry their signals to the spinal cord which then stimulates the parasympathetic system. These signals set up strong peristaltic waves that can effectively empty the entire large bowel. Other processes that are part of the reflex response involve increasing the intra-abdominal pressure by taking a deep breath, closing the glottis, and contracting the abdominal muscles and the pelvic floor muscles. In infants and people without conscious control, this process proceeds naturally to defecation. However, in toilet trained children and healthy adults, the time for defecation is determined voluntarily, despite the defecation reflex.

In addition to several other reflex systems, the gastrointestinal tract has an intrinsic nervous system of its own called the enteric nervous system. It begins at the esophagus and extends all the way to the anus. This system particularly controls gastrointestinal movements and secretions. However, the degree of activity of the enteric nervous system can be altered strongly by both parasympathetic and sympathetic nervous system signals from the brain (see Chapter 12). The neurons of the parasympathetic system generally enhance activity of most gastrointestinal functions. Sympathetic branch stimulation has the opposite effect of inhibiting activity of the tract. Strong stimulation of this branch can totally block the movement of food. Understanding the relationship of these processes within the individual as a thinking and feeling being is useful in assessing problems of elimination and in planning nursing care.

Process of Urinary Elimination

The structures of urinary elimination include the kidneys, ureters, bladder, and urethra. One function of this system, to balance body fluids and electrolytes, is discussed in Chapter 11. The second function of these structures is the excretion of most of the end products of body metabolism. The intact operation of both of these functions contributes to internal homeostasis and to the regulation of body processes. As Marieb and Hoehn (2007) pointed out, "Much like a water purification plant that keeps a city's water drinkable and disposes of its wastes, the kidneys are usually unappreciated until they malfunction and body fluids become contaminated" (p. 998). The nephron is the basis for understanding renal function. The two kidneys together contain more than two million nephrons, each of which is capable of forming urine by itself. The nephron cleans, or clears, the blood plasma of unwanted substances as it passes through the kidney. The nephron's filtering process prevents waste substances from being reabsorbed. These unwanted substances, such as urea, creatinine, uric acid, and urates, are end products of metabolism. The needed substances such as water and electrolytes are reabsorbed into the plasma. In addition, the nephron clears the plasma of excesses of substances that tend to accumulate in the body, such as ions of sodium, potassium, chloride, and hydrogen. The unwanted portions of the fluid from the nephron filtration process are passed into the urine. The principles of urine formation and the mechanisms of metabolism in the kidney are discussed further in basic physiology texts.

As urine collects in the kidneys, pressure increases and initiates a peristaltic contraction of the ureter to move the urine into the bladder. The ureters are small smooth-muscle tubes that pass downward from the kidneys to the bladder. The ureters have both sympathetic and parasympathetic nerves, as well as other nerve fibers, along their entire lengths. The urinary bladder is composed of smooth muscle and has two principal parts: the body, where the urine collects; and the neck, a funnel-shaped extension of the body. The muscle of the bladder neck is referred to as the internal sphincter. It is an involuntary sphincter and it acts to keep the urethra closed. Beyond the bladder neck, the urethra passes through a layer of muscle called the external sphincter of the bladder. This is a voluntary skeletal muscle. As with the gastrointestinal tract, this voluntary sphincter is under the control of the central nervous system and can be used consciously to prevent urination. Micturition, also called voiding or urination, is the process by which the urinary bladder is emptied. This process involves two sets of reflexes, the storage and micturition reflexes. The storage reflex initiates the voiding process as follows. Urine accumulation causes bladder distention. Receptors on the bladder wall are activated that stimulate spinal cord reflexes. These keep the internal sphincter closed and contract the external sphincter. The storage reflex controls continence and starts the micturition reflex. The action of this second reflex has the following pattern. As the bladder continues to distend, the spinal cord sends a message to the brain to initiate the opening of the internal sphincter and relaxation of the external sphincter. If the micturition reflex does not result in emptying the bladder, then the nervous system structures remain inhibited for at least a few minutes, to as long as an hour, before another micturition reflex occurs. With an increasingly distended bladder, the micturition reflexes occur more frequently and powerfully. Eventually, when urine volume is greater than 500 mL, the micturition reflexes will result in the elimination of urine.

COMPENSATORY ADAPTIVE RESPONSES

Viewed as an adaptive system, the individual has innate and acquired ways of responding to the changing environment. Further, Roy conceptualizes these complex adaptive dynamics for the individual as the coping processes of the regulator and cognator subsystems. The basic life processes described in this chapter are intestinal and urinary elimination. However, when the processes of elimination are not integrated, then the regulator and cognator control mechanisms activate processes of compensation. Here we return to Canon (1932), the physiologist who used the term "the wisdom of the body" to describe the automatic self-regulation of physiologic processes. This is a useful phrase when studying Roy's concept of the regulator subsystem. Further, the thinking and feeling individual, by way of cognator activity, can do much to affect any need of the physiologic mode, elimination included. Regulator and cognator abilities, then, are important internal stimuli for the individual. These subsystems initiate compensatory adaptive responses that extend the effectiveness of behavior in reaching the goals of adaptation, including higher adaptation levels.

Compensatory abilities that respond to elimination needs include both automatic homeostatic functions of the regulator and voluntary, or conscious, activities of the cognator. The nurse needs to understand as fully as possible the wisdom of the body to identify and interpret changes in the patient's condition. Study of physiology and pathophysiology are important to this understanding. One particular illustration of a regulator activity described by Marieb and Hoehn (2007) underscores the importance of a high-fiber diet for GI health. A high-fiber diet promotes the positive processes of GI elimination. It increases the stool mass, which increases churning and then water absorption. This decreases the amount of time for the stool to pass through the colon. The bulky stool mass enlarges the diameter of the colon and stimulates sensory nerve fibers that carry signals to the spinal cord which then stimulates the parasympathetic system. As noted, these signals set up strong peristaltic waves that can effectively empty the entire large bowel. The opposite is true for diets with low fiber intake.

An illustration of a compensatory response to the need for elimination by way of the cognator is the conscious cognitive process through which an individual voluntarily controls intestinal elimination. We are familiar with the processes undertaken to toilet train young children. Before bowel training can begin, the sphincters have to mature (von Gontard & Neveus, 2006). In a toddler, the nervous system develops to the point that the child learns to control both urinary and intestinal elimination. Given the physiologic development, during bowel training the child learns to inhibit contraction of the external anal sphincter and thereby allows defecation to occur. Conversely, the child can contract the sphincter if the time is not socially acceptable for defecation to occur. If the sphincter is kept contracted, the defecation reflex can die out after a few minutes. Usually it does not return until an additional amount of feces enters the rectum, possibly several hours later. In some situations where people have lost control over their elimination processes, through either disease or injury, it is possible to implement bowel training, often in combination with bladder training. Here, individuals learn to regulate their elimination by understanding their normal pattern of defecation, regulating the amount of fiber and fluid in their diet, and using perineal exercises (Ash, 2005). Many have been able to regulate their elimination patterns through cognitive mechanisms even though they have lost the ability to neurologically control these processes.

COMPROMISED PROCESSES OF ELIMINATION

Changes in adaptation levels and adaptation problems can be caused by difficulties in any or all of the processes of elimination. Intestinal and urinary elimination and other means of elimination of wastes from the body are all interdependent. Two specific examples of compromised processes of elimination, symptoms of Crohn's disease and urinary retention, will be discussed.

Symptoms of Crohn's Disease

Crohn's disease is one of the inflammatory bowel diseases (IBD). The prevalence of Crohn's disease in the United States is approximately 162 cases per 100,000 as of 2001, according to the National Institute of Diabetes and Digestive and Kidney Diseases (NIDDK) statistics. It develops around the age of 15 to 30 years, equally affects both genders, and can result in many complications. Although it mostly affects the terminal ileum and proximal colon, Crohn's can involve any part of the GI tract. In some people, the disease can even manifest itself in other parts of the body, including the kidneys, skin, and joints (Smith & Watson, 2005). Crohn's disease is characterized by inflammation to the GI tract lining, distinct small ulcerations, and fistula formation. It most commonly presents as diarrhea and bloody or mucousy stools. The inflammation can potentially affect all layers of the intestinal lining with healthy bowel layers among the diseased layers. Although the cause of Crohn's disease is not proven, Marks et al. (2006) believe that the disease is caused by the immune system attacking itself, as well as a genetic component. This inflammatory process leads to white blood cell accumulation resulting in chronic inflammation, ulcerations, and ultimately bowel injury. Those suffering from the disease have many life-altering symptoms, including abdominal pain, diarrhea, rectal bleeding, poor nutritional absorption, and many others. Crohn's disease patients often have periods of remission followed by exacerbations; discouragingly, the changes in the disease pattern are unpredictable. As a result, a diagnosis of Crohn's disease lends itself to many psychosocial problems. Since Crohn's disease is an inflammatory process, the pharmaceutical agents used to treat the disease involve anti-inflammatory drugs and suppressing the immune system, as well as symptom management (NIDDK, 2006). Often a goal of therapy is to allow the bowel to rest during an exacerbation of the disease. However, maintaining proper nutrition is vital for the healing process. Patients will often require nutritional needs to be met via enteral or parenteral routes. Unfortunately most Crohn's disease patients require some type of surgical intervention. It is important for nurses to understand this compromised state of the body and the symptoms involved, in order to best care for the individual with Crohn's disease.

Urinary Retention

The inability to void, with accumulation of urine within the bladder, is known as urinary retention. Urinary retention is normally a result of the bladder muscles not contracting properly or the sphincter muscles not relaxing (National Institute of Diabetes and Digestive and Kidney Diseases, 2005); in the pediatric population it can also occur because of nerve damage or a congenital anomaly. The absence of voided urine related to retention is to be distinguished from anuria, complete suppression of urine formation by the kidneys, or oliguria, diminished urine secretion in relation to fluid intake. Possible causes of urinary retention include obstruction at or below the bladder outlet, spinal or general anesthesia, muscular tension, emotional anxiety, and medications such as sedatives, opiates, psychotropic drugs, and antispasmodics, which interfere with the normal neurologic function of the voiding reflex. Besides the absence of voided urine, the nurse may assess a distended bladder in an individual with urinary retention. As the bladder fills with urine, it rises above the level of the symphysis pubis and can be displaced to either side of the midline. The individual may report increasing discomfort and pain, which can be accompanied by increased blood pressure. The life-threatening condition of autonomic dysreflexia (or hyperreflexia) can occur in people with a spinal cord injury above T6 when the body cannot properly respond to stimuli (often a distended bladder or rectum) and leads to severe hypertension. Patients who are unable to communicate or are confused may become restless. When the cause is neurologic dysfunction, the individual may not sense the fullness of the bladder. Nursing activities related to urinary retention are focused on prevention and reduction of risk, particularly as related to postoperative patients. Measures including encouraging postoperative physical activity, positioning, allowing adequate time, relaxation exercises, running water, positive reassurance, or warm water poured over the perineum may promote urination and prevent retention. When preventive nursing measures are unsuccessful, one-time catheterization may be required to prevent subsequent complications. If urinary retention is a chronic problem, it is important to determine the cause and treat accordingly.

NURSING PROCESS RELATED TO ELIMINATION

Intestinal and urinary elimination are priority needs for the individual's physiologic adaptation. In applying the nursing process, the nurse makes a careful assessment of behaviors and stimuli related to these basic processes. In assessing factors influencing intestinal and urinary elimination, regulator and cognator effectiveness in initiating compensatory processes is considered. Based on thorough first- and second-level assessment, the nurse makes a nursing diagnosis, sets goals, selects nursing intervention, and evaluates care.

Assessment of Intestinal Behavior

The formation of a positive nurse–patient relationship is essential to collect data about an individual's elimination patterns. Since the topic of bodily secretions is considered personal by many, the nurse is aware of the privacy needs of the individual and one's own reaction when inquiring about another's elimination pattern. In addressing elimination, the nurse establishes privacy and an intrusion-free environment. The nurse's interaction with the patient considers the individual's language level and communication skills, as influenced by cultural and educational background. Main aspects of assessment include characteristics of stool, bowel sounds, presence of pain, and laboratory findings.

CHARACTERISTICS OF STOOL   When assessing intestinal elimination, the nurse observes the following behaviors. Stool is described by stating the amount, color, consistency, frequency, odor, and effort. Normally, the stool that is evacuated is soft, formed, and brown in color for adults. The frequency of a bowel movement varies with each individual, although one bowel movement a day is average. In healthy people, variations can range from stool evacuated twice a day to stool evacuated every 2 to 3 days. When making a judgment as to whether the frequency is adaptive or ineffective, the nurse assesses if the observed behavior represents a change from the individual's normal pattern. One author noted that "Contrary to popular belief, not everyone needs to have a bowel movement once a day" (Bisanz, 2007, p. 72D). Stool is to be passed with ease without straining or discomfort when the defecation reflex is first felt. Stool containing any unusual matter such as blood, mucus, pus, or intestinal worms is also noted. A careful, exact description of the stool is essential when blood is present. Observe whether the blood appears on the surface of the stool or if it is mixed throughout. If the female is menstruating, this may be the source of bright red blood on the surface of stool. Normal stool has a characteristic odor caused by bacterial action on the foods that are eaten. Any unusual odor should be noted, for it can have clinical significance.

BOWEL SOUNDS   Bowel sounds indicate the movements within the small and large bowel. In assessing these, the nurse notes the presence, frequency, or absence of bowel sounds. The abdomen is auscultated in all four quadrants proceeding in a clockwise fashion. The right lower quadrant is often the most prominent because the ileocecal valve, where the small intestine meets the large intestine, is located in this area. Using the diaphragm part of the stethoscope, the nurse listens in each quadrant, changing the auscultatory site 2 or 3 inches with each move. It is important to remove the stethoscope completely from the abdomen when changing locations, for pulling the stethoscope across the abdomen will produce interfering sound, can cause involuntary muscle spasms, and can be uncomfortable for the individual. Normal bowel sounds will be high-pitched, gurgling noises usually occurring five or more times a minute. Ineffective bowel sounds include extremely weak or infrequent sounds, or a complete absence of sounds. This can indicate bowel hypomobility or immobility. Before a determination of bowel sounds can be made, the abdomen is auscultated for at least 5 minutes. Bowel sounds indicating possible hypermotility of the bowel will be heard as frequent rushes of loud, high-pitched sounds. Passage of gas is a good indication that peristaltic movement is occurring.

PAIN   Pain related to bowel elimination is included as assessment of behavior by listening to what the individual says regarding discomfort and pain on evacuation of the bowel or the excessive accumulation of flatus or gas in the intestines. All verbal and nonverbal behaviors and the location, severity, duration, and onset of the pain are noted. Pain with intestinal elimination can be indicative of many things from hemorrhoids to malignancies.

LABORATORY FINDINGS   In completing the behavioral assessment of the bowel elimination component of the physiologic adaptive mode, laboratory results related to stool are checked when available. Specimens of the feces may be tested for occult blood when intestinal bleeding is suspected, but gross blood is not visible on inspection. Stool can also be assessed for many different pathogens such as bacteria, viruses, and parasites. *Clostridium difficile* colitis (a complication of a toxic strain of the bacteria) has become more common with the increased use of antibiotics. It is difficult to treat and easily spread in the health care setting (Sunenshine & McDonald, 2006). In the United States, the public media has covered the rise of colorectal cancers and with that has come a great increase in the number of colonoscopies done each year. At this time, the American College of Gastroenterology recommends everyone over the age of 50 have a routine colonoscopy. Laboratory values and procedures for assisting with these tests are available from reliable texts.

Assessment of Urinary Behavior

Similar to assessing intestinal elimination, the nurse must be cognizant of the personal nature of urinating and provide privacy for the individual's comfort. First-level assessment of behaviors of urinary elimination includes the nurse's observations of amount and characteristics of urine, frequency, urgency, pain, and laboratory findings.

AMOUNT AND CHARACTERISTICS OF URINE   The amount of urine per voiding and the total urinary output for 24 hours is recorded. The color and transparency, odor, frequency, urgency felt, and effort are noted as well. Normally, the amount of urine voided by the average adult will vary from 1,000 to 2,000 mL in a 24-hour period. Urine is normally pale yellow or amber in color because of the presence of the yellow pigment urochrome. In healthy individuals, urine that is pale and almost colorless is probably very dilute with a low specific gravity, while urine that is darker in color may have a higher specific gravity. Freshly voided urine has a clear transparency; cloudy urine or urine containing sediment can represent a disease state. This change in transparency could be caused by a reactional change of the urine if left standing for a period of time, as the pH changes from acidic to alkaline. The odor of fresh-voided urine is aromatic. When left standing, urine may develop an ammonia smell caused by the decomposition of urea by bacteria.

PRESENCE OF FREQUENCY OR URGENCY   The frequency of urination, urgency felt, and effort in starting and stopping the flow of urine can depend on many factors. For behaviors indicating retention, incontinence, difficulty starting or stopping the stream of urine, or dribbling, the effect of these alterations on the individual's activities of daily living and social relations is assessed. In general, the musculature of the bladder is capable of distending to the approximate capacity of 200 mL before the urge to void is felt. This begins the process of the micturition reflex described earlier. The stretch receptors in the bladder being stimulated, together with involuntary and voluntary control of the sphincters located at the opening of the bladder into the urethra, permit the flow of urine.

PAIN   The nurse assesses any pain related to urinary elimination. This includes pain or burning sensations prior to, during, or after urination. Normally, the individual will void with ease, without pain or discomfort. As an example, renal calculi (or kidney stones) can cause severe pain during normal activity and/or during urination.

LABORATORY FINDINGS   Laboratory data are useful, especially in comparing the findings in a routine urinalysis and findings of specific blood tests with normal values. The general characteristics and measurements of urine have been noted above. Chemical and microscopic examinations of routine urinalysis include findings related to glucose, ketones, blood, protein, bilirubin, red blood cells, crystals, white blood cells, and epithelial cells. In addition, valuable information about the kidney's ability to remove metabolic wastes is provided by blood tests. Substances examined in blood tests include blood urea nitrogen, creatinine, sodium, chloride, potassium, carbon dioxide, calcium, phosphate, uric acid, and pH. Further discussion is included in Chapter 11, Fluid, Electrolyte, and Acid–Base Balance, and in laboratory manuals.

Assessment of Stimuli for Intestinal and Urinary Behavior

With the assessment of stimuli, the nurse gathers data about factors influencing the behaviors identified in the first level of assessment of the adaptation nursing process. This includes the important factor of the body's adaptive ability to maintain integrated processes of elimination, as well as the coping strategies the individual uses to maintain or change behaviors. As the basic processes operate, both forms of elimination are influenced by the same categories of stimuli. Specifically, the following are factors to be considered in the assessment of stimuli for bowel and urinary elimination.

INTACT HOMEOSTATIC PROCESSES Homeostasis comprises the steady physiologic states that enable people to counteract changes both in external conditions and in internal bodily functions. The intact homeostatic process is particularly relevant for bowel elimination and is primarily responsible for adaptive intestinal elimination behaviors. As noted earlier, the digestion of food is completed in the small intestine as it absorbs nutrients from the ingested substances. Segmentation pushes the substance through the ileocecal valve into the large intestine, which absorbs a high percentage of the liquid as well as salts from the wastes. Intestinal contents are then propelled toward the rectum for evacuation. For urinary elimination the homeostatic processes of the filtration by the kidneys to eliminate wastes from the blood have been described.

DIET The type and amount of diet are important influences in bowel elimination, and to some extent urination. The nurse notes the individual's present daily nutritional intake and evaluates whether or not these foods provide roughage and bulk, such as high-fiber foods or fresh fruits and vegetables; contain natural laxative effects that promote normal stool consistency, such as prunes and brans; influence the production of excessive intestinal gas, such as cabbage and beans; and influence the color or consistency of stool. For example, the high milk intake of an infant can cause light-colored stool, and intolerance to certain foods can promote diarrhea. Many fruit and vegetables, such as watermelon and lettuce, have high water content, and therefore will increase the amount of urine. Conversely, foods with high sodium content could decrease the amount of urine secondary to the sodium–water balance. The ingestion of some foods, such as asparagus, will create a change in odor to urine. The nurse also notes the individual's diet to understand the associated cancer risks. Researchers found a significant increase of colon cancer in individuals consuming large amounts of alcohol (Su & Arab, 2004). Diets with a large amount of red meat, animal fats, and dairy products have been shown to increase a man's risk of prostate cancer (Key, Schatzkin, Willet, Allen, Spencer, & Travis, 2004). Conversely, a large consumption of fruits and vegetables is believed to protect against many cancers.

FLUID INTAKE Assessment of stimuli influencing elimination includes fluid intake. The nurse notes the amount of fluid the individual is taking, both orally and intravenously. Intake naturally influences the amount of urine excreted. Insensible loss of water through the skin and lungs are considered in relation to urinary output. Basically, when evaluating intake and output for 24 hours, these values will be approximately equal, allowing for some margin of difference. In some instances such as heart or renal failure that are critical to the maintenance of health, a basic measurement of fluid loss or gain is taken by weighing the individual at the same time each day. Related to fluid balance, the individual is assessed for conditions that can affect the fluid and electrolyte balance of the body. Examples are losses of fluids via other routes such as liquid stools, nasogastric tube drainage, emesis, or insensible loss occurring with high body temperature. Decreased fluid intake can promote stool that is dry and hard, and increase the risk for constipation. Fluid, electrolytes, and acid–base balance are discussed in Chapter 11.

IMMEDIATE ENVIRONMENT The immediate environment contributes to adaptation in this mode component as it does in others. This would include whether or not the individual can maintain or lacks privacy for his or her toileting needs. Many individuals report being too embarrassed to defecate in public bathrooms. They "hold it" until they are in more private settings. This pattern over time can put an individual at risk for many complications including constipation (Akpan, Gosney, & Barrett, 2006; Bisanz, 2007; Streeter, 2002). In assessing the immediate environmental stimuli, the nurse observes for factors that can influence the temperature and comfort of the room; convenience of the toilet, bedpan, or urinal; and the position the individual needs to eliminate either feces or urine. For example, the male who is unable to stand to void may have difficulty adapting his usual pattern within this environmental change. The individual immobilized in traction who uses a bedpan while in the reclining position may have difficulty expelling stool.

PAINFUL CONDITIONS When the individual has pain or discomfort with moving the bowels or urinating, the nurse assesses both the factors influencing the pain and the coping strategies the individual uses to deal with the pain. The nurse validates with the individual the cause of any pain influencing elimination. Possible causes that could cause bowel pain include the presence of conditions such as hemorrhoids, anal fissure, or abdominal cramping caused by excessive intestinal gas. The presence of a urinary tract infection can also be a source of pain with urination and interfere with initiating micturition. The coping strategies the individual uses for the pain are also assessed. For example, with hemorrhoids, the individual may use sitz baths, ointments, or special skin care for the irritated skin around the anus. Sitz baths may also be used to assist in resolving urinary retention. The nurse assesses how behaviors such as urinary retention or frequency have affected the voiding pattern and how the individual is coping with the problem. Predisposing factors that make behaviors better or worse are noted. For example, urinary incontinence may be precipitated by laughing, coughing, stress, activity, and so forth. The nurse assesses what coping strategies are being used presently and if the individual feels that they are effective or ineffective.

ELIMINATION HABITS A key assessment factor is the individual's usual bowel and urinary elimination pattern. The usual pattern is noted and its effect on and comparison with the behaviors observed are assessed. The nurse assesses if the individual has a routine schedule or time set aside each day for a bowel movement. A change in the present pattern from the individual's normal patterns is particularly important. The nurse notes factors that maintain or increase peristalsis, such as the individual's daily activity level or pattern of exercise, and factors that may increase urinary frequency or urgency. Determinants that decrease peristalsis include bed rest, immobility, or recent anesthesia, which can also induce urinary retention. The coping strategies that the individual uses to maintain elimination are identified. These could include drinking a hot liquid or the use of laxatives, enemas, or suppositories; or the use of diuretics. The frequency that they are utilized is also investigated, in particular for those at risk for bulimia nervosa or others on crash diets. Whether the individual thinks the strategies used are effective or ineffective is important to note.

STRESS Stress may be present as a focal or contextual stimulus in the daily pattern or for a currently observed behavior. The nurse thus assesses for physical or psychological states that can stimulate or hinder urination or defecation. Awareness of signs of physical and psychological stress, such as anxiety or illness, is part of the nursing assessment as these factors influence elimination behaviors. For example, under anxious or stressful situations, an individual may notice a feeling of urgency to void, although the bladder has just been emptied. Another example is fear of a recurring painful experience from urinating. In this case, the individual develops muscular tension, which inhibits relaxation of the perineal muscles that promote urination. Smith and Watson (2005) observed that, "Patients with irritable bowel syndrome commonly report exacerbation of symptoms at times of emotional stress" (p. 80).

FAMILY OR CULTURAL BELIEFS   Family or cultural beliefs concerning elimination begin early in childhood and can involve specific views about the need and schedule to eliminate wastes. The expected schedule of elimination may be related to beliefs about health. These background factors are relevant information, and the nurse identifies these beliefs as contextual stimuli.

DEVELOPMENTAL STAGE   Age is another contextual stimulus that the individual brings to the situation. The age of the individual is noted, since this will influence both types of elimination. For example, the young child may lack sphincter control and may have difficulties with toilet training. When assessing children it is particularly important to use language that they are familiar with to obtain a proper assessment (von Gontard & Neveus, 2006). During pregnancy, the enlarged uterus stretches the pelvic floor muscles and weakens the external sphincter, resulting in temporary urinary incontinence. With the normal aging process, the GI tract activity slows down and blood flow to the kidneys can be diminished related to a decrease in cardiac output; therefore, renal function may decrease. There is a decreased amount of pancreatic and stomach secretions, decrease in small intestine mucosal surface area, and colonic mucosal atrophy. These changes result in many pathological changes in the elderly. Increased risk of developing gastrointestinal problems such as malignancies, ulcerations, and diverticular disease occurs with older adults (Meiner, 2004). With aging, the pelvic floor muscles become weakened and the supporting connective tissue alters, causing the bladder to become funnel shaped. This change can result in bladder wall irritability. There can also be decreased bladder capacity related to its inability to elongate, but with increased residual urine after voiding. Therefore, the aging individual may be more likely to present with behaviors of frequency, incontinence, retention, and dysuria. None of these conditions are normal and should be further assessed. Another example would be an elderly male who has frequency of voiding accompanied by problems in initiating and ending the stream of urine. This can be related to prostatic enlargement with resultant urinary retention. Also, the elderly female with relaxation of the perineal muscles may present behaviors of stress incontinence or rectal prolapse.

PRESENCE OF DISEASE   The nurse identifies whether behaviors observed are related to a disease process, a surgical procedure, or trauma, which affects the normal structure, function, or regulation of the urinary or GI system. Examples for the urinary system include infections; disturbances of the central nervous system pathways, causing loss of voluntary control; tissue damage to the sphincters; and relaxation of the perineal structures from childbirth. Other factors that will be examined include the presence of an enlarged prostate gland or sexually transmitted diseases. Examples of diseases that affect bowel elimination include such conditions as ulcerative colitis, intestinal obstructions, and fistulas. Both the GI tract and the urinary system are very susceptible to many types of malignancies. More diseases are explained in general textbooks on pathophysiology.

MEDICATIONS AND TREATMENTS   Other factors in the immediate situation that influence elimination are medications, treatments, or tests. The nurse notes specific medications that the individual may be taking that influence stools or the color or amount of urine. For example, iron can cause dark, hard stools; certain vitamins and Pyridium can cause dark orange urine; narcotics can cause constipation; and diuretics increase the amount of urine excreted and often lighten the color. Sensitivities to certain other drugs, particularly antibiotics, can cause diarrhea and antibiotics will often change the odor of the urine as well. Any treatments or tests influencing elimination behaviors, such as a barium enema, cystoscope, or radiation therapy, are identified as well. Of particular significance is any altered means of elimination, such as a urinary catheter or a colostomy.

Nursing Diagnosis

Assessment data of behaviors and related stimuli are interpreted and used in establishing a nursing diagnosis. The nurse prepared to use the Roy Adaptation Model of nursing can state diagnoses as specific behaviors with the stimuli that are most relevant. Some examples have already been given, such as the example of involuntary release of urine related to relaxed muscles in an elderly person. Roy has developed a typology of indicators of positive adaptation related to intestinal and urinary elimination (see Table 3–1). Included in the typology are effective homeostatic bowel processes, stable pattern of bowel elimination, effective processes of urine formation, stable pattern of urine elimination, and effective coping strategies for altered elimination. Chapter 3 demonstrated the importance of recognizing situations of effective adaptation so that these can be maintained or enhanced. A nursing diagnosis addressing an indicator of positive adaptation could be, "stable pattern of urine elimination following surgery related to early ambulation and relaxed surroundings."

Commonly recurring adaptation problems as defined within the Roy Adaptation Model include diarrhea, bowel or urinary incontinence, constipation, urinary retention, flatulence, and ineffective coping strategies for altered elimination. Diarrhea is defined as a state in which the individual experiences a change in normal bowel habits characterized by the frequent passage of loose, fluid, unformed stools. When the individual presents with behaviors of diarrhea, abdominal cramping and rectal bleeding may also occur. Frequently, diagnostic procedures or laboratory tests may be necessary to determine the exact cause, such as Crohn's disease, and other related influencing factors. Bowel and bladder incontinence refers to the involuntary passage of stool or urine. Excessive gas in the stomach and intestines is termed flatulence and may be accompanied by abdominal distention. Certain foods contribute to the formation of excessive gas and should be reduced or eliminated from the diet.

The use of a summary label to develop a nursing diagnosis when more than one mode is being affected by the same stimulus is often an effective way of communicating a cluster of behaviors to experienced nurses. For example, "urinary incontinence related to spinal cord damage" might be such a diagnosis. The nurse would be immediately aware that the individual's physical self-concept, role function, and interdependence modes also would be involved. After extensive, successful rehabilitation, an individual with such injuries might have the diagnosis of, "effective coping strategies for altered elimination related to successful bladder and bowel training." In Table 7–1, the Roy model nursing diagnostic categories for the physiologic need of elimination are shown in relation to nursing diagnosis labels approved by the North American Nursing Diagnosis Association (NANDA International, 2007). Consider the following example. Mr. Beard is a 72-year-old man with a medical diagnosis of benign prostatic hypertrophy. This is a noncancerous enlargement of the prostate gland that has necessitated surgical intervention of a transurethral prostatectomy. Following the surgical procedure, he had an indwelling Foley catheter that

TABLE 7–1 Nursing Diagnostic Categories for Elimination

Positive Indicators of Adaptation	Common Adaptation Problems	NANDA Diagnostic Labels
• Effective homeostatic bowel processes • Stable pattern of bowel elimination • Effective processes of urine formation • Stable pattern of urine elimination • Effective coping strategies for altered elimination	• Diarrhea • Flatulence • Bowel incontinence • Constipation • Urinary incontinence • Urinary retention • Ineffective coping strategies for altered elimination	• Bowel incontinence • Diarrhea • Constipation • Risk for constipation • Perceived constipation • Impaired urinary elimination • Urinary retention • Total urinary incontinence • Functional urinary incontinence • Stress urinary incontinence • Reflex urinary incontinence • Risk for urge urinary incontinence • Readiness for enhanced urinary elimination • Overflow urinary incontinence

was in place for 48 hours and has been removed in preparation for discharge. It has been 6 hours since the catheter removal and he has not yet voided. He is expressing anxiety about the situation, is experiencing some pain, and his bladder is now palpable above the symphysis pubis. A nursing diagnosis could be, "urinary retention following catheter removal possibly related to urethral edema."

Goal Setting

Based on thorough assessment and understanding of adaptation problems related to elimination, the nurse sets goals in terms of outcomes in collaboration with the individual. A complete goal statement includes the behavior of focus, the change expected, and the time frame in which the goal is to be achieved. For example, for the individual experiencing the adaptation problem of constipation related to poor fiber intake, the long-term goal may be, "within 2 weeks, the individual will establish a regular pattern of bowel movements." An initial short-term goal could be that during the next week, the individual would identify foods high in fiber. To assist this individual in reaching this goal effectively, the nurse may need to include nutritional teaching as part of the plan of care. This will hopefully facilitate normal bowel elimination on 3 days of the week for the individual. In the previous example of Mr. Beard, the goal would focus on the behavior of urinary retention. A short-term goal may be, "in the next 30 minutes, Mr. Beard will have passed at least 30 mL of urine." The behavior in this goal is passing urine, the change relates to the amount of 30 mL as opposed to none, and the time frame is within 30 minutes.

Nursing Intervention

The nursing intervention step of the nursing process according to the Roy Adaptation Model depends on the identified stimuli as the nurse either promotes or reinforces the stimuli or takes action to change or delete them. In some instances, direct nursing intervention by way of the regulator and cognator processes is possible. Nursing interventions for the common adaptation problems related to elimination will be discussed in this section.

For the problem of symptoms of Crohn's disease, general nursing interventions include increasing psychosocial support, medical management, nutritional therapy, and potentially surgical management (Hall, 2007). These nursing interventions will require a multidisciplinary team approach with the nurse working closely with the patient. The goal of treatment for an individual with Crohn's disease is to induce and maintain remission (Hall, 2007). Drug therapy is often indicated and for long term. Thus, minimizing adverse side effects and increasing knowledge of the medications is paramount to successful treatment. Nutritional teaching is critical for an individual with Crohn's. As Hall (2007) stated, "Patients with Crohn's disease should be advised about diet, especially during a relapse where it is important to ensure adequate calorie and protein intake" (p. 18). Psychosocial support should also be a significant part of the nursing care given, especially at the time of diagnosis but also throughout the plan of care.

Crohn's disease is a specific disease process that causes diarrhea; however, many individuals experience diarrhea and can benefit from nursing care. Nursing interventions should be directed toward those identified causes when intervening for the problem of diarrhea. Other nursing interventions include avoidance or elimination of allergic dietary substances or drugs that promote loose, watery stools. Many people are aware of the foods that cause diarrhea, for example, alcoholic beverages, highly caffeinated liquids such as coffee, or rich pastries high in sugar content. With mild cases of diarrhea, nothing but clear liquids, such as water, tea, carbonated beverages, bouillon broth, and electrolyte-replacing drinks, is taken during the first 12 hours. Citrus juices are avoided, as well as cold liquids and concentrated sweets, which are poorly tolerated. During the next 12 hours, more foods, such as toast, soda crackers, and uncreamed soups, may be added. After the stool begins to firm, other bland foods can be added, with gradual advancement to the individual's regular diet.

With more severe cases of diarrhea, fluid and electrolyte replacement may be necessary, or the individual may need administration of medication to decrease peristalsis and relieve abdominal cramping. The individual with diarrhea is provided with an atmosphere conducive to relaxation and rest. The anal region is cleansed with mild soap and water after each movement to reduce local irritation and discomfort. When bowel incontinence (the inability of the rectal sphincter to control the passage of stool) is present, a bowel training program may be initiated. It is important to set aside a consistent time for evacuation. Ash (2005) discussed some different elements of bowel management for spinal cord injury patients, including abdominal massage, followed by a glycerine suppository, or for some, the insertion of a gloved finger into the rectum for stimulation. The individual should then attempt evacuation and allow adequate time.

Incontinent people may be embarrassed and have emotional distress. Special nursing care includes support and understanding, as well as measures to reduce possible skin irritation, odor, and the soiling of clothing and linen.

For urinary retention, as in Mr. Beard's situation, nursing interventions include early ambulation following surgery, putting in a sitting position or a standing posture for the male, providing the individual with privacy, listening to the sound of running water, dangling the hands in warm water, pouring warm water over the perineum or sitting in a warm bath to promote perineal muscle relaxation, or any other measure that might promote relaxation. If these measures fail, medications can be employed to promote the ease of voiding. Ultimately, bladder catheterization may be required. A complete diagnostic workup is done to identify the causative and contributing stimuli for the adaptation problem of incontinence. If stress incontinence is present, the individual tries to avoid excessive straining or conditions such as chronic coughing. Weight reduction and pelvic exercises are helpful in regaining bladder control. Kegel exercises increase the tone of the perineal muscles. Instruct the individual to contract the perineal muscles as though trying to stop the flow of urine. This should be done 10 times per session 3 times a day (NIDDK, 2005). Also, the individual should try to start and stop the stream of urine when voiding. A bladder training program may be required, which includes an adequate intake of fluids, strengthening exercises for the perineal muscles, and a definite schedule set aside for voiding. The intake of fluids should be carefully spaced throughout the day and limited before sleep to promote adequate rest. The individual is encouraged to void every 30 minutes to 2 hours, and as the program progresses, the urine is held for longer periods of time. As with anal incontinence, nursing care should include supportive measures to decrease emotional stress and possible skin irritation. Additional information on nursing management of incontinence is found in basic nursing texts and in textbooks on neuroscience nursing and care of the elderly.

Evaluation

Evaluation involves judging the effectiveness of the nursing interventions in relation to the individual's adaptive behavior. Whether or not the patient has attained the behavior stated in the goal is identified. The nursing interventions would be identified as effective if the individual's behavior is in accordance with the stated goal. If the goal has not been achieved, the nurse identifies alternative interventions or approaches by reassessing the behavior and stimuli and continuing with the other steps of the nursing process. Consider the example given earlier of a short-term goal set for the individual with constipation. In 1 week, the individual has identified foods high in fiber that are desirable, such as whole wheat toast with breakfast and lunch, an apple with lunch, and legumes with dinner. During the week, he had four bowel movements in the morning that were hard but eliminated without undue difficulty. At this point, another short-term goal would be set. This would be to add other contextual factors to create good bowel habits, such as drinking more fluids and increasing exercise. In Mr. Beard's situation, evaluation of the success of nursing interventions would be focused on his ability to void within the 30-minute time period. If he has been able to produce at least 30 mL of urine, the goal would have been achieved and a new goal established to continue to monitor the situation. If he was not able to void, another nursing intervention may be initiated such as a one-time catheterization.

Summary

This chapter focused on the application of the Roy Adaptation Model to the physiologic need of elimination with particular attention to intestinal and urinary elimination. An overview of these basic life processes was provided. Illustrations of adaptive compensatory processes related to elimination were described. Examples of two compromised processes, symptoms of Crohn's disease and urinary retention, were provided. Finally, guidelines for planning nursing care were described through identification of behaviors and stimuli for assessment along with formulation of nursing diagnoses and goals, and exploration of nursing interventions and evaluation.

Exercises for Application

1. Assess the bowel elimination behaviors of a child, adolescent, adult, and elderly person. Relate the stimuli of age for each individual to the assessed behaviors.

2. Develop a teaching plan to help an individual utilize strategies to cope with the adaptation problem of urinary retention.

Assessment of Understanding

QUESTIONS

1. Designate each of the following statements as related to either intestinal elimination (I) or urinary elimination (U).
   (a) _____ elimination of fluid wastes and excess ions
   (b) _____ defecation reflex and conscious sphincter control
   (c) _____ works to balance body fluids and electrolytes
   (d) _____ expulsion of undigestible substances
   (e) _____ excretion of the end products of body metabolism

2. Label the following compensatory processes as indicative of regulator (R) or cognator (C) activity.
   (a) _____ narrowing of colon in response to diet lacking in bulk
   (b) _____ voluntary control of micturition
   (c) _____ powerful contraction of circular muscles of the colon
   (d) _____ bowel training after spinal cord injury
   (e) _____ regulation of elimination patterns through diet and exercise

3. Name and describe one situation of compromised elimination.

4. List third first-level assessment behaviors that are related to intestinal elimination and three related to urinary elimination.
   (a) _____
   (b) _____
   (c) _____
   (d) _____
   (e) _____
   (f) _____

5. Discuss stimuli that can influence peristalsis and relate these to your understanding of the processes involved in movements of the intestines.

6. State a potential nursing diagnosis related to urinary elimination for a patient after surgery.

7. Identify two nursing interventions that help an individual cope with increased flatulence.
   (a) _____
   (b) _____

8. If a suggested nursing intervention has not been effective in meeting the goal established with the patient to meet elimination needs, discuss how the nurse will proceed based on the Adaptation Model nursing process.

FEEDBACK

1. (a) U, (b) I, (c) U, (d) I, (e) U
2. (a) R, (b) C, (c) R, (d) C, (e) C
3. One example of compromised elimination is urinary retention. This means that the individual is unable to void urine that has been collected in the bladder. Possible causes include obstruction at or below the bladder outlet, spinal or general anesthesia, muscular tension, emotional anxiety, and medications.
4. Intestinal elimination behaviors: (a) amount and characteristics of stool, (b) bowel sounds, (c) pain. Urinary elimination behaviors: (d) amount and characteristics of urine, (e) frequency and urgency, (f) pain.
5. Factors that maintain or increase peristalsis include the individual's daily activity level or pattern of exercise. Factors that decrease peristalsis include bed rest, immobility, or recent anesthesia. Movements of the intestines are both mixing and propulsive types. Mixing movements aid in absorption functions and propulsive movements move waste products toward elimination. General increase of muscle activity and related neurologic activity promotes such movement, thus facilitating bowel elimination.
6. Example of a nursing diagnosis: Urinary retention related to recent anesthesia.
7. Any of the following: reduce or eliminate foods that contribute to flatus formation such as beans, cabbage, onions, cauliflower, and milk products; avoid carbonated beverages; avoid swallowing excessive air; and increase activity level.
8. The nurse will return to the earlier steps of the process to see if the assessment is accurate and complete, the diagnosis is appropriate, the goal is realistic, and the nursing interventions are adequate.

References

Akpan, A., Gosney, M. A., & Barrett, J. (2006). Privacy for defecation and fecal incontinence in older adults. *Journal of Wound, Ostomy, and Continence Nursing, 33*(5), 536–540.

Ash, D. (2005). Sustaining safe and acceptable bowel care in spinal cord injured patients. *Nursing Standard, 20*(8), 55–64.

Bisanz, A. (2007). Chronic constipation. *American Journal of Nursing, 107*(4), 72B–72H.

Canon, W. (1932). *The wisdom of the body.* New York: Norton.

Hall, A. (2007). Diagnosis and current management of Crohn's disease. *Gastrointestinal Nursing, 5*(2), 11–20.

Key, T. J., Schatzkin, A., Willet, W. C., Allen, N. E., Spencer, E. A., & Travis, R. C. (2004). Diet, nutrition and the prevention of cancer. *Public Health Nutrition, 7*(1A), 187–200.

Marieb, E. N., & Hoehn, K. (2007). *Human anatomy and physiology* (7th ed.). San Francisco: Pearson Benjamin Cummings.

Marks, D. J. B., Harbord, M. W. N., MacAllister, R., Rahman, F. Z., Young, J., Al-Lazikani, B., et al. (2006). Defective acute inflammation in Crohn's disease: A clinical investigation. *Lancet, 367*, 668–678.

Meiner, S. E. (Ed). (2004). *Care of gastrointestinal problems in the older adult.* New York: Springer Publishing Company, Inc.

NANDA-International. (2007). *Nursing diagnoses: Definitions and classifications, 2007–2008.* Philadelphia: NANDA-I.

National Institute of Diabetes and Digestive and Kidney Diseases. (2005). *Nerve disease and bladder control* (NIH Publication No. 05–4560). Bethesda, MD: The National Digestive Diseases Information Clearinghouse.

National Institute of Diabetes and Digestive and Kidney Diseases. (2006). *Crohn's disease* (NIH Publication No. 06–3410). Bethesda, MD: The National Digestive Diseases Information Clearinghouse.

Smith, G., & Watson, R. (2005). *Gastrointestinal nursing.* Oxford: Blackwell Publishing.

Streeter, B. L. (2002). Teenage constipation: A case study. *Gastroenterology Nursing, 25*(6), 253–256.

Su, L. J., & Arab, L. (2004). Alcohol consumption and risk of colon cancer: Evidence from the national health and nutrition examination survey 1 epidemiologic follow-up study. *Nutrition and Cancer, 50*(2), 111–119.

Sunenshine, R. H., & McDonald, L. C. (2006). *Clostridium difficile*-associated disease: New challenges from an established pathogen. *Cleveland Clinic Journal of Medicine, 73*(2), 187–197.

Von Gontard, A., & Neveus, T. (2006). *The management of disorders of bladder and bowel control in childhood*. London: Mac Keith Press.

Additional References

American College of Gastroenterology- www.acg.gi.org

Colwell, J. C., Goldberg, M. T., & Carmel, J. E. (2004). *Fecal & urinary diversions: Management principles*. St. Louis, MO: Mosby.

Cotter, V. T., & Strumpf, N. E. (2002). *Advanced practice nursing with older adults: Clinical guidelines*. New York: McGraw-Hill.

Ignatavicius, D. D., & Workman, M. L. (2006). *Medical-surgical nursing: Critical thinking for collaborative care* (5th ed.). St. Louis, MO: Elsevier Saunders.

Jarvis, C. (2004). *Physical examination & health assessment* (4th ed.). St. Louis, MO: Saunders.

McCance, K. L., & Huether, S. E. (2002). *Pathophysiology: The biologic basis for disease in adults and children* (4th ed.). St. Louis, MO: Elsevier Saunders.

National Institute of Diabetes and Digestive and Kidney Diseases- www.niddk.nih.gov

NIDDK stastitics-http://digestive.niddk.nih.gov/statistics

Porth, C. (2005). Pathophysiology: Concepts of altered health status. Philadelphia: Lippincott.

CHAPTER 8

Activity and Rest

Activity and rest are basic needs in the physiologic mode. Through activity, people carry out daily living and present themselves to others within the environment. Activity also provides the physical stresses on body structures that promote normal growth and development. Rest, on the other hand, provides periods of restoration, repair, renewal of energies, and effectiveness of life processes. Two basic life processes that act to maintain an appropriate balance in both activity and rest are mobility and sleep. These two processes are the focus of this chapter. Innate and learned compensating strategies that act to maintain adaptation and health in this basic need are discussed. Examples of compromised processes of activity and rest are identified, with particular focus on the effects of immobility and sleep deprivation. To plan nursing care, assessment of behaviors and stimuli related to the needs for activity and rest are outlined based on an understanding of the two life processes. Guidelines for diagnoses, goals, and nursing interventions and evaluation are described. Emphasis is placed on the overall goal of preventing problems with activity and rest and promoting health in this physiologic mode component.

OBJECTIVES

After studying this chapter, the reader will be able to do the following:

1. Describe the basic life processes associated with activity and rest.
2. Describe one compensatory process related to the needs of activity and rest.
3. Name and describe two situations of compromised processes of activity and rest.
4. Identify important first-level assessment behaviors for the needs of activity and rest.
5. List second-level assessment common stimuli affecting activity and rest.
6. Develop a nursing diagnosis, given a situation related to activity and rest.
7. Derive goals for an individual with ineffective activity and rest in a given situation.
8. Describe nursing interventions commonly implemented in situations of ineffective activity and rest.
9. Propose approaches to determine the effectiveness of nursing interventions.

KEY CONCEPTS DEFINED

Activity: Body movement that serves various purposes such as carrying out daily living chores and protecting self or others from injury.

Activity intolerance: A state in which an individual has insufficient physiologic or psychological energy to endure or complete required or desired daily activities.

Disuse consequences: Changes in major body functions that result from a period of physical inactivity.

Disuse syndrome: The potential negative effects of curtailed physical activity, particularly when imposed by medical restrictions.

Gait: The manner of walking; the basic means of moving around from place to place.

Limbic system: Brain structures that govern basic biologic drives and emotional behavior by controlling neuroendocrine and autonomic systems through the hypothalamus.

Mobility: The basic life process for activity whereby one moves or is moved.

Nonlimbic structures: The sensory and motor cortex and associative systems.

Posture: Anatomic arrangement of body parts in a given position.

Recreation: A change in activity in which one becomes renewed for other activities.

Rehabilitation: An active and dynamic process through which an individual achieves optimal physical, emotional, psychological, social, and vocational potential.

Rest: Changes in activity in which energy requirements are minimal; more generally, refreshing relaxation.

Sleep: The basic life process for rest in which most of the body's physiologic activities slow down to allow renewal of energy for future activity.

Sleep apnea: The periodic cessation of breathing during sleep.

Sleep pattern disturbance: A compromised process of rest that includes inadequate amount of sleep and fragmented sleep.

BASIC LIFE PROCESSES OF ACTIVITY AND REST

Both activity and rest are key to human survival. The associated basic life processes include mobility and sleep. Activity refers to body movement that serves various purposes such as carrying out activities of daily living and protecting self or others from bodily injuries. Mobility is the basic life process for activity whereby one moves or is moved. Recreation is a change in activity in which one becomes renewed for other activities. Rest, on the other hand, involves changes in activity in which energy requirements are minimal; more generally, refreshing relaxation. During rest, energy is conserved and restored. Sleep is the basic life process for rest in which most of the body's physiologic activities slow down to allow for renewal of energy for future activity. Processes of mobility are an important focus for nursing care with more of the population at risk for concerns related to activity. This is because more of the population is made up of elderly, people with chronic illness, or those seriously ill. At the same time, there are increasing numbers of individuals in society whose lifestyle leads to stresses that interfere with getting adequate sleep and rest. Because of increasing difficulties in meeting the needs for activity and rest in today's society, the nurse is concerned with assisting people in meeting these needs. The aim is to promote effective mobility and sleep processes.

Process of Mobility

Mobility is the process whereby one moves or is moved. To move is to change location or position. The body structures of normal movement are the voluntary and autonomic neuromuscular and skeletal systems. About 50% of body mass is composed of muscle and 25% of bone and connecting structures (Burrell, Gerlach, & Pless, 1997). Muscles act through tension applied at the points of attachment to bones, which serve as levers. Muscles and bones combine with neurologic inputs to provide locomotion and activity. Nurses note that in addition to intact neuromuscular systems, mobility also involves the motivation to move and a free, nonrestrictive environment in which to move (Bronstein, 2001). In terms of brain function, limbic and nonlimbic structures are involved (Figure 8–1). The limbic system is made up of brain structures that govern the basic biologic drives and emotional behavior by controlling the neuroendocrine and autonomic systems through the hypothalamus, as noted in Chapter 12. A need for motion is generated, and influenced, by the sensorimotor part of the brain. The nonlimbic structures consist of sensory and motor cortex and associative systems.

The neural basis of movement has evolved into a hierarchy of increasingly complex action. The highest level operates in the association areas of the cerebral cortex and elaborates perceptions and overall motor plans or strategies. As part of this process, the limbic system denotes what is relevant to the perceived needs of the body. The middle level of the command hierarchy is where strategies are converted into motor programs or tactics. This level involves the sensorimotor cortex, cerebellum, basal ganglia, and brain stem. These programs correlate

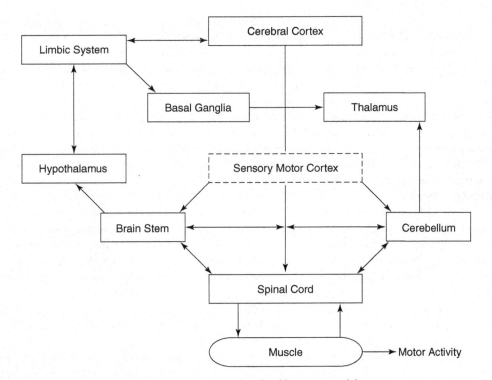

FIGURE 8–1 Central nervous system structures involved in motor activity.

body equilibrium, movement directions, force, and speed. In addition, they control mechanical stiffness of the joints, that is, whether the joints move or are held in one position. Natural movements of everyday life involve several joints and are composed of a series of simple movements that affect only one joint. The lowest level of control is the spinal cord, which translates commands into muscular activity. The spinal cord also regulates movement through stretch reflexes. (Chapters 10 and 12 further describe related sensory and neurologic processes and relevant discussions are found in basic anatomy and physiology texts.) The result of all these structures working in coordination is motor activity.

All of these processes are integrated so intricately that human movement has not yet been duplicated in efforts to build robots. This remains the case even as researchers are teaching robots to express emotion. In an early article in a popular science journal (Dworetzky, 1987) noted:

> It's no wonder movie makers still use people dressed up in robot suits instead of using the real thing. Today's commercial robots don't walk like men [sic], actually balancing their bulk, but stay on their feet statically, like tables on wheels. They're incapable of counter-balancing, of shifting their center of gravity to make lifting or pushing more efficient, so they must be over-engineered into glorified forklifts in order to work without toppling over. (p. 18)

This type of robot movement was evident to the world in the media coverage of the mechanical success of the rovers Sojourner and Phoenix even as they carried out the extraordinary missions of exploring Mars.

For the individual, the stress caused by physical movement is essential in maintaining all major body functions. Bones themselves are dynamic tissues that undergo continuous remodeling. Where bone experiences stress, it will increase osteoblastic activities to increase ossification. Bone that is not stressed will have increased osteoclastic activity and bone resorption. Therefore, the musculoskeletal system maintains its bone strength, as well as muscle tone, only if adequate stresses are imposed regularly, as through physical exercise. Physical movement also promotes the normal oxygenation process by stimulating cardiovascular circulation and proper lung expansion with mobilization of its secretions. Skeletal movement promotes normal urinary tract flow and stimulates gastric mobility that is essential for proper digestion of foods. It also has a positive effect on bowel elimination. Maintenance of normal metabolic rate requires adequate physical stresses to maintain proper equilibrium between catabolic and anabolic activities.

One author sees exercise as a vital component to an individual's well-being, particularly for older patients (Anderson, 2007). Regular exercise can not only help prevent boredom, but also osteoporosis, diabetes mellitus, and heart disease. Physical activity can help manage pressure ulcers, arthritis, depression, obesity, and psychosocial health. It can also improve joint mobility, insomnia, indigestion, constipation, and the majority of pulmonary conditions. However, only 23% of adults perform enough regular, sustained exercise to have significant health benefits. Rather 70% to 75% of the adults in the United States are sedentary and report no leisure-time activity or are not regularly active (USDHHS, 2000). The goals set in Healthy People 2010 are aimed at reversing the sedentary lifestyle.

The human dimensions of what it means to an individual to plan and carry out movement is noted in a neurologist's account of witnessing patients become suddenly mobile, after years of virtual immobility. The situation involved receiving a new treatment for parkinsonian symptoms induced by encephalitis. In his widely read book, Sacks (1983) called what he saw in patients "awakenings." He commented that we are critically dependent on a continual flow of impulses and information to and from all the sensory and motor organs of the body. More poignantly he states, "We must be active or we cease to exist: activity and actuality are one and the same" (p. 302).

Process of Sleep

The need for rest is as important as the need for activity, and sleep is an important life process for obtaining rest. Rest generally means changes in activity in which energy requirements are minimal. It is the prelude to sleep. However, rest also can be thought of in a broader context of refreshing relaxation. In the latter meaning, rest is not defined as mere physical inactivity. Rest includes the quality of relaxation that comes with freedom from physical discomfort and psychological stresses such as anxiety. Most notably, rest is an individualized matter. What leads to relaxation and restoration of energy will vary from person to person. Rest may be changing activity, such as taking a walk during a lunch break at work. Vacation and other kinds of recreation also provide rest. For some individuals, rest is best attained while doing nothing—sitting outside watching the ocean, beside a fireplace indoors in winter, or watching raindrops on the window in spring. During rest, physiologic processes slow down to allow renewal of energy. Physiologically, heart rate recovery is greatest at the beginning of a rest period. Thus, it is suggested that several short rest periods rather than one long, extended period are more effective. Many offices have adopted napping policies for their employees, allowing them to take time out for a brief rest during the workday. Industrial studies suggest that 15% of work time be given to rest, with increases of 20% to 30% in evenly distributed times for strenuous workloads.

Sleep is the process by which most rest is accomplished, with human beings spending an average of one third of their lives sleeping. Behaviorally, rest becomes sleep when the ability to respond to environmental stimuli is diminished. However, in this partial state of unconsciousness the individual can be easily aroused by stimulation. Sleep is a rhythmic and active process with defined stages. There are five stages and two major types of sleep differentiated by the frequency and amplitude of electroencephalogram (EEG) waves. Through most of a typical night of 7–8 hours of sleep, the individual alternates between non-rapid eye movement (NREM) sleep and rapid eye movement (REM) sleep. This pattern of recurring sleep cycles, including occurrence, timing, and duration of stages, is called the architecture of sleep. Generally, the night's sleep begins with the lights out and less than 20 minutes of awake time. A period of drowsiness, stage 1, follows and will reoccur at intervals throughout the night, especially to begin a new sleep cycle. During the first 30 to 45 minutes of the sleep cycle, the individual passes through four stages of NREM sleep. This culminates in slow-wave sleep. In deeper sleep, the frequency of EEG waves decreases and the amplitude increases. In about 90 minutes, after stage 4 sleep has been attained, the EEG pattern changes abruptly. The waves become irregular and seem to backtrack through the stages until alpha waves appear. This is the onset of REM sleep. On the EEG, REM sleep looks much the same as the awake state. However, the characteristic eye movements appear and can be observed through the closed eyelids. Other bodily changes accompany REM sleep.

As noted, the sleep cycles during the night typically alternate between REM and NREM with occasional partial arousal. After each REM episode, the individual returns to stage 4 again. REM sleep occurs about every 90 minutes. The length of REM sleep gets longer with each cycle. The first REM period lasts 5–10 minutes and the last one 20 to 50 minutes. Since most dreaming occurs during REM sleep, the longest dreams occur just before awakening. Brain stem mechanisms, including the control of specific neurotransmitters, regulate the stages of sleep. For example, the reticular activating system maintains the awake state, but also mediates some sleep stages, especially dreaming sleep. The hypothalamus controls the timing of the sleep cycle. The hormone melatonin helps set the sleep–wake cycles. Serotonin prepares the brain for slow-wave sleep. In addition to the nightly cycle, the daily alternating cycles of sleep and wakefulness reflect a natural circadian or 24-hour rhythm.

During sleep, the individual's physiology differs significantly from that when awake. The cardiovascular, respiratory, and gastrointestinal systems are most affected. Other alterations include cerebral blood flow, metabolism, temperature regulation, and endocrine and renal function. These effects differ in the various stages of sleep and are based on the characteristics of sleep. For example, with the loss of wakefulness, neural control of respiration changes as the cortical component is lost and metabolic control predominates. The result may be normal variations, such as rapid or irregular breathing, or abnormal responses such as snoring or obstructive apnea. Beginning in stage 1, there is decreased activity in vital bodily functions such as heart rate, temperature, respiration, and basal metabolic rate. During the deep sleep that starts with stage 3, the basic metabolic rate is decreased by 10 to 20 percent. This is demonstrated by a drop in body temperature, heart rate, and blood pressure. Muscle tone becomes atonic. The skin may become flushed and warm, with mild diaphoresis. Blood pressure decreases during stages 3 and 4. During stage 4, growth hormone is released and there is a decreased concentration of corticosteroids. These changes seem to promote protein synthesis, which can assist in restoration and repair of biologic structures and functions.

During REM sleep most of the body's skeletal muscles go limp and are actively inhibited. It may be that this temporary paralysis prevents us from acting out our dreams while the eye movements may be following the visual images of the dreams (Marieb & Hoehn, 2007). Variability of both blood pressure and heart rate is increased during REM sleep, possibly related to other changes such as decreased cardiac output. During this stage, there is an overall but transient increase in physiologic activities in the body. This may result from marked but brief cutaneous vasoconstriction, a reduction in urine volume, and possibly, an increased level of plasma catecholamines. Body temperature, heart rate, and blood pressure are all increased, sometimes even to above the level of the individual's waking state. An increase in cerebral activity is indicated by increased cerebral blood flow. When awakened during this stage, many people report vivid dreams. Nocturnal attacks of conditions such as anginal pain, gastric pain, and asthma can be triggered during this stage. Although REM sleep is included within each cycle, since the cycles occurring later in the sleep period have more REM sleep there is greater vulnerability to these attacks around 5 or 6 a.m.

Sleep researchers postulate that NREM sleep is an anabolic state and responsible primarily for physiologic restoration. This is supported by the fact that NREM sleep takes precedence over REM sleep when an individual is recovering from sleep deprivation. Still, more is known about the description and mechanisms of sleep than about its functions or how it acts to renew the individual for another day's activities. In discussing theories of why we need sleep, Wickens (2000) noted that the fact is that all animal species simply have to sleep. He provides the example of the Bottlenose dolphin which must continually break the surface of the water to breathe. These animals sleep with one hemisphere at a time, that is, the two sides of the brain take turns to sleep with one hemisphere always remaining awake to direct behavior. Thus sleep provides a vital need.

COMPENSATORY ADAPTIVE PROCESSES OF ACTIVITY AND REST

Many compensating strategies for activity and rest are embedded in an understanding of mobility and sleep and rest processes. Some of these are innate, some are learned, and some are a combination of both. Combining innate responses with learning is an important approach for nurses in promoting patient adaptation. Two examples of combined compensating strategies are the use of feedback in movement and the learned relaxation response to promote rest and sleep.

Use of Feedback in Movement

The command hierarchy for movement described earlier makes it possible for the individual to complete simple tasks, such as casually throwing a piece of paper into the wastebasket and very complex tasks, such as feeding oneself. In the first action, the individual uses a ballistic control system. Prior to movements, a precise sequence of motor commands is worked out to produce the correct pattern of muscular contractions that are needed to achieve the goal of hitting the basket. It is clear that, once the paper leaves the hand, no amount of sensory feedback about its trajectory is going to enable an individual to modify the flight. In the example, the individual begins with the desired result, and translates this into an appropriate pattern of commands, drawing on a library of motor programs suitable for different acts. These commands produce the actual result through their effect on the body's muscles. If the program is a good one, the actual result is the same as the desired result, that is, the paper lands in the basket.

This type of movement, however, is not efficient in most human action because an individual cannot have an infinite number of motor programs to draw upon. Also, noise, that is, unpredictable additional sensory input, is always present. The system needs to cope with the problem of noise, such as the slightest breeze blowing from an air conditioner. It also must make complex computations in advance including the nature of the load to be moved and a host of internal factors such as body temperature, the degree of fatigue, and the amount of energy available. Feedback control systems are the answer. These operate on the same general principles as the adaptation level described for the individual as an adaptive system. In a motor control system, the possibility of using feedback greatly improves the functioning of the system. A simple feedback control system starts with the desired result and, at every moment, compares this with the actual result. This comparison is made by sensory information feedback, and the difference between the two is a measurement of error. The smaller the error, or the difference between actual and desired result, the more nearly the individual succeeds in accomplishing the task. The error signal is used to generate motor commands to reduce the difference between the desired and actual results. The computation of correcting commands is a much simpler process than the calculations needed in a ballistic system.

An additional capability of the human motor feedback control system is that of learning. When this feature is added, the system is a sort of compromise between a guided and a ballistic system. The main forward pathway is the same as in a ballistic system in that the desired result is again converted into a suitable pattern of output commands by means of stored programs. What is new about this system is that it also incorporates feedback about the actual result, which is compared with the desired result to provide an error signal. However, this error signal, instead of being used to generate commands directly in the course of the movement, is used instead to modify the parameters of the program for movement. The system learns by experience, and faulty programs are altered for future successful motor activity. This behavior is highly characteristic of human motor systems learning to execute complex actions. An individual throwing darts at a target for the first time may use a preexisting program from throwing a ball, or initially from tossing toys on the floor from a high chair. As the individual practices, the feedback from each throw is used to reduce error and gradually evolve an accurate program for dart throwing.

Another positive feature of the motor feedback control system is that at times it is difficult to obtain feedback about actual results quickly enough for them to be of use during an action like throwing the dart. However, it may be possible to use internal feedback to predict the result of a particular motor command before the actual result is known. From a general sensory knowledge of the mechanical properties of the hand and arm, and information about the kinds of loads that are present, an individual can form an estimate of what position the limb will adopt in response to any particular pattern of motor commands. This estimate is formed entirely within the brain; it is available long before any feedback from the actual movement has returned from the peripheral sensory motor system. In the internal feedback control system, the desired result is not compared with the actual result, but with the predicted result. The prediction is derived by sending a copy of the motor commands to a neural model of the mechanical properties of the body, which is used to predict the probable result. Again, actual results are compared with the predicted result. Errors are used to correct the model itself, thus improving the accuracy of the predictions. Learning motor skills, then, becomes a matter of learning to predict the behavior of the body. The compensating strategy of using feedback in making mobility more effective is particularly important in rehabilitation.

Learned Relaxation Response

It has been noted that life stresses and worries can interfere with restful sleep. The relaxation response can be a learned compensatory process that enhances an innate, autonomic response to promote rest and sleep. In this response, the individual is alert, but the body processes slow down as sympathetic nervous system arousal is decreased and the individual feels a sense of calmness. The relaxation response has been studied extensively by Benson (1975) and colleagues. It is used as complementary treatment of serious health conditions such as cardiac disease and cancer. There are many possible approaches to elicit the relaxation response. In 1988, Benson and colleagues founded the Mind/Body Medical Institute at the New England Deaconess Hospital and the Harvard Medical School. It was there that they derived the following method of eliciting the relaxation response. The current website of the Benson-Henry Institute for Mind Body Medicine lists the process as follows:

> Step 1: Pick a focus word or short phrase that's firmly rooted in your personal belief system. For example, a nonreligious individual might choose a neutral word like "one" or "peace" or "love." A Christian individual desiring to use a prayer could pick the opening words of Psalm 23, "The Lord is my shepherd"; a Jewish individual could choose "Shalom."
>
> Step 2: Sit quietly in a comfortable position.
>
> Step 3: Close your eyes.
>
> Step 4: Relax your muscles.
>
> Step 5: Breathe slowly and naturally, repeating your focus word or phrase silently as you exhale.
>
> Step 6: Throughout, assume a passive attitude. Don't worry about how well you're doing. When other thoughts come into your mind, simply say to yourself, "Oh well," and gently return to the repetition.

Step 7: Continue for 10 to 20 minutes. You may open your eyes to check on the time, but do not use an alarm. When you finish, sit quietly for a minute or so, at first with your eyes closed and later with your eyes open. Then do not stand for 1 or 2 minutes.

Step 8: Practice the technique once or twice a day.

Another simple approach that nurses can use in many clinical situations is progressive muscle relaxation, which was introduced in the 1920s by American physiologist Edmund Jacobson. The rationale for the effectiveness of this approach is that the stress response cannot exist when the muscles of the body are relaxed. The purpose of teaching progressive muscle relaxation is to provide a sense of control and to minimize the effects of stress, rather than to directly affect stress and illness. The relaxation response benefits the individual by decreasing the anxiety associated with strange environments and stressful or painful situations; increasing the effect of pain medications and helping the patient to dissociate from pain; decreasing fatigue by interrupting protective muscle tensing; increasing relaxed breathing to replace shallow breaths that result from anxiety and fear; providing periods of rest that are as beneficial as a nap and are preparation for restful sleep; decreasing heart rate, blood pressure, and respirations; and improving effectiveness of the endocrine and immune systems (Dossey, Buzzetta, & Kenner, 1992).

In teaching progressive muscle relaxation, the nurse keeps in mind four basic components of relaxation techniques:

- A quiet environment that deletes most noise and distractions.
- A comfortable position, such as sitting or lying without undue muscle tension.
- Focusing on muscle groups as a mental device to shift the mind from logical, externally oriented thoughts.
- Use of the principle that a muscle will relax when it is let go after being tensed.

Progressive relaxation consists of tensing and relaxing muscle groups and focusing on the feelings of relaxation. After discussing the approach with the patient, the nurse leads the individual to develop the relaxation response by instructions to assume a comfortable position and to begin by focusing on breathing easily. For each muscle group, the muscles are tensed for 5 to 7 seconds and then relaxed completely. The individual then focuses for about 10 seconds on the sensations of the relaxed muscles, such as warmth, tingling, and lightness. Sequential tensing of the following muscle groups has been found to be effective.

1. Hands, arms, and shoulders. Clench fists, extend the arms in a slightly raised position, and pull the shoulders tight.
2. Outer face. Raise eyebrows to hairline and protrude the lower jaw.
3. Inner face. Squeeze eyes tightly closed, wrinkle nose, purse lips.
4. Neck. Rest ear on right shoulder, then left shoulder.
5. Shoulders, chest, and abdomen. Push shoulders back and chest forward, with abdomen pulled in.
6. Trunk, legs, and feet. Pinch buttocks together raising slightly, extend legs and flex feet, pointing toes upward.

The nurse coaches the individual through this sequence and observes for effectiveness of the teaching. Nurses can practice progressive muscle relaxation exercises and teach them to colleagues. Cues that the relaxation response has been learned include changes in breathing from slower, deeper breaths to slow, somewhat more shallow and more audible breathing as relaxation deepens; fluttering of the eyelids; relaxing of jaw tension, sometimes to the extent that the lips part and the jaw drops slightly; lack of muscle holding. Lack of holding is demonstrated by lifting the arm gently by the wrist without detectable resistance. In addition, the arm moves as easily as an object of similar weight (Dossey et al., 1992).

As an aid to rest and sleep, the nurse can suggest that, once learned, the relaxation response can be practiced twice a day for 20 minutes. Time spent in sensing the feelings of relaxation are an integral part of the exercise and receive about twice the amount of time as the muscle tensing. Between focusing on different muscle groups, the individual is directed to return to being aware of breathing easily. Abbreviated forms of the muscle relaxation exercises can be repeated in any stressful situation and can be done before preparing to go to bed for sleep.

COMPROMISED PROCESSES OF ACTIVITY AND REST

There are many situations in both health and illness when an individual's needs for activity and rest are not being met and when compensatory processes are not adequate for adaptation. The result can be compromised processes of mobility and sleep. Adaptation problems can result when any of the processes related to activity and rest are disrupted. Two specific examples of compromised adaptive processes related to activity and rest are discussed in this section. Disuse syndrome is the term used for the potential negative effects of curtailed physical activity, particularly when imposed by medical restrictions. Sleep pattern disturbance is a commonly occurring compromised process associated with the need for rest.

Disuse Syndrome

A major issue of physical immobility is disuse syndrome. The North American Nursing Diagnosis Association defines "high risk for disuse syndrome" (NANDA International, 2007) as a state in which an individual is at risk for deterioration of body systems as the result of prescribed or unavoidable inactivity. There are many neuromuscular, skeletal, and other conditions that lead to inactivity. A fractured bone may require a period of immobile therapeutic alignment preoperatively to prevent further damage to the fractured bone or the surrounding soft tissues. Postoperatively, immobility can promote proper healing of the repaired fracture. In the case of a patient who is suffering acute cardiac insufficiency, limited activity is an important part of the therapeutic regime. This measure is to conserve the oxygen and energy consumption required by nonpriority physical activity, minimizing the cardiac load for the damaged heart muscle. The same principle applies when the nurse places a patient with a fever on bed rest. An elevation of 1 degree in body temperature will require a 7% increase in basic metabolic rate, or energy needed. The nurse uses bed rest to prevent further exhaustion of the already stressed body. At the same time, the risks of immobility must be addressed by recognizing the potential for disuse syndrome. Some specific consequences of physical inactivity are listed in Table 8–1. The first two columns are organized by changes in major body functions that result from a period of physical inactivity. The behavioral effect of these changes, termed disuse consequences, is summarized in the third column. Changes from inactivity can further affect adaptation related to the physiologic need for activity and rest. For example, a deficit in muscle mass, tone, and strength indicates muscle atrophy, which is a part of the disuse syndrome. In turn, the atrophied muscle is less effective in performing physical activity. The older person is especially prone to disuse syndrome when immobilized.

TABLE 8–1 Consequences of Physical Inactivity–Disuse Syndrome

Body Function	Underlying Changes	Disuse Consequences	Preventive Interventions
Musculoskeletal	Muscles: Autolysis of unused muscles	Muscular atrophy with weakness and decreased endurance	Muscle conditioning exercises: isometric, isotonic, resistive
	Bones: Increased osteoclastic process due to lack of physical stresses of weight bearing on the bones leads to increased urinary excretion of calcium	Osteoporosis and vulnerability to pathologic fracture	Physical activities that would produce the stresses of weight bearing: standing and walking, pushing and pulling
	Joints: Decreased pliability and increased density of the collagen meshwork leads to fibrous formation and shortening of the muscle fibers	Joint contractures with permanent loss of joint mobility	ROM (range-of-motion) exercises: active, assisted, passive
	Nerves: Denervation due to prolonged compression of nerve fibers and decreased circulation	Paralysis, foot drop, and wrist drop	Frequent change of position, use of foot board
Circulatory	Cardiac overload due to central pooling of the circulatory volume	Deconditioning leads to poor exercise tolerance	Frequent change of position; including sitting up and standing positions, if possible
	Loss of regulatory mechanism to maintain central BP (normally with position change to sitting up, the splenic and peripheral vessels constrict to maintain the central blood volume)	Postural hypotension, dizziness, and fainting in upright position	
	Sluggish venous return due to lack of pumping mechanism generated by muscular contractions of physical activity	Dependent (local) edema, especially of the lower extremities	Muscle exercises to stimulate the circulation
	Hypercoagulability of blood due to injury or surgery combined with physical inactivity	Thrombus formation leads to pulmonary embolism	Well-fitting antiembolic stockings

(continued)

TABLE 8–1 (*continued*)

Body Function	Underlying Changes	Disuse Consequences	Preventive Interventions
Pulmonary	Limited expansion of lungs due to arms crowding chest and diaphragm not dropping	Hypoventilation	Positions of maximum chest expansion
	Medium for infection due to stasis of secretions in lungs and poor pulmonary circulation	Hypostatic pneumonia	Frequent change of positions, and deep breathing and coughing exercises
Metabolic	Increased catabolic processes lead to increased excretion of nitrogen via gastrointestinal and urinary tract combined with poor protein intake due to poor appetite	Negative nitrogen balance leads to poor tissue healing	Ensure adequate intake of dietary protein
Eliminative	Urinary stagnation due to lack of natural position of gravity in recumbent position and loss of proprioception	Urinary retention Urinary tract infection	Frequent encouragement to void, providing adequate toilet facility and position of comfort; ideal position for male client is standing up, while sitting up is ideal for female client
	Increased calcium content in the urine	Nephrolithiasis	Ensure adequate fluid intake with cranberry juice to acidify the urine pH level
Integumentary	Inability to carry out daily personal hygiene measures and prolonged compression of tissues, resulting in decreased circulation	Pressure sores and decubiti ulceration formation with secondary infection	Frequent change of position; use of protective devices (pillow, padding); frequent massaging of all bony prominences
Sensory-perceptual	Decreased environmental stimuli lead to decreased sensory stimulation; changed perceptual axis with recumbent position; inability to manipulate own environment	Anxiety, disorientation, loss of proprioception; change in body image; boredom; egocentricity	Environment structuring to provide meaningful stimuli; use of calendar, radio, TV, and wall clock can be helpful

TABLE 8-1 (*continued*)

Body Function	Underlying Changes	Disuse Consequences	Preventive Interventions
			Provide opportunity to carry out meaningful conversations with others
			Visits from family and friends are very important

Source: Cho, J. S. (1984). Activity and rest. In S. C. Roy (Ed.), *Introduction to nursing: An adaptation model* (pp. 141–143). Englewood Cliffs, NJ: Prentice Hall.

From the perspective of the Roy Adaptation Model, physical inactivity affects the total person as well. The nurse uses knowledge of the adaptive modes to recognize that the inability to move about and interact with people and the environment in one's usual pattern greatly affects the individual's self-concept, role function, and interdependence (see Chapters 14, 15, and 16). The effect on the other modes takes place through the sensory perceptual processes that involve, in particular, anxiety, change of body image, and egocentricity. All four adaptive modes are affected by the stimulus of inactivity. Disuse syndrome refers to the potential negative effects of curtailed physical activity, particularly when imposed by medical restrictions. This is a diagnostic term broad enough to include these effects, particularly when viewed from the perspective of a specific nursing model such as the Roy Adaptation Model and from an understanding of the research related to this concept.

Sleep Pattern Disturbance

It is estimated that more than one half of all adults cite difficulties with sleeping at some time in their lives. Sleep problems are often overlooked in health care settings because other symptoms are given higher priority. However, inadequate sleep leads to an increased risk for accidents, inefficiency at work, irritability in social relations, and exacerbation of other health problems. The nurse is frequently the individual with whom the patient talks about sleep disturbance. Careful assessment of the problem can be useful in helping the individual get the help that is needed. A conceptual model of impaired sleep was created by the Nursing Sleep Curriculum Task Force in 2002 (Figure 8–2). The model distinguishes between sleep deprivation and sleep disruption. Inadequate amounts of sleep can occur for many reasons from simply delaying bedtime or early wake time to jet lag and shift work. Sleep disturbance involves fragmented sleep related to factors such as breathing problems or other health conditions such as pain and discomfort. The model shows how such sleep pattern disturbances can lead to adverse health outcomes for the individual on a physiologic, cognitive/behavioral, emotional, and/or social level.

Risk factors for impaired sleep are divided into three main categories: environmental, personal, and developmental (Lee, 2003). Environmental factors such as unexpected noise or light can cause fragmented sleep, or repeated arousal during sleep, which is also known as maintenance insomnia. Other factors that cause this kind of impaired sleep are frequent

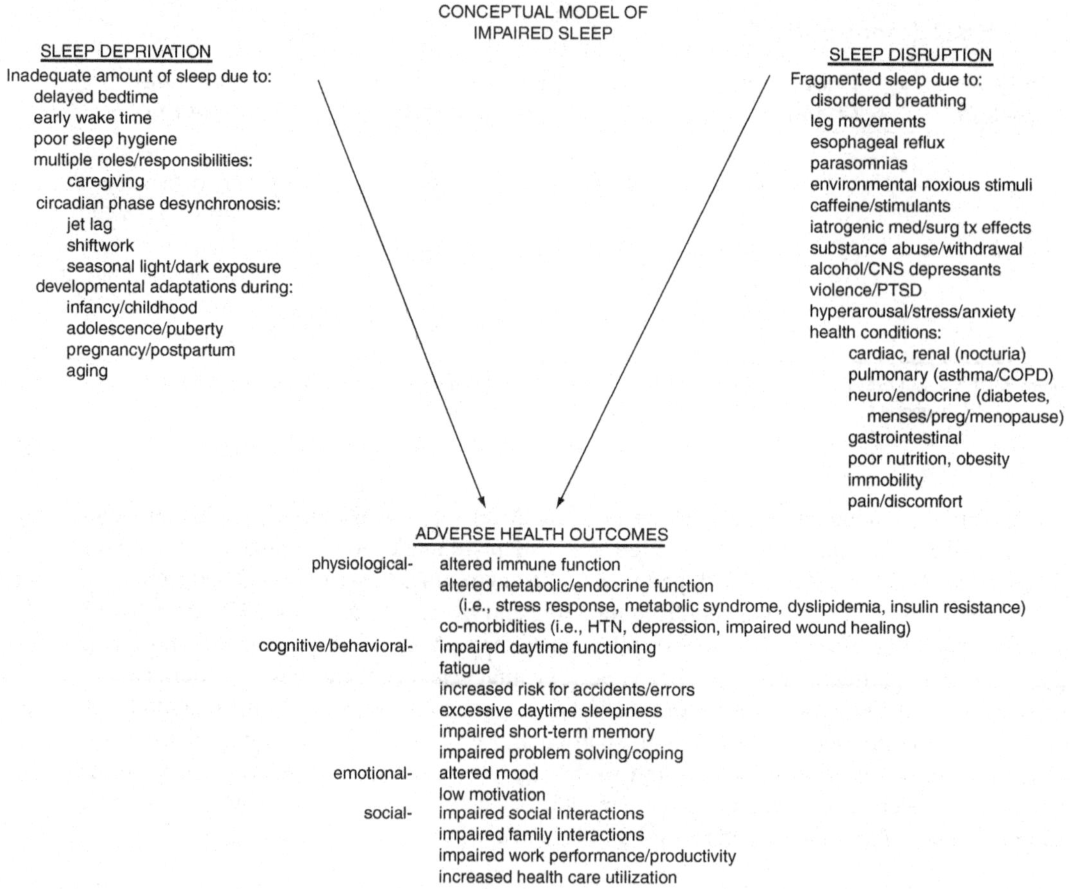

CONCEPTUAL MODEL OF
IMPAIRED SLEEP

SLEEP DEPRIVATION

Inadequate amount of sleep due to:
 delayed bedtime
 early wake time
 poor sleep hygiene
 multiple roles/responsibilities:
  caregiving
 circadian phase desynchronosis:
  jet lag
  shiftwork
  seasonal light/dark exposure
 developmental adaptations during:
  infancy/childhood
  adolescence/puberty
  pregnancy/postpartum
  aging

SLEEP DISRUPTION

Fragmented sleep due to:
 disordered breathing
 leg movements
 esophageal reflux
 parasomnias
 environmental noxious stimuli
 caffeine/stimulants
 iatrogenic med/surg tx effects
 substance abuse/withdrawal
 alcohol/CNS depressants
 violence/PTSD
 hyperarousal/stress/anxiety
 health conditions:
  cardiac, renal (nocturia)
  pulmonary (asthma/COPD)
  neuro/endocrine (diabetes,
   menses/preg/menopause)
  gastrointestinal
  poor nutrition, obesity
  immobility
  pain/discomfort

ADVERSE HEALTH OUTCOMES

physiological- altered immune function
        altered metabolic/endocrine function
         (i.e., stress response, metabolic syndrome, dyslipidemia, insulin resistance)
        co-morbidities (i.e., HTN, depression, impaired wound healing)
cognitive/behavioral- impaired daytime functioning
        fatigue
        increased risk for accidents/errors
        excessive daytime sleepiness
        impaired short-term memory
        impaired problem solving/coping
emotional- altered mood
        low motivation
social-   impaired social interactions
        impaired family interactions
        impaired work performance/productivity
        increased health care utilization

FIGURE 8–2 Conceptual Model of Sleep. (Lee, K.A. Nursing Sleep Curriculum Task Force. In Lee, K.A. (2003). Impaired sleep. In: Carrieri-Kohlman, V., Lindsay, A.M., & West, C.M. (Eds.). (2003). *Pathophysiological phenomena* in *nursing* (3rd ed.). Philadelphia: WB Saunders. (pp. 363–385). Used with permission).

urination, diarrhea, or nausea and vomiting. Personal factors include physiologic and psychological stressors stemming from poor nutrition, personal crises, too much or a lack of physical activity, disease, or medical treatments that may even include hypnotic agents. Developmental risk factors result from unhealthy lifestyle behaviors that developed early in an individual's life as a response to stressors and unrecognized sleep disorders such as narcolepsy or delayed sleep phase syndrome. Additional lifestyle choices that compound impaired sleep include drinking caffeinated beverages close to bedtime, consuming alcoholic beverages in an attempt to fall asleep, or using one's bed for other purposes than sleep or sexual activity, such as watching TV.

Nurses can help the individual establish good sleep habits and possibly prevent sleep pattern disturbance. Adequate time, an appropriate environment, and freedom from worry all contribute to good sleep habits. Taylor, Lillis, and LeMone (2001) stated that a nurse also can act as a role model in helping a patient achieve better sleep habits. It is more difficult for a patient to establish a good routine when the nurse appears and behaves in a way that indicates a lack of adequate sleep. Nurses should not merely concentrate on their patients' well-being; rather, they should also focus on their own lifestyles for effective health teaching. Nurses can incorporate principles of good sleep hygiene into their own health routines.

NURSING PROCESS RELATED TO ACTIVITY AND REST

Meeting activity and rest needs is important for the physiologic adaptation of the individual, as well as for integrity of the other adaptive modes. With an understanding of mobility and sleep processes, and related compensatory and compromised processes, the nurse can complete a holistic first- and second-level assessment for an individual's activity and rest needs. Based on judgment about nursing care needs, the next step of the nursing process is the nursing diagnosis. The assessment and diagnoses are then used to set goals with the patient, to select nursing interventions, and to evaluate the outcomes of care.

Assessment of Behavior for Mobility

Given the importance of mobility to the individual's physical and psychological integrity, the nurse assesses activity needs based on understanding mobility as a human life process. Specific assessment factors are examined to determine the adequacy of mobility level and to identify any existing adverse consequences of immobility. Two major categories of assessment are considered. The first category is the frequency, intensity, and duration of daily physical activity carried out by the individual. The second is the assessment of the individual's motor function status, which depends on muscle and joint mobility, posture and gait, and coordination.

PHYSICAL ACTIVITY   The benefits of physical activity for fitness have been widely recognized since the 1950s, when President Eisenhower called attention to this need. Regular exercise continues to be a target for the health of the nation as noted in the Healthy People 2010 goals for physical activity (USDHHS, 2000). Some progress has been made in decreasing the number of people who die from coronary artery disease. The number of people who have regular moderate and vigorous physical activity and strength training activities has increased as well. The goal has been exceeded in the number of work site fitness programs. However, the tendency to be sedentary continues to increase with age. Current studies show that the majority of people, particularly women, children, low-income populations, and minorities, still do not get enough regular exercise. Obtaining information on the individual's patterns of daily physical activity is important in planning care to avoid the consequences of inadequate activity and to promote health, fitness, and well-being. By observing, discussing, and recording the frequency, intensity, and duration of physical activity, the nurse can judge the adequacy of activity level in relation to the individual's total physical condition.

MOTOR FUNCTION   Through assessment of motor function, the nurse determines the type of physical activity the individual is capable of performing and identifies consequences of inactivity.

Functional Assessments   Functional abilities relate to the individual's ability to carry out activities of daily living such as bathing, dressing, feeding, and walking. In addition, the skills needed to live independently include using the telephone, shopping, preparing food, and doing basic housekeeping. A number of assessment tools are available for use by rehabilitation nurses, physiatrists, or therapists. Ignatavicius & Workman (2002) noted that Functional Independence Measure (FIM) is a uniform data system used for outcome measurement across the United States. The FIM seeks to quantify what the individual actually does and does not focus on the specific impairment. The functions for assessment are self-care, sphincter control, mobility and locomotion, communication, and cognition. The FIM is particularly useful in rehabilitation, but has been modified for use in acute care and home care as well.

Muscle Mass and Tone   All active movements, such as lifting, pushing, and pulling, require muscle contractions. Muscle mass (size) and tone (firmness) are assessed by grasping the center of the muscle and feeling that it is firm, supple, and full-bellied. In the older person, it is expected that there is less shape and contour of major muscles. In the child, muscles are softer and have less mass.

Muscle Strength   Muscle strength varies widely according to age and training. Strength is tested by asking the individual to move using certain muscles, using resistance, or holding an instrument still while the examiner tries to move it. An example is testing flexion and extension at the elbow by having the patient pull and push against the examiner's hand. Levels of strength are commonly scaled from 0 (no muscular contraction either seen or felt) to 5 (normal muscle strength). Table 8–2 describes commonly used levels of strength. Generally, a muscle strength rated below 3 is considered indicative of disability.

Joint Mobility   Joint mobility is assessed by an active or passive demonstration of each joint's range of motion. The range of motion is the direction and degree a joint is capable of moving. This varies for different joints, for example, the ankle moves by flexing about 50° and extending about 20°, whereas the hip can flex as much as 135°, extend 28°, abduct 50°, and adduct about 30° as well as rotate (Figure 8–3). Some expected limitation of joint mobility occurs with aging. When there is good mobility, bones move freely and smoothly without pain.

Posture   The anatomic arrangement of body parts in a given position is called posture. Correct posture is a factor in physical safety since inappropriately aligned muscles and joints during activity can result in injury or deformity. Good posture is body alignment that permits optimal weight balance and operation of motor function. In the upright standing position, the head, shoulders, and pelvis are aligned; the arms hang freely from the shoulders; and the feet are aligned with toes pointing straight ahead (Figure 8–4). An individual's preferred posture is a significant behavioral indicator since deviations from good posture may be indicative of some dysfunction. For example, an individual with obstructive lung disease tends to lean forward with arms braced.

TABLE 8–2 Levels of Muscle Strength

Grade	Strength
5	Free range of motion against normal resistance and gravity
4	Full range of motion against moderate resistance and gravity
3	Full range of motion against gravity only
2	Full range of motion with gravity eliminated
1	Slight muscle contraction palpable, but no movement noted
0	No visible or palpable contraction; paralysis of limb

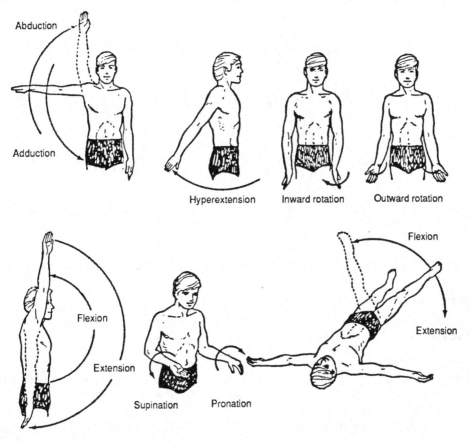

FIGURE 8–3 Range of motion movements.

Gait   Gait is the manner of walking and provides the basic means of moving around from place to place. The nurse assesses whether or not the individual walks easily and comfortably, with self-assurance, good balance, and symmetry of movement. Is there the presence of a limp, pain or discomfort, fear of falling, loss of balance, difference in movement from one side to the other, or unusual movements? A deviation in gait can impose undue stress on certain musculoskeletal parts and, in time, lead to deformity. For example, when a patient is using a "swing through" gait on crutches, the movement is not the same as normal walking; it will eventually result in weakening of the lower extremities. A proper gait with good posture will allow a safe and optimal level of mobility.

Motor Coordination   Good motor coordination requires both intact neurologic and musculoskeletal function and will have an effect on the individual's activity status, particularly self-care activities. Coordination is easily tested by having the individual perform rapidly alternating movements such as placing one foot on the opposite knee and sliding it down that shin to the big toe or moving a finger from the examiner's finger to one's own nose. A child as young as 6 years can easily do these tasks. Further details on assessing each of these aspects of motor function can be found in texts on physical assessment.

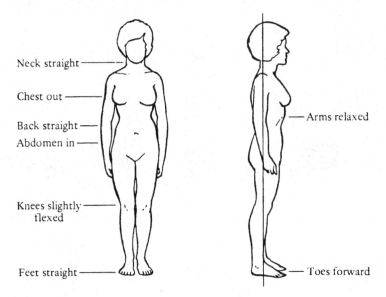

Neck straight

Chest out

Back straight

Abdomen in

Knees slightly
flexed

Feet straight

Arms relaxed

Toes forward

FIGURE 8–4 Correct standing position.

Assessment of Behavior for Sleep

Sleep and rest are important to the individual's physical and psychological integrity. Behavioral observations of adequacy of meeting sleep and rest needs, and background knowledge in this area, provide the basis for planning nursing care. The nurse examines specific assessment behaviors based on understanding the processes related to these needs. For rest and sleep, the following are assessed: quantity and quality of daily rest, sleep pattern, and signs of sleep deprivation.

QUANTITY AND QUALITY OF DAILY REST   Behavior related to rest can be assessed simply by observing and recording rest periods throughout the day. The need for daily rest periods other than nightly sleep depends on an individual's physical and psychological condition in a given situation. However, for most hospitalized patients, deliberately planned rest periods may be a necessary part of total care. Continuous tossing and turning while resting in bed or fidgeting of hands may indicate restlessness. The mere absence of physical activity may not provide effective rest for an individual who is under mental stress. People with activity intolerance may show one or more of the following behaviors: exertional discomfort, difficulty completing activities, and verbal report of being easily fatigued. The individual's assessment of being "well rested" or "tired" is the most important behavior for the nurse to note.

SLEEP PATTERN   An individual's sleep pattern is assessed by recording observations or reports of how long it takes to fall asleep, restlessness during sleep, number of arousals during each sleep period, early awakening, and sleepiness during the day. Understanding the individual's usual pattern of sleep in relation to any recent change is important in the assessment. A thorough sleep history includes questions in the following areas: bedtime problems, excessive daytime sleepiness, awakenings during the night, regularity and duration of sleep, and sleep disordered breathing. A sleep log or diary may be helpful. This is the individual's own written account of sleep experience for 2 weeks. Sample forms are available to give the individual.

SIGNS OF SLEEP DEPRIVATION   Behavioral cues of sleep deprivation include reddened eyes, puffy eyelids, dark circles around the eyes, and frequent yawning. Humans, unlike animals, can deliberately postpone the initiation of sleep. It has been reported that the record for sleep postponement is about 10 days (Friedman, 1993). The effects of sleep on physiologic and psychological integrity have been studied by observing and recording behavioral changes that occur following a period of sleep deprivation. These studies indicate that loss of sleep brings changes in brain function and causes alteration in biochemical processes in the body. Sleep loss causes not only physical fatigue and poor neuromuscular coordination, but also signs of psychological dysfunction which are manifest as general irritability, inability to concentrate, disorientation, and confusion. The severity of these effects depends on the degree and length of deprivation and the individual's pre-deprivation condition. Additional behaviors that may indicate sleep deprivation are reduction in one's role performance at work, school, or home; increasing irritability, restlessness, and disorientation; listlessness; slight hand tremors; expressionless face; and thick speech with mispronounced and wrong choice of words. The individual's sense of having enough sleep is the important behavior to assess regardless of additional data from observation. More extensive assessment tools for clinically evaluating sleep and rest have been developed. Major medical centers have sleep disorder clinics where patients can be referred to receive diagnostic evaluation and treatment. This may involve sleep laboratory studies to make an accurate diagnosis of a sleep disorder.

Assessment of Stimuli for Activity and Rest

Along with the behavioral assessment of activity and rest needs, the nurse assesses the stimuli affecting these needs and how they are being met. Some of the categories of possible stimuli relate to both activity and rest and some are more relevant to one or the other. The categories discussed here include physical condition, psychological condition, environment, developmental stage, and personal habits related to activity and sleep. These factors act together and are assessed as the pattern of stimuli affecting the individual.

PHYSICAL CONDITION   For activity needs, disruptions in the structure and function of the musculoskeletal system are physical conditions that act as key focal stimuli affecting the individual. Such disruptions can occur by either direct physical injuries to muscles and bones or by central nervous system disorders. Regardless of the underlying causative factor, a dysfunctioning musculoskeletal system will cause a direct and immediate effect on motor function. A fractured bone will inevitably necessitate a limitation of physical activity related not only to the loss of function, but also to the discomfort and pain experienced. An individual with an illness, depending on the nature and severity of the condition, will limit physical mobility either voluntarily or because of medically imposed restrictions. Bed rest is often an integral part of therapeutic treatment because rest provides a period of restoration and repair. Particular concerns for planning nursing care when limited activity is part of the plan of care will be addressed later in this chapter.

Rest and sleep particularly are influenced by the physical stresses experienced at a given time. The extent of illness is assessed as affecting rest and sleep. The more serious the illness, the more time an individual will need to spend in rest and sleep. Levels of daily physical activity also are assessed. Whereas vigorous physical activity tends to lengthen the deep-sleep cycle, a lack of physical activity will result in a feeling of unsatisfied sleep caused by lack of deep sleep. Physical discomfort and pain are other common causes that reduce the level of satisfactory rest and sleep. Travel by jet airplane across time zones or working shifts that rotate can alter the body's rhythmic sleep–wake cycle.

PSYCHOLOGICAL CONDITION Psychological condition in a given situation and at a given time has an effect on both activity and rest. Further, it was noted earlier that activity involves the motivation to move. Motivation is a psychological condition and includes knowledge about activity and its beneficial effects for health. A situation in which misinformation is a focal stimulus for inactivity is that of a new mother on a postpartum unit who does not get out of bed to take a shower. With further assessment, the nurse might learn that the mother's cultural background taught her not to move out of bed for several days following giving birth. Psychologically depressed people tend to reduce their physical activity to a bare minimum. The catatonic state of a psychotic individual exemplifies this case to the extreme. In a catatonic state, the individual is not able to initiate body movements, even though physical and physiologic dysfunction cannot be demonstrated. Since sorting and consolidating daily living experiences seems to be done by the brain during sleep, an individual who is under psychological stress has increased need for rest and sleep. However, the increased cortical activity of stress and worry can also disrupt the individual's normal sleep pattern, inducing a feeling of unsatisfied sleep need. It is not uncommon for a psychologically stressed individual to wake up with disturbing dreams and complain of unsatisfactory rest and sleep even after spending many hours in bed.

ENVIRONMENT A free, nonrestrictive environment in which to move is required for physical activity. A suitable environment for activity includes availability of space and adequate physical and personal assistance. Unsuitable factors, such as adverse environmental temperature and surroundings, will act to restrict the individual's activity. For example, encouraging daily walks for an individual after a heart attack will be ineffective if the individual is contending with severe winter weather conditions and has no indoor alternative, or if the neighborhood seems to be an unsafe place to walk. Lack of privacy can also be a focal or contextual stimulus. An individual may be reluctant to do exercises on a mat or in a swimming pool of a busy physical therapy department. A child placed in a playpen will have a restricted range of physical activity which, over time, could affect the child's normal growth and development.

The immediate environment affects rest and sleep. Since human beings require an average of one third of their total lifetime for sleep, each individual develops unique habits and patterns related to the immediate environment for sleep. Through the years, these individualized patterns take on the character of ritualistic habits. It is not uncommon for an individual to experience difficulties in falling asleep, or staying asleep, if the usual sleep habits cannot be followed, or if the bedtime schedule of activity is altered. An unfamiliar or unsuitable environment also disrupts rest and sleep. Such stimuli as unpleasant noise, light, odor, and room temperature can be disturbing factors. This was likely a factor in an early study that recorded the EEGs of intensive care patients for 48 hours. In these patients, only 50% to 60% of total sleep during a 24-hour period occurred at night. The remaining 40% to 50% occurred during the day. Patients also had less total sleep time than they would have usually had at home (Hilton, 1976). The timing for normal sleep is regulated further by external factors such as sunrise, sunset, and length of day; ambient temperature; physical activity and rest; timing and type of meals; and timing of social cues such as increased morning noise from traffic or farm animals.

PERSONAL HABITS   Any motivational or conditional factors that last over a period of time can affect the individual's personal habits related to activity. The effect of a habit, or accustomed pattern of behavior, can be a strong influence in a given situation. If a health care worker has the habit of doing physical aerobic exercise every day, finding a way to exercise when away from home for business or a vacation will be a high priority. Helping others to overcome poor habits related to levels of activity is an important health promotion effort for the nurse. As noted, sedentary style of life has grown among the general population in the United States and persists even with broad public education on the benefits of exercise. This habit within the culture is based on the following circumstances: machines do the work and provide transportation; increased computer time at work and home; decreased financial resources in schools, colleges, and communities for physical activity instruction, playgrounds, parks and recreation facilities, and after-school sports programs and staff; and children spending increased time watching television and playing video games (USDHHS, 1995).

An individual's habits related to the use of drugs and alcohol can act as a stimulus for sleep and rest. An individual who is sedated with medications, or consuming large amounts of alcoholic beverages, will not be ready, either physically or psychologically, to be involved in physical activity. In turn, changes in activity levels then influence the quality of sleep. Alcoholic beverages and drugs such as barbiturates and opiate derivatives may be effective for initiating sleep and rest on a temporary basis. However, over time, they actually induce sleep deprivation because of their tendency to suppress REM sleep. These substances are habit forming, and as an individual develops a tolerance, they become ineffective with prolonged use.

DEVELOPMENTAL STAGE   Another contextual stimulus for both activity and sleep is age. It takes some developmental maturity to master the psychomotor skills for self care activities. Similarly as one ages independent living depends upon some physical activity ability. With an increasing aging population, more options are available to match services to changing level of abilities. Examples are living communities that offer independent living, assisted living, and long-term care.

Related to sleeping, generally younger people sleep longer, until the individual reaches young adulthood. The average time spent for sleep in different age groups can be summarized as 22 hours for the neonate, 14 to 16 hours for infants, 10 to 12 hours for toddlers and preschoolers, and 8 to 10 hours for schoolchildren. Young adults, those in middle years, and elderly individuals spend an average of 7 to 8 hours daily for sleep. Recent studies have demonstrated that elderly men and women have multiple miniature arousals to stage 1 or awake during the normal night's sleep. The teen years can be a time of risk for sleep deprivation as young people take on work as well as school and social activities.

Nursing Diagnosis

As noted in Chapter 3, the data from the nursing assessment of behaviors and stimuli are interpreted in the statement of a nursing diagnosis. The statement includes a clustering of the observed behaviors with the most relevant influencing stimuli. A nursing diagnosis related to adequate activity may be stated, "Good muscle tone and 4+ muscle strength in major muscle groups of all four extremities related to knowledge of health benefits of fitness and commitment to regular exercise program."

In situations where there are problems related to needs for activity and rest, the nursing diagnosis will convey the essence of the problem in a way that will direct the subsequent steps of the nursing process. This clarity of communication is facilitated by using the approach recommended by the Roy Adaptation Model for stating the diagnosis, that is, a statement of observed behaviors with the most relevant influencing stimuli. For example, the nurse may see a young professional woman in an outpatient department who says that she must have a virus because she is not feeling well. In assessing activity and rest needs, the nurse notes the following data. The individual reports difficulty falling asleep and frequent arousals from sleep during the night. Her eyes are reddened with puffy eyelids and dark circles under the eyes, and she states she knows she is not sleeping well. She also mentions concerns about the responsibilities associated with a job promotion. The diagnosis can be stated as, "Reports of poor sleep pattern, with eyes showing evidence of sleep deprivation, related to a recent change in job responsibilities."

Another way of stating a nursing diagnosis is to use a summary label from an established classification system that best identifies the nurse's judgment of the clinical situation. In earlier discussion of the Roy model, two classification lists were described: one for indicators of adaptation and one for commonly recurring adaptation problems (see Chapter 3). In Table 8–3 the Roy model nursing diagnosis categories for the physiologic mode need of activity and rest are shown in relation to nursing diagnosis labels approved by the North American Nursing Diagnosis Association (NANDA International, 2007). For experienced nurses, a summary diagnostic label can convey a behavioral pattern when more than one mode is being affected by the same stimulus. Consider the following illustration. A 28-year-old male was involved in a car accident with resultant paraplegia (loss of voluntary muscle control and sensation of the lower extremities). He is involved in aggressive physical and occupational therapy to learn to care for himself while in a wheelchair. Nurses on the 24-hour-care unit, where the patient stays, use knowledge of movement processes to make the following diagnosis, "High potential for disuse

TABLE 8–3 Nursing Diagnostic Categories for Activity and Rest

Positive Indicators of Adaptation	Common Adaptation Problems	NANDA Diagnostic Labels
• Integrated processes of mobility • Adequate recruitment of compensatory movement processes during inactivity • Effective pattern of activity and rest • Effective sleep pattern • Effective environmental changes for altered sleep conditions	• Immobility • Activity intolerance • Restricted mobility, gait, and/or coordination • Disuse syndrome • Inadequate pattern of activity and rest • Sleep deprivation • Potential for sleep pattern disturbance	• Risk for disuse syndrome • Impaired physical mobility • Impaired bed mobility • Impaired wheelchair mobility • Impaired transfer ability • Impaired walking • Delayed surgical recovery • Sedentary lifestyle • Sleep deprivation • Readiness for enhanced sleep • Insomnia • Energy field disturbance • Fatigue

syndrome related to prolonged immobility and paralysis." As noted earlier, immobility has a profound effect on the physiologic needs of the body. At the same time, the individual's feelings about self and what he is able to do in social roles is greatly affected. The nursing diagnosis with the summary diagnostic label "disuse syndrome" conveys this complex interrelationship.

Activity intolerance has been defined by NANDA as a state in which an individual has insufficient physiologic or psychological energy to endure or complete required or desired daily activities. This diagnosis can be related to such factors as anxiety, acute and chronic pain, weakness and fatigue, sedentary lifestyle, deconditioned status, and pathology such as cardiac arrhythmias and circulatory or respiratory problems. These factors result in an imbalance between oxygen supply and demand. This condition can be recognized by behaviors of complaints of fatigue and weakness, abnormal heart rate or blood pressure in response to activity, and exertional discomfort or dyspnea.

Sleep apnea is the periodic cessation of breathing during sleep. Further, neurologic, respiratory, and cardiovascular systems are also involved. Because sleep apnea results in frequent awakenings, irritability and daytime drowsiness can result. For this reason, sleep apnea can be a dangerous sleep disorder for the community as well as for the individual. Motor vehicle accidents can occur when the individual experiences daytime sleepiness. The nurse can be helpful in identifying people who need immediate diagnosis and treatment. Often the first manifestation of a problem is a complaint from a spouse, family, or significant other about loud, irregular snoring. Obese males are particularly prone to this disorder because fat deposition in tissues can reduce the diameter of the oropharynx and diminish upper airway exchange. Following a careful assessment of activity and rest needs and deriving a nursing diagnosis, the fourth step of the nursing process, goal setting, is carried out.

Goal Setting

In using the Roy Adaptation Model, goal setting is the stating of clear outcomes for the individual as a result of nursing care. As noted, a complete goal statement contains the behavior of focus, the change that the nurse and patient together expect, and the time frame in which the goal can be achieved. Depending on the situation, the goal may be long term or short term. Consider the individual with the diagnosis of "good muscle tone and 4+ muscle strength in major muscle groups of all four extremities related to knowledge of health benefits of fitness and commitment to regular exercise program." If this individual suddenly is hospitalized with a fractured pelvis suffered in a motor vehicle accident, an appropriate goal in the new situation of immobility is, "Upper extremity muscle tone will be maintained at a good level and strength will be increased from 4+ to 5+ during the 4 weeks of acute care." This goal is influenced by the need to prepare the individual for use of the arms to bear weight on crutches during rehabilitation. In the case of the individual who reports a poor sleep pattern, with eyes that show evidence of sleep deprivation related to a recent change in job responsibilities, a short-term goal is, "In the next week, the individual will identify in writing early in the day the two major responsibilities that are of most concern, and for the concern that is most distressing, consider several alternate ways of dealing with it."

Within the activity and rest component of the physiologic mode, the general overall goal is to promote adequate activity and rest for normal growth and development and for restoration, repair, and renewal of energies and effective life processes. Balance is the goal. Activity is balanced with the need for activity, and rest is balanced with the need for rest. These goals are made specific in the many situations that nurses encounter that can interfere with meeting these needs for activity and rest. For example, the individual's rest needs may be adequately met in terms of length and quality of sleep, but if the individual's ongoing physical stress level is beyond the available energy level, a negative energy balance indicates the need to set a goal related to increasing the quality and quantity of rest. Similarly, in earlier examples of the individuals with heart disease or a fever, the need for rest increases; providing more rest becomes part of the goal of nursing care to achieve balance of this need. Since nurses often see patients during times of change that affect their activity and rest, they are in a position to develop preventive goals rather than allow consequences of imbalances in activity and rest to occur. Based on knowledge related to movement and sleep processes, and the specific goals for the individual, the nurse plans appropriate nursing interventions.

Nursing Intervention for Activity and Mobility

Each step of the nursing process provides direction for the nursing intervention stage. The goal focuses on the behavioral description of the patient situation. The nursing interventions address the context of the behaviors, that is, the focal, contextual, and residual stimuli, and the individual's ability to cope with these using regulator and cognator processes. Understanding this combined effect on individuals and their abilities is the basis for helping the individual to handle the experience in the direction of positive adaptation. Nursing measures used to promote adequate activity include health teaching to promote physical activity that maintains physical fitness, removing any discomfort or restriction that is unnecessarily limiting movement, providing timely feedback in reestablishing neurologic control of movement, and careful planning of preventive measures for those who must be immobilized. Two nursing interventions are significant in promoting health for individuals and the community as a whole.

HEALTH TEACHING   Health teaching to promote exercise for physical fitness involves both information and motivational factors. It has been noted that, although exercise is recognized as enhancing health, many people in the United States do not include enough physical activity in their daily lives. In health teaching, the nurse acknowledges with the individual the difficulties of establishing and maintaining an adequate exercise program and identifies with the individual the particular barriers and positive influences. The benefits of exercise are stressed, and accurate information is provided about exercise recommendations. Just as immobility affects all body systems and the four adaptive modes, so, too, does physical activity benefit the individual as a whole being. Positive effects have been shown on the functioning of the cardiovascular, respiratory, and musculoskeletal systems, as well as improved metabolism, nutrition, and bowel elimination. In addition, exercise positively affects self-esteem, intellectual activity, and social and emotional status. Evidence shows that a primary benefit of regular physical activity is protection against coronary artery disease. Likewise, regular exercise appears to provide some protection against such chronic conditions as hypertension, adult-onset diabetes, some cancers, osteoporosis, and mental health changes such as depression. The nurse can teach the individual to assess physical fitness in relation to needs for activity using five criteria: cardiovascular endurance, muscle strength and endurance, joint flexibility, body weight and composition, and motor performance skill. The nurse helps the individual to use insight into personal needs, to problem solve, and to plan within the given social context to create a healthy lifestyle. The following recommendations for exercise have received backing from the U.S. Centers for Disease Control and Prevention and the American College of Sports Medicine.

1. Individuals should engage in a total of 30 minutes of moderate-intensity exercise over the course of most days of the week. The individual is not required to do all 30 minutes during one session, but can accumulate this total throughout the day. Walking, gardening, dancing, and walking up stairs rather than taking the elevator are all ways to incorporate more physical activity into daily life. People can also fulfill this recommendation through planned exercise or recreation such as tennis, swimming, or cycling.
2. People who do no exercise should begin by incorporating even a few minutes of exercise into their daily routine with the goal of eventually reaching 30 minutes per day. Activities to increase joint flexibility and muscle strength should also be included.

PREVENTIVE MEASURES   Preventive measures for those who must be immobilized are important in care of hospitalized people, as well as for the elderly or debilitated at home or in long-term care facilities. Nursing intervention for disuse syndrome has general and specific aspects. The general aspect includes those preventive measures that promote maintenance of normal movement functions. By promoting an individual's movement, the nurse facilitates accomplishment of daily living tasks and also helps provide the body with the physical stresses that are essential in maintaining the internal physiologic functions. In planning preventive nursing interventions, the nurse takes the nature and extent of medically imposed restrictions into consideration. As noted earlier, at times, a period of complete bed rest or other limited movement is medically indicated; therefore, the nurse cannot manage the focal stimulus, that is, the enforced physical inactivity. However, other factors are managed through well-planned preventive measures so that disuse syndrome is avoided and the effects of immobility are minimized without impeding the purpose of the needed temporary immobilization. A similar situation exists when pathology of the neuromuscular skeletal system limits mobility, as in the case of paraplegia. General preventive nursing interventions include the following four major principles: maintenance of good body alignment, frequent change of positions, maintenance of joint mobility, and conditioning of muscles. These nursing interventions are summarized in column 4 of Table 8–1.

GOOD BODY ALIGNMENT   As noted, good body alignment is a body posture in which the body parts are arranged in an anatomically functional position and the weight distribution is well balanced in a stable manner. The normal functional standing position is shown in Figure 8–4. Good body alignment is assumed in all body positions. For example, in the supine, or lying position, the body is in full extension, resembling the upright position. Incorrect body alignment or posture will impose undue stresses on muscles, ligaments, and joints. Poor body alignment that is frequent or prolonged can leave permanent defects such as flexion contracture of the neck or foot drop. These outcomes are not uncommon among bedridden patients.

POSITIONING   Disuse syndrome is a direct result of static body positions for prolonged periods of time. Changing the patient's position is another way to manage the major stimulus for these consequences. The supine position is the most common position assumed by ill individuals. For some patients, this static position becomes prolonged without spontaneous body movements, for example, in situations of paralysis or unconsciousness. Frequent changes of position with proper body alignment are provided to prevent nerve damage in the pressure areas, joint contractures, pressure sores, and loss of the postural adjustment mechanism for the maintenance of central blood pressure in the upright position. Within mobility restrictions, body position can include many different positions including prone, that is, lying on the stomach. Frequent changes of position not only relieve the pressure of body weight, promoting general circulation, but the movement of changing positions also facilitates dislodging of bodily discharges, such as mucus secretions of the respiratory tract. An active change of position to a sitting-up position is effective in maintenance of the postural adjustment mechanism and consequently prevents the symptoms of postural hypotension (lowered blood pressure upon standing). At times, it is easy to think that sitting up in a chair is too big a task for a particular patient. However, the nurse knows that, although the process of struggling to get out of the bed and moving to a chair takes a lot of effort on the parts of both the patient and the nurse, the benefits of such movement, when within therapeutically indicated limits, are paramount. This activity provides almost all of the physical exercises that contribute to the prevention of disuse syndrome.

MOBILIZATION   To maintain joint mobility, either active or passive exercises are done. In active range-of-motion (ROM) exercise, the patient initiates and completes the full range of motion (see Figure 8–3). For an individual who is too weak or is partially paralyzed, assisted or passive ROM exercising is accomplished. In assisted ROM exercise, the individual initiates the movement but requires assistance to complete the full range of motion. For a paralyzed or unconscious individual, passive ROM exercises are done, that is, initiating and completing the full range of motion is accomplished by the nurse. The involved limb is supported at all times during the motion to prevent straining the muscles and ligaments. Passive limb movement does not involve muscle contractions as in active motion. Therefore, it does not achieve muscle conditioning but it is effective in preventing joint contractures. Joint motion exercise is never carried out beyond the point of pain or resistance.

MUSCLE CONDITIONING   There are several types of exercises that contribute to muscle conditioning. The primary purpose of muscle conditioning exercise is to prevent muscular atrophy and weakening. However, because muscle exercise provides physical stress on other structures, it aids, to some extent, in promotion of general circulation and prevention of osteoporosis. All active body movements, such as lifting and moving objects, induce isotonic exercise. In isotonic exercise, the muscle fibers shorten during the muscle contraction and the joint moves. This is distinguished from isometric exercise, which is performed to maintain muscle tone without moving the joint. A setting exercise is an example of an isometric exercise. Muscle setting is accomplished simply by purposefully contracting or hardening of a group of muscles for 10 seconds and then releasing to relax. This type of exercise is effective in conditioning the abdominal, gluteal, and quadriceps muscles. The use of isometric exercise requires a certain degree of caution. During the muscle-setting period, intrathoracic pressure increases due to the trapping of air against the closed epiglottis, a phenomenon called the Valsalva maneuver. The Valsalva maneuver can precipitate cardiac arrest in an individual who has a damaged heart. This untoward reaction occurs because the increased intrathoracic pressure prevents normal cardiac input, and subsequently decreases cardiac output and the coronary circulation. In any case, if this type of exercise is instituted, the individual is taught to exhale during the muscle-setting period.

Resistive exercise is another form of muscle conditioning. This exercise is done by pulling or pushing against a stationary object. Because of its pumping effect on the venous system, this type of exercise is effective not only for muscle conditioning, but also in stimulating venous return. Simple activity such as pushing the feet against a foot board is effective for conditioning the gastrocnemius and quadriceps muscles. Pulling on the trapeze bar is effective for conditioning the upper arms and shoulder muscles. Basic nursing skills textbooks provide detailed steps for instituting these exercises. Further, the nurse works with other members of the health care team including physiotherapists and occupational therapists who have special expertise in this area.

REHABILITATION   Nurses are involved in rehabilitation, a nursing intervention involving the whole individual and often focusing on activity needs. Rehabilitation is an active and dynamic process through which an individual achieves optimal physical, emotional, psychological, social, and vocational potential. Basic premises include maintaining dignity and personal wholeness in a life that is as independent and self-fulfilling as possible. The Association of Rehabilitation Nurses defines their practice as facilitating individuals, through optimum adaptation, to reengage in the mainstream of living whereby each individual functions maximally within the environment. Rehabilitation programs for cardiac, respiratory, and neuromuscular conditions are common. Cancer rehabilitation programs are less common but Beck (2003) pointed out that they need to be developed further because of the increase in diagnoses of cancer and the increase in the rate of survival. An individual's goals for rehabilitation may range from employment or reemployment for the handicapped person to the more limited achievement of developing self-care abilities. Restoration to former capacity may be possible in some situations such as a mild head injury or mild stroke. However, in other situations, such as severe head injury, paralyzing spinal cord injury, or major stroke, complete recovery of function may not be possible and permanent disability is likely. In this case, the individual and the family are helped to accept, adjust to, and compensate for the existing deficit and to establish an optimal level of function.

Nursing protocols during rehabilitation directed at preventing disability include skin care, positioning and alignment, frequent turning, and range-of-motion exercises. The nurse helps to maintain intact skills and functions by encouraging the patient to be as independent as possible in activities of daily living. The nurse's participation is key in exercise programs aimed at restoring functions, particularly mobility. Details of prevention, maintenance, and restoration protocols can be found in textbooks on rehabilitation. Rehabilitation programs include many health care providers working in collaboration with the patient and family. However, the nurse spends the most time with the patient on a daily basis and can help coordinate a schedule so that optimum benefit is derived from rehabilitation activities. The patient needs a high energy and motivation level for demanding activity such as learning ambulation. Nursing knowledge of mobility processes and of feedback as a compensatory process in learning efficient movement can be helpful throughout the rehabilitation process. An example of use of this knowledge may be with a patient who has neuromuscular deficits that affect mobility of one side. This may be the result of a stroke on the side of the brain that controls motor programs for the opposite side of the body. The patient may be receiving occupational therapy to learn to eat independently. In helping the patient with an evening meal, the nurse is aware of the need for added feedback to relearn motor movements. The patient is directed to visually scan the tray, and verbal cues are provided as the patient reaches for items on the tray. Past-pointing errors are common after certain types of brain damage, but can be overcome with coaching to relearn the motor program involved.

ILLUSTRATION OF NURSING INTERVENTIONS FOR ACTIVITY NEEDS   An illustration of specific planning of nursing interventions to meet activity needs is provided for an individual who suddenly is hospitalized with a broken pelvis suffered in an automobile accident. Two nursing diagnoses for this individual are: (1) good muscle tone and 4+ muscle strength in major muscle groups of all four extremities related to knowledge of health benefits of

fitness and commitment to regular exercise program; and (2) potential for disuse consequences related to sudden, therapeutically enforced immobility and age of 62 years. A number of long- and short-term goals are indicated, each with nursing interventions that identify
stimuli that can be managed to reach the goal.

For the first goal, the nurse plans a series of nursing interventions. The patient is involved in self-care activities as soon as possible after admission. Simple activities such as
participating in bathing, combing the hair, shaving, or putting on makeup in bed allows the
pulling and weight bearing of active movement. This is effective in muscle conditioning, as
well as stimulating general circulation and promoting mobility of joints. Even though the exercises done in the hospital will be different from the individual's usual pattern of exercise,
they are even more important at this time. The nurse describes the exercises and their specific
purpose, recognizing strengths within the individual such as knowledge of health benefits and
commitment to regular exercise. Then, the patient is involved in setting up a schedule of muscle strengthening exercises for the upper extremities that includes lifting on a trapeze bar, increasing the number of times and the frequency gradually. Since pushing and pulling against
a stationary object is important, the nurse can use ingenuity to provide such an object, such as
stabilizing the over-bed table.

To maintain an effective exercise program, the nurse focuses on the individual's
knowledge and commitment, the scheduled use of muscles that are the primary target, providing the equipment to complete the exercises, and providing an environment that does not
restrict the program, for example, conflicting schedule of therapies. For this particular
patient, a chart of progress of muscle strength can be made. The patient and the nurse will
recognize that some unavoidable muscle weakness can occur early in the program. However,
keeping the long-term goal in mind is useful. Knowing that, even if this goal is not achieved,
the individual will be better ready to undertake the next stage of rehabilitation than if the
muscle strengthening program had not been instituted and carefully carried out is encouraging for both patient and nurse.

Nursing Interventions for Rest and Sleep

Some general measures for promoting quality rest and sleep by managing the major stimuli
identified earlier include the following: provision of physical comfort, alleviation of psychological stresses, structuring daily activity schedule, structuring a restful environment, and
controlled use of hypnotic drugs and alcohol.

PHYSICAL COMFORT   Since physical pain and discomfort are among the most common
causes for disruption in rest and sleep, providing physical comfort is a method of relief from
the disruption. Good personal hygiene aids physical comfort and improves the quality of rest
and sleep. A warm bath can be relaxing. For some people, spicy food may interfere with
sleep. This possibility, as well as whether or not the individual is hungry, is discussed with the
individual and remedied as appropriate. Soothing backrubs can be comforting and effective in
inducing sleep. As noted earlier, mere physical inactivity does not provide good-quality rest.
In some situations, administration of an analgesic medication is indicated for relief of pain to
enhance comfort. Appropriate timing of analgesic administration is important. For patients in
pain, the nurse is not concerned with long-term drug dependency (see Chapter 10). However,
the choice of drug is made carefully so that the individual does not experience the consequences of REM sleep deprivation.

ALLEVIATION OF PSYCHOLOGICAL STRESS   Alleviation of psychological stress may be necessary to allow for rest and sleep. The nurse provides the individual with opportunities to ventilate feelings of fear, anxiety, and frustration. In a hospital setting, lack of knowledge or understanding of what is happening often generates feelings of powerlessness. These feelings can trigger anxiety (see Chapter 14). Sometimes it is a misperception or incorrect understanding that causes unnecessary anxiety. The nurse is in a position to check out the patient's understanding of the situation and its particular personal meaning. She is sensitive to the individual's subtle, as well as obvious, behaviors indicating distress and interfering with restful sleep. From the individual's perspective, then, the nurse can help in dealing appropriately with these factors, focal or contextual, that are interfering with rest and sleep.

For people in the hospital or at home, anxiety about not sleeping can be the psychological stress that is focal in disturbing sleep. Researchers have noted that trying too hard to sleep aggravates the problem. When struggling with the need for sleep and the inability to fall asleep, feelings of anxiety, frustration, and anger can trigger arousal and tension. Practical nursing interventions to deal with these situations have been suggested. They include going to bed only when sleepy and using the bed only for sexual activity and sleeping, not reading or watching television. If an individual is unable to fall asleep in about 20 minutes, getting up and going to another room until sleepy or turning the clock toward the wall may assist. With wakefulness during the night, likewise, it is suggested that the individual get up and return to bed only when sleepy. Finally, it is useful to awake at the same time every day and not to take daytime naps. Eventually, going to bed is associated with rapidly falling asleep.

PHYSICAL ACTIVITY   As noted earlier, physical activity induces NREM sleep; therefore, adequate amounts of physical activity, within the individual's restrictions, are worked into the daily schedule. However, any vigorous physical activity or events that trigger strong emotional responses are avoided near bedtime. Every effort is made to ensure that the sleep cycles can take their full course so that the individual will not suffer from REM sleep deprivation. Treatment procedures and other activities are grouped together in such a way that the number of interruptions is kept to a minimum. Each sleep cycle takes 90 or more minutes. Therefore, scheduling the interruptions at about 2-hour intervals will allow each sleep cycle to take its full course. A large amount of food and fluid taken in the late evening will require unnecessarily frequent arousals caused by increased gastrointestinal and bladder stimulations. Any drugs that have a diuretic effect are not administered at bedtime. For healthy people, moderate exercise used consistently can lengthen and deepen sleep.

RESTFUL ENVIRONMENT   In structuring a restful environment, the nurse takes into consideration the individual's personal habits and bedtime routine. The environment in general is to be free of all kinds of noxious stimuli. Room temperature, light, noise, and odor are checked out for suitability. Unavoidable, but unpleasant, noise can be disguised by pleasant music. People will differ in the degree of quiet needed for restful sleep. Some need absolute quiet and others prefer some background noise. Increasingly, it is possible to arrange the environment differently for each patient as more hospitals have private rooms. The effect of a strange environment on an individual's sleep usually does not last more than 3 or 4 days. This information can help the individual control anxiety about changes in sleep pattern in the hospital. Special care units present problems in establishing a restful environment by reason of their equipment and activities. Nonetheless, the nurse strives to make this environment as conducive to rest and sleep as possible. The nurse can emphasize a sense of security in the constant watchfulness of the individual's condition throughout the night. The careful scheduling of activities as noted is particularly relevant in these settings. In this case, however, activity for one patient may affect another patient more readily because of the physical setup of many units. Sometimes it is staff conversation, a stimulus easily managed by the nurse, that is most disturbing to the patient.

HYPNOTIC DRUGS Lastly, hypnotic drugs are controlled carefully and used in selected situations for sleep since they have been identified as related to quality of sleep and rest. The same is true of alcohol, particularly when it is used habitually for sleep. The nurse explains that such substances are effective on a short-term basis only and that they tend to suppress restful or REM sleep. The individual is encouraged to restrict their use. The nurse then assists the individual to find alternate means to promote sleep. Given the scope and variety of settings and situations that call for individually designed nursing interventions to assist people with activity and rest needs, careful evaluation of the effectiveness of these nursing interventions is particularly important.

Evaluation

As in each of the modes of adaptation, with the physiologic need for activity and rest, the evaluation phase of the nursing process reflects the behavioral assessment. In the example given earlier, an individual who reported poor sleep pattern, with eyes showing evidence of sleep deprivation, related to a recent change in job responsibilities, returns to the clinic with the same behaviors that the nurse noted 1 week earlier. That is, the individual reports difficulty falling asleep and frequent arousals from sleep during the night, as well as having reddened eyes, puffy eyelids, dark circles under the eyes, and feelings of poor sleep. This individual also reports continuing concerns about the responsibilities associated with the job promotion. As related by the patient, these concerns have been intensified by difficulty in identifying in writing the 2 major responsibilities that are of concern and frustration in trying to develop strategies to handle this part of the job. The individual is also more anxious about the sleep disturbance and struggles with efforts to go to sleep and with concern about meeting the short-term goal set for beginning to handle the difficulty. The nurse notes evidence of unclear and slightly confused thinking (see Chapter 12), possibly related to ongoing sleep disturbance.

Since the behaviors of interest have not changed and the nurse is concerned about the increasing behavioral signs of the problem worsening, she provides the individual with specific instructions for moderate active exercises at noontime and relaxation exercises to use at bedtime. She also decides to have the patient evaluated for the prescription of a short-term hypnotic. The nurse then asks the individual to come back for a morning appointment in 3 days, after getting some sleep, so that they can work together on the problem. The goals of identifying in writing the two major job responsibilities that are of most concern and developing several alternate ways of dealing with the most distressing concern will again be attempted. The nurse will provide guidance in the use of a problem-solving process. This example shows a revision in the nursing intervention plan based on evaluation of an ineffective nursing intervention and assessment of additional behaviors.

Summary

In this chapter, the Roy Adaptation Model was used as a perspective from which to view activity and rest needs. The theoretical basis related to this need was developed that includes the processes of mobility and sleep. Related compensatory adaptive processes were identified, as well as examples of compromised processes. Each step of the nursing process was discussed and demonstrated with examples of behavior and stimuli, of nursing diagnoses, goals, and nursing interventions as well as evaluation of the effectiveness of nursing care.

Exercises for Application

1. Identify the focal and contextual stimuli that influenced the amount of physical activity you engaged in on a particular day in the past week.
2. Develop a tool that can be used in the assessment of rest and sleep. In your tool consider both the usual pattern and current condition.
3. Using the tool developed in item 2, assess the rest and sleep needs of one person under 25 and one person over 60 years of age.

Assessment of Understanding

QUESTIONS

1. The basic life process associated with activity is (a) _____ and with rest is (b) _____. Describe each of these concepts.
2. Describe a compensatory process associated with the need for activity and rest that was not included in the discussion in the chapter.

SITUATION:

Mrs. Liu is a 73-year-old widow with a social history of no known relatives or close friends who can visit her during her hospital stay. While waiting for a major surgical procedure for a fractured left femur, she is placed on the activity restriction of complete bed rest. Without a properly planned preventive nursing intervention, Mrs. Liu likely will develop some of the very serious disuse consequences.

3. For Mrs. Liu identify the disuse consequences that can occur in 3 of the following bodily functions: metabolic, musculoskeletal, circulatory, pulmonary, eliminative, integumentary, and sensory perceptual.

4. Label the following first-level assessment behaviors as to whether they are associated with the need for activity (A), rest (R), or both (B).
   (a) _____ 24-hour pattern of activities
   (b) _____ self-report of status
   (c) _____ muscle mass and tone
   (d) _____ joint mobility
   (e) _____ lifestyle
   (f) _____ gait
   (g) _____ irritability and restlessness
5. Name 3 contextual stimuli that affect activity and rest.
6. Formulate a nursing diagnosis for Mrs. Liu.
7. Develop a short-term and a long-term goal statement for Mrs. Liu.
8. Understanding that repair and restoration take place during rest and sleep, you are trying to improve the quality of sleep for Mrs. Liu. List at least 2 major nursing interventions to accomplish this.
9. What would be the behavior that would indicate that Mrs. Liu had achieved the goals developed in your answer to question 7?

FEEDBACK

1. (a) Mobility: the process whereby one moves or is moved.
   (b) Sleep: the process whereby most of the body's physiologic activities slow down to accomplish renewal of energy for future activity.
2. Examples: At times, it is important to stay awake rather than fall asleep, for example, if you have to drive a distance. Some people use caffeine, loud music, or conversation to help them avoid sleep when occasionally required. Stopping frequently to assess alertness is important.

   Some people find a repetitive activity (counting "sheep") is helpful to divert their mind and induce sleep.

   When the ability to move about is limited, for example, when nurses in the operating room are "scrubbed" on a case or for chorus members during a lengthy performance, circulation in the leg muscles is maintained by repeatedly moving the toes.
3. Metabolic: negative nitrogen balance.
   Musculoskeletal: osteoporosis, joint contractures, denervations.
   Circulatory: postural hypotension, dependent edema, thrombosis.
   Pulmonary: hypoventilation.
   Eliminative: urinary retention, kidney stones, constipation.
   Integumentary: pressure ulcers.
   Sensory perceptual: disorientation, confusion, anxiety.
4. (a) B, (b) B, (c) A, (d) A, (e) B, (f) A, (g) R
5. Physical condition, psychological condition, environment, or personal habits.
6. Example of nursing diagnosis: Potential for disuse consequences related to the activity restrictions associated with bed rest.
7. Example of short-term goal: Prior to surgery, Mrs. Liu will be actively participating in range-of-motion exercises for unaffected muscle groups.
   Example of long-term goal: Within 3 hours of surgery, Mrs. Liu. will sit in a chair for 10 minutes, or within 5 days following surgery, Mrs. Liu. will achieve sufficient mobility to enable her to return home with assistance provided as required.
8. Any two of the following:
   Maintain physical comfort and freedom from pain.
   Maintain an adequate amount of physical activity in order to induce deep sleep.
   Limit nighttime interruptions to a minimum to allow full cycles of sleep to take place.
   Alleviate psychological stress, which may increase need for REM sleep.
9. Examples: Mrs. Liu demonstrates and reports doing the range-of-motion exercises for unaffected muscle groups at regular intervals.
   Mrs. Liu expresses understanding of the importance of early mobilization following surgery and accomplishes sitting in a chair for 10 minutes within the first 3 hours after surgery.
   Mrs. Liu is confident with her ability to get around and, with required assistance provided in her home, is discharged from the hospital in 5 days.

References

Anderson, M. A. (2007). Activity, rest, and sleep as criteria for health. In M. A. Anderson (Ed.), *Caring for older adults holistically* (4th ed., pp. 120–132). Philadelphia: F. A. Davis.

Beck, L. A. (2003). Cancer rehabilitation: Does it make a difference? *Rehabilitation Nursing, 28*(2), 42–47.

Benson, H. (1975). The Relaxation Response. New York: William Morrow and Company.

Benson-Henry Institute for Mind Body Medicine. (2006). *Elicit the relaxation response.* Retrieved from http://www.mbmi.org/basics/whatis_rresponse_elicitation.asp

Bronstein, K. S. (2001). Human mobility: An overview. In C. Stewart-Amidei & J. A. Kunkel (Eds.), *AANN's Neuroscience Nursing: Human responses to neurologic dysfunction* (2nd ed., pp. 407–424). Philadelphia: W. B. Saunders

Burrell, L. O., Gerlach, M. J. M., & Pless, B. S. (1997). *Adult nursing: Acute and community care* (2nd ed.). Stamford, CT: Appleton & Lange.

Dossey, B., Buzzetta, C., & Kenner, C. (1992). *Critical care nursing: Body-mind-spirit.* Philadelphia: Lippincott.

Dworetzky, T. D. (1987, October). The willowy six-footer that bends at the waist. *Discover, 18.*

Friedman, D. (1993). Sleep disorders. In B. Long, W. Phipps, & V. Cassmeyer (Eds.), *Medical-surgical nursing: A nursing process approach* (pp. 228–243). St. Louis, MO: Mosby.

Hilton, J. (1976). Quantity and quality of patients' sleep: Disturbing factors in respiratory intensive care unit. *Journal of Advanced Nursing, 1*, 453–468.

Ignatavicius, D., & Workman, L. (2002). Medical-surgical nursing: Critical thinking for collaborative care. (4th ed.) Philadelphia: W. B. Saunders Company.

Lee, K. A. (2003). Impaired sleep. In V. Carrieri-Kohlman, A. M. Lindsey, & C. M. West (Eds.), *Pathophysiological phenomena in nursing: Human responses to illness* (3rd ed.). St. Louis, MO: Saunders.

Marieb, E. N., & Hoehn, K. (2007). *Human anatomy and physiology* (7th ed.). San Francisco: Pearson Benjamin Cummings.

NANDA-International. (2007). *Nursing diagnoses: Definitions and classifications, 2007–2008.* Philadelphia: NANDA-I.

Sacks, O. (1983). *Awakenings.* New York: Dutton.

Taylor, C., Lillis, C., & LeMone, P. (2001). *Fundamentals of nursing: The art and science of nursing care* (4th ed.). Philadelphia: Lippincott.

U.S. Department of Health and Human Services. (1995). *Healthy people 2000: Mid-course review and 1995 revisions.* Washington, DC: Public Health Service.

U.S. Department of Health and Human Services. (2000, Jan.). *Healthy people 2010: Vol. 1 and 2* (Conference Edition). Washington, DC: Centers for Disease Control and Prevention, President's Council on Physical Fitness and Sports.

Wickens, A. (2000). *Foundations of psychology.* Harlow, England: Pearson Education Limited.

Additional References

Smith-Temple, J., & Johnson, J. Y. (2002). *Nurses' guide to clinical procedures* (4th ed.) Philadelphia: Lippincott.

CHAPTER 9

Protection

Protection is the fifth basic need identified in the physiologic mode of the individual person in the Roy Adaptation Model. This mode component includes important adaptation processes. Through life processes of defense, the body is protected against disease and integrity is maintained. The body has both nonspecific and specific protection processes. The nonspecific defenses include both surface membrane barriers and cellular and chemical defenses. However, it is the immune system that constitutes the specific defense process of the body. Working together, these complex processes serve a vital role in meeting the need for protection by providing lines of defense against the invasion of disease-causing substances. This protection against disease promotes adaptation.

In this chapter, the basic life processes associated with protection—nonspecific defense processes and specific defense processes—are addressed. Examples of compensatory and compromised processes related to protection are described. Finally, guidelines for planning nursing care are described including assessment of behaviors and stimuli, formulating diagnoses, establishing goals, selecting nursing interventions, and evaluating nursing care.

OBJECTIVES

After studying this chapter, the reader will be able to do the following:

1. Describe two basic life processes associated with the need for protection as presented in the chapter.
2. Describe one compensatory process related to each of the basic life processes associated with protection.
3. Name and describe two situations of compromised processes of protection.
4. Identify first-level assessment factors, that is, behaviors, associated with the need for protection.
5. For second-level assessment, identify common stimuli that affect protection.
6. Develop a nursing diagnosis, given a situation related to protection.
7. Derive goals for an individual with ineffective protection in a given situation.

8. Describe nursing interventions commonly implemented in situations of ineffective protection.

9. Propose approaches to determine the effectiveness of nursing interventions.

KEY CONCEPTS DEFINED

Antibody-mediated immunity: Specific defense processes involving antibodies in the body's fluids.

Antigens: Substances such as proteins, nucleic acids, large carbohydrates, and some lipids that trigger the immune system.

Antimicrobial chemicals: Nonspecific defense chemicals that include interferons, complement, and urine.

Cell-mediated immunity: Specific defense processes involving lymphocytes and macrophages.

Complement: A group of about 20 plasma proteins that causes destructive lesions in foreign cells and amplifies the inflammatory response.

Fever: Abnormally high systemic body temperature that inhibits multiplication of bacteria and increases metabolic rate to enhance repair processes.

Immune system: A functional system that recognizes foreign molecules (antigens) and acts to inactivate or destroy them (Marieb & Hoehn, 2007, p. 379).

Immunity: The ability of the body to resist disease-causing agents. Active immunity is produced by an encounter with an antigen. Passive immunity is short-lived immunity resulting from antibodies obtained from another human or animal donor; no immunologic memory is established.

Immunocompetent: The ability of lymphocytes to respond to a specific antigen.

Inflammatory response: The body's second line of defense; initiated when cells are injured. Inflammatory chemicals cause blood vessels to dilate, capillaries to leak, and neutrophils and monocytes to be attracted to the area.

Interferons: Antimicrobial chemicals released by virus-infected cells to protect uninfected cells from the virus and interfere with the ability of the virus to multiply within the infected cells.

Natural killer cells: Cells that attack and destroy virus-infected or cancerous body cells.

Nonspecific defense processes: Surface membrane barriers and cellular and chemical defenses that function to hinder pathogen entry, prevent the spread of disease-causing microorganisms, and strengthen the immune response.

Phagocytes: Defense cells (nonspecific) that engulf and digest pathogens that enter the body through the mechanical barriers.

Pressure ulcers: Any lesions resulting from unrelieved pressure that causes damage to underlying tissue.

Pus: A mixture of dead or dying cells and living and dead pathogens; often a product of the inflammatory response.

Specific defense processes: Defense processes that are targeted against specific antigens.

Surface membrane barriers: Intact skin and mucous membranes; the body's first line of defense.

BASIC LIFE PROCESSES OF PROTECTION

The physiologic need of protection is viewed as consisting of two basic life processes: nonspecific defense processes or innate immunity, and specific defense processes or adaptive immunity. Together these two functional defense systems work to protect the body from foreign substances such as bacteria, viruses, parasites, and abnormal body cells.

Nonspecific Defenses: Innate Immunity Processes

Innate immunity involves a nonspecific immune response, targeting a variety of different pathogens. The system is comprised of four defense mechanisms: anatomic, physiologic, phagocytic, and inflammatory, which work together to prevent the spread of disease and initiate the adaptive immune response (Goldsby, Kindt, & Osborne, 2000). These systems include both surface membrane barriers and cellular and chemical processes. The surface membrane barriers involve the skin and mucous membranes. The cellular and chemical defenses include phagocytes, natural killer cells, the inflammatory response, antimicrobial chemicals, and fever. According to Marieb and Hoehn (2007), the innate immune system functions "to reduce the workload of the second protective arm, the specific defense system, by preventing entry and spread of microorganisms throughout the body" (p. 373).

ANATOMIC BARRIERS Anatomic barriers, consisting of intact skin and mucous membranes, are the body's first line of defense. Unbroken skin forms a barrier against pathogens and other harmful substances. The skin's two distinct layers, the epidermis and dermis, work together to protect the body from pathogens. The epidermis creates the outer layer of the skin and consists of keratin, a tough, insoluble protein (Marieb & Hoehn, 2007). Keratin is an important aspect of protection, resisting acids, alkalis, and bacterial enzymes, thus preventing them from invading the body. The dermis contains blood vessels, sebaceous glands, and sweat glands enabling further protection against harmful substances. Another substance involved in protection is sebum, an oily substance secreted by the sebaceous glands that contains bacteria-killing chemicals and maintains the skin's pH between 3 and 5. This acidic epithelial surface environment protects against the growth of microbes providing further protection to the body. Additionally, the skin functions to protect deeper tissues from mechanical, chemical, and bacterial damage; ultraviolet radiation and thermal damage; and desiccation or drying out.

Sweat glands in the skin aid the body in heat loss and heat retention, and, through the process of perspiration, aid in the excretion of urea and uric acid. In addition, hairs and hair follicles provide minor protective functions while the nails protect fingers and toes. Mucous membranes, the second component of the anatomic barrier, also function as a physical barrier against pathogens for the body. Mucus in respiratory and digestive tracts traps microorganisms. Nasal hairs filter and trap microorganisms, and cilia in the lower respiratory passages propel debris-laden mucus toward the upper respiratory tract. Secretions in the stomach, vagina, oral cavity, and eyes either destroy pathogens or inhibit the growth of bacteria and fungi.

PHYSIOLOGIC BARRIER Numerous physiologic barriers exist within the body providing further protection against pathogens. These barriers include temperature, stomach pH, and various chemical mediators (Goldsby, Kindt, & Osborne, 2000). The body's normal temperature inhibits growth of certain pathogens. In addition, the extremely acidic gastric environment prevents most pathogens from surviving. The third physiologic component of the innate immune system involves a variety of soluble proteins involved in chemical processes of innate immunity including lysozymes, interferons, and the complement system (Goldsby, Kindt, & Osborne, 2000). Lysozymes are enzymes that can cleave to the bacterial cell wall preventing further invasion and destruction by the pathogen. Inteferons are proteins released by virus-infected cells that have the ability to stimulate the adaptive immune response and protect uninfected tissue (Marieb & Hoehn, 2007). An additional protein system facilitating innate response is complement. Complement, a group of 20 plasma proteins, causes destructive lesions in foreign cells and amplifies the inflammatory response (Marieb & Hoehn, 2007).

PHAGOCYTIC BARRIER Phagocytosis is an important part of the innate immune response and involves both macrophages and neutrophils. Phagocytosis involves the ingestion of pathogens, digestion of the ingested material, and final release of digested products from the phagocytic cell (Goldsby, Kindt, & Osborne, 2000). Phagocytosis is initiated when the macrophage or neutrophil recognizes nonself bodies. To ensure that the body does not destroy healthy cells, the phagocytic cell can distinguish nonself substances from self-substances by recognizing three common nonself characteristics: rough surfaces, lack of a protein coat, and presentation with an antibody/complement system (Guyton & Hall, 2000). Eosinophils also use phagocytosis to remove foreign material from the body; however, they tend to be weak phagocytes, involved in parasite removal (Guyton & Hall, 2000).

INFLAMMATORY BARRIER The inflammatory response is initiated when cells are injured, releasing inflammatory chemicals such as histamine and bradykinin. The substances cause blood vessels to dilate, capillaries to leak, and neutrophils and monocytes to be attracted to the area. The four signs of inflammation are redness, heat, swelling, and pain. As Marieb and Hoehn (2007) noted, the inflammatory response "(1) prevents the spread of damaging agents to nearby tissues, (2) disposes of cell debris and pathogens, and (3) sets the stage for repair" (p. 376). A product of the inflammatory response may be pus, a mixture of dead or dying cells and living and dead pathogens.

Specific Defenses: Adaptive Immunity Processes

The body's second line of defense is the immune system, the body's specific defense processes. Marieb and Hoehn (2007) described the immune system as "a functional system that recognizes foreign molecules (antigens) and acts to inactivate or destroy them" (p. 379). The action of the immune system is "targeted" against specific antigens. It protects the body against a wide variety of pathogens and abnormal body cells by recognizing foreign substances and mounting a systemic and targeted attack against them.

Authors have identified four important aspects of the immune response: antigen specificity, diversity, memory, and self/nonself recognition (Goldsby, Kindt, & Osborne, 2000, p. 10). Antigen specificity indicates that the adaptive immune system is able to recognize and act against particular foreign substances. Second, the adaptive immune system has diversity, an ability to identify a variety of different molecules and differentiate between various foreign antigens. The third aspect of immune response is that it has immunologic memory, recognizing previously encountered pathogens and initiating a stronger, heightened state of immune reactivity to later contacts. Lastly, the immune system is capable of self/nonself recognition, enabling recognition and distinction of self-molecules from foreign (nonself) molecules and establishing an attack only on molecules identified as nonself. These four characteristics allow for recognition of foreign molecules, initiation of an appropriate response from both the innate and specific immune systems, memory of the molecules for future response, and the protection of self molecules from potential destruction, resulting in successful protection for the body's overall health.

Adaptive, also known as specific, immunity consists of two populations of lymphocytes: B lymphocytes and T lymphocytes, creating two types of immune response (Goldsby, Kindt, & Osborne, 2000). B-cell lymphocytes are secreted from the bone marrow and released fully mature, whereas T-cell lymphocytes are produced in the bone marrow and then migrate to the thymus for maturation. Only as they mature do the cells become immunocompetent, that is, capable of responding to a foreign pathogen. It is understood that genes determine resistance to specific foreign substances. The B-cell lymphocytes make up antibody-mediated immunity while the T-lymphocytes create cell-mediated immunity.

Antibody-mediated immunity involves B cells and antibodies, a glycoprotein that recognizes a particular epitope on an antigen and facilitates clearance of the antigen (Goldsby, Kindt, & Osborne, 2000). Antigens, molecules that trigger an immune response, initiate antibody-mediated immunity. Antigens, presented to B cells via Antigen Presenting Cells (APC), include foreign proteins, nucleic acids, many large carbohydrates, and some lipids. The antigens evoke an immune response from the B cells. Two types of B cells respond to an antigen: antibody-secreting plasma cells and memory cells. The antibody secreted from the plasma cell recognizes specific antigens, binds to the antigens, and facilitates destruction and clearance of the foreign antigen from the body. The memory cells subsequently produce membrane-bound antibodies and work to facilitate a faster response to an antigen if presented to the body a second time. Antibody-mediated immunity can be acquired naturally or artificially and can be active or passive in nature. Naturally acquired active immunity occurs through contact with a pathogen or infection, while artificially acquired active immunity is generated artificially by the introduction of dead or attenuated pathogens. Passive immunity is acquired naturally when antibodies pass from the mother to the child either via the placenta before birth or through breast milk after delivery. Passive immunity is provided to an individual with the injection of immune serum (gamma globulin) containing antibodies capable of binding with a specific antigen.

The T-cell lymphocytes in cell-mediated immunity destroy a foreign substance in a different manner than the B-cell lymphocytes. However, the two systems have a collaborative relationship and work concurrently to destroy foreign pathogens in the body. Two types of T cells, the T-helper cell and the T-cytotoxic cell, work together with the B cells to identify and destroy foreign particles. T-helper cells recognize foreign antigens and respond by initiating cytokine secretion to facilitate a stronger immune response (Goldsby, Kindt, & Osborne, 2000). Alternatively, cytotoxic T cells respond to foreign antigens by killing the molecule. The cytotoxic T cells and helper T cells recognize antigens via their T-cell receptor (TCR) and an additional molecule: the major histocompatibility complex (MHC). There are differing presentations of antigens to the T-helper cells by the MHC (Goldsby, Kindt, & Osborne, 2000). Regardless of presentation, the antigen is recognized as foreign and subsequently destroyed.

The information provided in this chapter about nonspecific and specific defense processes related to the need for protection is designed as an overview. The reader is encouraged to seek more detailed information about these important human processes from anatomy and physiology resources. At this point, however, discussion turns to the Compensatory Adaptive Processes and Compromised Processes that occur related to protection. Nurses are aware of these processes to determine an appropriate plan and nursing intervention for the patient, enabling optimal adaptation and functioning.

COMPENSATORY ADAPTIVE PROCESSES

As described in this chapter, the need for protection is met through innate (nonspecific) and adaptive (specific) defense processes. However, when the processes of protection are not stable or adequate, compensatory adaptive processes occur. Viewed as an adaptive system (see Chapter 2), the individual has innate and acquired ways of responding to the changing environment. Further, Roy conceptualizes these complex adaptive dynamics of the individual as coping processes of the regulator and cognator subsystems. The thinking and feeling individual, by way of cognator activity, can do much to affect adaptation levels within the physiologic mode. Cognator and regulator subsystems provide compensatory adaptive responses that extend the effectiveness of behavior in meeting the goals of adaptation. Adaptation levels, as an internal stimulus, can be integrated, compensatory, or compromised.

Compensatory adaptation for protection includes, in many respects, what the nonspecific and specific defense processes are all about, that is, providing lines of defense against the invasion of disease-causing substances. However, under compromised situations, the defense systems are enhanced. The following examples demonstrate symptoms of enhanced inflammatory response. During times of tissue injury, the inflammatory response is initiated resulting in the following four signs: redness, heat, swelling, and pain. Another example of a compensatory adaptation level involves compensation through learning and relates to individuals traveling in a foreign country, particularly one in which the food and water supply is of questionable purity. Travelers have learned that it is important to carefully assess the food to be eaten for the possibility of contamination and to rely on a dependable supply of bottled water or other processed beverages for fluids.

The development and application of immunization programs represents an organized and massive undertaking to provide a compensatory adaptation level for entire populations. As described earlier, scientists have learned that it is possible to assist immune systems to develop protection against specific communicable diseases. Through immunization programs, many infectious diseases have been virtually eradicated. The immunization process for the individual and programs for the community can be regarded as a learned (cognator) activity indicative of compensatory adaptation.

COMPROMISED PROCESSES OF PROTECTION

When adaptation levels are neither integrated nor compensatory, compromise leads to adaptation problems. Adaptation problems can be caused by difficulties in any or all of the processes of protection. With respect to the need for protection, eight compromised processes are identified. They are disrupted skin integrity, pressure ulcers, itching, delayed wound healing, infection, allergic reaction, ineffective coping with changes in immune status, and ineffective temperature regulation. Three specific examples of compromised processes of protection are further explored: pressure ulcers, hyperallergic reaction, and ineffective coping with changes in immune status.

Pressure Ulcers

Pressure ulcers are any lesions resulting from unrelieved pressure that causes damage to underlying tissue. It is estimated that approximately 9% of all hospitalized patients and 23% of all individual care home residents are affected by pressure ulcers (Agency for Health Care Policy and Research, 1994). According to Pieper (2000), many factors contribute to pressure ulcer development including pressure, shear force, friction, moisture, nutritional debilitation, and lack of adequate tissue oxygenation. Prolonged localized pressure on bony prominences such as the sacrum, ischial tuberosity, trochanter, and calcaneus cause tissue necrosis, which results in ulceration. A broad range of tissue damage can occur in pressure ulcers as indicated by the National Pressure Ulcer Advisory Panel (NPUAP) staging system. Stage I involves a slight alteration in intact skin; Stage II involves a partial-thickness skin loss involving the epidermis, dermis, or both; Stage III is full-thickness skin loss with tissue damage that may extend down but not through the underlying fascia; and Stage IV involves a full-thickness skin loss with extensive destruction to muscle, bone, and supporting structure (Doughty et al., 2006). Tissue damage creates additional health care problems for the patient, altering the skin's ability to provide protection, adding additional stressors to the compromised system. In addition, pressure ulcers add additional burden to the health care system, requiring additional treatment and increasing cost. A review from the Agency for Health Care Policy and Research (AHCPR) indicates that pressure ulcers prolong hospitalization, increase health care cost, and decrease patient quality of life, thus the need for appropriate assessment and nursing intervention (Agostini, Baker, & Boagardus, 2001). Preventive measures will be addressed later in this chapter.

Hyperallergic Reaction

In some instances, the immune system elicits such a large response to foreign antigens that inflammation and tissue damage result, termed Hypersensitivity Disorders (Porth, 2005). As described by Porth (2005, p. 412), four types of hypersensitivity disorders exist. Type I hypersensitivity is an immediate hypersensitivity response, elicited by the IgE antibody, resulting in a massive release of mast cells. This type of hypersensitivity disorder is often coined an "allergic reaction." Bronchial asthma and food allergies are examples of Type I hypersensitivity disorder. Type II disorders involve the humoral immune response, and result in direct injury or destruction of cells. Blood transfusion reactions and drug reactions are examples of Type II disorders. Type III disorders involve antibody clumping, called immune complexes, which elicit complement response, neutrophil recruitment, and subsequent inflammation. Tissue injury and vasculitis result, causing the damage seen in autoimmune diseases such as systemic lupus erythematosus (SLE) and acute glomerulonephritis. Type IV is the last hypersensitivity disorder and is T-cell mediated. T cells elicit cytokines and elicit a massive immune response resulting in tissue damage. Contact dermatitis and hypersensitivity pneumonitis are examples of Type IV hypersensitivity reaction.

The nurse will be aware of the altered immune responses that result from hypersensitivity disorders. While a normal immune response results in better health outcomes, an excessive immune response can hinder the patient's health. The hypersensitivity disorders can greatly compromise the health of the patient. Further, these disorders are occurring more frequently. The Centers for Disease Control (CDC) reports that from 1980 to 1996 asthma prevalence among children increased 4.3% and was the third ranking cause of pediatric hospitalization in the United States (CDC, 2007). Additionally, irritant contact dermatitis is the most common occupational skin disease in the United States with a rise in incidence (National Institute for Occupational Safety and Health (NIOSH), 2007). The increased incidence and level of harm that result from hyperallergic reactions clearly indicates that nurses will be aware of compromised immune reactions and be able to assess, report, and provide appropriate nursing interventions to limit the immune response in these disorders.

Immunodeficiency

Ineffective coping with changes in immune status is particularly evident in immunodeficiency disorders. Defective function of one or more mechanisms of the immune system results in inadequate protection for the body against microbial infections or other antigens. These disorders are classified as either primary, when there is improper development of the immune system, or secondary, if it results from depression of the immune system from environmental factors or infection. Examples of primary immunodeficiency disorders include X-linked hypogammaglobulinemia, DiGeorge syndrome, and severe combined immunodeficiency (SCID), whereas examples of secondary disorders include Hodgkins disease and acquired immunodeficiency syndrome (AIDS) (Porth, 2005).

Of particular significance in the 1990s and early twenty-first century is acquired immunodeficiency syndrome (AIDS), described by the U.S. Secretary of Health and Human Services (Marieb & Hoehn, 2007, p. 366) as the "plague of the twentieth century." As of 2006, 39.5 million adults and children are living with HIV/AIDS throughout the world (UNAIDS, 2006). As Marieb and Hoehn (2007) described

> AIDS is characterized by severe weight loss, night sweats, swollen lymph nodes, and increasingly frequent infections, including a rare type of pneumonia...and a bizarre malignancy Kaposi's sarcoma, a cancer-like condition of blood vessels evidenced by purple lesions of the skin. Some AIDS victims develop slurred speech and severe dementia. The course of AIDS is grim, and thus far inescapable, finally ending in complete debilitation and death from cancer or overwhelming infection. (p. 394)

Recent research advances in improving health and prolonging life for people with HIV infection and AIDS have occurred in the area of drug therapies, for example, protease inhibitors and vaccines. However, as effectiveness of antiviral therapies increases, disease complexities increase as well. With the accumulation of new information about HIV infection and disease progression, the Office of AIDS Research of the National Institutes of Health (NIH) sponsored a panel to define principles of therapy of HIV infection in clinical practice. The panel defined 11 principles to provide the scientific basis for specific guidelines for the treatment of HIV-infected persons. The principles are being widely disseminated to health care providers in an attempt to keep treatment current with research (National Institutes of Health, 1998).

NURSING PROCESS RELATED TO PROTECTION

Protection is a priority requirement for the individual's physiologic adaptation. In applying the nursing process, the nurse makes a careful assessment of behaviors and stimuli related to the basic life processes of nonspecific and specific defense processes. In assessing factors influencing the need for protection, regulator and cognator effectiveness in initiating compensatory processes is also considered. Based on this thorough first- and second-level assessment, the nurse makes a nursing diagnosis, sets goals, selects nursing interventions, and evaluates care.

Assessment of Behaviors of Innate Immunity

The first level of assessment as it relates to the innate immune system provides the nurse with an indication of how the individual is managing to cope with factors affecting the anatomic, physiologic, phagocytic, and inflammatory barrier surface associated with protection. The nurse's background in anatomy, physiology, and pathophysiology provides the basis for decisions as to whether the observed behavior is adaptive or ineffective. As with assessment of other components of the physiologic mode, assessment related to the innate immune system involves observation, measurement, and subjective reporting.

HISTORY   The nurse initially obtains an understanding of the individual's history related to the innate immune system. This includes past medical history, family history, and psychosocial history including lifestyle.

SKIN   Inspection of the skin is primary in the initial phase of assessment. This includes a description of the skin's appearance in terms of color. For example, erythema (redness of the skin), cyanosis (dusky blue color), jaundice (yellowness of skin), and pallor (paleness of face, conjunctiva, and mucous membranes) are some terms that may be applicable. Any changes in the normal pigmentation should be noted. It is important for nurses to be knowledgeable of variations in skin appearance for racial groups commonly encountered in their specific area of practice. Initial assessment of the skin also includes a description of skin lesions that may be present, noting color, distribution, shape and arrangement, duration of presentation, and whether lesions appear to be primary (direct result of a causative factor) or secondary (resulting from changes in a primary lesion). Inspection and identification of lesions is particularly important to ensure proper nursing intervention and healing of the skin. Primary lesions include macules, papules, nodules, and wheals, requiring a range of nursing interventions from observation to medication administration (Bickley, 2000). Secondary lesions, including ulcers, fissures, and erosions, may require additional nursing interventions and may cause long-term damage to the skin and body's protection system if not properly addressed (Bates, 2000).

Vascularity of the skin is the third aspect to be addressed. Vascular lesions resulting from the dilation of small blood vessels may be apparent. Birthmarks, nevi, and scars should also be noted and recorded as to their location, their dimensions, and, in the case of scars, how they were acquired. Palpation of the skin provides further important information related to temperature, moisture, texture, mobility, turgor (elasticity of the skin), and skin thickness. Normal skin is warm to touch. Its texture is typically smooth and soft. Normal skin moves easily over most areas and, when pinched, should immediately return to its normal shape (turgor). Skin lesions related to sexually transmitted illness such as herpes genitalis are of significance to nurses and have public health implications because of their rising incidence. Herpes genitalis initially appears as a blister or pimple progressing to an ulcerated state. It is generally located on the vagina, cervix, and female or male external genitalia.

PAIN AND SKIN CONDITION RELATED TO AN OPERATIVE INCISION The nurse carefully assesses postoperative pain and skin condition as it relates to an incisional area. People who have had surgery are expected to experience some pain as a protective response following an incision. The duration of pain depends on the nature of the surgery and on the individual's tolerance of pain. The presence of pain is identified through the observation of activities such as crying, tense positioning, tightening of facial muscles, and through patient statements. In describing the pain experience, the nurse must note the type, duration, and location of the pain. The nurse recognizes the patient's right to effective pain management in the postoperative period. Further discussion of pain is found in Chapter 10. The nurse assesses skin integrity at the operative site by observing the color of the skin, whether the sutures or adhesive strips are intact, and the presence or absence of drainage. If drainage is present, the nurse notes the color, amount, and odor. The patient's phagocytic immune response and antibody-mediated immune response operate as protective functions, which cause the drainage and odor. Any signs of erythema, edema, increased pain, or temperature above 102.5°F should be noted and reported as these symptoms may indicate infection. With same-day surgery and early discharge of surgical patients, the nurse provides education to the patient and family about assessing wound healing.

HAIR AND NAILS Examination of the hair will address distribution, quantity, texture, and condition of the scalp. The scalp appears smooth, moist, and clean. The presence of cysts, dandruff, or scabs would be considered unexpected or ineffective behaviors. The distribution of the individual's hair is assessed, bearing in mind that there are many normal variations. Variations that warrant further assessment are alopecia, unexpected general or local hair loss; a noticeable change in the character of the hair; excessive hair growth in women; and the disappearance of body hair from an area where it normally is present. Observations are made about the cleanliness of the hair. The expected adaptive behavior is the presence of clean hair in normal distribution and consistency on the head, extremities, trunk, pubic area, and face. Nails are examined closely because they are useful in assessing the individual's general state of health. The nurse notes the color, shape, thickness, adherence to the nail bed, and presence of lesions. Normal nails are transparent with a translucent, white end. Assess the nails by asking whether the nails are soft, hard, brittle, peeling, pitted, or splitting. What is their color? Is the surface ridged and are there transverse lines indicative of injury or other pathologic processes? Clubbing of the fingers is indicative of decreased oxygenation and is an important indicator of cardiopulmonary disease.

PERSPIRATION AND BODY TEMPERATURE Sweat glands produce sweat in response to emotional stress or to regulate body temperature. Sweat glands exist on all body surfaces except for the palms of the hand and soles of the feet and consist of two types: eccrine and apocrine glands (Bickley, 2000). Located throughout the body, the eccrine glands work primarily to regulate body temperature, whereas the apocrine glands produce sweat in response to emotional stress and are located mostly in the axillary and genital regions (Bickley, 2000). The nurse assesses the quantity, color, and location of perspiration on the body. The adaptive behavior for perspiration is a musty, salty, or sour odor. Perspiration is termed "malodorous" if it is particularly offensive, a situation caused by the breakdown of bacterial products found on the skin.

Measurement of body temperature is an important indicator of the final component of the innate immune processes: fever. The definition of fever continues to evolve as research uncovers new information regarding the benefits of fever. However, fever is generally considered an increase in body temperature 1 degree Celsius above normal diurnal body temperature (Thompson, 2005). A fever occurs in response to an immune system threat, stimulating immune system activity including increased neutrophil migration, increased secretion of interleukin1, and proliferation of T-lymphocytes (Thompson, 2005). Endogenous and exogenous pyrogens initiate fever, inducing the release of prostaglandin E2. Subsequently, prostaglandin E2 binds to receptors in the hypothalamus increasing the set point, initiating shivering and vasoconstriction, resulting in fever (Kunert, 2008). Fever is self-limiting and the thermoregulatory response remains intact. This is contrary to hyperthermia where the thermoregulatory response does not remain intact and the thermoregulatory center is overwhelmed by either excess heat production, impaired heat loss, or excessive environmental heat, such as in heat stroke or heat exhaustion often requiring nursing intervention (Kunert, 2005). In contrast, hypothermia is a term used to describe body temperature below normal.

MUCOUS MEMBRANES   First-level assessment of mucous membranes includes the individual's description of, or signs of, pain or discomfort in oral and nasal mucous membranes, the eyes, or the vaginal mucous membranes. Aspects to be noted include excess or decrease in secretions, edema, color of membranes, and lesions. Assessment of the oral cavity should describe the presence of stomatitis, oral plaque, carious teeth, coated tongue, condition of the gingiva, or dry mouth.

GASTROINTESTINAL SYSTEM   As mentioned, the parietal cells of the stomach produce hydrochloric acid, maintaining an acidic environment. This acidic environment provides protection against various microorganisms and facilitates initial steps in food digestion. Assessment of gastric pH is essential when placing nasogastric tubes. Fluid collected from the stomach usually has a pH of 3; however, various internal and external stimuli may alter the pH including stress (lowers pH) and histamine antagonist acid reflux medications (increase pH) (Lehne, 2007).

INFLAMMATORY RESPONSE   Two types of inflammation occur in response to stimuli: acute and chronic. The acute response responds early to injury, occurring before a full immune system response, and limits the extent of injury (Porth, 2000). The acute response involves both vascular and cellular involvement. The vascular stage involves increased capillary permeability and vasodilation, whereas the cellular stage summons inflammatory mediators (histamine, plasma proteases, and cytokines) and inflammatory white blood cells (neutrophils, granulocytes, and mast cells) (Porth, 2000). The vascular and cellular responses result in leukocyte migration, enabling phagocytosis, opsonization, and intracellular killing, furthering the inflammatory process and immune system response (Porth, 2000). The acute inflammatory response results in the four well-known signs of inflammation: redness, heat, swelling, and pain. The chronic inflammatory response is a longer process, resulting in persistent inflammation. The chronic response may last for weeks to months, involve macrophages and lymphocytes, and often result in the formation of scar tissue (Porth, 2000). Assessment of an inflammatory response in a patient is imperative and careful description of location, appearance, and presence of discharge is done by the nurse.

LABORATORY EXAMINATION   Laboratory examination of blood, urine, and secretions provides important information about microscopic defense activities that are under way in the human body. The presence of bacteria, plasma proteins, or foreign cells and molecules contributes to the determination of specific factors that are contributing to behaviors associated with the cellular and chemical defense processes.

Assessment of Behavior Adaptive (Specific) Immune System

INDICATIONS OF THE IMMUNE RESPONSE   The nurse observes the individual for indications that the immune response is occurring. Low-grade fever is often indicative of the initial viral attack and the release of interferon by the damaged cells. Second, there may be localized swelling of lymph nodes progressing to local inflammatory signs, generalized inflammatory response, malaise, aches and pains, and further progression to nausea, vomiting, and diarrhea.

IMMUNOLOGIC STATUS   In assessment of an individual's status relative to communicable diseases, several areas of behavior are of concern. It is important to know which communicable diseases the individual has had or has been immunized against. In some chronic and degenerative diseases such as leukemia and acquired immunodeficiency syndrome (AIDS), the individual's immunologic protection is compromised. Additionally, recipients of organ transplants require immunosuppression medications, which greatly decrease their immunologic protection. The complications prompting the individual's need for care are a result of ineffective or absent immune responses of the body. The nurse anticipates that individuals with such diagnoses will demonstrate many ineffective behaviors related to the need for protection. For example, there may be evidence of infectious processes within the body such as symptoms associated with pneumonia.

LABORATORY EXAMINATION   Clinical indications of the immune response are also evident in laboratory findings related to blood cell counts, immunoglobulin levels, and serum complement level, for example. As the nurse identifies the individual's behaviors relative to the need for protection, an initial evaluation is made as to whether these behaviors are adaptive or ineffective. To guide this evaluation, the nurse uses knowledge related to normal physiologic functioning, established normal values, and the individual's report of what is personally "normal" or adaptive. In consultation with the patient or family, the nurse establishes the tentative identification of adaptive and ineffective behaviors. With the initial priorities being the ineffective behaviors, the nurse then proceeds to identify the related stimuli.

Assessment of Stimuli

In the second level of assessment, assessment of stimuli, the nurse gathers data about internal and external factors influencing the behaviors identified in the first assessment phase of the adaptation nursing process. This includes the body's adaptive ability to maintain the structure, function, and regulation of the protection component, as well as the coping strategies the individual uses to maintain or change behaviors.

ENVIRONMENTAL FACTORS   Many of the factors that influence the innate immune processes originate in the environment. According to the Roy Adaptation Model, Chapter 2, the environment is defined as "all conditions, circumstances, and influences that surround and affect the development and behavior of humans as adaptive systems, with particular consideration of person and earth resources" (p. 46). Therefore, environmental stimuli include natural elements such as the sun and oxygen; however, they also include nonnatural stimuli such as pharmaceutical agents and other interventions. Environmental stimuli affect all aspects of the innate immune system and must be assessed to determine appropriate nursing interventions to promote optimal patient functioning. The environment affects the skin on many levels. First, extreme temperatures may influence the color and integrity of the skin. Cold weather as an environmental stimulus contributes to dry skin, whereas exposure to the sun can burn the skin. Other environmental stimuli can also alter the skin. Poison ivy, urine, feces, soap, and some medications can irritate the skin and this can lead to the development of a rash. Chemical and mechanical irritants can interfere with the integrity of the surface membrane barriers and cellular and chemical defenses.

Second, excess sun exposure is an environmental stimuli that can negatively affect the skin, altering the integrity and causing bodily harm. Skin cancer is associated with excess sun exposure and is one of the most common cancers in the United States (Bickley, 2000). Excess sun exposure alters skin cell DNA resulting in abnormal and abhorrent cell growth or cancer. Three types of cancer may result: basal cell, squamous cell, and malignant melanoma. Other risk factors include family history of melanoma, light skin, atypical moles, and immunosuppression (Bickley, 2000). The nurse assesses all risk factors as additional stimuli that may affect skin integrity and subsequent body protection.

Patient positioning and oxygenation are other stimuli that affect skin integrity. Sitting or laying in the same position for a long time increases the risk of developing pressure ulcers, which greatly affect skin integrity, inhibiting the skin's ability to provide essential protection. In addition, lack of oxygen secondary to hypoxia or poor perfusion also alters skin integrity. Without adequate oxygenation, skin cells die, leading to necrosis and deterioration of the skin. Scars often are the result of injuries or previous surgical interventions. The factors causing scars often point the nurse in the direction of other physiologic problems that may or may not be of immediate concern. Skin piercing is a practice accepted by an increasing number of people. The practice is assessed as a factor interrupting skin integrity. Environmental factors influence other processes of the innate immune system, including body temperature and perspiration. For example, environmental stimuli that influence perspiration include room temperature, the amount of circulating air, and humidity. Factors that influence perspiration include the thickness of clothing worn and personal hygiene measures, such as frequency of bathing and the use of soaps and deodorants. Increased exercise or activity and stressful or anxiety-producing situations also contribute to increased perspiration and increased body temperature. The mucous membranes are also affected by environmental stimuli. Foods high in starch and refined sugar increase the amount of plaque present in the oral cavity, resulting in increased dental caries and potential gingivitis. The nurse will assess whether these stimuli are affecting the patient's mucous membranes and provide education accordingly to prevent further deterioration of the gums.

Pharmaceutical agents also affect the innate immune processes, making them significant stimuli for effective or ineffective immune responses. For example, it is well known that calcineurin inhibitors and steroids decrease the response of the innate and specific immune systems, deterring these processes from activating a full response to invading pathogens. In addition, gingival hypertrophy is a side effect of calcineurin inhibitors, altering the mucous membrane's ability to provide protection. As previously noted, antihistamine and gastrointestinal medications prevent parietal cells from releasing hydrochloric acid, increasing the pH of the gastric environment and inhibiting the gastrointestinal role in protection. It is evident that certain medications alter the innate immune response. Therefore, it is essential that the nurse obtain a thorough medication history with each patient to determine how medications influence each patient's innate immune response and how well their protection processes are functioning.

INTEGRITY OF THE MODES   Internal disruptions to other components of the physiologic mode, or self-concept, role function, and interdependence modes, may be manifest in the innate immune response through alterations in the internal physiologic process of the body. Generalized rise in body temperature may be an indication of an increased metabolic rate associated with medical conditions such as hyperthyroidism; or it may be the manifestation of fever, strenuous exercise, or sunburn. Localized rise in skin temperature may be indicative of injury or infection. Situations where skin temperatures are cooler than normal may be indicative of shock or arterial disease. Skin becomes drier as well as thinner as an individual ages. Dryness can also be associated with physiologic conditions such as dehydration, myxedema, and chronic renal disease. Texture of the skin, which is normally smooth and soft, can be influenced by local irritation, trauma, or a systemic problem. Mobility of the skin is decreased in situations of edema or with certain pathologic conditions such as scleroderma, an autoimmune disease that results in fibrosing of tissue. Turgor is also affected in situations of dehydration and with aging. Thickness of the skin is affected by disease conditions or frequent injection.

Alterations in the condition of hair and nails may be indicative of disease processes such as hormonal imbalance and endocrine problems, or indicative of a side effect of drugs. Although gray hair is normally associated with aging, it can result from local nerve injury. Alterations in nails may also be indicative of injury or disease processes. As noted, clubbing of the fingers is associated with cardiopulmonary disease, for example. It is also suggested that stress is a factor that can lead to cutaneous disorders such as pruritus, urticaria, psoriasis, dermatitis, and acne. Nutritional status affects the overall condition of the skin, hair, and nails. Pale-appearing skin may be related to anemia caused by a diet low in iron. Hair loss is evident in those suffering from some nutritional disturbances. Psychological disturbances are sometimes manifested through skin disruptions such as rashes, itching, and acne.

COGNATOR EFFECTIVENESS   One function of the cognator is for the individual to use judgment in the daily activity. The effectiveness of this central coping process is a factor that can influence the condition of the skin and mucous membranes by how it handles hygiene practices. Maintaining clean, dry skin is important to avoid infection. Effective oral hygiene maintains healthy mucous membranes and teeth. A well-balanced diet and adequate fluid intake are necessary for optimal general health, and for the health and functioning of the skin and mucous membranes in particular. There is increasing awareness of the importance of protection from sunlight. Exposure to chemical and physical agents is also an important consideration. These are factors that the individual makes judgments about using the cognator.

DEVELOPMENTAL STAGE   Aging is another factor that contributes to changes in the skin. Infants are prone to skin disorders because their skin structures are functionally immature. The infant dehydrates easily because the epidermis is very permeable. Milia and cradle cap are common protective behaviors caused by the increased activity of the sebaceous glands during late fetal life and early infancy. Temperature regulation is more labile in the neonate since the skin has an immature ability to shiver in response to cold or perspire in response to heat.

During the adolescent period, the sebaceous glands become highly active and increase in size. The condition of the skin can be disrupted by the development of acne. The behavioral manifestations of skin integrity for an elderly person are affected by the aging process. Skin pigmentation becomes uneven due to the clustering of melanocytes. The elasticity of the skin is decreased and the skin is more delicate as a result of decreased hydration and vascularity of the dermis. Lines and wrinkles appear as a result of the loss of subcutaneous fat. The hair becomes thicker in the nose and ears while the scalp hair grays and thins. The nails become hard and brittle. Steps can be taken to prevent many of these changes. Protection from undue exposure to risk factors, safety, and nutrition play important roles in the avoidance of injury to the skin.

Assessment of Stimuli for Specific Defense Processes

Many of the stimuli potentially affecting the specific defense processes of the immune system relate to the integrity of the modes, developmental stage, environmental considerations, and cognator effectiveness.

INTEGRITY OF THE MODES According to Burrell (1992, p. 164), stress is understood to make an individual more vulnerable to organisms in the immediate environment. Nutrition status also affects cell-mediated immunity; malnutrition and protein deficiency cause atrophy of the thymus and other lymphoid tissue.

DEVELOPMENTAL STAGE The immune system or the specific defense mechanisms are affected with aging, as are the nonspecific defense processes. The older individual encounters a greater number of infections, which are more severe in nature, and this may be the result of the body's inability to trigger an effective immune response. It appears that the production and function of the T- and B-cell lymphocytes are affected in some manner as the aging process proceeds. Additionally, young infants have an immature immune system. During gestation, the fetus receives antibodies from the mother via the placenta; however, a mature immune system does not occur until the infant is exposed and elicits a response to various foreign antigens. The mother can supplement the infant's immune system via breast-feeding, for breast milk contains numerous antibodies and infants who are breast-fed have greater protection from illness than non–breast-fed infants (Hanson & Korotkonva, 2002).

ENVIRONMENTAL FACTORS Environmental considerations include the use of tobacco, alcohol, and other drugs. Cigarette smoke suppresses T cell formation, and alcohol destroys lymphocytes. Antibiotics, cytotoxic drugs, and nonsteroidal anti-inflammatory drugs suppress the immune response, while corticosteroids and calcineurin inhibitors cause the destruction of T cells and inhibit protein synthesis in lymphocytes and phagocytes. Radiation also affects the immune process by killing lymphocytes and diminishing the number of cells able to replenish them. Surgical removal of the thymus, lymph nodes, or spleen can also seriously impair immune system functioning.

COGNATOR EFFECTIVENESS The individual's perception, knowledge, and skill are often factors that interfere with adaptation as related to protection. Good nutrition is necessary for a properly functioning immune system. According to Lehmann (1991), protein-calorie malnutrition is considered to be one of the most frequent causes of immunosuppression. Malnutrition can affect the functioning of the T cells, B cells, and macrophages. When the amount of protein is diminished, it causes a depressed antibody response, decreased numbers of T cells, and ineffective phagocytic activity. Research in the field of psychoneuroimmunology is exploring connections among psychological factors such as emotions and attitudes, the nervous system, and the immune system (Santrock, 2006). Relationships between emotional status and the immune system are being demonstrated. For example, depression is thought to adversely affect and suppress the immune system. Associated with cognator effectiveness is the individual's knowledge about prevention and early detection of disease processes. Increasingly, prevention and health promotion are becoming a major focus of health care systems throughout the world.

Immunization programs provide people with the opportunity to avoid many communicable diseases that in times past claimed many lives. For example, flu immunizations are available in many areas to prevent particular strains of influenza from infecting susceptible individuals in the population. Knowledge about communicability, diagnosis, and treatment of sexually transmitted illnesses is increasingly important. In many areas, programs are being developed to assist in the education of the public relative to prevention of and protection against this widespread health problem. Education of the public is important in the prevention and early detection of sexually transmitted diseases. It is important for the nurse to assess the individual's understanding and practice of preventive and health promotion activities related to the need for protection.

Nursing Diagnosis

The assessment information related to behaviors and stimuli are interpreted in the form of a nursing diagnosis. The statement of the diagnosis is formulated by considering the data of the first and second levels of assessment. The diagnosis includes a statement of observed behaviors with the most relevant influencing stimuli. Indicators of effective adaptation in protection are evident in nursing diagnosis statements such as "intact skin free of excoriation and lesions related to nutritious diet and hygiene patterns," or "profuse perspiration related to outside temperature of 102°F." In the latter situation, perspiration is the body's method of adapting to warm temperatures in the external environment. An alternate way of stating a nursing diagnosis is to use a summary label that best identifies the nurse's judgment of the clinical situation from an established classification system. The Roy model has two classification lists, one for indicators of adaptation and one for commonly recurring adaptation problems. The complete classification lists for the Roy model are included in Chapter 3. In Table 9–1, the Roy model nursing diagnostic categories for the physiologic need of protection are shown in relation to nursing diagnosis labels approved by the North American Nursing Diagnosis Association (NANDA-International, 2007).

Common adaptation problems or broad areas of concern within the component of protection include pressure ulcers (decubitus ulcers) and itching (pruritus). Pressure ulcers occur frequently in the elderly and those who are immobilized; they result from disrupted circulation to the affected tissue. (Issues related to immobility are discussed in Chapter 8.) A relevant nursing diagnosis for this adaptation problem could be "pressure ulcer, measuring 2.5 cm (width) by 5 cm (length) with no edema, erythema, or eschar, and edges intact, on left lateral ankle related to prolonged pressure and immobility." Indicators of positive adaptation related to the problem of pressure ulcers would include skin integrity with the absence of skin infection.

One alteration in comfort related to skin protection may be "itching." The focal stimulus for itching may be a skin disorder resulting from a systemic disease or pregnancy. An allergic

TABLE 9–1 Nursing Diagnostic Categories for Protection

Positive Indicators of Adaptation	Common Adaptation Problems	NANDA Diagnostic Labels
• Intact skin • Effective healing response • Adequate secondary protection for changes in skin integrity and immune status • Effective processes of immunity • Effective temperature regulation	• Disrupted skin integrity • Pressure ulcer • Itching • Delayed wound healing • Infection • Potential for ineffective coping with allergic reaction • Ineffective coping with changes in immune status • Ineffective temperature regulation • Fever • Hypothermia	• Impaired oral mucous membrane • Risk for perioperative positioning injury • Risk for falls • Risk for trauma • Risk for infection • Readiness for enhanced immunization status • Impaired skin integrity • Risk for impaired skin integrity • Impaired tissue integrity • Impaired dentition • Ineffective protection • Risk for self-mutilation • Self-mutilation • Risk for other-directed violence • Risk for self-directed violence • Risk for suicide • Risk for poisoning • Risk for contamination • Contamination • Latex allergy response • Risk for latex allergy response • Readiness for enhanced immunization status • Risk for imbalanced body temperature • Ineffective thermoregulation • Hypothermia • Hyperthermia

reaction (immune response), local lesion, dry skin, and emotional upset are other influencing factors. The time of day is a contextual stimulus since itching is often worse at night when there are fewer activities on which to focus. A warm environment also increases itching. A nursing diagnosis reflecting this adaptation problem is "itching related to contact with poison ivy." Once the nursing diagnoses have been established, the nurse proceeds to the next step of the nursing process, goal setting. The priority nursing diagnoses, those relating to the ineffective behaviors and the focal stimulus, would be given initial consideration, although the importance of maintaining adaptive behavior is acknowledged.

Goal Setting

In the fourth step of the nursing process as described in the Roy Adaptation Model, the nurse, in collaboration with the individual receiving care, establishes goals, that is, statements of behavioral outcomes of nursing care for the individual. The goal should address the behavior, the change expected, and the time frame in which the goal is to be achieved. Goals may be long term or short term, and these time frames are relative to the situation involved. In the example of the nursing diagnosis, "pressure ulcer, measuring 2.5 cm (width) by 5 cm (length) with no edema, erythema, or eschar, and edges intact," a relevant goal would focus on the pressure ulcer. A short-term goal could be, "Within 3 weeks, the pressure ulcer on the left ankle will decrease in diameter from 2.5 cm to 1 cm." In this goal, the behavior relates to the size of the pressure ulcer and the healing that is expected to occur, the time frame is "within 3 weeks", and the change is the decrease in the diameter of the ulcer.

Another example of goal setting shows the importance of maintaining effective adaptation. The situation relates to the postoperative condition of an incision, a disruption in skin integrity that could lead to ineffective adaptation if an infection develops. The nursing diagnosis notes that the patient has an incision with a dressing resulting from surgery to the abdomen. A goal statement focuses on the status of the incision: "Within 2 days, incision edges will be approximated with evidence of normal healing and the absence of infection." Here, the behavior focuses on the healing of the incision; the time frame is within 2 days; and the change expected is the evidence of normal healing, the approximation of the wound edges, and the absence of infection.

Although the goals described relate to situations in which skin integrity has been disrupted, it is important for the nurse to derive goals to preserve the protective functions of the body. Within this context are many preventive and health-promoting goals related to protection. One program aimed at prevention of HIV in young black women was developed by nurses who produced the film *Women's Voices Women's Lives* (Norris & DeMarco, 2005). The nurse scholars worked with HIV-infected, older black women in the community to develop a strategy to prevent HIV in younger women. The result was the HIV prevention film in which the women candidly told their stories. The film is the basis for prevention programs in the community. A population goal related to this particular initiative could be, "Within 3 years, the new cases of HIV infection in women between 15 and 30 years of age will be reduced from 2007 levels by 50%." Here, the time frame is 3 years, the measured behavior for the population is "new cases of HIV infection in women between 15 and 30 years of age," and the change expected is a 50% reduction.

Many preventive and health-promoting goals can be set within the need for protection. A nurse in a community agency may establish a goal for an infant that relates to immunization status at a particular age. For example, "At 4 years of age, the child will demonstrate active immunity against common communicable childhood diseases." The behavior associated with this goal is "immunity." Once the behavioral goals have been established, the nurse identifies the nursing interventions most likely to assist in the achievement of the desired outcomes.

Nursing Intervention

When the goals have been established for behaviors that will promote adaptation, the nurse determines the nursing interventions that will assist the individual in attaining the stated goals. Nursing interventions for the promotion of protection depend on the stimuli identified. The nurse manages the stimuli by either promoting or reinforcing them or by taking action to change or eliminate the stimuli. In addition, the nurse can affect the internal stimulus of adaptation level by nursing interventions that focus on the cognator or regulator processes. In the situation of a pressure ulcer, frequent positioning of the immobilized patient assists in promoting circulation by changing the pressure on the bony prominences. From a different perspective and situation, the body's internal protective response is facilitated through programs of immunization in the community agencies. Many health promotion programs have been designed to assist individuals in protecting and promoting their own health by early detection of disease processes. Each of these examples can be viewed as attempts to manage stimuli that compromise an individual's protective processes.

Many nursing interventions associated with aseptic technique are directed at control of microorganisms and the minimization of inflammatory and infectious responses of the body. For example, preoperative skin cleansing is an attempt to manage the opportunity for foreign substances to enter the site of the incision. Specific nursing interventions are directed at factors contributing to adaptation problems related to protection. Nursing interventions to control itching include soothing baths, trimming the nails, and the use of firm pressure instead of scratching. For localized itching, the application of cool, wet compresses may be used. Temperature control and the use of diversionary activities such as watching television are other suggested nursing interventions. The nurse routinely observes the skin color of the individual and notes localized areas of red, blue, or mottled skin, which indicate decreased circulation. Rubbing around these areas helps to restore circulation. If the skin integrity becomes disrupted, as in the case of a pressure ulcer, then other nursing interventions are necessary.

There are many nursing interventions applicable to the care of individuals with pressure ulcers. Once again, these nursing interventions are directed at the stimuli identified in the second level of assessment.

1. Nutritional status is addressed. Adequate dietary intake or supplementation is necessary if the individual is malnourished. This may require supplementation with vitamins or minerals if deficiencies are confirmed.
2. Tissue load (the distribution of pressure, friction, and shear on the tissue) will be managed. Positioning techniques include staying off the ulcer and using appropriate positioning devices. Pressure-relieving overlays, mattresses, and beds can be helpful adjuncts to turning every 2 hours.
3. Support surfaces including standard mattresses, foam, static flotation, alternating air, low-air loss, and air-fluidized mattresses are considered, along with cost and availability.
4. Care of the ulcer itself can involve debridement, wound cleansing, and application of dressing or other therapy. Debridement of necrotic tissue is necessary before

healing will occur. Wet-to-dry dressings are one method to accomplish this, as is enzymatic debridement.

5. Wound cleansing should be gentle and use of antiseptics should be avoided as these agents are cytotoxic and retard the healing process. Normal saline is the preferred choice.

6. Dressings should protect the wound, be biocompatible, and provide hydration.

7. Bacterial colonization and infection must be managed. Topical antibiotics may be indicated.

8. Patient education can enable people to become partners in the healing process, where possible. Information should include risk factors, pathology, principles of wound healing and nutrition, product selection, and assessment of healing.

Nursing interventions will be directed at the prevention of pressure sores. The identification of patients at risk can assist in this prevention. Sparks (1993) identified three factors that are suggested to be the best discriminators for pressure ulcer risk: friction, being dependent in self-care, and being confined to bed or chair. To decrease the stimulus of moisture on the skin, the patient and bed need to be clean and dry. Lifting when repositioning, instead of pulling, as well as keeping the bed wrinkle free, decreases the problem of friction. A diet high in protein and vitamins is essential to the repair of tissue. The application of lotion helps to keep the skin soft and intact.

Protection is a component of the physiologic mode where nursing interventions often focus on maintaining adaptive behaviors in an effort to prevent adaptation problems. Thus, many nursing interventions are protective and preventive in nature. Specifically, nurses are conscientious in their efforts to minimize the opportunity for infectious processes to enter the body. For example, herpes genitalis is a sexually transmitted disease and much can be done in the form of prevention. Nurses are often in positions where they can help to prevent the spread of such infections through programs of counseling and education. It is important that nurses maintain current knowledge regarding sexually transmitted diseases and their treatment.

Protective and preventive nursing interventions are particularly important related to the increasing incidence of AIDS. Nursing measures associated with the prevention of the spread of AIDS and the care of the increasing numbers of hospitalized individuals in the final stages of the disease are vitally important and have widespread implications for nurses functioning in all aspects of practice. Some years ago Rogers (1989, p. 254) pointed out, "prevention is the only approach to dealing with this epidemic [AIDS]." This nursing intervention includes information regarding protection from and prevention of the disease, particularly in relation to self, other patients, and staff. Standard precautions set forth by the Centers for Disease Control and Prevention include a two-tiered approach to infection control that is used in many settings for all patients and includes bloodborne, airborne, and epidemiologically important pathogens (West & Cohen, 1997). The success of the nursing interventions such as those described in assisting the individual to achieve the preset behavioral goals is determined through evaluation. This is the sixth step of Roy's nursing process.

Evaluation

Evaluation involves determining the effectiveness of nursing interventions related to the individual's behavior in terms of the preset goals. Was the goal that was set in the fourth step of the nursing process attained? To make this decision, the nurse assesses the behavior of the individual after the nursing interventions have been implemented. As in the initial assessment steps, observation, measurement, and subjective reporting are used. The nursing interventions are considered effective if the individual's behavior aligns with the preset goals.

Looking back to the goal related to the pressure ulcer, it was identified that the diameter of the lesion should reduce from 2.5 cm to 1 cm within 3 weeks. If the nursing interventions described were assisting with the healing process, it would be noted by the nurse that the size of the lesion had decreased. If no change was noted, the nurse would proceed through the nursing process again, perhaps establishing that the goal was unrealistic, that not all stimuli have been identified, or that there are other nursing interventions that may be appropriate to attain the goal. Expected outcomes for the protection component would be the maintenance of integrity of the nonspecific and specific defense processes. The individual's skin should be intact and free of discomforts such as itching. It may be helpful for the individual to acquire knowledge regarding skin care and its importance in the area of protection. Indicators of positive adaptation related to the problem of itching would include patient statements indicating relief of discomfort, a skin free from scratch marks and abrasions, and an intact skin surface. Indicators of positive adaptation related to the problem of pressure ulcers would be the maintenance of skin integrity with the absence of skin infections.

Once the effectiveness of the nursing intervention has been determined, the nurse returns to the first step of the nursing process to look more closely at behaviors that continue to be ineffective. It is important to recognize that the nursing process is ongoing and simultaneous. Although it is necessary to discuss each aspect of the nursing process as a separate entity, the nurse keeps in mind that each aspect is related to and affected by the other.

Summary

This chapter has focused on the application of the Roy Adaptation Model to the physiologic need of protection. An overview of the basic life processes, nonspecific and specific body defense processes associated with protection, was provided. Illustrations of innate and learned adaptive compensatory responses related to protection were described and examples of two compromised processes, pressure ulcers and ineffective coping changes in immune status, were provided. Finally, guidelines for planning nursing care beginning with identifying factors for assessment of behaviors and stimuli through the formulation of nursing diagnoses, goals, and nursing interventions were explored and evaluation of nursing care was described. In providing for the individual's need for protection by promoting and maintaining nonspecific and specific defense processes, the nurse contributes to the overall integrity of the individual.

Exercises for Application

1. Identify activities that you engage in, as a healthy adult, that are directed at your adaptation in the need for protection.
2. If you were a resident in a nursing home as a result of the progression of multiple sclerosis and immobilized in a wheelchair, what nursing interventions would you require to assist you in the maintenance of adaptation relative to protection?
3. You have an acquaintance who has offered to provide hospice care in her home for a friend with AIDS. What advice would you offer as to how she should protect herself and her family?

Assessment of Understanding

QUESTIONS

1. Classify the following components of protection as associated with nonspecific defense processes (N) or specific defense processes (S).
    (a) _____ antibodies
    (b) _____ phagocytes
    (c) _____ mucous membranes
    (d) _____ lymphocytes
    (e) _____ skin
    (f) _____ natural killer cells
    (g) _____ macrophages
    (h) _____ inflammatory response
    (i) _____ fever

2. Label the following compensatory adaptation level as indicative of regulator (R) or cognator (C) activity.
    (a) _____ wound healing process following incision
    (b) _____ universal precautions practiced by health care workers
    (c) _____ covering one's mouth when coughing
    (d) _____ swelling of tissue following an insect bite
    (e) _____ cold symptoms
    (f) _____ preoperative skin cleansing

3. Name and describe one compromised adaptation process of protection related to (a) nonspecific defense processes and one related to (b) specific defense processes.
    (a) _____
    (b) _____

4. In behavioral assessment of an operative site, which of the following factors would be important to note and measure?
    (a) approximation of wound edges
    (b) temperature of skin at wound edge
    (c) color of skin at wound edge
    (d) presence of discharge
    (e) pain in the incisional area

5. Developmental stage is an important stimulus affecting protection behaviors. Label the following behaviors according to the developmental stage to which they pertain: infant (I), adolescent (A), or older adult (O).
    (a) _____ uneven skin pigmentation
    (b) _____ epidermis very permeable
    (c) _____ nails become hard and brittle
    (d) _____ sebaceous glands active and increase in size
    (e) _____ temperature regulation labile

SITUATION:

A 45-year-old woman with multiple sclerosis has been admitted to a continuing care facility as a result of progression of the disease. Although she has limited movement of one arm, the rest of her body is paralyzed. Contractures have developed in her legs and arms and careful positioning is required. She has very limited ability to fulfill any of the activities of daily living and is catheterized intermittently for bladder control. She has developed a reddened area on her coccyx that is at risk for breaking down without careful attention.

6. Construct a nursing diagnosis focusing on the need for protection, with particular attention to the potential for disrupted skin integrity.

7. Develop a goal relative to the behavior of "reddened skin over coccyx." The goal should include the behavior of concern, the change expected, and the time frame involved.

8. Nursing interventions are focused on the stimuli causing the behavior of concern, in this situation, reddened skin over the coccyx. For each of the stimuli identified below, suggest a nursing intervention that could assist in dealing with the problem.

Stimuli	Nursing Intervention
(a) Continual pressure on coccyx from supine position	_____
(b) Friction on skin when moving up in wheelchair	_____
(c) Incontinence between catheterizations	_____
(d) Nutritional status less than body requirements	_____

9. Which of the following behaviors would indicate that the nursing intervention had been effective in goal achievement?
   (a) breakdown of skin over coccyx
   (b) increase in size of reddened area
   (c) disappearance of redness over coccyx
   (d) patient's report of pain and discomfort

FEEDBACK

1. (a) S, (b) N, (c) N, (d) S, (e) N, (f) N, (g) S, (h) N, (i) N
2. (a) R, (b) C, (c) C, (d) R, (e) R, (f) C
3. (a) A burn (disrupted skin integrity) is a situation in which the skin has been damaged by heat, friction, or chemicals. This results in disruption of the surface membrane barrier of the body.
   (b) A reaction to mismatched blood (ineffective coping with allergic reaction) is a situation in which the immune system mounts an attack on infused blood cells that are not appropriately matched to those of the individual.
4. a, c, d, and e
5. (a) O, (b) I, (c) O, (d) A, (e) I
6. Example of nursing diagnosis: "Potential for disrupted skin integrity (pressure ulcer) related to immobilization and pressure on coccyx."
7. Example of goal: "Within 2 days, the skin over the coccyx will be free of redness and irritation."
8. (a) management of tissue load to relieve pressure on the area at all times; repositioning every 2 hours
   (b) assistance with repositioning to avoid friction on the area
   (c) keep area clean and dry and exposed to air as much as possible
   (d) consultation with dietitian to ensure adequate intake and nutritious diet
9. c

References

Agency for Health Care Policy and Research. (1994). *Quick reference guide for clinicians: Pressure ulcer treatment.* U.S. Department of Health and Human Services. Washington, DC: (AHCPR Publication No. 95–1653).

Agostini J., Baker D., & Bogardus S. (2001). Prevention of pressure ulcers in older people. Shojania, K., Duncan, B., McDonald, K., & Wachter, R. AHRQ Publication No. 01-E058. 2001. Evidence Report/Technology Assessment No. 43, Making healthcare safer: A critical analysis of patient safety practices. P. 301–106.

Bickley, L. S. (2000). *Bates' guide to physical examination and history taking* (8th ed.). Philadelphia: Lippincott Williams & Wilkins.

Burrell, L. O. (1992). *Adult nursing in hospital and community settings.* Norwalk, CT: Appleton & Lange.

Centers for Disease Control and Prevention. (2007). Asthma's impact on children and adolescents, *Environmental Hazards and Health Effects.* Retrieved January 9, 2008, from http://www.cdc.gov/asthma/children.htm.

Doughty, D. Ramundo, J., Bonham, P., Beitz, J., Erwin-Toth, P., Anderson R., & Rolstad, B. S. (2006). Issues and challenges in staging of pressure ulcers. *Journal of Wound, Ostomy, and Continence Nurses Society, 33,* 125–132.

Goldsby, R. A., Kindt, T. J., & Osborne, B. A. (Eds.). (2000). *Immunology* (4th ed.). New York: W. H. Freeman and Company.

Guyton, A. C., & Hall, J. E. (Eds.). (2000). *Textbook of medical physiology.* Philadelphia: W. B. Saunders Company.

Hanson, L. and Korotkonva, M. (2002). Breastfeeding may boost baby's own immune system. *Pediatric Infectious Disease Journal,* 21. pp. 816–821.

Interagency Coalition on AIDS. (1996/97). New international network calls for urgent action on children and AIDS. *Canadian AIDS News, IX*(3), 2.

Kunert, M. (2008). Stress and adaptation. In C. M. Porth (Ed.), *Pathophysiology (3rd ed.)* (pp. 187–200). Philadelphia: Lippincott Williams & Wilkins.

Lehmann, S. (1991). Immune function and nutrition: The clinical role of the intravenous nurse. *Journal of Intravenous Nursing, 14*(6), 406–420.

Lehne, R. (2007). *Pharmacology for nursing care.* Philadelphia: W. B. Saunders Company.

Marieb, E. N. & Hoehn, K. (2007). *Human anatomy and physiology* (7th ed.). San Francisco: Pearson Benjamin Cummings.

NANDA International (2007). *Nursing diagnoses: Definitions & classification, 2007–2008.* Philadelphia: NANDA-I.

National Institutes of Health. (1998). Report of the NIH panel to define principles of therapy of HIV infection. *Annals of Internal Medicine, 128,* 1057–1078.

National Institute for Occupational Safety and Health. (2007). Allergic and irritant dermatitis: Additional information. Retrieved January 9, 2007, from http://www2a.cdc.gov/nora/NaddinfoAllergy.html.

Norris, A. E., & DeMarco, R. (2005). The experience of African American women living with HIV creating a prevention film for teens. *Journal of the Association of Nurses in AIDS Care, 16*(2), 32–39.

Pieper, B. (2000). Mechanical forces: Pressure, shear, and friction. In R. A. Bryant (Ed.), *Acute and chronic wounds: Nursing management* (pp. 221–264). St. Louis, MO: Mosby.

Porth, C. M. (Ed.). (2000). *Pathophysiology* (7th ed.), Philadelphia: Lippincott Williams & Wilkins.

Porth, C. (2005). Essentials of Pathophysiology: Concepts of Altered Health States (2nd ed.) Philadelphia: Lippincott Williams & Wilkins.

Rogers, B. (1989). AIDS and ethics in the workplace. *Nursing Outlook, 37*(6), 254–256.

Santrock, J. W. (2006). Life-span development. (11th ed.) Dubuque, IA: Brown.

Sparks, S. M. (1993). Clinical validation of pressure ulcer risk factors. *Ostomy Wound-Management, 39*(4), 40–41, 43–46, 48.

Thompson H. J. (2005). Fever: A concept analysis, *Journal of Advanced Nursing, 51*(5), 484–492.

UNAIDS. (2006). Global summary of the AIDS epidemic: December 2006, *UNAIDS/WHO AIDS Epidemic Update 2006.* Retrieved January 2, 2007, from http://data.unaids.org/pub/EpiReport/2006/02-Global_Summary_2006_EpiUpdate_eng.pdf.

West, K., & Cohen, M. (1997). Standard precautions—a new approach to reducing infection transmission in the hospital setting. *Journal of Intravenous Nursing, 20*(6 Suppl.), 7–10.

CHAPTER 10

Senses

The senses play an important role in adaptation. They are channels of input necessary for the individual to interact with the changing environment. The model of integrated cognitive processing presented in Chapter 12 indicates that immediate sensory experience is the focal stimulus to be processed. Sensations, and the resulting perceptions, are influenced greatly by who the individual is and their context, that is, environmental, cultural, and other background experiences. In the Roy Adaptation Model, these influences are contextual and residual stimuli, as is adaptation in the other modes. In turn, one's life functioning depends on intact sensory function and adapting to the effect of temporary or permanent disabilities related to sensation.The life processes related to primary senses of seeing, hearing, and feeling are explored in this chapter. Examples of compensatory adaptive strategies and compromised processes related to sensory processes are described. There is particular focus on the compromised sensory experiences of pain and hyperactivity, which nurses encounter frequently in clinical practice. The nursing process is explored as it relates to promoting adaptation related to the senses.

OBJECTIVES

After studying this chapter, the reader will be able to do the following:

1. Describe three primary senses associated with the complex process by which an individual receives and exchanges information as presented in this chapter.
2. Identify one compensatory process related to each of the primary senses.
3. Name and describe two situations of compromised processes of the primary senses.
4. Identify significant first-level assessment behaviors for each of the primary senses.
5. List second-level assessment common stimuli that affect primary senses.
6. Develop a nursing diagnosis, given a situation related to the primary senses.
7. Derive goals for an individual with adaptation problems associated with the primary senses in a given situation.
8. Describe nursing interventions commonly implemented in situations of adaptation problems associated with the primary senses.
9. Propose approaches to determine the effectiveness of nursing interventions.

KEY CONCEPTS DEFINED

Detectors: Sensory receptors that act to detect the presence or absence of some component of the environment.

Feeling: A complex process involving the somatosensory system whereby touch and pressure, position sense, heat and cold, and pain are detected, transmitted, and interpreted.

Hearing: A complex process involving the peripheral structure of the ear, auditory neural pathways, and the auditory areas of the brain whereby sound waves are detected, transmitted, and interpreted.

Hyperactivity: The general term given to a group of behaviors such as constant movement, short attention span, distractibility, and poor impulse control; also referred to by terms such as attention deficit disorder, hyperkinesis, or minimal brain dysfunction.

Kinesthesia: Position sense resulting from mechanical changes in the muscles and joints, both the sense of static limb position and the sensation of limb movement.

Pain: A biobehavioral, subjective, and personal experience of noxious stimuli, considered to be whatever the patient says it is and occurring whenever the patient says it does. Acute pain is short in duration, has an identifiable cause, and follows an expected time course depending on the cause. Chronic pain is persistent and does not have a predictable time limit.

Perception: The interpretation of a sensory stimulus and the conscious appreciation of it.

Sensation: Processes whereby energy (light, sound, heat, mechanical vibration, and pressure, for example) is transduced into neural activity that becomes perception.

Suffering: Endurance of a difficult state, physiologic, psychological, or both; a severe state of distress associated with loss or threat of loss of the integrity of the individual.

Transducers: Sensory receptors that act to sample a portion of the energy associated with a component of the environment and convert the sampled energy into an electrical signal containing information.

Vision: A complex process involving the peripheral structure of the eye, visual neural pathways, and the visual area of the cerebral cortex in the occipital lobe of the brain whereby light energy is detected, transmitted, and interpreted.

BASIC LIFE PROCESSES OF SENSATION

Sensation includes processes whereby energy, such as light, sound, heat, mechanical vibration, and pressure, is transduced into neural activity that becomes perception. A particular characteristic of sensation is that it can cause an immediate reaction or its memory can be stored in the brain for minutes, weeks, or years and then can help to determine the individual's reactions at some future date. Sensory experience initiates most activities of the nervous system (Guyton & Hall, 2006). The neurologic basis for sensory processes provides some common principles for understanding these processes. These have been identified by Kolb and Whishaw (1996) and can be summarized briefly as follows:

1. Receptors are specialized parts of cells that transduce sensory energy into neural activity and are designed to respond to a narrow band of energy.
2. Receptive fields are the specific part of the environment to which the receptor responds and locates sensory events in space.

3. Receptors may be rapidly or slowly adapting, that is, if the sensation fades quickly it is rapidly adapting.
4. Localization and detection are determined by receptor density and overlap.
5. Neural relays of three or four neurons, connected in sequence, get information from receptor cells to the cortex.
6. Information transmission involves the coding of action potentials from all sensory systems and the carrying of that information along nerves, then tracts of the brain and spinal cord.
7. Sensory subsystems include multiple pathways such as different pathways from the eye to the visual cerebral cortex for color perception and for tracking moving objects.
8. Each sensory field is represented multiple times in the cortex, and one is considered the primary area for that sensory field.

The senses reduce an enormous array of environmental factors and influences to the single common language of the nervous system. Some years ago researchers noted that this is a first and very important step in enabling an individual to cope with a highly complex world (Meiss & Tanner, 1982). There are a large variety of sensory receptors in the human body and a continuous stream of stimulation to these receptors. Sensory receptors act as both detectors and transducers. They detect the presence or absence of something in the environment. Then, as transducers, they sample a portion of the energy associated with the particular event and convert the energy sampled into an electrical signal containing information such as the intensity of sound. Sensation gives rise to perception, another complex process that involves the central nervous system. Perception is a process of the cognator subsystem identified in the Roy model (see Chapter 2). Perception is defined as the interpretation of a sensory stimulus and the conscious appreciation of it. A simple description is that sensation is a result of activity of receptors and their associated pathways and corresponding cortical sensory areas. Perception, in comparison, is the result of activity of cells in the cortex beyond the first synapse in the sensory cortex. From the perspective of the Roy Model and a nursing view of information processing (Roy, 2001), one considers that the immediate sensory experience is transformed into a perception in association with such factors as education and experience; that is, the focal stimulus is processed in the light of contextual and residual stimuli. Perception includes providing meaning to what is sensed. For example, knowing that one's house is located near a highway where road repairs are taking place, an individual will attach a nonthreatening meaning to the rapid-fire noise of a jackhammer. As noted earlier, previous sense experiences can be stored as part of the interpretation of a present sense experience.

The primary senses of seeing, hearing, and feeling are processes by which an individual receives and exchanges information needed for the activities of life, including relating to others. The sensory network initiates most neural activity with stimuli acting on the visual, auditory, tactile (on the surface of the body), or other kinds of receptors.

Vision Processes

In introducing the visual system, Wickens (2000) noted that for human beings this is a highly sophisticated system providing us with detailed information about the form and patterns of the environment. Ability of vision to detect changes in light may be our most important sense. Vision is a series of processes involving the peripheral structure of the eye, visual neural pathways, and the primary visual area of the cerebral cortex in the occipital lobe of the brain. Some optic nerve fibers send branches to the midbrain and the hypothalamus as additional visual areas. The retina of the eye is the visual receptor. Light enters the eye and is bent slightly by the cornea. It is then bent further by the lens so that images are focused on the receptors at the back of the eye. The human retina has photoreceptor cells that function to transduce light energy into action potentials. The rods are sensitive to dim light and used for night vision. The cones transduce bright light for daytime and color vision. The rods contain rhodopsin, the purple-colored visual pigment. The cones have three photopigments.

The photopigments trap light and initiate chemical activity. The axons of ganglion cells, the third type of cells, leave the retina to form the optic nerve. Axons from the inner half of each eye cross over in the optic chiasm and terminate in the opposite occipital lobe. The separate pathways formed deal with visual perception in the primary cortical area and with such functions as eye reflex activity in secondary areas. Different parts of the visual field are represented in different parts of the brain. Thus, an individual may have varying visual disturbances after brain damage, for example, from a stroke, depending on areas of the brain affected. If the stroke affects the left side of the brain, the individual may not be able to see in the right visual field. To understand how the brain cells representing vision act, researchers have used microelectrodes to record the activity of these cells in cats and monkeys under local anesthesia. Visual stimuli are presented on a screen placed in the animals' visual fields. Results from studies indicate that the cells seem to differ in two ways (Kolb & Whishaw, 1996). The receptive fields (areas of responding cells) seem to be larger at each succeeding level of cortex. Thus complexity increases at higher brain levels. Second, cells in different levels of the visual system respond to different properties of visual stimulation. For example, there are cells that respond to the corners of objects and others that respond to moving objects.

Hearing Processes

Hearing is defined as the complex process whereby sound waves are detected, transmitted, and interpreted. Sound waves consist of changes in air pressure. The anatomy of the ear provides the basis for understanding the process whereby the ear transduces sound waves into action potentials. The outer ear catches the waves of pressure and deflects them into the ear canal. They are slightly amplified and directed to the eardrum. The eardrum vibrates when sound waves strike it. Transmission of the vibrations is by way of three small bones in the middle ear to the fluid of the inner ear. One of the bones, the stirrup, drives the fluid back and forth in the rhythm of the sound waves. The movements of the fluid cause a thin membrane, the basilar membrane, to resonate. It is this movement of the basilar membrane that causes movements of the auditory receptors. These receptors are the hair cells in the organ of Corti, whose cell membrane potentials are altered, resulting in neural activity. Different frequencies of sound are coded by way of the structure of the spiral-shaped cochlea, which holds the basilar membrane and organ of Corti.

Axons of the hair cells leave the cochlea to form the major part of the auditory nerve, the eighth cranial nerve. After projecting to the level of the medulla in the lower brain stem, synapses are formed and two distinct pathways emerge. One pathway projects to the primary auditory cortex and the other to the secondary regions. Representation of each cochlea in both sides of the brain is one way these pathways differ from the visual pathways. Less is known about the auditory cortex than about either the visual or the somatosensory. In general, it appears that in each subfield that has been mapped, low tones are represented farther back, with high tones more forward. Single neurons in the auditory system code the frequency or pitch of sounds, with different neurons having their greatest sensitivity to different sound frequencies. Below the level of the cortex, generally, cells are responsive to a broader band of frequencies than are cells higher in the central nervous system.

Feeling Processes

Feeling is the common term given to the complex processes whereby sensation from the somatosensory system is detected, transmitted, and interpreted. The somatosensory system includes the nervous system mechanisms that receive information from the body. It is a multiple sensory system composed of the following submodalities:

1. Touch and pressure, which is elicited by mechanical movement of body tissue.
2. Position sense or kinesthesis, resulting from mechanical changes in the muscles and joints, including both the sense of static limb position and the sensation of limb movement.
3. Heat and cold, showing neural discharges related to skin temperature changes.
4. Pain that is activated mainly by noxious stimuli near levels that damage tissue.

The sensation of touch has at least 20 different types of receptor cells, each of which transforms a different type of energy. In describing the somatosensory pathways, the complexities involved are simplified by considering that there are two subsystems. The first is for fine touch, pressure, and kinesthesis. The second is for pain and temperature (Kolb & Whishaw, 1996). The first system has fibers that leave the receptors and ascend the dorsal columns of the spinal cord to synapse in the lower brain stem. These fibers cross over and terminate in the thalamus and from there projections go to several areas of the cortex.

The second subsystem follows a different pattern. The fibers related to pain and temperature leave the receptors to synapse in the dorsal horn of the spinal cord. These cells then cross over to the other side of the cord and form a new tract. This tract terminates primarily in two areas of the thalamus. Finally, projections go to various areas of the cortex, as is the case with the other sensory systems. The results of the work of numerous researchers have suggested that at least five basic sensations are coded in the somatosensory system: light touch to the skin, deep pressure to the fascia below the skin, joint movement, pain, and temperature. Specific cells in the thalamus respond to only one mode of stimulation. At the level of the cortex, there is response also to a specific stimulus, but a given cell is responsive to a smaller region, making it possible to locate the stimulus on the skin. Other cells, even at the skin surface, have more complex properties, such as those of the hand, which respond to movement and precise orientation of stimuli. These properties make it possible to explore shape tactilely and in three dimensions.

COMPENSATORY ADAPTIVE PROCESSES

According to the Roy Adaptation Model, compensatory adaptive processes are activated by way of the regulator and cognator subsystems. The processes of sensation provide many examples of compensatory adaptive processes. An example of an innate regulatory process related to vision is light and dark adaptation. It is a common experience that when entering a darkened area, such as a movie theater, or going outside after sunset without lighting, it takes time for the eyes to adapt. When going into bright light after being in a darkened area, light adaptation takes place more quickly. During light adaptation, the individual feels an uncomfortable brightness that makes vision less effective. Both the rods and cones of the eye structures are involved in light and dark adaptation. When bright light enters the visual system set for dim light, the compensation that occurs is that the rod system essentially turns off. The cones and retinal neurons rapidly adapt in about a minute. After being overexcited, they are sufficiently desensitized for usual visual acuity.

While adapting visually in a dark environment, the individual may lose balance and have trouble moving around effectively. Changes in the cones occur in the first 7 minutes in the dark environment and allow a small increase in visual acuity. This is followed by a less rapid, but quantitatively greater rod adaptation. Enough rhodopsin returns to the rods after 20 minutes in the dark for dim-light vision. Reflexive changes of the pupil dilating allow more light to enter and contribute to dark adaptation. Dark adaptation also can be assisted by learned behavior in conjunction with the compensatory processes. The individual entering a dark room can plan ahead to have one hand on the wall to assist with balance. Dark adaptation can be maintained when visual acuity in the dark is necessary. For example, the individual viewing fluoroscopy wears red goggles when going into a brightly lighted area. The wavelengths in the red part of the spectrum allow cone vision to continue while stimulating rods only to a small degree. Thus, the individual can avoid having to wait 20 minutes to repeat the whole process of dark adaptation.

COMPROMISED PROCESSES OF THE SENSES

Adaptation problems can be caused by difficulties in any of the sensory processes. The two examples of compromised processes related to sensation were selected because of both their high incidence and the importance of the nursing role in planning care. Hyperactivity and pain are discussed here. It is estimated that 3% to 5% of all children are affected by what is now called attention-deficit/hyperactivity disorder (ADHD), possibly as many as 2 million American children. Families face the challenge of helping the child to effectively integrate sensory input and to modulate a response appropriate to environmental information. Another specific compromised process of sensation is the adaptation problem of pain. The nurse constantly meets people in pain. Varying degrees of discomfort usually go along with conditions for which people seek health care. Although pain is increasingly understood, all the advances of science have not eliminated the experience of pain. Further, although many treatment options are available, undertreatment of pain remains a significant problem in health care.

Hyperactivity

The general term hyperactivity was given to a group of behaviors that now have specific meanings and diagnostic criteria. Both the International Classification of Diseases and the DSM-IV group symptom domains for Attention Deficit Hyperactivity Disorder (ADHD) and Hyperkinetic Disorder (HKD) under inattention, hyperactivity, and impulsivity. The disorders are usually diagnosed in childhood and may last into adulthood, although some experts note that motor hyperactivity usually lessens in adolescence. Differences in activity levels for infants and children are common. Texts in pediatric nursing caution about the need to determine medically whether the child is truly hyperactive or is just a very active child. Differences in activity levels of infants have been described as ranging from placid, easygoing infants to those who have periods of calm and periods of greater activity to those who are in constant motion. These differences can be as great as the most active infant having 300 times the motility of the placid baby. Rowland (2005) noted that Attention Deficit Disorder (ADD), with or without hyperactivity, may be evident in infancy by reduced need for sleep, later by difficulty falling asleep, waking too early, or by multiple awakenings during the night. Further, an infant who is hyperactive may squirm and fidget, be difficult to hold, resist being confined to a crib or playpen, rest infrequently, and not be able to sit quietly.

For the child, behaviors are impulsive and seem uncontrolled. The child's attention span is short and there is difficulty sitting still and responding to discipline. Fidgeting or excessive running may be noted. Sleep difficulties and difficulty learning are a part of the behavioral pattern. The effects of the behavioral pattern often are noted in parents and siblings who may have difficulty coping with the busy, intense activity of the child's boundless energy. Children with the disorder are described as restless as shown by going from one toy to another without getting engaged. At school they may get up from their seats and wander in the classroom. They tend to talk too much. One author (Rowland, 2005) pointed out that they are impulsive, disorganized, and forgetful, and sometimes emotionally labile. Most children with ADHD are of normal intelligence but their marked distractibility may interfere with learning. In children affected by this neurobehavioral pattern, in its entirety or in part, boys outnumber girls by about four to one.

More recent studies note that genetic factors contribute strongly to ADHD. As with other conditions, genetic and environmental interactions are considered. Genes may act to modify the individual's response to particular environmental influences. Some environmental stressors include prenatal alcohol, smoking, medicines or illegal drugs, low birth weight, lead exposure, and child neglect (Taylor, 2007). It is now known that ADHD is associated with subtle changes in the structure and function of the brain. In practice, the diagnosis is made based on clinical history and observation, not on psychological or biologic markers. Carson et al. (2007) noted that a change in the child's condition, based on genetics and environment, leads to the symptoms of ADHD that are likely to be associated with alterations in the brain structures and functions that regulate the control of attention and impulses. One hypothesis is that there is dysfunction of the prefrontal cerebral cortex. Neurochemical theories have focused on monoamine neurotransmitter pathways.

Through EEG and PET studies of adults and animals, it has been noted that getting ready to process a visual stimulus quiets the activity of neurons in the visual areas of the brain. When a stimulus appears, for example, an arrow on a screen, the brain's electrical activity in the visual area is increased in amplitude. These observations suggest that, in normal individuals, the act of preparing for a target quiets the sensory system. Accordingly, it is hypothesized that attention deficits result in part from a problem in the child's preparatory mechanisms for attention. If this is the case, the child would be less successful in amplifying relevant stimuli so that these stimuli stand out over distracting stimuli. The greater distractibility of the child with the disorder arises because the quieting mechanisms have failed and the important signals are not amplified. The child is distracted from important sensory cues more readily (Posner & Raichle, 1994). Given the effect of the disorder on a child's development, particularly academic and social, families are often in need of support and specific help in handling the child's behavior.

The Centers for Disease Control and Prevention (CDC, 2007) noted that it is normal for children, at one time or another, to have trouble focusing and behaving. However, deciding if a child has ADHD is a several-step process. There is no single test to diagnose the disorder, but one step of the process includes having a medical exam, including hearing and vision tests. This is done to rule out other problems that have similar symptoms. Secondly, a checklist is used for rating ADHD symptoms and taking a history of the child from the parents, teachers, and sometimes, the child. The CDC recommends that if a parent or doctor has concerns about ADHD, they can take the child to a specialist such as a child psychologist or developmental pediatrician. There are also local early intervention agencies for children under 3 and public schools for children over 3. The CDC sponsors a National Resource Center with information for both children and adults at www.help4adhd.org. The aim is to help each child reach his or her full potential by getting help as early as possible.

Pain

Pain involves input to certain sense receptors and deserves special consideration because the phenomenon of pain is one of the most significant areas of nursing practice. Constantly meeting people in pain, both from disease and from treatments, can be distressing for the nurse. However, the novice quickly realizes that the ability of the nurse to provide comfort and alleviate suffering is a fundamental component of nursing responsibility. The experienced nurse never forgets this responsibility and strives throughout a career to improve abilities to provide comfort-giving measures. Writings by McCaffery and colleagues (1979, 1997; McCaffery & Beebe, 1989; McCaffery & Robinson, 2002) have been influential in providing an in-depth and practical understanding of pain as a human experience. Basically pain is a sensory, affective, behavioral, and cognitive personal experience of noxious stimuli. Pain is considered to be whatever the patient says it is and occurs whenever the patient says it does (McCaffery, 1979). This definition emphasizes the subjective and personal nature of the pain experience. Another commonly used definition is that pain is "an unpleasant sensory and emotional experience associated with actual or potential tissue damage, or described in terms of such damage" (International Association for the Study of Pain, 1979).

Significant evidence from research opens new perspectives on understanding the experience of pain. The reader is referred to McCaffery's seminal work and more recent publications by this and other experts for continuing to learn about topics related to pain. In its simplest form, pain acts as a protective mechanism to warn the individual of actual and potential sources of tissue damage. An example is withdrawing a hand quickly from a hot stove. This example illustrates the elements of sensation from specialized receptors, transduced into neural activity, then neural relays through the spinal cord, and finally, the involvement of specialized brain centers in interpretation of the pain stimulus. However, because of its complex biobehavioral nature, and the difficulty of contexts in which it occurs, pain more often loses its compensatory function and becomes a compromised process of sensation. The nurse learns to help the individual deal with pain that continues long after its adaptive purpose has been achieved.

The gate control theory of pain (Melzack & Wall, 1965, 1970, 1989) changed the focus of pain research. The shift from peripheral factor to CNS mechanisms also received wide attention in practice because the concepts have been useful in treating pain. In this theory, both the peripheral and central nervous systems are involved. However, the brain is important as a system that filters, selects, and modulates inputs. The higher CNS processes can deliver descending inhibitory messages to influence the spinal gate control system. The concept of neural plasticity was added to the theory (Turk & Melzack, 2001). It uses the idea that the nervous system is not totally hard-wired; rather it interacts with other inputs and can modify over time its own structure and functioning (see Chapter 12). Although the model may not be complete, it helps to understand the biobehavioral nature of pain, and contextual factors influencing this experience. This knowledge provides a basis for effective nursing intervention.

Pain processing occurs as other sensory processing and involves receptors, transduction, transmission, modulation, and perception. The receptors that transmit noxious stimuli (pain) are called nociceptors. These nerve endings are undifferentiated or free nerve endings and are found in nearly every tissue of the body. The nociceptors respond to thermal, chemical, and mechanical stimulation. For example, pressure is one type of mechanical stimulation. The response is release of chemical mediators such as cytokines and neuropeptides. Certain neurotransmitters, such as bradykinin, histamine, serotonin, and substance P, may be important in sensitizing the nerve endings and enhancing transmission of pain (Thorpe, 1990). Transduction, that is the generation of impulses, occurs by way of the A-Delta and C-fibers. The extensive supply of A-delta myelinated (fast) fibers, larger C unmyelinated (slow) fibers, and large A fibers on the skin result in the ability to localize pain when a finger is cut with a sharp object, for example. This combination of fibers also accounts for the initial stinging, sharp pain, and the slightly delayed throbbing and more diverse pain. In contrast, the viscera has fewer A-delta fibers and large A fibers. Thus, it is difficult to localize intra-abdominal pain. Transmission is the process of the electrochemical impulses being relayed to the CNS. Different types of nerve fibers and special spinal tracts form a complex network for relaying the pain sensation. Complex biochemical reactions occur throughout the process. Neurotransmitters can increase or decrease transmission of impulses from pain receptors. There may even be different receptors and different neurotransmitters for acute and chronic pain (Puntillo, Miaskowski, & Summer, 2003).

The primary processing area, or gate for pain, is located in the dorsal horn of the spinal cord. Groups of nerve cells lie in layers of the central portion of the gray matter of the spinal cord. Each group of nerves has a different function in relaying pain sensation messages. For example, one group is called lamina V and seems to be the key area for transmission of nociceptive stimuli from the dorsal horn to the opposite side of the spinal cord, where an ascending pathway transmits the sensation to the thalamus. The specialized ascending spinal tract is supplied with A-delta fibers and has only two synapses. Pain sensation by this route is sharp, well-localized, and relayed rapidly. Another ascending tract originates in the dorsal horn of the spinal cord and transmits impulses to the thalamus and limbic system. It travels close to the other ascending tract, but differs in that it has many synapses and mainly C fibers. Consequently, transmission of nerve impulses by this route is slower and more diffuse. Another tract, the dorsal column, also originates in the dorsal horn, but ascends dorsally and does not cross until the medulla and then synapses at the thalamus. Sensations received by way of this column specifically help the individual locate an injury.

The ascending spinal tracts carry the varying pain sensations to the thalamus, from which other neurons send the impulses to the cortex. The central mechanisms of pain involve the brain structures of the thalamus, limbic system, and reticular formation. The thalamus is a relay station, but also seems to play an important role in translating the sensation to a perception. Interactions of the ascending spinal tracts with the limbic system can be the source of fear, anxiety, and attention to pain in the individual experiencing pain. Within this system, the hippocampus and amygdala seem to be structures for translating short-term memory into long-term memory. This is an important factor in the management of pain. The reticular formation, and in particular the reticular activating system (RAS), influences the individual's level of arousal, including anxiety and distractibility. Further, the role of the cerebral cortex in memory and learning is significant for purposes of managing pain.

While various categories of pain are recognized, the focus here is on pain felt as a physiologic process that affects the other three adaptive modes, self-concept, role function, and interdependence. The physiologic process of pain can be acute or chronic, and the assessments and nursing interventions are different. Acute pain is short in duration, has an identifiable cause, and follows an expected time course depending on the cause. Acute pain goes away as healing occurs. Acute pain serves a useful purpose when it alerts an individual to an illness or injury. The symptom of pain may aid the health care personnel to determine the nature of the problem. Short-term pain can also accompany many therapies and diagnostic procedures. Perhaps the most common example of this is postoperative surgical incision pain. Chronic pain is persistent and does not have a predictable time limit. Approximately 10% to 20% of patients in primary care report chronic pain as a chief complaint (Marcus, 2005). Sometimes chronic pain is referred to as pain lasting longer than 3 months. However, rather than using an arbitrary time limit, the nurse focuses on the characteristics of chronic pain. When pain is chronic, it serves no useful purpose and may or may not have an identifiable cause that can be dealt with directly. The persistence of chronic pain is a constant source of suffering for the patient, and a challenge for the nurse in helping the patient with pain management. Patients who report chronic pain also experience psychological distress and disability that sometimes result in difficulties with relationships.

Understanding some common terms used in relation to the pain experience—pain levels, threshold, tolerance, and suffering—can be useful in nursing practice. However, using the subjective definition given by McCaffrey (1979) and the premises of holistic and individualized nursing care ensures that the terms are used correctly and avoids negative judgment on any individual's experience and interpretation of it. Pain levels means simply that various stimuli provoke varying amounts or degrees of pain. For example, a small area of burned tissue does not hurt as much as more extensive burn trauma. Similarly, although a surgical incision can always be uncomfortable, a chest wall incision that is aggravated by breathing and coughing can produce a more intense level of pain than an abdominal incision. Pain threshold is the level of intensity of the stimulus that causes the sensation or perception of pain. Given the same intensity of a noxious stimulus, the awareness of the beginning of the pain experience varies from individual to individual.

Pain tolerance is the amount of pain an individual can endure at a given time. Two people may experience pain at the same threshold, but the higher pain-tolerant individual may more readily incorporate the pain into overall sensations at the time without it becoming a major focus of attention. Further, for a given individual, pain tolerance will vary in different situations. An example is the patient with a severe headache who told the nurse, "I can stand a lot of pain, except if it is in my belly; my mother died of ovarian cancer." Finally, suffering relates to endurance of a difficult state, physiologic, psychological, or both. Suffering has been defined as a severe state of distress associated with loss or threat of loss of the integrity of the individual (Cassell, 1989). Although pain and suffering are not the same human experience, they are frequently linked. Experts noted that the suffering accompanying pain includes interpersonal, economic, and occupational issues as well as a myriad of other factors that are associated with the interpretation and subsequent response to the perception of pain (Turk & Melzack, 2001). Given the individual nature of pain, the nurse can be unjust to patients if she compares the pain experience of one individual with another, or uses a personal standard of expected responses to pain stimuli. Rather, the nurse will accept the challenge of learning more about the complexity of pain and the individual's experience of it.

NURSING PROCESS RELATED TO THE SENSES

Any loss of sensory function can affect the individual greatly, that is, a change in this physiologic mode component, affects all the adaptive modes. However, as the Roy Adaptation Model clearly emphasizes, people have great capacities to adapt to both internal and external changes. The nurse understands the processes by which the senses act to perceive and interact with the world and the related compensatory and compromised processes. Based on this understanding, the nurse can more competently assess people and plan care to promote sensory adaptation. It is possible, then, to assist individuals with temporary or permanent sensory losses to achieve and maintain the highest level of adaptation of which they are capable. In addition to the effect a sensory loss may have on the individual, loss of a functioning sense can change the way others, including health professionals, view an individual. For example, legally blind individuals often report that store clerks, waiters and waitresses, and others rarely address them directly when they are accompanied by a sighted person. In the hospital, a hard-of-hearing person may be labeled as confused or disoriented when he or she does not give what are considered appropriate responses to the queries of hospital staff. The confusion suddenly clears when the nurse recognizes the individual's hearing limitation and makes efforts to compensate for the loss.

The application of the nursing process is the formalized way that the nurse makes assessments and plans appropriate care to promote adaptation, mastery, and human and environment integration related to the senses. In dealing with the complex processes of the senses, as in other adaptive mode components, the nurse makes careful assessment of behaviors and stimuli. Diagnosis and mutual planning to set goals and select nursing interventions are based on the assessment. Evaluation then compares the reassessment of behaviors with the established goals.

Assessment of Behaviors for Processes of Vision

Behavioral assessment of vision involves physical assessment skills using both observation and measurement. In addition, the nurse uses sensitive interviewing, intuition, and perceptiveness. At times the nurse may conduct baseline assessments, for example, performing vision screening tests for schoolchildren. At other times, these assessments may be more precise and complete, for example, when visual field tests are done by a nurse practitioner in the annual physical examination of an individual who is a pilot.

FUNCTIONAL EXAMINATION   The external, or functional, examination of the eye includes its ability to move in its orbit and the reaction of the pupil to light and accommodation. Visual acuity refers to the ability of the eye to form an image in the finest detail. Visual acuity is measured for distance or far vision and for reading or near vision. Far vision can be tested by use of a Snellen chart. The individual is asked to identify letters or objects of varying sizes in a well-lighted area. The acuity of each eye is measured separately while the other eye is covered with an opaque card. The expected response is that the individual can identify letters of the 20 line at 20 feet when asked to read the chart. The term 20/20 is used for normal vision. Test cards for near vision are made for the individual with normal vision to read at 14 inches. Legal blindness usually involves visual acuity in the better eye, corrected with glasses, between 20/200 and 20/400. Reading is possible with this level of visual acuity, but high-powered magnifiers are needed and speed and endurance are limited. Gross orientation and mobility are usually adequate, but traffic signs are difficult to see. Near blindness means that the individual can count figures at 4 feet. Vision is reliable only under ideal circumstances and nonvisual aids are used. Total blindness means that the individual has no light perception and must rely entirely on other senses (Burrell, Gerlach, & Pless, 1997).

Usually there is greater importance placed on clarity of central vision. However, losses of peripheral or color vision can also be incapacitating. A perimeter is the instrument used to test peripheral vision. This indicates how far to the side the individual can see without moving the eye. The test is conducted with the individual's vision fixed with test objects moved in from the far periphery. Sometimes this can be done electronically with lights on a 360° field on the wall. Other times, the moving object is a piece of chalk on a string so that a mark is made on the spot where the individual first reports seeing the object in the line of vision. Normally, the individual can report visualizing objects in each of the four visual quadrants. To test color vision, the individual is asked to identify colored figures or test plates having a background of colored dots with a superimposed figure or number that can be discriminated only if the individual has the ability to identify colors. Referral to an ophthalmologist is indicated if the individual notices vision problems, there is unexplained or unnoticed vision loss of 20/30 or more, or upon examination the individual has losses in given visual fields or fails the test for color vision (Burrell, Gerlach, & Pless, 1997).

INTERNAL EXAMINATION   Internal examination of the structure of the eye is done in several ways. A tonometer is used to measure the intraocular pressure, which normally is 11 to 22 mmHg. The interior of the eye can be seen with an ophthalmoscope, which directs a small beam of light through the pupil. Refraction tests ascertain the ability of the lens and cornea to focus on the retina. Again, a referral to a physician is made if the nursing assessment reveals evidence of eye pathology.

Assessment of Behavior for Hearing Processes

Determining the degree and type of auditory processing and whether or not an individual has hearing loss is done by a careful history of complaints of hearing difficulties, physical exam to confirm intact structures, and hearing tests. Indications of hearing difficulty that the nurse may observe are such comments as "You are speaking too softly; I don't understand you," or, "They just mumble; the words are loud enough but I can't make out what they are saying."

Screening for hearing loss can be done with an audioscope to assess the individual's ability to hear pure tones at the frequencies of usual speech. If the individual has difficulty hearing these tones, a referral for an audiogram is warranted. The exam is done by an audiologist using specialized equipment to produce and control sounds. Auditory brain stem evoked responses (ABRs) provides a noninvasive way to record responses in certain parts of the central auditory pathways (Porth, 2005). An ABR measures the electrical responses arising from the auditory neural pathway. The test uses electrodes applied to the scalp and a series of clicks emitted at a rapid rate through earphones. The electrical activity detected by the electrodes following stimulation by clicks is delivered to a computer that extracts the acoustic response from ongoing neural activity. The acoustic response is then transferred to paper, as in an EEG or EKG, and the resultant waveforms can be studied. The test is useful to identify hearing threshold and to distinguish between cochlear and retrocochlear pathology.

Selecting an auditory screening test depends on the age of the individual. Any hearing loss for a child can have a major impact on development, particularly of language and learning. Estimates of varying degrees of hearing loss in newborns range from 1 to 4 per 1000. Early identification through screening programs is advocated and required by many states in the United States. The tests used are evoked otoacoustic emissions (EOAE) or the ABR. Both tests are noninvasive, easy to perform, and generally take less than 5 minutes. Both tests are ways of measuring responses to clicks or tones. If hearing loss is identified for the newborn or young child, full developmental and speech and language evaluation is needed (Porth, 2005). As individuals age, degenerative hearing loss is common. About 40% of the population over 75 years is affected and an estimated 23% between 65 and 75 years. Although a common problem, many older people do not get appropriate assessment for hearing loss. An audiogram is done to determine the loss in various frequencies. High frequencies are affected first.

There are two additional tests related to hearing function. The Rinne test is used to compare bone conduction with air conduction of sound. The tone produced by the tuning fork is generally heard approximately twice as long by air as by bone conduction. Weber's test is used to compare hearing in the two ears. In this test, the tone produced by the tuning fork is heard with equal loudness by both ears. In addition to the behaviors noted on testing, the nurse is also alert to other behaviors that may indicate difficulty hearing such as faulty speech, inattentiveness, unresponsiveness, strained or intense facial expression, and a tendency toward withdrawal in social situations.

Assessment of Behavior for Feeling

Assessment of somatosensory processing has many facets. These relate to the five basic sensations previously identified and are assessed for intact sensation and symmetry of feeling.

SENSATION   Light touch is tested by touching the skin with a wisp of cotton. With eyes closed, the individual states when and where he or she is being touched. Joint movement is tested by having the individual identify the position of fingers as up or down as the examiner moves them. The sense of pain is estimated by pinprick, occasionally substituting the blunt end of a safety pin. The individual reports whether the stimulus is sharp or dull. Two test tubes filled with hot and cold water can be used to test temperature. As the individual reports temperature changes, the examiner charts any areas of loss with oblique lines, one way for heat and the other direction for cold.

SYMMETRY   The ability to perceive the stimulus is the basic behavior assessed in sensory processing within each of the modalities of seeing, hearing, and feeling. Bickley and Szilagi (2007) make some general suggestions about assessment of feeling and sensory processing. The first is to compare the symmetry of sensation on the two sides of the body. With pain, temperature and touch compare distal and proximal areas of the extremities. If vibration and position are normal in the fingers and toes, then it can be safely assumed that the more proximal areas will also be normal. The examiner scatters the stimuli and varies the pace of testing so that most major peripheral nerves are covered and so that the patient does not merely respond to a repetitive pattern of testing. If an area of sensory loss or hypersensitivity is detected, the examiner maps out the boundaries in detail. Textbooks on physical assessment and general clinical nursing practice are available to provide additional details on assessment of feeling.

Assessment of Behavior for Pain

The assessment of pain merits particular attention given its significance in nursing practice. Some basic guidelines for assessment of pain can be followed even though the phenomenon is complex and presents itself in multiple forms. Whether the situation involves a school nurse and a 10-year-old child complaining of a stomachache, a hospital nurse responding to a patient in the postanesthesia room, or a home care nurse visiting an individual with chronic rheumatoid arthritis or terminal cancer, certain information is useful to plan for promoting adaptation. In a keynote address, the president of the American Pain Society promoted "Pain as the Fifth Vital Sign" (Campbell, 1995). The purpose was to increase awareness of pain assessment among health professionals. As in assessment of the senses in general, the nurse obtains a behavioral description of the individual's pain experience and the factors influencing it.

RAPPORT   Initially in assessing pain, the nurse establishes rapport with the patient and believes the report of pain, recognizing that the patient is the only authority on the pain being felt. The patient's report of pain is accepted in a caring manner. The nurse listens without interrupting and uses accepting nonverbal communication, such as making eye contact and touching the patient. Repeating and clarifying information show concern and are helpful in making an accurate assessment.

DESCRIPTION OF PAIN   The next step in pain assessment is to describe the pain: location, quality, intensity, onset, and duration. Although the location of pain may seem apparent, such as from an obvious problem such as a fracture or deep cut, the fact is that nurses sometimes erroneously assume that they know the source of an individual's pain complaint. For example, a 65-year-old man recovering from laminectomy surgery complained of being miserable and was grimacing. The nurse assumed that he was experiencing pain related to the surgical incision site and administered the potent intramuscular analgesic that was prescribed. After the injection, the patient commented "At home I just take a couple of aspirin when I have a headache like this." It is also common for an individual to have pain in more than one location at the same time. It is important that the nurse confirm the source of the individual's pain during each assessment of the situation. Whenever possible, ask the individual to indicate exactly where each pain is. The individual who complains of stomach pain may point to the left lower quadrant. A headache may turn out to be cervical neck pain when the site is demonstrated. In addition, even pain in an expected location can also indicate a newly developing problem. One example is an individual with a fracture who mentions increased pain in the cast area. The nurse may discover, by careful questioning regarding the exact location of pain, that a new concern is a developing infection under the cast.

The nurse assesses the quality of the pain by asking the patient to describe the pain in words. Words commonly used include sharp, dull, stabbing, cramping, aching, gnawing, burning, throbbing, tender, heavy, "feels like a boil," and "feels like a lot of pressure." The nurse suggests words only if the patient is having difficulty describing the pain and always gives a choice of terms: "Would you describe it as a sharp pain or a dull pain?" Be alert to references or comparisons to past episodes of illness or pain: "It's a lot like the last time I came to the emergency room," or, "Once I had distress like this after a big Italian meal," or, "Of course, I've had stomach problems all my life, but this time it's pretty bad." These kinds of comments can be followed through to obtain a thorough assessment and can help establish whether the individual's pain experience is acute or chronic in nature.

Intensity of pain is also described from the patient's perspective. The nurse lets the patient describe how strong the pain experience is, for example, mild, moderate, or severe. In addition, the nurse can use a numeric scale of 0 to 10, with 0 meaning no pain and 10 being the worst possible pain. The advantage for using a scale is that it is generally understood by the individual and provides an individualized measure of pain that the nurse can use to judge pain relief or the worsening of pain for that individual. Further, once the scale has been explained, it takes less energy for the patient in pain to respond to the question of where on the scale to make the current rating of pain. For example, the patient who has multiple fractures of one arm may report pain at 7 on the scale. Following administration of an analgesic, when the nurse returns to assess the effectiveness of the nursing intervention in relieving pain, the patient responds to the question by changing the rating to 2 on the scale. Faces on pain scales can be used with children. Such scales consist of a series of different facial expressions. The nurse explains to the child that each face is for an individual who feels happy because there is no pain, or hurt, or sad because there is some or a lot of pain. The child is asked to choose the face that best describes the pain experienced.

An approach similar to the faces scale can be used with some adults for whom communication is difficult. However, explanation of the use of the faces scale requires some language and cognitive competency. Nursing research recently has focused on how to assess pain in those who cannot self-report, such as people with cognitive impairment and the critically ill. Health care accrediting bodies issued pain-management standards in 2000. Most facilities have devised policies and procedures for obtaining pain-intensity ratings as part of routine care. McCaffery and Pasero (2005) clarified that pain behavior scales and pain behavior checklists can be useful if used appropriately. However, it is important to remember that they are not equivalent to the patient's report of pain intensity. For patients who cannot self-report, the recommendations by McCaffery and Pasero have been included in a position paper of the American Society for Pain Management in Nursing (Herr et al., 2006). Recommendations are made in the categories of persons with advanced dementia, infants and preverbal toddlers, and intubated and/or unconscious persons. The recommendations have some points in common: (1) Attempt self report, (2) document potential causes of pain, (3) observe patient behavior, (4) use surrogate reporting, and (5) attempt an analgesic trial.

Assessment of pain includes noting the onset and duration of pain. This is especially important during initial assessments to determine the acuteness or chronicity of the pain but can also elicit helpful information whenever a complaint of discomfort is voiced. The simple question, "When did you start noticing the pain?" may prompt the individual to relate a certain position in bed or the ingestion of a particular food or medication to the discomfort he or she is feeling. An aspect that is related to onset and duration is the constancy of the pain, and the individual is certainly the best judge of this. An individual being treated for severe diarrhea and fluid and electrolyte imbalance complained of pain around the site of an intravenous infusion. There was no problem apparent to the nurse, but when the question of whether it hurt all the time was asked, the puzzle was solved. It was related that the discomfort started when the most recent intravenous feeding bottle was hung, but was not present when the arm was held in a slightly bent position. The nurse realized that the higher dose of potassium in the most recent bottle was causing the pain, and it was relieved when the individual bent his arm and so slowed down the rate of infusion. Rather than subjecting the individual to an unnecessary intravenous restart, communication showed that a slower infusion rate, which the physician approved, kept the individual comfortable.

AGGRAVATING FACTORS   In assessing pain, the next step following a thorough description of the pain is to identify the aggravating and alleviating factors. Aggravating factors are those that make the pain worse, while alleviating factors are those that reduce pain. The individual may be able to identify certain activities, positions, temperatures, or times of day that tend to make the pain more intense. In identifying factors that reduce pain, the nurse will ask what specific pain relief methods the individual has used and what has worked for him or her in the past.

SIGNS OF OTHER PHYSIOLOGIC CHANGES   Next, the nurse examines the site that the individual indicates is painful. Examination is done to look for other signs such as heat, redness, swelling, tenderness, abnormal position, or factors that may be causing local irritation. For example, a postoperative patient who complains of pain in the calf of the leg may show additional signs on examination. If a red, firm, tender area is noted, this is reported to the physician for diagnosis of a possible thrombophlebitis.

SIGNS OF BEHAVIORAL CHANGES   In the next step of assessing the pain experience, the nurse describes the behavioral response to pain. In acute pain, the individual may be restless, thrashing, rubbing the body part, pacing, tensing muscles, grimacing, wincing on movement, and making other facial expressions of discomfort. Physiologic responses to acute pain include increased heart rate and respirations, as well as increased blood pressure. With an individual in chronic pain, the behavioral response is more likely to include a tired-looking, masked facial expression; quiet; increased sleep and rest; and diverted attention. An individual in chronic pain will not likely have changes in vital signs. People who have long endured chronic pain, even when it is severe, may have accommodated to the feeling of pain and therefore demonstrate little outward response. Depression often accompanies chronic pain, and this can serve to drain energy. Consequently, the individual tends to avoid both displays of pain and speaking of it related to feelings of helplessness, taking on an "Oh, what's the use" attitude. Sometimes there may not be any identifiable affected body part. For example, the pain connected with some disorders of the pancreas is of such a chronic nature that an individual may be observed watching television or talking casually on the phone even while experiencing severe pain.

Individuals in acute or chronic pain are likely experiencing anxiety. However, manifestations of anxiety, as well as the other behavioral responses to pain, will be individualized by the person. Another point in assessing pain is that some people with acute or chronic pain may not volunteer information about pain, as they assume that the nursing staff knows their situation and need. It may, in fact, be puzzling to patients that some nurses will question them about pain and others never mention it. One individual being observed for a kidney stone thought that he was expected to have pain only in the late afternoon and evening hours, as the nurses there in the evening were the only ones who frequently checked his level of comfort. Other people will not rely on the solicitude of the nursing staff and will readily share their response when they are hurting. The nurse incorporates into the assessment an understanding of the individualized experience of pain, and also the very individualized methods of expressing it. The nurse's own behavioral response also affects the patient's expression of pain.

VALIDATION OF FOCAL STIMULUS   The final step of assessment of the pain experience is to compare the nursing judgment with the individual's impression to see if both people have the same idea as to the cause of the pain. This has been discussed earlier in this text as validating the focal stimulus. An example of this process might be as follows. The nurse says to the patient: "It seems to me that you're a little more uncomfortable today. Is it because you didn't rest well last night?" The patient responds: "Well, that is partly it, but they were just in to remove all my dressings and drains and I just haven't been able to settle down since." This is also the time to check what the individual thinks will give relief. Recalling that pain is a subjective experience and recognizing that the individual is the only authority about his or her pain, the nurse also knows that the patient is the only one to tell whether or not techniques intended to bring comfort have been effective. When people are hurting, many aspects of normal physiology and human activity and interaction such as eating, moving, walking, sleeping, communicating, and sexual function can become less effective. Thus, pain reflects a compromised adaptation level affecting the other physiologic mode components and adaptive modes. Behavior observed can involve any of the modes. The nursing diagnosis, however, will focus on the pain. Goals and nursing management for addressing all modes affected will be aimed at the relief of the pain.

Assessment of Stimuli

In nursing assessment both physical assessment skills and interviewing methods are used. Specific interview questions are useful in assessing factors influencing sensory processes. This is the second-level assessment to identify stimuli. The introduction to sensory processing has highlighted the fact that sense experience becomes perception in the context of an individual's total life experience. As with each mode of the Roy Adaptation Model, in addition to assessing the behaviors, the nurse looks carefully at the context, or total life experience, relative to adaptation of the senses. Guidelines for assessing focal, contextual, and residual stimuli for all sensory processes are summarized in six basic questions (Table 10–1). Each question can help the nurse assess the individual's life experience. These questions are discussed for the sensory impairments of seeing, hearing, and feeling.

IMPAIRMENT TEMPORARY OR PERMANENT   An important factor influencing the individual's adaptation is whether the impairment is temporary or permanent, or if this is an unanswerable question at the current time. An example is a nurse's encounter with three people newly admitted to a hospital neurologic unit. They all have paralysis and loss of sensation in their right arms and hands. In reviewing the medical reports and in interviewing these people, the nurse determines by first- and second-level assessment (see Chapter 3) that one of them probably has a correctable situation. He has been admitted for a workup before brain tumor surgery, which is thought to have good possibilities for correcting the loss of arm sensation. The second individual sustained the loss of sensation in a skydiving accident 5 years ago, and the loss appears permanent. The third individual had a cerebral vascular accident 2 days ago, and it is uncertain at this time whether or not sensation will return to the right limb. It is clear that without incorporating this kind of information in assessment data, it would be difficult to complete the remaining steps of the nursing process with these people.

TABLE 10–1 Questions for Nursing Assessment of Stimuli for Sensory Impairment

1. Is sense impairment temporary or permanent?
2. Is impairment recent or long standing?
3. Is more than one impairment present?
4. How does the person view the loss of function?
5. How is the person affected in the current environment?
6. What is the person's level of knowledge, the knowledge needed, and readiness for teaching?

IMPAIRMENT RECENT OR LONG STANDING The second question closely follows the first, as it is fundamental to assessment. Is the impairment recent or long standing? When an 80-year-old man casually comments that he has not been able to hear anything with his left ear since he was young, the nurse may register this information with a sense of significance different from the response to another individual's complaint of sudden loss of hearing after a period of unconsciousness caused by a malfunction of scuba diving equipment.

MORE THAN ONE IMPAIRMENT The third question raises the concern of whether or not one or more than one impairment is present. Perhaps an individual with diabetes is learning to adjust to paresthesia (loss of feeling) affecting both feet, but is also experiencing retinal degeneration causing pronounced loss of vision.

INDIVIDUAL'S VIEW OF LOSS OF FUNCTION Throughout the assessment, the nurse is incorporating information regarding the fourth question, how does the individual view the loss of function? There is a wide range of reactions regarding both old and new problems involving the major senses, and these reactions are based on all the contextual and residual factors that make the individual unique. For example, the slightest danger of a potential loss of hearing could be very threatening to a musician, whereas an individual who works around jet aircraft might take it in stride as an expected component of the job. Nurses assess how individuals feel about newly developed losses, and also try to understand how people are coping with long-standing incapacities. Does the blind individual confront the loss of vision with continued anger, forced resignation, or matter-of-factness? Some people, for example, may still require a great deal of help in reaching a level of adaptation many years after becoming blind, while others may be at a stage of knowing they have met such a challenge with the best possible adaptation.

EFFECT IN CURRENT ENVIRONMENT The nurse deals with the fifth question and considers it of immediate relevance in all nursing encounters. How is the individual affected in the current environment of home, work, school, clinic, or hospital and moving from one place to another? The individual's comfort in these settings is very important. Even more fundamental are safety factors. The nurse is very careful to assess any loss of sensation with a view to potential safety problems. To what degree does the individual not see, hear, or feel, and what hazards does this present? Can the schoolchild with retinitis pigmentosa safely play sports in the bright sunlight, or would school gym sports such as tumbling and swimming be better choices? Does the hard-of-hearing, hospitalized individual tend to smile and nod even when addressed by a name other than his own? Does the patient with cataracts see well enough to ambulate safely around obstacles in the long-term care facility? The nurse learns quickly that nursing according to the Roy Adaptation Model fosters and encourages physical independence. However, responsibility in assessing the sensory processes is rooted in a sharp awareness of potential situations that could result in harm to the individual. In particular, the combination of a new environment, as when an individual is admitted to the hospital or has to travel to visit a clinic, and the stress of illness may change the context so as to reduce the safety level for a usually adapted individual.

LEVEL OF AND NEED FOR KNOWLEDGE AND READINESS FOR TEACHING The sixth assessment question follows naturally from the other five, and helps the nurse finalize the assessment. What is the individual's level of knowledge, the knowledge needed, and readiness for teaching? Is teaching for long-range purposes needed, as, for example, the proper method for inserting contact lenses, or how the newly diagnosed glaucoma patient will instill eye drops daily? Is the concern for short-term specific bits of information, such as safety precautions while one eye is bandaged? Is it appropriate for one nurse to conduct the teaching, or do notes need to be made on charts, care plans, or home care flowcharts so that more than one nurse can contribute to teaching information, reinforcing the learning that has been accomplished and reassessing learning needs? Are individuals significant to the patient also involved in health teaching? How much can the individual be expected to absorb, and on which senses can one rely? The nearly blind individual will learn little from a teaching film, and the individual who is in the process of adapting to a hearing aid will profit little from a small-group discussion. From the data that are generated by these questions, the nurse can identify which factors are most immediately influencing the individual, that is, what is focal and what is contextual or contributing to adaptation of sensory processes, and any alterations in their functioning. Finally, the nurse can note stimuli that need further assessment because they may be affecting the individual's ability to respond positively to the situation, but they have not yet been verified by the nurse or the patient.

Basically, many of the problems of altered sensation are medical problems with associated medical interventions to treat the many possible disruptions to the underlying neurologic pathways. Understanding of neuropathology is one way the nurse uses a broad knowledge base in clinical practice. The nurse's total assessment of the individual's behavior and context related to all the senses provides the understanding of the individual's life experience from which the nursing diagnoses are derived and plans for nursing care implemented.

Nursing Diagnosis

Diagnosis in the physiologic mode component of the senses proceeds in the same way as discussed throughout this text. The data from the nursing assessment of behaviors and stimuli are interpreted in the statement of a nursing diagnosis. One method for stating a nursing diagnosis according to the Roy model is for the nurse to identify a cluster of observed behaviors and the most relevant stimuli. An example of a nursing diagnosis for a 5-year-old boy who has just started kindergarten is: "child will not stay seated in the classroom, runs constantly at recess, does not follow directions, and sometimes falls asleep related to probable medical diagnosis of attention deficit hyperactivity disorder and inconsistency in child care while single mother works." Another way of stating a nursing diagnosis is to identify a summary label from an established classification list. Using the diagnostic label, the nurse communicates the judgment regarding the clinical situation in a way that most clearly represents the essence of the problem. In Chapter 3, two classification lists based on the Roy Adaptation Model were described, indicators of positive adaptation and commonly occurring adaptation problems. In Table 10–2, the diagnostic categories based on the Roy model for the senses are related to the diagnostic labels approved by the North American Nursing Diagnosis Association (NANDA International, 2007). The most common diagnosis related to the senses from the NANDA list is sensory–perceptual alteration (specify as to visual, auditory, kinesthetic, tactile, or olfactory). In a given clinical situation, each summary label can be described better by adding a statement of the relevant stimuli. For example, a school-aged child may have a diagnosis of "altered visual sensation related to recent, sudden, and permanent loss of sight in one eye by

TABLE 10–2 Nursing Diagnostic Categories for the Senses

Positive Indicators of Adaptation	Common Adaptation Problems	NANDA Diagnostic Labels
• Effective processes of sensation • Effective integration of sensory input into information • Stable pattern of perception, that is, interpretation and appreciation of input • Effective coping strategies for altered sensation	• Impairment of a primary sense • Potential for injury • Loss of self-care abilities • Stigma • Sensory overload and deprivation • Sensory monotony or distortion • Potential for distorted communication • Pain • Acute • Chronic • Perceptual impairment • Ineffective coping strategies for sensory impairment	• Risk for injury • Acute pain • Chronic pain • Readiness for enhanced comfort • Stress overload • Disturbed sensory perception • Impaired verbal communication • Readiness for enhanced communication

being struck with a baseball that caused retinal damage." In time, a positive adaptation diagnosis for a hyperactive child may be "increasing effectiveness of integrating sensory input related to consistent plan for quieting techniques used by mother, teacher, and grandmother."

Sometimes an experienced nurse makes a nursing diagnosis based on the Roy Adaptation Model by using a commonly accepted term that summarizes a behavioral pattern when more than one mode is affected by the same stimuli. An example is: "sensory disturbance of overload related to same-day surgery." Sensory input, that is, all the stimuli received by the senses, varies in both amount and predictability. Continuous input of meaningful sense cues is necessary for adaptive human behavior. Sensory disturbance occurs when an individual is receiving cues at either end of the continuum of absolute reduction in sensory stimulation (sensory deprivation) or increased stimulation to the point of too much (sensory overload). Qualitatively, input ranges from stimuli that have no order or predictability (distortion) to stimuli that are never-changing, repeated, and continuous (monotony). The amount of deprivation, overload, distortion, or monotony that affects a given individual depends on the individual and the other factors of the situation. In Roy model terms, this means the effect of sensory input depends on the individual's integrity of adaptive modes, adaptation level, and other stimuli.

Specific examples of variation of sensory input (focal stimuli changes) that nurses may encounter are deprivation (blindness, eye patches, deafness, isolation, and immobility), distortion (one eye patched, scarred cornea, partial deafness, tinnitus, and strange hospital noises), overload (same-day surgery and special intensive care units), monotony (same position and respirator). Behavioral responses to sensory deprivation extend from mild to extreme. Mild reactions to reduced or increased sensory input include boredom, restlessness, irritability, fatigue, drowsiness, mental confusion, and occasional anxiety. In more extreme cases—for example, when researchers have placed subjects in a black, soundproof box—drastic cognitive responses include delusions, primary process thinking, and inability to think. Emotionally, the participants became labile, or unstable. Perceptual hallucinations were frequent. One important contextual factor influencing the behavioral response to variation in sensory input was the amount of concurrent social contact. In the black box experiments, the participants had less drastic effects if they were in audio contact with the experimenter.

If input through one modality is reduced, for example, if the eyes are patched, then input in other modalities are contextual stimuli. One researcher found that eye-patched patients with hearing impairments had greater reactions to the deprivation than eye-patched patients with normal hearing. Others have noted that immobility at the time of deprivation increases its effect. Some studies have shown that certain drugs have been precipitating factors in responses to deprivation. Investigators have validated the expectation that length of time of deprivation is significant. For patients whose eyes were patched for less than 24 hours, only 35% had one or more mental symptoms. However, when the time was increased, 100% had one or more symptoms of deprivation. This is considered in situations such as the case of long-term healing of a serious eye injury. One study found that knowledge of the anticipated length of time of deprivation also lessens the symptoms. Residual factors that may possibly affect behavioral responses to variations in sensory input are age (older individuals seem more susceptible), gender (women seem to tolerate disturbance longer than men), and personality factors (for example, the compulsive individual has a greater need to structure the environment).

Goal Setting

In setting goals using the Roy Adaptation Model, the nurse makes a clear statement of outcomes expected for the individual as a result of nursing care. This statement is mutually developed when possible and stems from the nursing diagnosis. A clear goal statement is one that contains the behavior of focus, the change or stability expected, and the time frame for achieving the goal. In dealing with altered sensation, the nurse considers both short- and long-term goals. Often a long-term goal is made up of several successive short-term goals. Given an example of a child with blindness in one eye, the clinic nurse may establish with the child and his mother the goal that he will travel to and from school safely by himself 1 day in a given week. The long-term goal is that he will be independent in participating safely and effectively in classroom and school activities. For each goal, the nurse establishes appropriate strategies planned to meet the goal. The outcome criteria established by the American Association of Neuroscience Nurses (AANN, 2001) for individuals with uncompensated sensory deficits, particularly of vision, hearing, and tactile sensation, are as follows:

- The individual communicates a sense of comfort and security within the environment.
- The individual uses assistive devices and compensatory techniques correctly.
- The individual sustains no burns, falls, wounds, or pressure injuries.

The nurse then proceeds to develop and implement appropriate strategies to address each goal.

Nursing Intervention

The goal of the nursing care plan focuses on the behaviors noted in the nursing assessment. In the next step of the nursing process, interventions are based on the stimuli related to the behaviors assessed. Management of the focal stimulus is a preferred method of promoting adaptation. With this physiological mode component, a loss may be the focal stimulus, and many sensory losses cannot be altered. Nursing interventions thus deal with the individual's total experience, comprised of focal, contextual, and residual stimuli. These are the stimuli that affect the individual's experience of altered sensation. In understanding the individual's total experience, the nurse can better design appropriate interventions. One example of nursing intervention relates to the stimuli involved in the diagnosis for the 10-year-old boy with recent loss of vision in one eye and the goal to facilitate safety and independence in traveling to and from school. Nursing approaches could include providing the child and his parents with a booklet with CD on safety for the partially sighted, determining the distance and terrain to be covered on the way to school, 10 minutes a day practice walking in an area with obstacles, and having his brother accompany him on the first few walks. For individuals with one or more sensory impairments, the AANN lists the following general nursing measures:

- Orient the individual to the environment, utilizing the intact senses.
- Modify the environment and daily routines to include such things as permanent placement of furniture and articles and adaptation of the telephones, doorbells, and warning devices.
- Provide detailed information and instruction related to the disability and appropriate compensatory approaches.
- Institute appropriate safety precautions such as providing assistance and supervision and eliminating or reducing environmental hazards.

In considering nursing interventions for adaptation problems stemming from sensory deprivation and overload, a tangible and immediate change in or management of stimuli is used. Situations in which an individual is deprived of adequate sensory input include a blind or deaf individual placed in an isolation room, immobilized in traction, or on a respirator. The nurse makes direct use of personal contact on a scheduled basis. Television and radio, music personally selected on a digital player, and careful choice of roommates and room location are some nursing interventions designed to increase stimulation. If the adaptation problem stems from overstimulation, as can occur with same-day surgery, prolonged outpatient testing procedures, a noisy location on the unit, or intensive-care unit situations, the nurse again intervenes. This time the plan may provide for uninterrupted rest periods, a move to a quieter location, providing a quiet place for patients to rest between tests, and similar measures designed to reduce the amount of new experiences with which the individual is confronted in a given time period. This can be especially important for an older individual or a person who is confused (see Chapter 12). To this point, the presentation of nursing interventions has focused on sensory disturbance. Further discussion of nursing interventions focuses on the compromised adaptive processes discussed previously, hyperactivity and pain.

HYPERACTIVITY Managing the environment of a hyperactive child involves interventions that are both preventive and reactive. Preventive nursing interventions are environmental modifications used to reduce stimuli that can contribute to the problem behavior. Some contextual stimuli that can be managed for the hyperactive child include amount of noise, movement, or other individuals who may be particularly stimulating. The nurse can help families provide a home atmosphere that has decreased stimuli; for example, busy wallpapers, curtains, and fabrics are best avoided. Sparse, smooth-lined furnishings can be helpful. Reactive nursing interventions teach the child more appropriate ways to deal with his or her own behavior. Strategies include learning self-regulation, listening, and problem-solving skills. For example, for children of school age, it is particularly important that nurses, parents, physicians, and teachers work together in assessing the child's needs and planning a consistent approach to care. Teamwork is facilitated by common understandings of the nature of the problem and the plan for care. The nurse can provide encouragement and support during diagnosis and the time it takes to develop, modify, and maintain an effective plan for care.

Although education about ADHD is the foundation for an effective treatment plan, Brown (2000) noted that it does not change the underlying impairments resulting from chemical problems in the brain. Well-managed medication brings improvement in about 85% of children, according to most drug studies. Medication management requires working with dosage to get therapeutic responses and to minimize side effects. Medication alone is not enough. Medication can enhance effectiveness of behavioral and cognitive approaches. Manuals of nursing interventions are available for both teachers and parents that list specific nursing interventions for given behaviors. An example of the goals and objectives set up for the specific behavior "Does not listen to what other students are saying" is as follows:

- Goals: (1) The student will improve listening skills in nonacademic settings. (2) The student will attend to what other students say.
- Objectives to meet the goals include: (1) The student will maintain eye contact when other students are speaking on two out of three occasions. (2) The student will listen quietly when other students are speaking on one out of two occasions. (3) The student will repeat what other students have said with 25% accuracy. (4) The student will respond appropriately to what other students say on one out of four occasions.
- For this behavior, one manual (McCarney, 1994) lists 21 nursing interventions, with the first being to make certain that the student's hearing has been recently checked. It is then recommended that the student be reinforced for listening when spoken to by other students, for example, making eye contact, putting aside materials, answering students. The student may be given a tangible reward such as classroom privileges, line leading, passing out materials, or 5 minutes free time. The student may also be given an intangible reward such as praise, a handshake, or a smile for listening to what other students are saying. A third nursing intervention is to reinforce the students in the classroom who listen to what other students are saying. The fourth nursing intervention directs the teacher or parent to speak to the student to explain what the student is doing wrong (for example, failing to listen to what other students are saying) and what the student should be doing (for example, listening to other students when they speak to him or her and listening to other students when they speak to a group). Further approach are listed.

Given the complexity and constancy of intervention plans, the parents need constant support and encouragement. The nurse can suggest safe, age-related play and social activities. Reassurance that the child's behavior is not willful and that the hyperactivity may decrease in adolescence can be comforting to parents. Adolescence presents the challenge of developing strategies to facilitate independence seeking and continue development of self-management of modulating. Parents sometimes need release time provided by a reliable substitute caregiver. Three or four hours, a couple of times a week, may decrease the frustrations of parents who are constantly implementing a plan for given behaviors of hyperactivity. Referral to national and local support groups and online resources from the CDC as noted may be helpful as parents can offer much support and firsthand suggestions for these families.

PAIN   Unrelieved and undertreated pain remains a public health problem despite nearly 30 years of efforts by health professionals including nurses as well as lay organizations. In an influential paper, Melzack (1990) noted that undertreatment leads to the tragedy of needless pain and suffering. The author pointed out that one reason, fears about addiction, was not valid. Concern over addiction led many nations in Europe and elsewhere to outlaw virtually any uses of morphine and related substances. There is a high social concern for drug abuse and its consequences. However, such fears by the patient in pain or health care workers planning pain relief interventions are generally misplaced. Many caregivers in countries where morphine is legal for medical therapy, including the United States and Great Britain, fear turning patients into addicts and therefore deliver amounts that are too small or spaced too widely to adequately control pain. Based on numerous studies that validate the distinction, Melzack urges health care workers to distinguish between the addict who craves morphine for its mood-altering properties and the psychologically healthy patient who takes the drug only to relieve pain.

Studies that document undertreatment identify groups most at risk as older adults, minorities, and addicts. One study found that 40% to 85% of nursing home residents had pain that was undertreated. The findings of another study showed that Hispanics with pain were half as likely as white patients to receive analgesics (Ignatavicius & Workman, 2006). Pain can be a frightening, frustrating, and at times overwhelming experience, not only for the suffering individual, but also for others involved in the situation. As difficult as it may be to witness suffering, people in pain cannot be helped when caregivers avoid them. Feeling confident regarding what is effective nursing care for people experiencing pain helps alleviate the nurse's own apprehensions. The nurse will continue to search for individualized interventions among many possible approaches until adequate pain relief is reported by the individual. It was noted earlier that the gate control theory of pain links the physiologic and psychological events of pain. The resulting explanation for the holistic human experience provides several approaches to nursing intervention in managing pain. At the site of the pain receptors, other receptors can be stimulated to override the nociceptive, or painful messages. Pain impulses can also be altered in what has been termed the physiologic "gate" in the dorsal horn of the spinal cord. The interconnections of spinal nerve fiber tracts, thalamus, reticular formation, and cortex are the mechanisms for messages to open or close the "gate."

There are a number of approaches available when relief from pain and discomfort is the goal. Based on the cause of the pain, the nurse selects one or more interventions. Common approaches to pain relief are listed in Table 10–3. We can view each approach as a particular way of managing the focal and contextual factors contributing to the pain experience. It should be emphasized that the importance of more than one nursing intervention is often overlooked. The individual with incision site pain from a bowel resection may require an intramuscular analgesic, but a short ambulation to relieve gas accumulation also may be warranted. A refreshing bath, a lotion back rub, and some local heat or cold application may be the best combination for an individual experiencing a flare-up of spinal osteoarthritis.

The context in which the pain management strategies are presented is important to their effectiveness. People want relief and the nurse always suggests interventions to the patient in a positive manner, conveying the idea that pain relief is the specific goal. Even when individuals have to be denied what they see as a relief measure, a positive approach can help, as in the following

TABLE 10–3 Approaches to Pain Relief

1. General comfort
   - Repositioning person in bed or wheelchair
   - Tightening sheets, realignment of pillows, covers
   - Changing dressings
   - Warm or cool baths or showers
   - Back rubs
   - Ambulation
2. Other physical
   - Heat or cold local application
   - Massage
   - Exercise
   - Immobilization
   - Transcutaneous electrical nerve stimulation
3. Behavioral–Cognitive
   - Relaxation exercises
   - Imagery and biofeedback
   - Presence, distraction, touch, and reassurance
   - Education and instruction—pain and pain relief
   - Music therapy
   - Hypnosis
4. Opioids
   - Agonists: morphine, fentanyl, hydrocodone, hydromorphone, meperidine, methadone, codeine
   - Agonists/Antagonists: pentazocine, butorphanol, nalbuphine, buprenorphine
5. Non-opioids
   - Acetaminophen
   - NSAIDs (nonselective): aspirin, ibuprofen, naproxen, etodolac, ketoprofen, piroxicam, salsalate
   - Cox-2 Inhibitors: Celebrex, Bextra
6. Local and regional anesthetic blocks
7. Adjuvant analgesics

example. An individual was seen in the emergency room at 2:00 a.m. with the medical diagnosis statement, "rule out appendicitis." The emergency room physician wrote orders for close observation, intravenous fluids, and "no pain medication until seen at 6 a.m. by surgeon." The patient asked the nurse for a shot for pain. Instead of responding flatly that she could not give the medication, the nurse carefully explains that potent medications would mask symptoms and make the process of medical diagnosis more difficult. Other measures that the nurse could use include staying with the patient for several minutes and incorporating such comments as the following in their conversation: "You'll be able to rest better now that the initial diagnostic work is finished. I'll check on you frequently throughout the night, but I feel that you'll be able to sleep now. You were dehydrated and the intravenous fluid will take care of that problem."

Drug therapy is often used in control of pain. Concern for patient safety in drug administration has led to considering the "five rights." The five are: the right drug, the right dose, the right time, the right route, and the right client (Kazanowski & Laccetti, 2002). Often nurses make judgments, or help patients learn to make judgments, about drug management. This includes deciding which drug, which route of administration, what dose, and how doses will be timed. The nurse combines teaching about medication with teaching related to other pain-relieving approaches. Analgesics are common drugs of choice when pain relief is the goal, even though they treat only the symptom of pain and not the cause. Analgesics are classified in several ways: non-opioids, opioids, local and regional anesthetics blocks, and adjuvant analgesics. Drugs may also be addictive or nonaddictive, prescription or over-the-counter, strong or weak, and peripheral or central acting. An ideal analgesic would have the strength matched to the intensity of the pain, be nonaddicting, and have few side effects. Peripheral-action drugs interfere with the transmission of painful stimuli from body sites, whereas central-acting drugs alter perception of and consequently responses to pain on a cortical level.

Opioids, such as morphine, are the more potent of the oral, intramuscular and epidural agents. They interact with the opiate receptors in the body. The nonopioid agents, such as acetaminophen (Tylenol, Datril, Tempra), and nonsteroidal anti-inflammatory drugs (NSAIDs) such as aspirin and ibuprofen (Motrin, Advil, Nuprin), are considered less strong and do not have opiate receptor affinity. Newer drugs are selective NSAIDS called Cox-2 inhibitors (such as Celebrex and Bextra). The specific anti-inflammatory properties of these drugs make them effective for certain painful conditions, arthritis, for example. The nurse is aware of potential side effects of all drugs. Aspirin and other NSAIDs require particular vigilance for gastric discomfort or bleeding. With the search for more effective drugs for pain relief, sometimes new medications are in use before the side effects are known fully. The nurse continues to be aware of developing research in the area. More detailed information about the properties of analgesics and about other drug therapies for pain can be found in pharmacology resources and pain management texts. As discussed above, concern for drug addiction limits appropriate clinical judgment for use of pain medication. Based on this concern, the U.S. Agency for Health Care Policy and Research (AHCPR) issued a set of guidelines related to the management of acute pain. These recommendations are summarized in Table 10–4.

Nursing judgment of a high order is used when medications are part of planned interventions for pain relief. This is especially true when several options are prescribed. There may be oral, intramuscular (IM), and intravenous (IV) preparations ordered. Several different drugs or various doses for the same drug are ordered at the same time. Patient-controlled-analgesia (PTA) with an IV infusion or internal pump and epidural analgesia are often used for better pain control, particularly in postoperative patients. The patient adjusts the dose of the drug on the basis of the level of pain and response to the drug. A lock is set so that the patient cannot accidentally overdose. The advantages are more consistent pain relief and more control by the patient. In regard to clinical judgments by the nurse, consider the case of a 34-year-old man admitted to an orthopedic unit after sustaining several fractures and various lacerations during a motorcycle accident. After surgery to insert a pin and cast application, his pain relief medication orders were as follows: Demerol 75 to 100 mg IM every 3 to 4 hours for severe pain, Demerol 50 to 75 mg IM every 3 to 4 hours for moderate pain, Visteril 50 mg IM may be added to Demerol doses as needed, Tylenol 10 mg orally every 4 hours as needed, and Mylanta 30 cc orally every 4 hours as needed.

TABLE 10–4 AHCPR Summary Recommendations for Acute Pain

---

1. *Promise patients attentive analgesic care.* Patients should be informed before surgery, verbally and in printed format, that effective pain relief is an essential part of their treatment.

2. *Chart and display assessment of pain and relief.* A simple assessment of pain intensity and pain relief should be recorded on the bedside vital sign chart or a similar record that encourages easy, regular review by members of the health care team and is incorporated in the patient's permanent record.

3. *Define relief levels to trigger a review.* Each institution should identify pain intensity and pain relief levels that will elicit a review of the current pain therapy, documentation of the proposed modifications in treatment, and subsequent review of its efficacy.

4. *Survey patient satisfaction.* At regular intervals defined by the clinical unit and quality assurance committee, each clinical unit should assess a randomly selected sample of patients who have had surgery within 72 hours. Patients should be asked their current pain intensity, the worst pain intensity in the past 24 hours, the degree of relief obtained from pain management interventions, and satisfaction with relief and the staff's responsiveness.

5. *Analgesic drug treatment should comply with several basic principles.*

   a. Nonopioid "peripherally acting" analgesics: Unless contraindicated, every patient should receive an around-the-clock postoperative regimen of an NSAID.

   b. Opioid analgesics: Analgesic orders should allow for the great variation in individual opioid requirements, including a regularly scheduled dose and "rescue" doses for instances in which the usual regimen is insufficient.

6. *Specialized analgesic technologies*, including systemic or intraspinal, continuous or intermittent opioid administration or patient-controlled dosing, should be governed by policies and standard procedures that define acceptable levels of patient monitoring and appropriate roles and limits of practice.

7. *Nonpharmacologic interventions.* Cognitive and behaviorally based interventions include a number of methods to help patients understand more about their pain and to take an active part in its assessment and control. These interventions are intended to supplement, not replace, pharmacologic interventions. Staff should give patients information about these interventions and support patients in using them.

8. *Monitor the efficacy of pain treatment.* Periodically review pain treatment procedures.

Source: Acute Pain Management Guideline Panel, 1992. Used with permission.

Judgments involve differentiating between moderate and severe pain, deciding if Vistaril will be of help to this individual, administering Tylenol and Mylanta when the need is assessed, and determining the appropriate interval between each injection of Demerol in the context of the pain experience at that time. In addition to assessing the kinds of discomfort the individual is experiencing at a given time, other factors are relevant to nursing judgments. They are the exact hour and amount of the last pain medication and how it affected him, how he perceives the pain, and his size. The typical as-needed drug order essentially means that the drug is given only after the pain returns. Evidence demonstrates that this approach, based on the fear of addiction, is not valid (Melzack, 1990). Rather, there is another, more humane way to treat pain, which was pioneered in the treatment of cancer patients and is gaining broader acceptance. In this approach, the pain is controlled continuously by doses that are given regularly, according to a schedule that has been determined to prevent recurrence of the individual's pain. With this preventive administration of medication before pain becomes extreme, patients require fewer doses and are better able to resume regular activities earlier.

Other nursing interventions for pain include general comfort measures, such as positioning and warm or cool baths or showers. Other physical approaches for pain relief include local applications of heat and cold, massage, and exercise. Many protocols for behavioral-cognitive interventions have been demonstrated to be effective, such as to the presence of the nurse for encouragement, distraction, relaxation exercises, and imagery and biofeedback. For some individuals, referral to a pain clinic is the best option. These programs integrate many of the above approaches. They aim to foster independence and self care while promoting pain control and improving quality of life.

Evaluation

The effectiveness of nursing interventions is evaluated by determining whether or not the goals of the plan for care have been accomplished. The preset goals identified the behavior of focus, the change or stability desired, and the time frame. Consider the goal described earlier for the child with a recent loss of sight in one eye: "The child will travel to and from school safely by himself 1 day this week." The behavior of interest is the child's trips to and from school. If he has, in fact, made at least one trip by himself this week without injury, the goal has been accomplished. If this goal was not accomplished, the nurse will assess the situation further to see if all relevant factors in designing the nursing intervention have been considered. For example, in spite of his stated eagerness to try this task, the child may be more afraid than he will admit, particularly if he thinks older children will take advantage of his vision limitation. Another possibility is that the nursing interventions have not been used long enough. The child may need more practice navigating on his own street with someone nearby to give feedback and warn him if he is about to make a mistake.

In evaluating nursing interventions for pain, the main criterion is pain relief. As indicated earlier, the patient is the authority on the pain experience and the report of relief is the most important behavioral indicator. The individual is also observed for decrease in nonverbal cues of discomfort, for example, clenched teeth, tightly shut lips, furrowed brow, biting the lower lip, grimacing, and rhythmic or protective body movements. Relief may be partial and the intervention may need to be modified in some way. For example, the individual may require a larger dose of analgesic, increased ambulation, more frequent position changes, reinforcement of relaxation techniques, or a combination of nursing interventions to obtain more complete relief. In addition, the nurse will evaluate whether or not the individual is experiencing any negative side effects from the intervention, such as decreased respirations from an analgesic or pressure on a body part from special positioning.

Summary

This chapter has focused on the senses as a component of the physiologic mode and channels for receiving information and thus interacting with the environment by way of complex neurologic networks. The theoretical basis for understanding the basic life processes of the senses, particularly vision, hearing, and feeling, were presented briefly. Compensatory processes of sensation were identified and two examples of compromised processes, pain and hyperactivity, were discussed. The nursing process based on the Roy Adaptation Model was described. Behaviors and stimuli for assessment were identified and nursing diagnoses related to the senses, goal setting, interventions, and evaluation were described.

Exercises for Application

1. For 2 hours, restrict the use of one of your senses by patching one eye. Go about your usual activities and after the 2 hours, write down any difficulties you had. Include any particular emotional reactions related to these difficulties or the experience in general.

2. Spend a few minutes reflecting on the greatest intensity or degree of physical pain you have ever felt. Describe this experience to a friend.

3. Devise a way to assess pain in a school-aged child.

Assessment of Understanding

QUESTIONS

1. The three primary senses described in this chapter were vision (V), hearing (H), and feeling (F). Label each of the following statements according to the primary sense to which they apply.
   (a) _____ somatosensory pathways
   (b) _____ occipital lobe of the cerebral cortex
   (c) _____ pain
   (d) _____ kinesthesia
   (e) _____ primary auditory cortex
   (f) _____ rods and cones
   (g) _____ touch and pressure

2. Identify one compensatory process related to each of the primary senses.
   (a) Vision:
   (b) Hearing:
   (c) Feeling:

3. Identify three commonly recurring adaptation problems that apply to all three primary senses.
   (a) _____
   (b) _____
   (c) _____

4. Name two first-level assessment behaviors for each of the three primary sense processes.
   (a) Vision: _____ and _____
   (b) Hearing: _____ and _____
   (c) Feeling: _____ and _____

5. In this chapter, six questions for general assessment of stimuli related to sensory processing were presented. What were those questions? List the six questions.
   (a) _____
   (b) _____

   (c) _____
   (d) _____
   (e) _____
   (f) _____

SITUATION:

A patient has just had surgery to remove a tumor between the inner ear and the brain stem (vestibular schwannoma or acoustic neuroma). He has lost hearing on the affected side. He complains of distorted sound, being unable to tell the direction of sound, being fearful of adequately monitoring his environment, and difficulty in relating to his grandchildren because he cannot understand what they are saying.

6. State a nursing diagnosis for this patient.
7. Derive a goal statement that contains the behavior of focus, the change expected, and the time frame involved.
8. Give at least five basic considerations for nursing judgment when administering medication for pain relief.
   (a) _____
   (b) _____
   (c) _____
   (d) _____
   (e) _____

9. Which is the most important criterion for evaluating whether or not nursing interventions have achieved the goal of pain relief?
   (a) the individual's statement of comfort
   (b) the time and amount of medication given

FEEDBACK

1. (a) F, (b) V, (c) F, (d) F, (e) H, (f) V, (g) F
2. (a) prescribing of glasses, use of large-print books
   (b) lip reading or sign language
   (c) using oven mitts when removing hot objects from the oven, wearing rubber gloves in hot dishwater, good skin care processes for people with reduced feeling in hands and feet
3. Any three of: impairment of a primary sense, potential for injury or loss of self-care abilities, potential for distorted communication, stigma, sensory monotony or distortion, sensory overload or deprivation, acute pain, chronic pain, perceptual impairment, ineffective coping strategies for sensory impairment.
4. (a) Vision: Two of: visual tests, functional examination, internal examination.
   (b) Hearing: Two of: auditory screening tests to measure sensitivity and discrimination, evidence of other difficulties (faulty speech, inattentiveness, unresponsiveness, withdrawal in social situations).
   (c) Feeling: Two of: sensation behaviors (response to light touch, joint movement identification, pinprick and dull object to test pain sensation, test of temperature detection, test for symmetry of sensation).
5. (a) Is the impairment temporary, permanent, or is this unanswerable at the current time?
   (b) Is the impairment recent or long standing?
   (c) Is more than one impairment present?
   (d) How does the individual view the loss of function?
   (e) How is the individual affected in the current environment of home, work, school, clinic, or hospital and moving from one place to another?
   (f) What is the individual's level of knowledge, the knowledge needed, and readiness for teaching?
6. Examples of nursing diagnoses: Uncompensated auditory deficit, or, stated difficulty dealing with environment and important relationships related to sudden, recent, and permanent loss of hearing in one ear.
7. Example of a goal: Within the next week, the patient will report enjoying a visit with his grandchildren when he gave them the opportunity to be at the level of his hearing ear and to see his new device for transmitting sound from the deaf side to the hearing ear.
8. Any of the following: the location of the pain, the source, onset and duration, constancy, intensity, and type as reported by the individual, individual's experience of this pain and previous experiences, whether a combination of approaches can bring relief, size of the individual, exact time and amount of last pain medication administration, as well as evaluation of relief obtained, and the type of medication available.
9. a

References

Agency for Health Care Policy and Research. (1994). *Quick reference guide for clinicians: Pressure ulcer treatment.* U.S. Department of Health and Human Services. Washington, DC: (AHCPR Publication No. 95–1653).

American Association of Neuroscience Nurses. (2001). Stewart-Amidei, C., Kunkel, J., & Bronstein, K. (Eds.). *AANN's neuroscience nursing: Human responses to neurologic dysfunction* (2nd ed.). Philadelphia: W. B. Saunders.

Bickley, L. S., & Szilagi, P. G. (Eds.). (2007). *Bates' guide to physical examination and history taking* (8th ed.). Philadelphia: Lippincott.

Brown, T. E. (2000). *Attention-deficit disorders and comorbidities in children, adolescents, and adults.* Washington, DC: American Psychiatric Press, Inc.

Bullock, B. L., & Rosendahl, P. P. (1992). *Pathophysiology: Adaptations and alterations in function* (3rd ed.). Philadelphia: Lippincott.

Burrell, L. O., Gerlach, M. J. M., & Pless, B. S. (1997). *Adult nursing: Acute and community care* (2nd ed.). Stamford, CT: Appleton & Lange.

Campbell, J. (2001). Pain as the fifth vital sign. In D. C. Turk & R. Melzack (Eds.), *Handbook of pain assessment* (2nd ed.). New York: Guilford Press.

Carson, M., Metzger, L., Lasko, N., Paulus, L., Morse, A., Pitman, R., & Orr, S. (2007). Physiologic reactivity to startling tones in female Vietnam nurse veterans with PTSD. *Journal of Traumatic Stress 20(5): 657–666.*

Cassell, E. J. (1989). The relationship between pain and suffering. In C. S. Hill & W. S. Fields (Eds.), *Drug treatment of cancer pain in a drug-oriented society: Advances in pain research and therapy* (Vol. 11, p. 61). New York: Raven Press.

Centers for Disease Control and Prevention. (2007). What Is Attention-Deficit/Hyperactivity Disorder (ADHD)? Retrieved February 1, 2008, from http://www.cdc.gov/ncbddd/adhd/what.htm

Guyton, A., & Hall, J. (2006). *Textbook of medical physiology* (11th ed.). Philadelphia: W. B. Saunders Company.

Herr, K., Coyne, P. J., Key, T., Manworren, R., McCaffery, M., Merkel, S., Pelosi-Kelly, J., & Wild, L. (2006). Pain assessment in the nonverbal patient: Position statement with clinical practice recommendations. *Pain Management Nursing,7(2) 44–52.*

Hill, C. (1987). Sensory functions and alterations. In J. Servonsky & S. Opas (Eds.), *Nursing management of children* (pp. 1221–1261). Boston: Jones and Bartlett.

International Association for the Study of Pain. (1979). Subcommittee on taxonomy of pain teams: A list with definitions and notes on usage. *Pain, 6,* 249–252.

Ignatavicius, D., & Workman, M. L. (Eds.). (2006). *Medical-surgical nursing: Critical thinking for collaborative care* (5th ed.). St. Louis, MO: Mosby.

Kazanowski, M. K, & Laccetti, M. S. (2002). *Nursing concept: Pain.* Boston: Jones & Bartlett.

Kolb, B., & Whishaw, I. (1996). *Fundamentals of human neuropsychology* (4th ed.). New York: W. H. Freeman and Company.

Marcus, D. (2005). *Chronic pain: A primary care guide to practical management.* Totowa, NJ: Humana Press.

Marks, R. M., & Sachar, E. J. (1973). Undertreatment of medical inpatients with narcotic analgesics. *Annals of Internal Medicine, 78,* 173.

McCaffery, M. (1979). *Nursing management of the patient with pain* (2nd ed.). Philadelphia: Lippincott.

McCaffery, M. (1997). Pain management handbook. *Nursing 27(4),* 42–45.

McCaffery, M., & Beebe, A. (1989). *Pain: A clinical manual for nursing practice.* St. Louis, MO: Mosby.

McCaffery M., & Pasero, C. (2005). *Pain: Clinical manual* (2nd ed.). St. Louis, MO: Mosby.

McCaffery, M., & Robinson, E. (2002). Your patient is in pain. Here's how you respond. *Nursing 32*(10), 36–45.

McCarney, S. B. (1994). *The attention deficit disorders intervention manual.* Columbia, MO: Hawthorne Educational Services.

Meiss, R., & Tanner, G. (1982). Sensory receptors. In E. Selkurt (Ed.), *Basic physiology for the health sciences* (pp. 115–159). Boston: Little Brown.

Melzack, R. (1990, February). The tragedy of needless pain. *Scientific American,* 27–33.

Melzack, R., & Wall, P. (1965). Pain mechanisms: A new theory. *Science, 150,* 971.

Melzack, R., & Wall, P. (1970). Psychophysiology of pain. *International Anesthesia Clinics, 81*(1), 3.

Melzack, R., & Wall, P. (1989). *The challenge of pain* (rev. ed.). New York: Penguin.

Mitchell, P. H., Hodges, L. C., Muwaswes, M., & Walleck, C. A. (Eds.). (1988). *American Association of Neuroscience Nurses' Neuroscience nursing: Phenomena and practice* (pp. 501–515). Norwalk, CT: Appleton & Lange.

NANDA International (2007). *Nursing diagnoses: Definitions & classification, 2007–2008.* Philadelphia: NANDA-I.

Porth, M. C. (2005). *Pathophysiology concepts of altered health states* (7th ed.). Philadelphia: Lippincott.

Posner, M. I., & Raichle, M. E. (1994). *Images of mind.* New York: Scientific American Library.

Puntillo, K. A., Miaskowki, C., & Summer, G. (2003). Pain. In V. Carrieri-Kohlman, A. M. Lindsey, & C. M. West (Eds.), *Pathophysiological phenomena in nursing: Human responses to illness* (pp. 235–254). St Louis, MO: W. B. Saunders Company.

Rantz, M. J., & LeMone, P. (Eds.). (1997). *Classification of nursing diagnoses.* Proceedings of the 12th conference NANDA. Glendale, CA: CINAHL Information Systems.

Rowland, L. P. (2005). *Merritt's textbook of neurology* (11th ed.). Philadelphia: Lippincott Williams and Wilkins.

Roy, C. (2001). Alterations in cognitive processing. In C. Stewart-Amidei, J. Kunkel, & K. Bronstein (Eds.), *American Association of Neuroscience Nurses' Neuroscience nursing: Human responses to neurologic dysfunction* (2nd ed., pp. 275–323). Philadelphia: Saunders.

Servonsky, J., & Opas, S. (Eds.). (1987). *Nursing management of children.* Boston: Jones and Bartlett.

Taylor, E. (Ed.). (2007). *People with hyperactivity: Understanding and managing their problems.* London: Mac Keith.

Thorpe, D. M. (1990). Comprehensive pain care: The relief of pain and suffering. *Dimensions of Oncology Nursing, 4*(1): 27–29.

Turk, D. C., & Melzack, R. (Eds.). (2001). *Handbook of pain assessment* (2nd ed). New York: Guilford Press.

Wickens, A. (2000). *Foundations of biopsychology.* Harlow, UK: Prentice-Hall.

CHAPTER 11

Fluid, Electrolyte, and Acid–Base Balance

The maintenance of fluid, electrolyte, and acid–base balance is identified in the Roy Adaptation Model as one of four complex processes associated with the physiologic mode. Keeping fluids and chemical substances in correct proportion is vital for the integrity of the individual. In this chapter, the basic life processes associated with fluid, electrolyte, and acid–base balance are addressed. Many body systems are involved in these processes. However, the key activity of the kidney in maintaining balance through the processes of filtration, reabsorption, and secretion is addressed. In particular, the complex processes associated with the maintenance of fluid balance, electrolyte balance, and acid–base balance are the topics of focus. Illustrations of compensatory and compromised processes are also discussed. The assessment of behaviors and stimuli affecting these complex processes is explored. Finally, guidelines for planning nursing care by formulating nursing diagnoses, establishing goals, selecting nursing interventions, and evaluating nursing care are described.

OBJECTIVES

After studying this chapter, the reader will be able to do the following:

1. Describe the basic life processes associated with the need for fluid, electrolyte, and acid–base balance as presented in this chapter.

2. Describe one compensatory process associated with fluid, electrolyte, and acid–base balance.

3. Name and describe two situations of compromised processes of fluid, electrolyte, and acid–base balance.

4. Identify important first-level assessment behaviors of the basic life processes associated with fluid, electrolyte, and acid–base balance.

5. List second-level assessment common stimuli that affect fluid, electrolyte, and acid–base balance.

6. Develop a nursing diagnosis, given a situation related to fluid, electrolyte, and acid–base balance.

7. Derive goals for an individual with ineffective fluid, electrolyte, or acid–base balance in a given situation.

8. Describe nursing interventions commonly implemented in situations of ineffective fluid, electrolyte, and acid–base balance.

9. Propose approaches to determine the effectiveness of nursing interventions.

KEY CONCEPTS DEFINED

Acidosis: A decrease in arterial blood pH below 7.35 (excess of hydrogen ion concentration) related to accumulation of acid or loss of base.

Alkalosis: An increase in arterial blood pH above 7.45 (deficit of hydrogen ion concentration) related to accumulation of base or deficiency of acid.

Calcemia: Relating to calcium in the blood.

Electrolytes: Substances (salts) that break down into ions when in solution.

Filtration: A passive process occurring in the glomerulus of the kidney wherein blood plasma is filtered and proteins and blood cells, too large to pass through the membrane, remain behind.

Fluids: Internal body fluids located within (intracellular) and outside (extracellular) body cells in various parts of the body not available for general body use, for example, joint fluid or pericardial fluid (third space fluids).

Homeostasis: The maintenance of stable internal environment of the body.

Hyper: A prefix meaning excess or above normal value.

Hypo: A prefix meaning deficit or below normal value.

Kalemia: Relating to potassium in the blood.

Natremia: Relating to the sodium in the blood.

Osmolarity: Concentration of solutes in a solvent as expressed per unit of weight (kg) of the solvent.

pH: The concentration of hydrogen ions; refers to how acid or alkaline a solution is.

Reabsorption: The reclamation of useful substances (for example, water, glucose, amino acids, ions) from the filtrate back into the blood during the process of blood purification in the kidney.

Secretion: The movement of substances (hydrogen and potassium ions, creatinine, ammonia) from the blood into the filtrate (reabsorption in reverse).

COMPLEX PROCESSES OF FLUID, ELECTROLYTE, AND ACID–BASE BALANCE

Adaptation concerning fluid, electrolyte, and acid–base balance is referred to as the process of homeostasis. Marieb and Hoehn (2007) defined homeostasis as the maintenance of a stable internal environment of the body. A wide variety of body systems including the respiratory, circulatory, gastrointestinal, renal, nervous, and endocrine systems are involved in regulating the maintenance of fluid, electrolyte, and acid–base balance. However, the major responsibility rests with the kidneys. The reader is referred to texts on anatomy and physiology for basic information about the physiologic structures addressed in this chapter. The kidneys function to maintain the purity and constancy of internal fluids. They process gallons of fluid each day, filtering out wastes and excess ions and returning needed substances to the blood. They regulate the volume and chemical makeup of the blood by achieving proper fluid, electrolyte, and acid–base balance.

Filtering of blood and the formation of urine is carried out by three processes. The processes are filtration, reabsorption, and secretion. Every day the kidneys filter nearly 2,000 liters of fluid from the bloodstream. Filtration takes place through glomeruli into the tubules. The tubules process the filtrate by taking substances out of it (reabsorption) and adding substances to it (secretion). Filtration is a nonselective, passive process that occurs in the glomerulus. The filtration membrane filters blood plasma; proteins and blood cells are too large to pass through and remain behind. Normal blood pressure is required to force plasma out of the blood and into the tubules in filtrate formation. Reabsorption pertains to the reclamation of useful substances (for example, water, glucose, amino acids, ions) from the filtrate back into the blood. Reabsorption begins and is mostly accomplished in cells of the proximal convoluted tubule. Although some reabsorption occurs by osmosis, most depends on an active transport process.

Very selective membrane carriers are used. There are many carriers for substances needing to be retained, such as glucose and amino acids. On the contrary, there are few for waste products, such as urea, creatinine, and uric acid. The ions retained or excreted depend on the body's needs at the time with respect to pH and electrolyte composition of the blood.

Secretion relates to movement of substances such as hydrogen and potassium ions, creatinine, and ammonia from the blood into the filtrate. This is reabsorption in reverse. The process is important for ridding the body of substances, for example, certain drugs, that have not been filtered already.

The kidneys have four key activities associated with fluid and electrolyte balance.

• The excretion of nitrogen-containing wastes, urea, uric acid, and creatinine
• Maintaining water balance
• Maintaining electrolyte balance
• Maintaining acid–base balance of the blood

Excretion was reviewed in Chapter 7. In this chapter, the remaining three processes are reviewed.

Fluid Balance

Fluids within the body can be intracellular, extracellular, or third space fluids. For the body, water serves as the universal solvent in which electrolytes and nonelectrolytes are dissolved. The concentration of solutes in water influences fluid balance between intracellular and extracellular compartments. The kidneys are signaled to absorb more or less water and ions in response to two particular hormones. The antidiuretic hormone (ADH) increases water reabsorption and conserves body water. Aldosterone increases tubular reabsorption of sodium and water and decreases tubular reabsorption of potassium. Third space fluids refer to those that are extracellular and have collected in various parts of the body. This is a result of injury, infection, or compromised circulation. These fluids are not available for body functions. For example, in ascites fluid collects in the peritoneal cavity.

The mechanisms for fluid balance of the body include the thirst center that affects fluid intake, ADH secretion, and urinary output. Water is taken into the body as liquids and food. A small amount of fluid is added as the by-product of cellular metabolism of solid food. Water is lost from the body through excretion of urine and feces, perspiration, and respiration. The thirst mechanism regulates liquid intake. Plasma osmolarity, the concentration of solutes as expressed per unit of weight (kg) of solvent, triggers the thirst mechanism and the release of ADH from the hypothalamus. As noted, output of water is regulated by the kidneys. As Burrell, Gerlach, and Pless (1997) pointed out, "Regardless of large variations in intake, individuals with normal kidney function are able to maintain normal water balance by secreting either dilute or concentrated urine" (p. 112).

Electrolyte Balance

Electrolytes are substances (salts) that break down into ions when in solution. Thus, electrolyte balance addresses concentrations of salts within the body. The major elements forming salts within body fluids are sodium, potassium, and calcium. Sodium plays a central role in fluid and electrolyte balance by controlling extracellular fluid volume and water distribution in the body. Changes in plasma sodium levels affect plasma volume and blood pressure as well as the volumes in the intra- and extracellular fluid compartments. Sodium regulation involves a variety of neural and hormonal mechanisms. Aldosterone from the adrenal cortex constitutes a complex hormonal influence in the process of sodium balance by enhancing sodium reabsorption by the kidneys. Recall that water follows the movement of sodium by osmosis. Antidiuretic hormone (ADH), produced in the posterior pituitary and stimulated by the hypothalamus, increases the permeability of the collecting tubules of the kidney and enhances water reabsorption. In addition, pressoreceptors in the heart respond to changes in blood volume and stimulate the hypothalamus and posterior pituitary in the production of ADH.

Potassium is required for normal neuromuscular functioning and metabolic activity. The role of potassium in the synthesis of protein is particularly important. Even a slight alteration in potassium levels affects neurons and muscle fibers. In turn, there can be profound effects on other body functions such as cardiac muscle function and cognitive function. Regulation of potassium is accomplished primarily by renal mechanisms. When concentrations of potassium fall below normal levels, the kidneys conserve potassium by reducing its secretion. There is, however, limited ability of the kidneys to retain potassium. Thus, taking in appropriate levels of potassium is important. Three major factors determine the rate and extent of potassium secretion: tubule cell potassium content, aldosterone levels, and the pH of the extracellular fluid.

Most body calcium is found in the bones but a small percentage is required in the extracellular fluid for normal clotting of blood, cell membrane permeability, and secretory functions. Muscular excitability also is affected by calcium. Calcium is regulated by parathyroid hormone and its antagonist, calcitonin (produced by the thyroid gland). Parathyroid hormone affects calcium release from bone, absorption of calcium by the small intestine, and kidney reabsorption of calcium. Other minor elements such as magnesium and chloride have important functions within the body. Magnesium is a constituent of many coenzymes that contribute to normal muscle and nerve irritability. Chloride helps maintain the osmotic pressure of the blood. Further information about these elements and those previously described is contained in physiology resources.

Acid–Base Balance

The acid–base status of body fluids is related to the concentration of hydrogen ions and is described in terms of pH. The pH refers to how acid or alkaline a solution is. Normal values of pH of body fluids range from 7.35 to 7.45. There are three types of acid–base regulators in the body. Chemical regulators involve the carbonic acid–bicarbonate buffer system, which regulates the concentration of hydrogen ions in the blood. Biological regulation occurs by the absorption and release of hydrogen ions by cells. Lastly, physiologic buffering systems involve the lungs and the kidneys. Buffer systems are important in resisting a change in pH in one or more fluid compartments, while respiratory and renal mechanisms rid the body of excess acid or retain hydrogen ions. To maintain acid–base balance, the kidneys control reabsorption of excess bases by actively secreting excess hydrogen and by retaining bicarbonate ions. Chemical buffers temporarily tie up excess hydrogen or bases and the respiratory centers modify blood pH by retaining CO_2. This decreases the pH. The respiratory center can eliminate more CO_2 from the blood to increase blood pH. It is the kidney mechanisms that can remove metabolic acids and excess bases from the body.

Full discussion of the complex processes related to fluid, electrolyte, and acid–base balance is not within the scope of this text. Basic physiology sources, for example, Marieb and Hoehn (2007), review the intricacies of these processes.

COMPENSATORY ADAPTIVE PROCESSES

Roy's concept of the regulator subsystem can be described in the phrase "the wisdom of the body," which means the automatic self-regulation of physiologic processes. Further, the thinking and feeling person, by way of cognator activity, can do much to affect any component of the physiologic mode, and this includes the complex processes associated with fluid, electrolyte, and acid–base balance. Regulator and cognator abilities, then, are important internal stimuli for the individual. These subsystems activate compensatory adaptive processes that extend the effectiveness of behavior in reaching the goals of adaptation.

One particular illustration of a regulator activity relates to the functioning of the kidney. If large amounts of water are lost through the lungs, in perspiration, or in the stool, the kidneys compensate that loss by excreting less, more highly concentrated, urine. When intake is excessive, kidneys excrete generous amounts of diluted urine. When blood volume drops, related to hemorrhage, excessive sweating, or diarrhea, for example, arterial blood pressure drops and this ultimately results in a decreased amount of filtrate formed by the kidneys. The change in blood composition stimulates osmoreceptors in the hypothalamus, which in turn signal the posterior pituitary to release antidiuretic hormone, the effect of which is to prevent excessive water loss in the urine. As more water is returned to the bloodstream, blood volume and blood pressure increase to normal levels and only small amounts of very concentrated urine are formed.

An illustration of a compensatory cognator response associated with the complex processes of fluid, electrolyte, and acid–base balance is that of artificial renal dialysis. In some situations, the kidneys are unable to carry out their normal functions due to damaging kidney infections, physical trauma, chemical poisoning, or inadequate blood delivery to the kidneys in a condition such as arteriosclerosis. The body quickly becomes contaminated with poisonous wastes. In these cases, hemodialysis with the use of an apparatus called an artificial kidney can be used to prevent death; peritoneal dialysis is another option. Some people who cannot regain kidney function may become candidates for the more definitive treatment of a kidney transplant. In the meantime they are totally dependent on dialysis and, as a result, are very knowledgeable about the process. They know when it is indicated and how their lifestyle is adapted to accommodate this compensatory adaptive process.

COMPROMISED PROCESSES RELATED TO FLUID, ELECTROLYTE, AND ACID–BASE BALANCE

Fluid Imbalance

Disturbances of fluid balance in the body can be described in terms of excessive water loss (dehydration), excessive intercellular water retention, and accumulation of fluid in the interstitial compartments (edema). Water volume is closely tied to sodium levels since sodium functions as a magnet for water, controlling extracellular fluid volume and water distribution in the body.

Electrolyte Imbalance

Disturbances in electrolytes are described with combinations of prefixes and root words. Hyper means excess or above normal, and hypo means deficit or below normal. Kalemia relates to potassium; natremia relates to sodium; and calcemia relates to calcium. A decrease in sodium ion concentration in the blood, hyponatremia, inhibits the release of antidiuretic hormone and allows more water to be excreted in the urine. An increase in sodium levels, hypernatremia, such as caused by decreased blood volume, stimulates the release of antidiuretic hormone and results in less water in the urine. Potassium excess in the extracellular fluid, hyperkalemia, increases neuron and muscle fiber excitability and causes depolarization. Deficits, hypokalemia, cause hyperpolarization and nonresponsiveness. Both situations can lead to abnormal cardiac rhythm and cardiac arrest. Confusion is the manifestation in the brain of these situations of potassium imbalance. Low levels of calcium, hypocalcemia, result in increased excitability and muscle tetany. High levels, hypercalcemia, inhibit neuron and muscle cell activity.

Acid–Base Imbalance

Abnormalities in acid–base balance are of two types. The respiratory system control of pH can lead to respiratory acidosis or alkalosis. Metabolic acidosis and alkalosis are due to nonrespiratory controls of pH. Acidosis is a decrease in arterial blood pH below 7.35. This represents a higher than optimal hydrogen concentration for the functioning of most body cells. Alkalosis occurs whenever the pH of arterial blood rises above 7.45, representing an abnormally low hydrogen ion concentration in the extracellular fluid. Respiratory acidosis occurs when gas exchange in the lungs is hampered by disease or inadequate inspiration. The result is the accumulation of carbon dioxide in the blood. Alkalosis occurs when carbon dioxide is released in excessive amounts, for example, through hyperventilation. Acidosis results in central nervous system depression and can result in coma and death. Alkalosis results in overexcitement of the nervous system and can lead to muscle tetany, extreme nervousness, convulsions, and respiratory arrest leading to death.

NURSING PROCESS RELATED TO FLUID, ELECTROLYTE, AND ACID–BASE BALANCE

Fluid, electrolyte, and acid–base balance are priority requirements for an individual's physiologic adaptation. In applying the nursing process, the nurse makes a careful assessment of behaviors and stimuli related to these complex processes. In assessing factors influencing fluid, electrolyte, and acid–base balance, regulator and cognator effectiveness in initiating compensatory processes is also considered. Based on this thorough first- and second-level assessment, the nurse makes a nursing diagnosis, sets goals, selects nursing interventions, and evaluates care.

Assessment of Behavior

The nurse in practice in all settings will have an understanding of behavioral norms indicating fluid, electrolyte, and acid–base balance. Further, the nurse is a skilled observer to recognize behaviors indicating changes in balance. Due to frequent contact with the individual, the nurse is in an excellent position to assess both subtle and overt behaviors and changes in behaviors indicating ineffective body responses. It is easier to prevent imbalances if the nurse has knowledge of stimuli that influence these intricate processes. The nurse then uses this knowledge to predict and monitor the individual for potential imbalances. After reviewing the individual's history, the nurse proceeds with a systematic assessment of fluid, electrolyte, and acid–base balance. In this case, the basic needs and complex processes associated with the physiologic mode of the Roy Adaptation Model serve as a guideline for the assessment.

OXYGENATION   Related to the need for oxygenation are behaviors indicative of respiratory and circulatory function within the body. The particular behavioral manifestation will depend on the stimuli. For example, cardiac arrhythmia can be a manifestation of potassium excess in the blood. Problems with blood volume are manifest in the characteristics of the pulse and blood pressure. Therefore, assessment of fluid, electrolyte, and acid–base balance as related to the need for oxygenation would involve assessment of the pulse, blood pressure, respirations, and change in skin color.

NUTRITION   Associated with nutrition need and related to fluid, electrolyte, and acid–base balance are appetite, thirst, symptoms of nausea and vomiting, and the condition of the tongue. Increased thirst can indicate excessive amounts of sodium or potassium in the body. A dry, furrowed tongue signals a deficit in fluid volume in the body.

ELIMINATION   The amount and characteristics of urinary output, intestinal output, and bowel activity are important behaviors related to fluid, electrolyte, and acid–base balance. Urinary output is an important indicator of fluid volume while diarrhea can influence both fluid volume and electrolyte balance. Levels of intake and output are important behavioral indicators in assessing fluid, electrolyte, and acid–base imbalance. A decrease in bowel sounds heard on abdominal auscultation can indicate problems with potassium levels in the body.

ACTIVITY AND REST   Imbalances in fluid, electrolyte, and acid–base balance will also affect the individual's need for activity and rest, and their report of how they are feeling. Complaints of fatigue, malaise, drowsiness, restlessness, agitation, and irritability may be behavioral indicators of ineffective adaptation related to electrolytes, particularly calcium levels. Disruptions in bone integrity also can indicate calcium problems.

PROTECTION   Related to the processes of physiologic protection is the condition of the skin, and the skin, in turn, reflects fluid, electrolyte, and acid–base balance. The nurse would expect to find abnormalities in skin temperature, turgor, and color in situations of fluid volume alterations. Peripheral and perioral sensation can be affected by calcium deficits, with patients reporting "tingling" of fingers or lips. Expected findings with decreases in fluid volume are diminished reflexes and decreased tearing and salivation.

NEUROLOGIC FUNCTION   Fluid, electrolyte, and acid–base imbalance can result in neurologic manifestations including belligerence, apathy, confusion, disorientation, and headache, and progressive alteration in the functioning of the central nervous system.

LABORATORY EXAMINATION   An important behavioral assessment of fluid, electrolyte, and acid–base balance is the results of laboratory tests. In particular, the nurse examines findings related to concentrations of elements and ions in the blood and urine. Urine is normally clear, yellow, and usually slightly acidic, but its pH value varies widely. Substances normally found in urine are nitrogenous wastes, water, and various ions, always sodium and potassium. Substances not normally found in urine include glucose, albumin or other blood proteins, blood, pus, white blood cells, and bile. Hemoglobin and hematocrit levels are important indicators of blood volume. Specific gravity of urine is an important indicator of body sodium level.

Once the nurse has completed the behavioral assessment of fluid, electrolyte, and acid–base balance, a tentative judgment is made as to whether the behaviors are adaptive or ineffective. As identified in Chapter 3, normal values are available to guide this judgment, as are general expectations relative to the identified behaviors. In other situations, pronounced regulator activity with cognator ineffectiveness may provide the key to the identification of ineffective adaptation. By obtaining an indication of whether the individual is maintaining an appropriate balance of fluids, electrolytes, and acids and bases, priorities can be established for the next level of nursing assessment, namely, the assessment of stimuli.

Assessment of Stimuli

With the assessment of stimuli, the nurse gathers data about the factors influencing the behaviors identified in the first-level assessment of the adaptation nursing process. This includes the important factor of the body's adaptive ability to maintain the regulatory processes of fluid, electrolyte, and acid–base balance as well as the coping strategies the individual uses to maintain or change behaviors.

INTEGRITY OF THE PHYSIOLOGIC MODE   Of the common stimuli affecting fluid, electrolyte, and acid–base balance, lack of integrity of some aspect of the physiologic mode is the most common source of disruption. In particular, disease pathology associated with acute or chronic illness or injury is frequently the focal stimulus causing ineffective processes of fluid, electrolyte, and acid–base balance. Consider the example of disruption of skin integrity from a burn. The subsequent loss of extracellular fluid and release of cellular potassium has pervasive effects on body homeostasis. Excessive calcium in the body can result from the breakdown of bone calcium in pathologic conditions such as metastatic cancer of the bone, multiple myeloma, or leukemia. With renal disease, the kidney has limited or no ability to excrete hydrogen ions, potassium, or water. Diabetes is another chronic condition that can adversely affect hydrogen ion concentration within the body. Deficient aldosterone production by the adrenal glands is an acute condition that results in loss of sodium and conservation of potassium. Each of these situations has a profound effect on fluid, electrolyte, and acid–base balance and adaptation. Stimuli that produce significant changes in blood pressure and volume include, for example, prolonged vomiting or diarrhea, excess perspiration, blood loss, severe burns, wound drainage, and pathologic vasodilation associated with bacterial shock. These stimuli serve to increase blood osmolarity. Through increased concentration of urine and increased water reabsorption, the body attempts to adapt by increasing blood volume.

ENVIRONMENTAL FACTORS   Environmental factors such as intense heat or inaccessibility of water also affect the body's ability to maintain fluids, electrolytes, and acids and bases in appropriate proportion. The nurse can provide advanced teaching for people to anticipate their fluid and related needs when planning to be in extreme environments.

MEDICAL INTERVENTIONS   Fluid, electrolyte, and acid–base imbalance may be instigated by the administration of medications or other treatment regimens. For example, excessive administration of intravenous solutions can overload the body with fluids. Use of potent or inappropriate diuretic medications results in loss of fluid, potassium, and sodium, especially without fluid replacement. To assist with this problem, some diuretics have been developed with the feature of enabling potassium conservation within the body. Overuse of antacids and laxatives can disrupt electrolyte balance by inhibiting the absorption of vital elements needed for balance. Gastrointestinal suctioning also can disrupt balance contributing to excessive loss of fluid and electrolytes.

COGNATOR EFFECTIVENESS   Cognator effectiveness, as associated with the individual's knowledge level, may constitute a stimulus contributing to the fluid, electrolyte, and acid–base imbalance in situations where there is inappropriate use of the medical interventions. For example, an individual may be precipitating excessive intestinal absorption of calcium with the overuse of vitamin D. Or the individual's dietary intake may be deficient in one or more of the vital elements, either because of lack of knowledge about a balanced diet or misguided fad dieting practices.

DEVELOPMENTAL STAGE   In the very young and the elderly, fluid, electrolyte, and acid–base balance are particularly influenced by body size and makeup, as well as developmental changes. In children, as compared with adults, water accounts for a greater proportion of total body mass, which makes it easier for them to lose fluid. In the neonate, 75% of body weight is body water, and the proportion of extracellular to intracellular fluid is greater. Further, on a weight basis, the turnover of water in children is five times greater than that of adults. In addition, the surface area to volume ratio is proportionally greater in children. Thus, fluid loss through evaporation is potentially greater for children. Older adults may lack essential electrolytes because of poor nutrition related to a variety of factors. Some factors of concern are inadequate dental care, decreased salivation, limited budget for food, and social isolation. In addition, water intake can also be a problem because the thirst mechanism becomes less effective with age. Older people may also limit fluid intake in the late afternoon and evening in an attempt to avoid having to get up to go to the bathroom at night.

Once the stimuli influencing fluid, electrolyte, and acid–base balance have been identified, the nurse proceeds to suggest whether they are focal, contextual, or residual in their effect on the individual's physiologic integrity. The focal stimulus is the one most immediately confronting the individual. The stimuli identified represent possible focal stimuli for the complex processes influencing fluid, electrolyte, and acid–base balance. Contextual stimuli are all other internal or external stimuli evident in the situation and contributing to the behavior following the focal stimulus. Residual stimuli represent the stimuli whose affect on the individual has not or cannot be validated.

Within the processes of influencing fluid, electrolyte, and acid–base balance, certain behaviors can be stimuli for other behaviors in some situations. For example, vomiting can be classified as a behavior since it constitutes an action under specified circumstances. However, vomiting can also be considered a stimulus where fluid, electrolyte, and acid–base balance is concerned since persistent vomiting can lead to excessive fluid loss and imbalance in vital elements needed by the body. At times, it may not be clear as to whether a particular activity is a behavior or a stimulus and, in many cases, it may indeed be both. Since the remainder of the nursing process is contingent on factors identified in first- and second-level assessment, it may be of value to document the factor as both a behavior and a stimulus to ensure that the concept is not lost as the nursing process proceeds. Experience will clarify the most appropriate method of documenting when such dilemmas are encountered in the assessment of the patient.

Nursing Diagnosis

Assessment data of behaviors and related stimuli are interpreted and used in establishing a nursing diagnosis. By using the Roy Adaptation Model, the nurse can state diagnoses as specific behaviors with the stimuli that are most relevant or may employ summary labels to convey complex concepts in abbreviated terms. Roy has developed a typology of indicators of positive adaptation related to fluid, electrolyte, and acid–base balance (see Table 3–1). Included in the typology are stable processes of water balance, stability of electrolytes in body fluids, balance of acid–base status, and effective chemical buffer regulation. It is important to recognize situations of effective adaptation so that these can be maintained or enhanced. In fluid, electrolyte, and acid–base balance, a nursing diagnosis illustrating adaptation could be, "stable processes of fluid, electrolyte, and acid–base balance related to adequate hydration, good nutritional status, and integrity of other physiologic components."

Commonly recurring adaptation problems defined within the Roy Adaptation Model include dehydration; edema; intracellular fluid retention; shock; hyper- or hypocalcemia, -kalemia, or -natremia; acid–base imbalance; and ineffective buffer regulation for changing pH. In situations of fluid, electrolyte, and acid–base disruption, it is important that the essence of the disruption be conveyed in the nursing diagnosis. The diagnosis then provides direction for subsequent steps of the nursing process. This is facilitated by identification of the specific behaviors that are of concern and the relevant stimuli that are influencing them. An example of this type of nursing diagnosis could be, "urinary output of 5 mL in 8 hours related to no oral fluid intake, traumatic injury to leg with excessive loss of body plasma, and lack of fluid replacement."

A disruption in fluid, electrolyte, and acid–base balance would likely yield many nursing diagnoses relating to each of the ineffective behaviors. A detailed approach, as described, may facilitate thorough interpretation of the data. The use of a summary label to develop a nursing diagnosis is often an effective way of communicating a cluster of behaviors to experienced nurses. The concept of "shock" might be such a diagnosis, for example. The diagnosis statement could be, "shock related to hemorrhage from gastric ulcer." Much information is contained using the terms "shock" and "hemorrhage" that would provide meaningful direction for the experienced nurse, but may be less meaningful and provide less direction for the individual with less clinical and theoretical background. In Table 11–1, the Roy model nursing diagnostic categories for the complex processes of fluid, electrolyte, and acid–base balance are shown in relation to nursing diagnosis labels approved by the North American Nursing Diagnosis Association (NANDA International, 2007).

In situations of fluid, electrolyte, and acid–base imbalance, it is easy for the nurse to focus on the pathophysiology involved rather than the behaviors and stimuli that are related to what is happening physiologically in the individual's body. Knowledge of pathophysiology is important to assist the nurse in the identification of behaviors and stimuli related to fluid, electrolyte, and acid–base balance. However, with the framework that the Roy Adaptation Model provides, behaviors and stimuli pertain to the individual's behavioral manifestation of the problem and the factors that appear to be affecting it. In turn, the nursing diagnosis also focuses on behaviors and stimuli rather than on the pathophysiologic condition(s). Once the nursing diagnosis is formulated, the nurse proceeds to the fourth step of the nursing process, goal setting.

Goal Setting

Based on thorough assessment and understanding of adaptation problems related to fluid, electrolyte, and acid–base balance, the nurse sets goals in terms of outcomes for the individual. A complete goal statement includes the behavior of focus, the change expected, and the

TABLE 11–1 Nursing Diagnostic Categories for Fluid, Electrolyte, and Acid–Base Balance

Positive Indicators of Adaptation	Common Adaptation Problems	NANDA Diagnostic Labels
• Stable processes of water balance • Stability of electrolytes in body fluids • Balance of acid–base status • Effective chemical buffer regulation	• Dehydration • Edema • Intracellular water retention • Shock • Hyper- or hypo-calcemia, -kalemia, or -natremia • Acid–base imbalance • Ineffective buffer regulation for changing pH	• Deficient fluid volume • Risk for deficient fluid volume • Excess fluid volume • Risk for imbalanced fluid volume • Readiness for enhanced fluid balance

time frame in which the goal is to be achieved. Depending on the situation, goals may be long term or short term. In the example provided, a patient was observed to have only 5 mL of urinary output in an 8-hour period. This is considered to be ineffective behavior when compared to the normal and expected urinary output of a healthy individual. A goal for this individual could be, "The patient's urinary output will increase within the next hour." This would constitute a short-term goal, the behavior of which is "urinary output," the change expected is "increase," and the time frame is "the next hour."

Consider a situation where an individual has been diagnosed with "diarrhea related to excessive use of laxatives." A long-term goal in this situation may be, "The individual will have regular bowel functioning without the use of laxatives within a 2-week period." Here the behavior is "bowel functioning," the expected change is designated by "regular" and "without the use of laxatives," and the time frame is "within a 2-week period." Generally, the goal of the nurse relative to fluid, electrolyte, and acid–base balance is to reestablish an adaptive state of balance. This goal is operationalized by the identification of the specific goals that address each of the ineffective and potentially ineffective behaviors identified. Another goal during the acute phase of fluid, electrolyte, and acid–base imbalance is to protect the individual from any potential injury or untoward occurrence. In this respect, the importance of anticipating potential problems associated with the individual's condition is evident. The necessity of involving the individual, where possible, in the establishment of the goals is a principle that must be remembered. This is important if the goals are to be realistic, and the individual is to be committed to their attainment. The nurse then proceeds to identify and implement nursing interventions to assist the individual in achieving the behavioral goals.

Nursing Intervention

The nursing intervention step of the nursing process according to the Roy Adaptation Model depends on the identified stimuli as the nurse either promotes or reinforces the stimuli, or takes action to change or delete them. Just as the focus of goal setting is the individual's behavior, the focus of nursing intervention is the stimuli influencing the behavior. Thus, according to the Roy Adaptation Model, nursing intervention is the management of stimuli and involves altering, increasing, decreasing, removing, or maintaining them. In the previous situation involving the patient with limited urinary output in 8 hours, nursing interventions could focus on the oral fluid intake, the injury to the leg, and the lack of fluid replacement. All of these are stimuli identified in the nursing diagnosis. By identifying and analyzing possible approaches, the nurse selects the approach with the highest probability of achieving the goal. Administering oral fluids may resolve the problem but if surgery is imminent, oral intake may jeopardize scheduling the procedure.

It so happens that the injury to the leg is scheduled for surgical repair. To assist with the management of this stimulus, the nurse would be involved in preparing the individual for the operating room. Intravenous fluids are started immediately. The nurse is involved in initiating the infusion and in monitoring its administration and subsequent effect on the patient.

In many situations of fluid, electrolyte, and acid–base imbalance, the nurse will be involved in the administration of parenteral replacement. Types of replacement include parenteral nutrition (PN), IV fluid and electrolyte solutions, blood, and blood components. The type of fluid, its rate of administration, and the additives will depend on the patient's situation, condition, size, and cause of the problem. For example, Ringer's lactate is a multiple electrolyte solution frequently administered for hypovolemic shock. The intravenous site must be carefully prepared and then monitored to ensure that the apparatus is intact and that direct access to the circulatory system is maintained. In addition, the site of access must be given meticulous care since it is a direct point of entry for bacteria into the bloodstream. In compromised fluid, electrolyte, and acid–base balance, ongoing monitoring of the individual in all aspects of the physiologic mode is of utmost importance. As medications are administered, alertness for reactions and drug interactions must be maintained. These actions point to the importance of initial assessment for allergies or chronic conditions for which medications are taken. Intake and output of fluids must be carefully monitored and recorded, and symptoms associated with the underlying physiologic disorder are assessed. This situation illustrates once again that the nursing process is ongoing and simultaneous, with nursing interventions being carried out as first and second levels of assessment are in progress.

Throughout the care process, emotional support is provided for the individual and family. Situations of fluid, electrolyte, and acid–base imbalance are urgent and involve other health team members in the assessment and treatment of the physiologic disruption causing the problem. It is important for the nurse to keep in mind and respond to the individual's needs and to function as a coordinator and integrator of the activities taking place. In the linear description of the nursing process, following implementation of nursing interventions, their effects on the individual's behavior are evaluated. This is accomplished in the sixth and last step of the nursing process, evaluation.

Evaluation

Evaluation involves judging the effectiveness of the nursing interventions in relation to the individual's adaptive behavior, that is, whether the individual has attained the behavior stated in the goals. The nursing interventions are identified as effective if the individual's behavior is in accordance with the stated goal. If the goal has not been achieved, the nurse identifies alternative nursing interventions or approaches by reassessing the behavior and stimuli and continuing with the other steps of the nursing process. In considering the previously identified goal, "The patient's urinary output will increase within the next hour," the nurse, in evaluating the effectiveness of the nursing intervention, would measure the urinary output within the hour. Had there been no urinary output, the absence of urine would be an indication that the patient was not progressing toward the goal and that the behavior continued to be ineffective. This would necessitate immediate action on the part of the nurse with prompt and continued reassessment and further intervention. In this situation, the patient was scheduled for surgical intervention. It would be important that the concern about urinary output be communicated to the care team in the operating room, so that the observation initiated on the unit would continue during the surgical procedure. This points to the importance of effective communication, verbal and written, so that continuity of care is maintained even though the involved health care team members change.

Summary

This chapter has focused on the application of the Roy Adaptation Model to the complex physiologic processes associated with fluid, electrolyte, and acid–base balance. An overview of these basic life processes was provided. Illustrations of innate and learned adaptive compensatory responses related to fluid, electrolyte, and acid–base balance were described and examples of compromised processes were provided. Guidelines for planning nursing care were outlined beginning with the assessment of behaviors and stimuli. Formulation of nursing diagnoses, goals, and nursing interventions were explored, and evaluation of nursing care was described.

Exercises for Application

1. Develop a tool to assist you with the assessment of fluid, electrolyte, and acid–base balance. In the tool, address important behavioral indicators and stimuli that commonly affect fluid, electrolyte, and acid–base balance.

2. Using the tool developed in exercise 1, assess your own status relative to fluid, electrolyte, and acid–base balance. Reread the relevant sections of this chapter to identify the adequacy of your tool.

Assessment of Understanding

QUESTIONS

1. The kidneys play a major role in the maintenance of fluid, electrolyte, and acid–base balance within the body. Which of the following constitute functions of the kidney?
   (a) the excretion of nitrogen-containing wastes
   (b) maintaining water balance
   (c) maintaining electrolyte balance
   (d) maintaining acid–base balance

2. Label the following compensatory processes as indicative of regulator (R) or cognator (C) activity.
   (a) _____ the commitment to drink eight glasses of water each day
   (b) _____ adherence to a sodium-restricted diet
   (c) _____ decrease in filtrate formation in kidney
   (d) _____ continuous ambulatory peritoneal dialysis (CAPD)
   (e) _____ thirst

3. In list A are compromised processes of fluid, electrolyte, acid–base balance. Match them to the descriptors in list B.

   List A
   (a) _____ acidosis
   (b) _____ hypocalcemia
   (c) _____ dehydration
   (d) _____ alkalosis
   (e) _____ hypernatremia
   (f) _____ edema
   (g) _____ hyperkalemia

   List B
   1. excess level of potassium in the blood
   2. sodium values of blood above normal
   3. calcium level in blood is below normal range
   4. accumulation of fluid in interstitial compartments
   5. excessive water loss
   6. a decrease in arterial blood pH
   7. accumulation of base in arterial blood

4. In assessment of behavior related to the complex physiologic processes of fluid, electrolyte, and acid–base balance, which mode(s) is (are) of particular concern?

5. List five common stimuli that lead to fluid, electrolyte, or acid–base imbalance.
   (a) _____
   (b) _____
   (c) _____
   (d) _____
   (e) _____

SITUATION:

Joe is a 20-year-old diabetic patient admitted to the hospital after having "24-hour flu" with nausea, vomiting, and headache. On assessment, the nurse identifies that he has not eaten or had anything to drink in 2 days. He reports scant urinary output twice in the last 24 hours.

6. Construct a nursing diagnosis consisting of a statement of behavior within one mode with its most relevant influencing stimulus.

7. Derive a goal related to the nursing diagnosis you developed in item 6.
8. Management of which stimulus(i) might assist in achievement of the goal set in the previous item?
   (a) The management of the nausea and vomiting by securing an order for antiemetic medication.
   (b) The management of the diabetic condition by investigating blood sugar level.
   (c) The management of intake with intravenous infusion.
9. If the goal developed in item 7 was "The patient will have a urinary output of 50 mL within 4 hours," what would be the key to evaluating the effectiveness of the nursing intervention?

FEEDBACK

1. a, b, c, and d
2. (a) C, (b) C, (c) R, (d) C, (e) R
3. (a) 6, (b) 3, (c) 5, (d) 7, (e) 2, (f) 4, (g) 1
4. the physiologic mode
5. (a) integrity of the physiologic mode
   (b) medical interventions
   (c) cognator effectiveness
   (d) developmental stage
   (e) environmental factors
6. Example of nursing diagnosis: "Decreased urinary output related to inadequate intake of fluids," or "Inadequate intake related to nausea and vomiting."
7. Example of goal: "The patient will have increased urinary output within 8 hours."
8. Any or all responses may apply.
9. The measurement of urinary output in 4 hours.

References

Burrell, L. O., Gerlach, M. J., & Pless, B. S. (1997). *Adult nursing: Acute and community care.* Stamford, CT: Appleton & Lange.

Marieb, E. N., & Hoehn, K. (2007). *Human anatomy and physiology* (7th ed.). San Francisco: Pearson Benjamin Cummings.

NANDA-International. (2007). *Nursing diagnoses: Definitions and classifications, 2007–2008.* Philadelphia: NANDA-I.

Additional References

Guyton, A. C., & Hall, J. E. (Eds.). (2000). *Textbook of medical physiology.* Philadelphia: W. B. Saunders Company.

Porth, C. M. (2000). *Pathophysiology.* Philadelphia: Lippincott Williams & Wilkins.

CHAPTER 12

Neurologic Function

Neurologic function plays an important role in an individual's adaptation. Both the regulator and the cognator subsystems are based on the processes of neurologic function. Intact neural channels affect regulator processing. Similarly, the cognator processes of perceptual and information processing, learning, judgment, and emotion have neurologic bases. Understanding of the complexities of neurologic processes is rapidly growing in the multidisciplinary neurosciences. This chapter focuses specifically on how this knowledge can help the nurse understand the thinking, feeling, moving, and interacting individual who is adapting within the changing world. This physiologic mode component contributes to the holistic functioning of the individual. We discuss two basic life processes key to neurologic function, cognition and consciousness. Compensatory strategies that act to maintain neurologic function are identified. Examples of compromised processes are discussed with a focus on memory deficits and decreased level of consciousness. Planning nursing care begins with assessment of behaviors and stimuli. Assessment related to cognition and consciousness is outlined in this chapter. Nursing diagnoses, goals, nursing interventions, and evaluation are described for this physiologic mode component. Emphasis is placed on promoting integrated thinking and feeling processes to promote health.

OBJECTIVES

After studying this chapter, the reader will be able to do the following:

1. Describe the basic life processes associated with the neurologic function as presented in this chapter.
2. Describe one compensatory process associated with neurologic function.
3. Name and describe two situations of compromised processes of neurologic function.
4. Identify important first-level assessment behaviors associated with neurologic function.
5. List second-level assessment common stimuli that affect neurologic function.
6. Develop a nursing diagnosis, given a situation related to neurologic function.
7. Derive goals for an individual with ineffective neurologic function in a given situation.

8. Describe nursing interventions commonly implemented in situations of ineffective neurologic function.

9. Propose approaches to evaluate the effectiveness of nursing interventions.

KEY CONCEPTS DEFINED

Action potential: Rapid changes in the cell membrane potential of the neurons associated with potassium within the cell and sodium outside the cell.

Cognition: A broad term encompassing the human abilities to think, feel, and act.

Coma: The state of unconsciousness from which an individual cannot be aroused to make purposeful responses.

Consciousness: Level of arousal and awareness, including orientation to the environment and self-awareness.

Integrated neural functioning: Integrated brain activity that is a result of centers for many functions being widely distributed and interconnected throughout the brain.

Memory deficit: Decrease in ability to process one's experience by storing and retrieving information.

Neural plasticity: The adaptive capacities of the central nervous system; the ability to modify its own structural organization and functioning.

Neuron: Structural and functional unit of the nervous system that carries information in the form of impulses.

Synapse: The junction point of one neuron to the next; site of neurotransmitter activity.

COMPLEX PROCESSES OF NEUROLOGIC FUNCTION

All neurologic functioning depends on the neuron as the structural and functional unit of the nervous system. Messages are carried throughout the body in the form of impulses through a succession of neurons. Anatomically, the links between neurons are highly organized in the complex structures of the nervous system. Figure 12–1 illustrates the major components of the central nervous system (CNS), the brain, the brain stem, and the spinal cord. These structures carry out the integration and command functions of the nervous system. In addition, the structures of the peripheral nervous system (PNS) are made up of 12 pairs of cranial nerves and 31 pairs of spinal nerves (Table 12–1). The function of the PNS is to provide communication lines that link all parts of the body. The peripheral nervous system has two functional divisions, the sensory or afferent and motor or efferent. The afferent division conducts impulses from the receptors to the CNS. The efferent or motor division has two parts. The somatic motor nerve fibers conduct impulses from the CNS to the skeletal muscles. Secondly, the autonomic nervous system (ANS) consists of visceral motor nerve fibers activated mainly by centers located in the spinal cord, brain stem, and hypothalamus. The ANS regulates the activity of smooth muscles, cardiac muscles, and glands. It is commonly considered the essential neurogenic regulatory system for maintaining the internal environment of the body at an optimal level, called homeostasis. The significance of the autonomic activity can be seen in Table 12–2, which describes the effects of ANS sympathetic and parasympathetic action on the body organs.

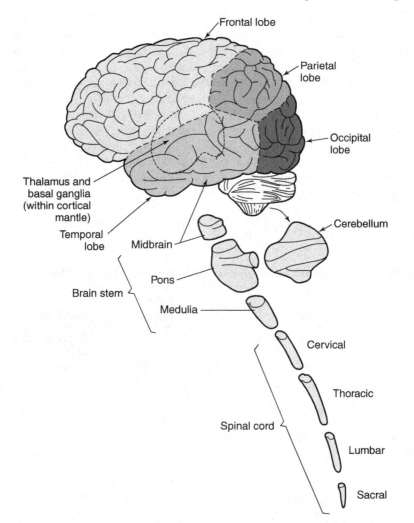

FIGURE 12–1 Major components of the central nervous system. (From Cohen, D. H., & Sherman, S. M. (1998). The nervous system. In Berne, R. M., & Levy, M. N. (Eds.), *Physiology* (p.74). St. Louis: Mosby. Redrawn from Kandel, E. R. & Schwartz, J. H. (1981). *Principles of neuroscience*. New York: Elsevier Science Publishing Co. Used with permission.)

In considering neurologic functioning, Marieb and Hoehn (2007) noted that neurons use changes in their membrane potential as communication signals for receiving, integrating, and sending information. Changes in membrane permeability result in cell depolarization and repolarization. These create graded and action potentials, the mechanisms of nerve impulse conduction. The flow of information is transmitted to their eventual destination across the synapses. The synapse is the junction point from one neuron to the next. Synapses are of two types, electrical and chemical. The electrical synapses are designed for rapid transmission across the synapse. The chemical synapses are specialized for the release and taking up of chemical neurotransmitters. The process is comparatively slow as it includes neurotransmitter release, diffusion, and binding. Electrical signals and neurotransmitters are called the "language" of the nervous system as they are used by each neuron to communicate with others to send messages to the rest of the body. Some of the most significant discoveries in the neurosciences recently relate to the identification of neurotransmitters and their actions. Marieb and Hoehn (2007) reported that more than 50 neurotransmitters or candidates have been identified. Neurologic function is carried out by way of complex networks of neuronal circuits or functional groups of neurons. These groups are organized into integrated hierarchies that contribute to broader neural functions. One way to examine the general design of this complex network is to look at the major functions it fulfills. These include the sensory division (see Chapter 10), the motor division (see Chapter 8), the division for processing of information, and the division for storage of information. The latter two divisions are discussed in this chapter as the process of cognition. Further, human consciousness is described as a related life process.

TABLE 12–1 Summary of Cranial and Spinal Nerves and Their Functions

Cranial Nerves	Function	Spinal Nerves	Function
I. Olfactory	Sense of smell		Sensation, movements and sweat secretions by muscles in regions
II. Optic	Visual acuity		
III. Oculomotor	Pupils and extraocular eye movement (EOM)	C1–5 Phrenic Plexis	Neck Diaphragm
IV. Trochlear	Eye movements	C5–7	Shoulder, arm
V. Trigeminal	Facial sensation and jaw movement; Corneal reflex (used more frequently in assessing the comatose patient)	C5–8 C7–8 L1–5 and S1 L2–5 and S1,2	Forearm Hand Pelvis Thigh
VI. Abducens	Eye movements	L4–5 and S1,2 S1,2	Leg Foot
VII. Facial	Facial movement and taste sensation (anterior two thirds of tongue)	S3,4,5 S2,3	Perineum Bladder
VIII. Acoustic	Gross hearing		
IX. Glossopharyngeal	Gag reflex and ability to swallow		
X. Vagus	Cardiac regulation Gastric secretion		
XI. Spinal accessory	Head movements		
XII. Hypoglossal	Tongue movements		

TABLE 12–2 Autonomic Effects on Various Organs of the Body

Organ	Effect of Sympathetic Stimulation	Effect of Parasympathetic Stimulation
Eye		
Pupil	Dilated	Constricted
Ciliary muscle	Slight relaxation (far vision)	Constricted (near vision)
Glands	Vasoconstriction and slight secretion	Stimulation of copious secretion (containing many enzymes for enzyme-secreting glands)
Nasal		
Lacrimal		
Parotid		
Submandibular		
Gastric		
Pancreatic		
Sweat glands	Copious sweating (cholinergic)	Sweating on palms of hands
Apocrine glands	Thick, odoriferous secretion	None
Blood vessels	Most often constricted	Most often little or no effect
Heart	Increased rate	Slowed rate
Muscle	Increased force of contraction	Decreased force of contraction (especially of atria)
Coronaries	Dilated; constricted	Dilated
Lungs		
Bronchi	Dilated	Constricted
Blood vessels	Mildly constricted	Dilated
Gut		
Lumen	Decreased peristalsis and tone	Increased peristalsis and tone
Sphincter	Increased tone (most times)	Relaxed (most times)
Liver	Glucose released	Slight glycogen synthesis
Gallbladder and bile ducts	Relaxed	Contracted
Kidney	Decreased output and renin secretion	None
Bladder		
Detrusor	Relaxed (slight)	Contracted
Trigone	Contracted	Relaxed
Penis	Ejaculation	Erection
Systemic arterioles		
Abdominal viscera	Constricted (adrenergic)	None
Muscle	Constricted Dilated (adrenergic) Dilated (cholinergic)	None
Skin	Constricted	None
Blood		
Coagulation	Increased	None
Glucose	Increased	None
Lipids	Increased	None

(continued)

TABLE 12–2 *(continued)*

Organ	Effect of Sympathetic Stimulation	Effect of Parasympathetic Stimulation
Basal metabolism	Increased up to 100%	None
Adrenal medullary secretion	Increased	None
Mental activity	Increased	None
Piloerector muscles	Contracted	None
Skeletal muscle	Increased glycogenolysis Increased strength	None
Fat cells	Lipolysis	None

Source: Guyton, A. C. and Hall, J. E. (2006). *Textbook of medical physiology* (p. 754). Philadelphia: Elsevier Saunders. Used with permission.

PROCESS OF COGNITION

In today's society, the processing of information is a major resource for individuals and any group. The world is changing rapidly and societies of developed countries have opened wide the information highway. Human ability and health is influenced and potentially enhanced in the information-processing society. Purposeful interactions and responses are needed. The human nervous system acts as a control mechanism for such interactions and responses. It receives literally millions of bits of information from different senses, integrates and interprets these, and initiates a response. The incredible speed of the processing is seen at every level of function. Examples include the pupillary reflex of the eye, quick evasive action when spotting a hazard on the road, and sensing of the tone of a group on entering a room. A further illustration of the complexity of processing is seen in a nurse caring for a dying patient. The nurse is able to take in more than bits of information; rather, the nurse experiences with the individual the range of emotions that lie in the meaning of life and its ultimate purpose for both of them. The complex transmitting of signals described earlier is just the beginning of human activities that provide meaning to life experiences. The integrated higher process of cognition that emerges makes it possible for one to connect past experiences with the present and relate both past and present to the future. This process is particularly important since it acts as the guide of life events. Furthermore, in the Roy Adaptation Model, understanding cognitive and emotional processing by the cognator subsystem is essential to understanding and relating to the adapting individual.

Cognition is a broad term for the human abilities to think, feel, and act. It is most frequently described as information processing. Models of information processing have developed from early applications such as telephone switchboards in the 1940s to wireless computerized data exchange in the early 21st century. A branch of computer science has been studying for the last half century what is called artificial intelligence exhibited by machines. The position taken by Das (1984) is still relevant today. He made an effective argument that if we wanted to understand how information is processed by human beings we must figure out how processing occurs in the brain rather than the computer. Computer programs have been able to simulate many parts of human information processing and are faster at some aspects such as searches for specific bits of information. However, the self-organizing and reflective nature of human processing makes it possible to reorganize stored information based on the context, make decisions, change them, and translate them into action. Black (1991) argued that the computer analogy of the brain is misleading because in life systems higher levels continually transform the lower. People constantly redefine and transform stimuli, their knowledge base, and the goals of activity. Just consider how the human brain of a freshman college student takes in and handles the events of the first day of classes.

Basically, information processing models for humans are described as having input, central processing, and output stages. A given model may emphasize one stage more than another depending on the purpose of the model. Das and colleagues (Das, Kar, & Parrila, 1996; Das, Kirby, & Jarman, 1979) developed a model of integrated cognitive processes based on three functional units of the brain. These units were derived from the work of Luria (1973, 1980). The first unit regulates cortical arousal and attention; a second unit codes information using simultaneous and successive processes; and a third provides for planning, self-monitoring, and structuring of cognitive activities. The functional units have both depth in the cortical layers and spread across brain hemispheres. This holistic view of brain functioning is in keeping with the developing neuroscience literature on brain mapping. The derived model blends understanding of the structure and functional units of the brain, neuropsychological processes, and it also provides ways to measure the processes.

Roy (1988, 2001) developed a related nursing model for cognition (Figure 12–2). This model draws from knowledge in the neurosciences and from observations in neuroscience

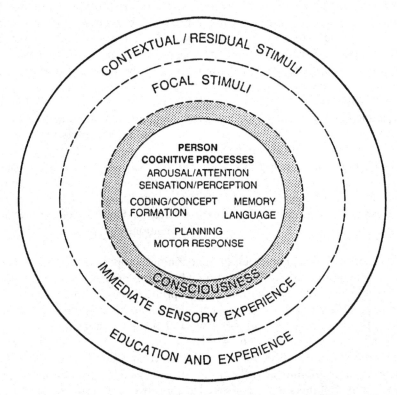

FIGURE 12–2 Nursing model for cognitive processing. (From Roy, C. (1988). Alterations in cognitive processing. In Stewart-Amidei, C., & Kunkel, J.A. (Eds.) (2001). *American Association of Neuroscience Nurses' Neuroscience nursing: Human responses to neurologic dysfunction.* Norwalk: Appleton & Lange. Used with permission.)

nursing practice. The inner circle lists basic internal processes of arousal and attention, sensation and perception; coding and concept formation, memory and language; and planning and motor response. These functions are dependent on the brain structure neurologically and neurochemically. The model shows that the basic cognitive processes occur within a field of consciousness. Consciousness (discussed in detail later in the chapter) is characterized by both arousal and awareness, particularly awareness of self. The environment for cognitive processing is based on an understanding of environment as defined in the Roy Adaptation Model. More specifically, the environment for cognitive processing includes focal stimuli as serial and concurrent input, and contextual and residual stimuli, considered primarily in terms of knowledge base. The broken lines in the figure indicate the permeability between the stimuli fields.

The circles of the model highlight contemporary views in both nursing and cognitive science that the individual is a participant and partner in the developmental process. Cognitive processing abilities throughout the life span are subject to interactions and involve multiple mutual influences. Development includes biologic aspects, or maturation, and environmental factors, such as learning opportunities. Research evidence has shown how sensory and motor maps in the cortex can be modified with experience (Gazzaniga, Ivry, & Mangun, 2002). Rather than age affecting development at a steady pace, this interactive model implies social, biologic, and environmental influences. Children and the elderly have a much greater degree of variability in expression of cognitive abilities. Their cerebral organization for cognitive processes is inherently more difficult to understand. More recently there has been increased study of these groups. Children are subject to growth spurts and developmental stages and lags. Changes associated with aging can be primary and nonpathologic, such as alterations in sensory functioning. They may also be secondary and pathologic, such as changes associated with Alzheimer's disease.

A principle basic to Roy's cognitive processing model is integrated neural functioning. This principle notes that brain activity is integrated due to centers for many functions being widely distributed and interconnected throughout the brain. Integrated neural functioning is manifested in several ways. Knowledge of exactly how thinking and feeling processes occur at the neurologic level is increasing with advances in brain imaging techniques. Scientists generally come to one major conclusion, that it appears that many brain areas participate and interact in these processes. Cortical and subcortical areas are involved, and processes of consciousness, attention, and perception are intimately interrelated.

The principle of integrated neural functioning is operating when the individual selects important stimuli from among all possible stimuli present and then channels these stimuli to the relevant brain centers for an appropriate response. Increasingly, data show that relevant brain centers for many functions are distributed throughout the brain. Mountcastle (1997) reviewed a century of work that used various approaches to obtain functional maps of the brain, and then made conclusions based on data from newer methods of brain mapping. Mountcastle recognized that each area of the cortex has distinctive layers and columns of cells; however, each also has its own unique set of extrinsic connections. Columns in areas located at some distance from one another, but with some common properties, may be linked by long-range connections within the cortex. Through these widely and reciprocally interconnected systems, integrated activity is the very essence of brain function. Mountcastle's conclusion supports Luria's (1980) insights noted above gained from 40 years of working with head-injured patients from World War II. The principle of integrated neural functioning calls into question the notion of localization (functions located in specific structures), lateralization (separate functions for each cerebral hemisphere), and stimulus–response learning (responses from reflexes chained together).

The brain's unique power is due mainly to its ability to store information, that is, to code a representation of experience for future use. An early scientist in the field, Lashley (quoted in Pribram, 1969), reviewed the experimental evidence related to how the brain goes about storage and retrieval. Lashley concluded, somewhat wryly, that on the basis of available evidence, learning and remembering were obviously impossible. Recent contributions to understanding memory demonstrate a number of distinctly different systems for memory. There is the possibility of discovering even more memory systems, each with its own relatively discrete structures and neurotransmitters. Different models of taking in and the stages of processing information have led to at least 134 different named types of memory (Lezak, Howieson, Loring, Hannay, & Fischer, 2004).

From what is known about higher processing functions, the storage of information is a function of the brain as a whole. What is called long-term memory results from the interaction of multiple networks, some known and some unknown. These are distributed throughout the nervous system and are activated by experiences distributed across time. The nursing student has strong memories of the motor task of giving an intramuscular injection. If she later learns that the faculty who taught her the skill has now written a book on introduction to nursing, her activated memory is restored as an enriched experience. Some authors have noted that theories of the consolidation phase of memory propose a gradual transfer of memory that uses processing from hippocampal and medial temporal lobe structures to the neocortex for longer term storage. For this reason, storage of information is influenced not only by the brain itself, but also by the individual's changing environment. The holistic formulation of cerebral function is useful in nursing assessments and nursing interventions related to cognition.

PROCESS OF CONSCIOUSNESS

Consciousness has many definitions. There is agreement that it involves an awareness of the internal and external environment. This awareness provides a readiness to act and also includes the human possibility of reflecting on one's actions. For clinical purposes, consciousness includes two components: arousal, the awakeness of the individual; and content, the awareness and interpretation of the internal and external environment. Consciousness also is a significant process associated with the individual's ability to adapt or self-regulate. This significance is based on the role of consciousness in the perception of sensory input and the central process of registering or coding information. Human activity is much more than output of a highly complex physical system. It cannot be understood solely in terms of musculature and neurocircuits. Activity stems from what is called intentionality. An individual's intentions stem from such things as needs, motives, values, and beliefs that are built into human consciousness.

Growing understanding of the many systems of the brain has led to beginning knowledge about consciousness as a process. No one structure or function can be equated with the process because consciousness is a composite produced by all cortical areas and their connections (Kolb & Whishaw, 1996). The basis for consciousness involves interactions of the cerebral cortex, subcortical structures including the hypothalamus, and brain stem centers. If any of these structures is damaged or disconnected from the other two, an altered state of consciousness results. The alert state requires the neural activity of the ascending reticular activating system of the brain stem communicating with both cerebral hemispheres. Similarly, feedback from the cerebral cortex of both hemispheres into the reticular activating system of the brain stem is necessary for consciousness.

There is much about human consciousness that still is considered unknown in terms of scientific explanation. Yet what began as a philosophic debate has been studied in many related sciences. The result is encouraging progress in understanding the importance of consciousness—of self, values, and action. One respected statement (Eccles & Robinson, 1984) noted that there is strong support for the hypothesis that the supplementary motor area of the brain is the sole recipient area for mental intentions that lead to voluntary movements. However, other authors insist that consciousness is a mode of action of the brain as a whole rather than a subsystem. The philosopher Kant (Kemp, 1979) described an individual as a subject who is responsible for one's actions. Self-consciousness is necessary to monitor and regulate behavior. To be self-conscious is to have knowledge of oneself. Self-consciousness involves knowledge, not just of one's physical state, but also of inner reality. Consciousness as an awareness of an inner reality includes the reality of mental states and activities. People can recognize that they are angry, happy, or believe or hope in something. However, there are different degrees of self-consciousness, since the ability to discriminate subtly different types of mental states presumably improves with practice and increasing experience. From the perspective of transpersonal psychology, Wilber (1997) presented a model of a spectrum of consciousness that moves from basic levels of matter to body, mind, soul, and then to spirit. As people move from one level to another, they enter into new, deeper, and wider spheres of consciousness at each stage.

The expansion of introspective consciousness is generally viewed as good both for the individual and for the society. As noted earlier, nurse-authors such as Newman (1994) view health as expanding consciousness. Scientists such as Wilber suggest how one might improve or enhance introspective access. Eccles describes the two-way flow of consciousness in a discussion of voluntary movement, freedom of will, and moral responsibility. Eccles (Eccles & Robinson, 1984) cites a transcendent importance of recognizing that by using thought, the individual can influence the operation of the neural mechanisms of the brain. In this way people can bring changes in the world for good or ill. Eccles uses the simple metaphor that the conscious self is in the driver's seat. Life can be regarded as successive patterns of choice that lead to the feeling of fulfillment, with resulting happiness that comes to a life centered on meaning and purpose. The Roy Adaptation Model's philosophic assumptions clearly recognize the ideal that each individual is to have the maximum freedom to realize her or his potential. This ideal stems from the belief that human life has common meaning, purpose, and destiny.

COMPENSATORY ADAPTIVE PROCESSES

A major compensatory adaptive process to preserve cognitive and neurologic functioning is neural plasticity. Plasticity refers to modification of structures with functional changes. Neural plasticity refers to the adaptive capacities of the central nervous system—its ability to modify its own structural organization and functioning. One can think of plasticity as a second fundamental property of the nervous system. According to the first property, a nerve excitation makes a rapid change that leaves no trace. Plasticity, on the other hand, permits enduring and functional changes to take place. The enduring changes of the developing nervous system have three specific characteristics. These plasticities occur at critical periods, can last over a lifetime, and seem to lack what is usually defined as motivation and reinforcement for their establishment. A well-studied example of molding the structure and function of the nervous system by environmental changes is the development of vision and hearing in animals. Limiting sensory input at a given time can result in lack of later ability to have full use of a given sense. Plasticity is greater in early years, with multiple new patterns of structure and function possible. The reservoir of plasticity decreases across the life span. Still, recent studies are focusing on plasticity of the adult brain, the aging brain, and particularly the person with brain injury.

There is evidence of greater potential for retaining and restoring nervous system functional effectiveness than was previously thought. Gazzaniga, Ivry, and Mangun (2002) cited experiments that show cortical areas fill in and take over areas not receiving innervation because of interruptions to somatosensory, visual, and auditory systems. The authors noted that this functional plasticity "suggests that the cortex of adults is a dynamic place where changes can still happen" (p. 648).

Many mechanisms of neural plasticity have been identified, including sprouting of remaining nerve fibers after injury. Following acute injury to the central nervous system, there are immediate decreases in the function of neurons in other areas of the brain or spinal cord caused by decreased input, shock, and other factors. Functional recovery from these remote effects is possible as a result of synaptic reactivation of neurons and this is facilitated by rehabilitation (Gouvier, Ryan, O'Jile, Parks-Levy, Webster, & Blanton, 1997). Though study in this area is incomplete, the knowledge that neural plasticity exists provides incentive for nursing research and practice in this area of promoting adaptation with neurologically injured patients at all phases of recovery.

COMPROMISED PROCESSES OF NEUROLOGIC FUNCTION

Adaptation problems can result when any of the processes related to neurologic function are disrupted. Two specific examples of compromised adaptive processes related to neurologic function are discussed here. Memory deficit is a commonly occurring problem associated with cognitive processes. Similarly, decreased level of consciousness is a significant compromised process of neurologic function.

Memory Deficit

A deficit in the ability to process experience by storing and retrieving information is generally termed memory deficit. Memory deficits stem from the complex working systems for reception, coding, and storage of information, as well as retrieval of information. As noted earlier, brain structures such as the hippocampus are involved in particular stages. This includes, for example, sorting, assembling, and supplying information that is emotionally significant. Short-term changes in synaptic function have been identified in work on habituation and conditioning, but how such changes might be converted into long-term memory lasting for years is not known. The role of metabolic activity, protein synthesis, and neurotransmitters in these processes are broad areas of study. It has been noted that an overriding principle of cognitive processing is the integrated functioning of the brain as a whole. This characteristic makes the memory storage and retrieval processes most sensitive to changes that occur throughout the brain.

Focal stimuli for memory deficits include metabolic changes, infection, tumors, seizures, stroke, and toxic reactions. The retrieval process seems most affected by these pathologies. The memory disturbance that generally follows closed head injury has particular characteristics. These patients may have a period of coma followed by a period of confusion. During the length of these two intervals, current events have not been stored. This time frame is commonly called the period of posttraumatic amnesia, and its duration is often used as an index of closed head injury severity.

Degenerative brain pathology, as sometimes occurs in alcoholism and other drug use, has long been known to produce defects of memory. Korsakoff's syndrome in long-term alcoholism has been studied extensively because these individuals have global amnesia and are readily available. The symptoms provide examples of memory deficits. The characteristics of this type of pathology are as follows (Kolb & Whishaw, 1996).

1. Anterograde amnesia, in which patients are unable to form new memories.
2. Retrograde amnesia, that is, the patients have global impairment of remote memory for most of their adult life.
3. Confabulation, where information is made up to cover up memory loss.
4. Meager content in conversation indicated by little spontaneous conversation.
5. Lack of insight that is particularly difficult because patients are virtually unaware of their memory deficit.
6. Apathy manifested by indifference and incapacity to persevere in ongoing activities.

Alzheimer's disease is another degenerative brain disorder that has generated interest for both clinical and scientific reasons. It accounts for about 60% of the dementias occurring in people over age 65 years, and it provides a good model for the study of senility in general. Dementia of the Alzheimer's type occurs less frequently in 40- and 50-year-olds. Changes in the brain structures include neuronal loss resulting in marked cerebral atrophy. The areas most affected are precentral gyrus of the frontal lobe, superior temporal gyrus, hippocampus, and substantia nigra. Microscopic changes include neurofibrillary tangles, senile or neuritic plaques, and granulovacuolar degeneration. Besides the structural changes, research has shown neurochemical changes, particularly abnormalities of the neurotransmitters. This condition leads to marked deficits in memory, judgment, language, and visuospatial perception, as well as symptoms of depression and other personality changes. Losses generally occur in stages of mild, moderate, and severe.

Individuals with memory deficits can be deprived of the richness of their own past. They can feel lost in the unfamiliar world of the here and now. They are suspicious of what may happen to them because of the inability to understand and predict events as yet unfolding. Adaptation problems related to memory can occur transiently, as in concussion, or for a prolonged period, as with Alzheimer's disease. The deficit can be continual or intermittent. It can have qualitative aspects such as defective spontaneous recall, lack of ability to integrate information into a whole as a basis for a modulated response, or conceptual inflexibility. In working with individuals with a diagnosis of memory deficit, the nurse recognizes that observations of behaviors and stimuli, together with updated knowledge in the field, provide the basis for planning care.

Decreased Level of Consciousness

Changing pressures within the cranium affect the level of consciousness because the skull is a nonflexible bony structure. The brain takes up 80% of the space inside the skull. Cerebrospinal fluid and the blood in the cerebral arteries and veins occupy the remainder of the space. A change in the volume of any one of these components brings about compensatory changes to maintain intracranial pressure (ICP) at a normal level. If pressure within the skull increases, however, there is little room to accommodate the change. Increased intracranial pressure (IICP) refers to an increase in pressure in the subarachnoid space where cerebrospinal fluid (CSF) circulates around the brain and spinal cord and in the ventricles. One bodily mechanism to attempt adaptation by immediately relieving IICP is brain herniation, that is, the brain protruding into another compartment or area, taking advantage of any spaces where brain structures meet. The brain itself is not rigid and can make shifts with fairly predictable patterns, each associated with characteristic clinical signs. This compensation is usually short lived, however, and quickly becomes life-threatening.

The several compartments of the cranium are separated by sheets of dura. Pressure shifts brain tissue from one area where pressure is high to another where pressure is lower. There are three major patterns of brain shift. Shifts across the intracranial cavity force the brain tissue under the dura that divides the two hemispheres (midline shift). In downward displacement, the hemispheres and the basal nuclei go through the tentorium where the midbrain passes (central herniation). Displacement and compression of blood vessels further contribute to disturbance of ICP and to cerebral hypoxia. Severe brain stem changes result. Finally, there is herniation through the foramen magnum where all the structures are being pulled downward (uncal herniation). The latter is signaled by warnings from structures that lie outside the brain parenchyma. Of particular clinical importance is the fact that the third cranial nerve, which controls pupil response and extraocular eye movements (EOM), may be caught between swollen structures and ligaments. Thus, the lethal effects of compression of the medulla can be prevented by the nurse's observation of a change in the size of the pupil of the eye. Mitchell (2001) discussed nursing assessment of potential brain herniation as consisting of serial monitoring, as discussed later, with the goal of earliest possible detection and referral for neurosurgical management.

A patient can have the diagnosis of decreased level of consciousness related to increased intracranial pressure. The anatomic basis for consciousness is divided into two regions: the cerebral hemispheres above the tentorium and the reticular formation of the brain stem extending from the midpons through the diencephalon. Understanding this problem requires an understanding of the condition of increased intracranial pressure (IICP). This condition can be seen in many neurologic disruptions, such as central nervous system tumors, brain abscess, hydrocephalus, aneurysms, and traumatic brain injury with contusions or hematoma.

NURSING PROCESS RELATED TO NEUROLOGIC FUNCTION

Neurologic function is important for an individual's adaptation in all of the four modes. In applying the nursing process, the nurse makes a careful assessment of behaviors and stimuli related to the complex processes of cognition and consciousness. In assessing factors influencing neurologic function, regulator and cognator effectiveness in initiating compensatory processes is considered. Based on a thorough first- and second-level assessment, the nurse makes nursing diagnoses, sets goals, selects nursing interventions, and evaluates care.

Assessment of Behavior: Cognition

Assessments of neurologic function, and cognition in particular, are at times subtle. This finely tuned assessment can be critical for the goals of adaptation from survival to the individual and environment transformations of increasing adaptation. The detail and outcome of an initial cognitive assessment varies according to the individual's condition. For example, a nurse in the emergency room may assess confusion and unclear speech in an elderly person with other significant neurologic signs and summon a neurologist for diagnosis of a stroke. The nurse in a well-baby clinic may be observing the developing integrated neural activity of a child over time, making detailed assessments of sensory, motor, and cognitive functioning, and using these data in planning care with the family.

In assessing the basic life process of cognition, the major concepts in Roy's nursing model of cognition in Figure 12–2 can be helpful. The model of cognition forms the structure for assessment of input, central processing, and output processes. Consciousness and sensory and motor evaluation are also important components in the assessment of neurologic function. These are described elsewhere: consciousness in the next section of this chapter, and sensory and motor evaluation in Chapters 8 and 10.

Ways to assess information processing and storing of memories are diverse. Each approach is based on understanding the organization of cognitive functions and of how these processes take place. Major functions of cognition are outlined in Table 12–3, based on the nursing model for cognitive processing. The nurse collects meaningful data using interview and observation. A careful history of change in cognition over time is important. Behaviors for each processing function are noted in a global way. Family members' reports and patient observations of functioning provide important clinical data needed for nursing care planning as well as for medical diagnosis. Nursing assessments related to integrated neurologic functioning lead to identifying dysfunctions that have an impact on daily living. Specific deficits and behavioral manifestations of each of the functions listed in Table 12–3 are described in detail by Roy (2001).

INPUT PROCESSES   Behavioral assessment of input processes focuses on two major areas: arousal and attention, and sensation and perception.

Arousal and Attention   Behaviors associated with arousal and attention tend to be apparent during the history-taking process. The individual's orientation is evident in responses to such questions as "What is your name?" and, "Where do you live?" Other behavioral aspects include selective attention, the speed with which the individual processes information, and the alertness demonstrated with such behaviors in response to direct commands.

Sensation and Perception   Sensation and perception include behaviors related to primary sense processing, pattern recognition, and naming and association. The assessment of primary senses has been addressed in other chapters, particularly Chapter 10. Pattern recognition can be assessed by asking the individual to select specific shapes to fit into containers of the same shape, for example. Naming and association can be assessed by asking simple questions to test for recognition of objects or pictures.

CENTRAL PROCESSES   The second assessment area associated with the cognition model is that of central processing. The four aspects included in this area are coding, concept formation, memory, and language.

TABLE 12–3 Major Functions of Cognitive Processing Within a Nursing Model

---

Input Processes

Arousal and attention
    Selective attention
    Speed of processing
    Alertness
Sensation and perception
    Primary sense processing
    Pattern recognition
    Naming and associating

Central Processes

Coding
    Registration
    Consolidation
    Synthesis
Concept formation
    Integrated recognition
    Abstraction and flexibility
    Calculation
Memory
    Simultaneous
    Successive
Language

Output Processes

Planning
Motor response
    Motor planning
    Initiating action
    Regulating action

Coding   Coding includes the registration, consolidation, and synthesis of information. Are the events underway being noticed by the individual and is the response within the realm of expectations under the circumstances? Is the individual able to perform direct commands and is there evidence of spatial orientation?

Concept Formation   Evidence of concept formation is associated with integrated recognition, abstraction and flexibility, and calculation abilities. To what extent can the individual comprehend the complexities of what is occurring in the environment? Abstraction and flexibility can be assessed by asking the individual to explain a proverb or to identify similarities or differences between two objects. The ability to perform mathematical calculations is a further indication of the individual's cognitive processing of concepts.

Memory   Memory can be viewed in terms of simultaneous and successive memory. Evidence of the individual's memory processing will be evident during the history-taking process shown in the ability to relate past medical problems. A test of memory is the individual's ability to repeat four numbers in reverse order. Remembrance of significant dates can also be an indicator of integrity of the individual's memory.

Language The individual's language capabilities are an important indicator of cognition. What are the characteristics of speech—flowing, spontaneous, rhythmic, clear enunciation, normal tone? Is the use and understanding of vocabulary at an expected level?

OUTPUT PROCESSES The third assessment area of cognition is output processes. Included in this is the assessment of the individual's capabilities associated with planning and with motor responses.

Planning Planning involves the ability of the individual to anticipate future possibilities and to appropriately determine actions required to effectively adapt. Evidence of judgment and insight would be indications of intact planning processes leading to realistic and achievable actions. The individual's inability to act in terms of the future would indicate ineffective cognition as it relates to the ability to plan.

Motor Response Motor response includes the aspects of motor planning, initiating action, and regulating action. Is the individual able to appropriately sequence motor activities to accomplish a task? Do his or her extremities respond to intentions formulated in the mind? For example, an individual might intend to move the right arm, but does that action happen physically as planned? At times, the debilitated elderly require prompting to help with initiating action. They may appear unable to feed themselves, but when helped to initiate the activity, are able to carry on independently. Regulation of action deals with the ability to appropriately sequence motor activity and to perform the action in consecutive and consistent steps. Many people with degenerative disease of the nervous system, such as Huntington's chorea, are unable to regulate their physical movements, with resulting jerky and random physical actions.

An assessment is made of each one of these functions by observing the individual involved in one ordinary task. For example, the nurse assesses the normal cognitive processing of a toddler when the child reaches out and calls for mother. The mother has been selected out from other stimuli in the room; the child perceives that she is there, recognizes a pattern, and makes an association. Coding, early concept formation, memory, and language have all been involved and the motor response follows. For more specific screening of level of functioning, a number of tests exist that are appropriate for clinical use. One test frequently used is the Mini-Mental State (MMS) (Anthony, LeResche, Niaz, Von Korff, & Folstein, 1982; Folstein, Folstein, & McHugh, 1975), which tests orientation, registration, attention, calculations, recall, and language. It takes 5 minutes to administer and has proven reliable in identifying dementia and psychiatric disorders. By noting subtle difficulties that an individual is having in information processing, the nurse can identify needs for formal neuropsychologic evaluation. The individual's frustration in ordinary situations or making excuses for simple mistakes can be initial cues of difficulties with cognition.

Assessment of Behavior: Consciousness

Unequivocally, the major assessment factor to determine neurologic status is level of consciousness. It has been said, "The brain does not fail unannounced." Rather, a predictable set of behaviors occurs and can be identified. Slight changes in level of consciousness are significant. Increasing forgetfulness or slight lethargy may be the first behavioral indicators of increasing intracranial pressure.

LEVEL OF CONSCIOUSNESS Level of consciousness can be classified in a number of ways. Mitchell (2001) noted that the amount and kind of stimulus required to arouse an individual and the nature of the response are basic dimensions used in all classifications. Therefore, these are the key factors to assess. The most frequently used approach in the acute care setting to quantify arousal is the Glasgow Coma Scale, or GCS (Jennett & Teasdale, 1977). The behaviors noted at regular intervals are eye opening, verbal response, and motor response. The examiner's voice is the stimulus, but if there is no response, then pressure can be applied to the individual's fingertip. The best response in a given time period determines the score because this has been found to be the most reliable score. The maximum cumulative score of 15 indicates a fully conscious, alert individual, whereas the minimum score of 3 indicates coma. Coma is described as the state of unconsciousness from which an individual cannot be aroused to make purposeful responses. Figure 12–3 shows how an individual's GCS can be noted on a flow sheet and the level of progress determined and evaluated over time. If the nurse notes a decrease in score, she recognizes this as an indication of worsening neurologic status that requires rapid attention.

MOTOR RESPONSE The quality of motor response is an important behavioral indicator of neurologic status. Neurologic control of basic motor functioning is tested first by asking the individual to squeeze the examiner's two hands simultaneously. Then the individual is asked to push both feet against the nurse's hands (if in bed) and equality of strength is noted. The general equality of all movements is also noted, as decreased muscle strength is a frequent behavioral indicator of neurologic disruptions.

RESPONSE TO PAIN If consciousness is impaired, the quality of motor response to pain is particularly important. This can be evaluated during a routine procedure that includes the use of a noxious stimulus, such as endotracheal suctioning. The following possible responses to pain are listed in order of increasingly disrupted neurologic functioning.

1. Purposeful movement. Movement is made away from the pain stimulus.
2. Nonpurposeful movement. A random movement is made in response to pain.
3. Decorticate rigidity. The legs extend and rotate internally with the feet plantar flexed. The arms adduct and are pulled in to the chest with the wrists and fingers flexed. This indicates the interruption of cortical motor fibers but intact pathways through the brain stem.
4. Decerebrate rigidity. As in decorticate posturing, the legs extend, the arms extend, the wrists and fingers are flexed. This indicates the disruption of motor fibers in the mid-brain and brain stem.

   Decorticate and decerebrate posturing may at first be unilateral and then become bilateral, the former being less serious. At first, the posturing may occur only with noxious stimulation. As the dysfunction increases, the posturing is continual. With severe neurologic dysfunction, there is no response to pain. This is usually a grave sign.

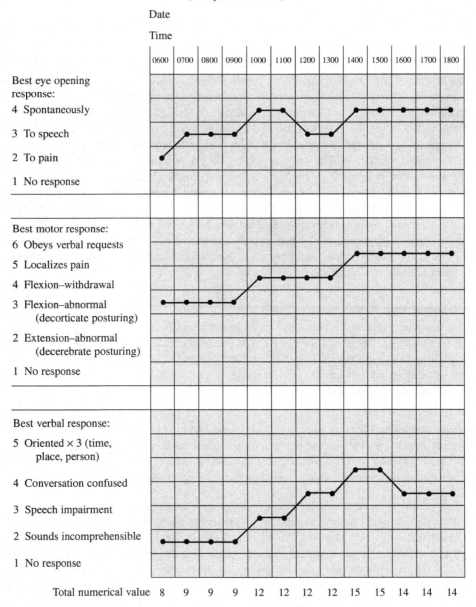

GLASGOW COMA SCALE
(Sample flow sheet)

FIGURE 12–3 Glasgow Coma Scale. (From Jennett, B., & Teasdale, G. (1977). Aspects of coma after severe head injury. *Lancet*, 1(8017), 878-881. Used with permission).

ORIENTATION AND LEVEL OF AWARENESS   Consciousness has been referred to as involving both level of arousal and awareness. Awareness includes the level of orientation and level of self-awareness. Oriented individuals know person, time, place, and purpose. They can respond with their name, what time of day it is, where they are, and why they are there. The confused individual appears dazed and in varying degrees, either continuously or intermittently, is not oriented to person, time, place, or purpose. Consciousness as self-awareness is reflected in the individual as an individual as well as in relationships with others. The nurse observes the individual's mood, expressions, grooming, mannerisms, and speech. Behaviors of the self-concept, role function, and interdependence modes are relevant for this assessment.

VITAL SIGNS Changes in vital signs are manifestations of changes in levels of consciousness, particularly when the situation becomes severe. Blood pressure initially demonstrates an increase in systolic pressure with widening of the pulse pressure. This is followed by a sudden decrease in systolic pressure. Pulse rate first slows but then becomes rapid and thready as increased intracranial pressure continues. Changes in respirations indicate deterioration in the patient's condition. Body temperature may vacillate between hyperthermia and hypothermia.

Assessment of Stimuli

The identification of factors that contribute to changes in neurologic status, cognition and consciousness in particular, is part of the nursing assessment of this physiologic mode component. As with behavioral assessment, the nurse can contribute significant information about the circumstances surrounding changes in neurologic functioning. On initial presentation, the nurse talks with the patient, family, or witnesses to the onset of ineffective behaviors. In the case of an automobile accident, did the individual lose consciousness first and then collide with another car? Was the homeless person found hallucinating on the street complaining of dizziness or deprived of meals with adequate protein? Did a painter simply fall from the ladder or did he clutch at his chest first? The focal and contextual stimuli can be related to the individual's medical condition or, in fact, stem from the individual in any of the four modes of adaptation. In the examples discussed, we see the kaleidoscopic characteristic of the model, with behaviors becoming stimuli and one stimulus affecting another.

PATHOPHYSIOLOGY Often a given neurologic medical diagnosis is the focal stimulus for the changes in cognitive behavior or consciousness observed by the nurse. For example, blood collecting in the subdural space from head trauma will affect the individual's ability to identify what day it is and where the individual is. Trauma, infection, neuromuscular disease, vascular disturbances, tumors, electrolyte imbalance, and developmental disorders result in varying degrees of deficits in cognition or consciousness. Degenerative diseases including Parkinsonism, Huntington's chorea, and Alzheimer's disease can affect the individual's level of consciousness and cognitive processing. If there is a sudden change in consciousness and the cause is not known, it is important that the patient be examined for signs of injury. Trauma to the brain can result from blunt force, penetrating wounds, contusion opposite a point of impact, or a fracture at the base of the skull. The resulting tissue damage can result in changes in level of consciousness and sometimes long-term consequences for cognitive processing. In some situations, the ingestion of noxious substances can be the cause of altered levels of consciousness with possible consequences for brain function long term. The individual's breath is smelled for the odor of alcohol, acetone, or other chemicals such as glue, kerosene, carbon tetrachloride, or gasoline. When drug use is suspected, it is important to establish when the last dose was taken. A vascular spasm may cause a brief and temporary headache that has little effect on the individual's cognition and adaptive potential. On the other hand, conditions such as cerebrovascular accidents (strokes) and multiple sclerosis can result in extensive changes that require great and prolonged efforts to maximize adaptive potential through the use of cognition.

IMMEDIATE SITUATION   On initial presentation, the nurse talks with the patient, family, or witnesses to the circumstance that prompted the change in level of consciousness or cognition. Was there a traumatic event? Did the individual express any perceptions, such as a severe headache, prior to the change? Or has the change been insidious and gradual? Responses to these questions can lead to further ideas about contributing factors. For example, it may be reported that the individual experienced a seizure just prior to the onset of the change in level of consciousness.

BLOOD GASES AND HEMOGLOBIN LEVELS   Two important internal factors that are noted by laboratory indicators are arterial blood gases and hemoglobin levels. Both have the greatest immediate effect on cognition and consciousness. The partial pressure of carbon dioxide ($PaCO_2$) in the arterial blood and oxygen (PaO_2) affect cerebral blood flow, which in turn influences alertness and the ability to process information. Similarly, if hemoglobin is low, the oxygen-combining capacity of the blood is reduced and cerebral hypoxia is exacerbated, with possible confusion. If the hemoglobin is above normal, there is a greater tendency for clot formation, resulting in vascular obstruction and, therefore, ischemia and changes in consciousness and cognition.

EFFECTS OF TREATMENT   The nurse recognizes that various treatment modalities, including medication and surgery, affect both consciousness and cognitive processes. Dramatic changes related to cognition follow certain forms of treatment. For example, surgical intervention can result in the cessation of formerly intractable seizures, with periods of inability to process information. Also, there is some swelling of the brain after neurosurgery and this can affect levels of consciousness for a limited period of time. Monitoring for signs of decreasing levels of consciousness is important during this period to identify any complications such as intracranial bleeding or infection.

Drugs categorized as anticonvulsants, cerebral vasodilators, and narcotic analgesics all affect level of arousal. The use of some sedatives such as tranquilizers and medications for sleep, particularly in the elderly, can inadvertently affect level of consciousness. Similarly, doses of steroids and anticonvulsants need to be monitored for the effect on the level of alertness and responsiveness. Sometimes coma is purposefully induced on a trial basis using barbiturates in a patient who has increased intracranial pressure that has not responded to conventional therapy. The therapeutic principle is that the immediate decrease in cerebral blood flow and brain metabolism will be beneficial. This treatment is reported useful in reducing intracranial pressure for patients with head injury, Reye's syndrome, encephalitis, and cerebral hemorrhage (Hickey, 1992). However, some authors noted that barbiturate coma remains a treatment option even through clinical trials have not yet clearly demonstrated its usefulness (Ignatavicius & Workman, 2006).

Altered cognition often results from changes in the physical environment. The environment can positively or negatively affect cognition. In the case of a disoriented individual, the hospital environment itself can greatly accentuate ineffective behavior. Artificial lighting, the noise of foreign machinery, and altered time schedules all contribute to an individual's confusion. Once such individuals are medically stable, returning them to the familiar surroundings of their homes can promote cognitive adaptation. Noise is an important stimulus, as it can further increase intracranial pressure. Even the lack of clutter in the environment serves as a stimulus. In the case of an individual who has had a cardiovascular accident, uncluttered surroundings in the home or hospital promote the behavior of orientation.

KNOWLEDGE ABOUT CONDITION Stress can result from inappropriately negative expectations of a neurologic medical diagnosis. If so, anxiety, fear, depression, and hopelessness may result. Expectancies are related to knowledge level. For example, a brain tumor erroneously signifies death to many. In fact, death occurs only in some cases. Paralysis may signify sterility, which is not usually the case in the female. It is therefore essential that the nurse have knowledge about the particular disruption being observed and understand the specifics of the individual case and medical prognosis. The effective exchange of information among doctor, nurse, patient, and family can be a key factor in the patient's developing realistic self-expectations.

For all neurologic conditions, the nurse asseses the patient's and family's understandings. Assessing this stimulus is important for the nursing intervention phase of planning care. Information is given according to the level of comprehension. Teaching is initiated when the acute period has subsided and learning readiness is evident—for example, when there is lack of denial of medical facts, lack of excessive anxiety, and pain is under control. Teaching measures include an exploration of what one should expect in terms of physiologic changes as well as modifications in self-concept, role function, and interdependence. To prevent complications or possible recurrence of the neurologic problem, the nurse informs the family and the individual of behaviors to report to the physician. Adjustments to changes in neurologic functioning can be made more successfully, and with less stress, when the individual can distinguish between expected bodily changes and indications of complications. The nurse helps clarify these expectations.

STRESS The stress of a neurologic condition also is a significant influencing stimulus. The neuroendocrine and behavioral response to stress is discussed in Chapter 13. Some specific applications of this concept as it affects consciousness and cognition are noted here. Stressors can take the form of painful procedures, emotional trauma, or a lowered body resistance from fatigue and malnutrition. Such stress factors serve as a stimulus for aggravating cognitive and neurologic changes. For example, the noxious stimulation such as suctioning or a venipuncture can cause intracranial pressure to increase. As this pressure increases, we see that behavioral manifestations of neurologic change may worsen, lethargy progressing to stupor, for example. In neuromuscular disruptions such as multiple sclerosis and myasthenia gravis, stress factors of fatigue; malnutrition; cold, damp weather; and even pregnancy can exacerbate the behavioral manifestations of those diseases and neuromuscular weakness.

NUTRITIONAL STATUS Nutritional status can affect cognition and neurologic functioning. For example, the nurse considers that obesity increases the risk of hypertension and having a cerebrovascular accident. Similarly, certain nutritional deficits affect neurologic status. For example, thiamine deficiency results in disturbances in the metabolism of nerve tissue. The tissue is then unable to appropriately utilize carbohydrates, resulting in the neurologic manifestations of weakness, muscle pain, and tenderness. The output part of cognitive processing is affected. Fluid intake can also affect neurologic status. For example, decreased fluid intake results in reduced intracranial pressure. Increased intake hastens recovery in certain neurologic infections. These changes can affect both alertness and cognitive deficits that have resulted from the pathology.

ACTIVITY AND REST   In neuromuscular disruptions, activity can either exacerbate or relieve particular behavioral manifestations of the condition. For example, tremors in Parkinson's disease decrease with activity and increase with rest. Increased muscular fatigability is a distressing feature of myasthenia gravis. It increases with activity and decreases with rest. Although coughing is an important activity after many surgeries, it is inadvisable in many cranial surgeries, because it increases intracranial pressure. Deep breathing and turning instead can promote adaptive ventilation. The nurse can use knowledge about positioning to enhance cognitive, neurologic, and adaptive functioning. For example, after a thrombotic or embolic cerebrovascular accident, keeping the patient in a side-lying position decreases the risk of aspiration. Keeping the head of the bed low for the first few days may promote cerebral circulation. Keeping the head of the bed slightly elevated and the head in alignment with the body are important for the patient with increased intracranial pressure. If the head is out of alignment with the body (that is, the body is flat and the head turned to the side), venous return from the brain is impaired and intracranial pressure increases further.

SELF-CONCEPT MODE   An adaptive self-concept is of utmost importance in dealing with chronic neurologic impairments, particularly those affecting cognition. Once the individual has been able to grieve the loss of function, integration of a new body image is essential. This reintegration is necessary to move forward with the tasks of rehabilitation. An adaptive body image can make the difference between one's relearning to walk, speak, and generally live up to one's potential, or being prone to progressive debilitation.

ROLE FUNCTION MODE   Within the role function mode, developmental level is considered a determinant of one's primary role. In the context of this chapter, specific neurologic conditions, and their effect on cognition, are more common at certain ages than others. For example, multiple sclerosis and head trauma occur most frequently in the young adult, whereas Parkinson's disease and cerebrovascular accident occur more frequently in the older adult. Disorientation is more prevalent in the elderly, due in part to sensory impairments, vascular degeneration, and selective changes in neurotransmitters.

INTERDEPENDENCE MODE   The interdependence adaptive mode highlights the importance of significant others and support systems in the life of an individual. For the individual with difficulties in cognitive functioning, family members hold unusual prominence in the individual's ability to cope with these changes. Many of the behaviors associated with changes in cognition are chronic. Situations of altered communication ability, muscular weakness, and disorientation require a great deal of patience. If the family or significant others offer support and understanding, this can act as a stimulus to enhance the individual's ability to cope. In some instances, the family may not be able to change a particular behavioral manifestation of neurologic dysfunction (such as progressive muscular weakness in Duchenne's muscular dystrophy), but their support can help prevent complications in all four adaptive modes. With the encouragement of the family, the individual may be better motivated to strengthen new muscle groups as other muscles are affected. This action not only affects the physiologic mode in helping to prevent the complications of inactivity, but the individual's self-concept is better maintained. Similarly, feelings of independence are encouraged as the individual is better able to carry out some of the responsibilities of previous roles by the simple fact of being more physically mobile.

Whenever possible, the nurse assists individuals with cognitive and neurologic impairments to maintain their role in the family. For the paralyzed individual, cognitive processes such as contributing to family decision making are promoted. The nurse assists the family in identifying the remaining adaptive behaviors and promoting these. If neurologic impairments are irreversible, the nurse assists the family in preventing complications, and if genetic influences are known, may discuss counseling with the family. The nurse who is assessing stimuli affecting an individual's processes of cognition and consciousness carefully considers the family and significant other relationships that are primary factors influencing how the individual will be able to deal with changes in function.

Nursing Diagnosis

Assessment data of behaviors and related stimuli are interpreted and used in establishing a nursing diagnosis. The nurse prepared to use the Roy Adaptation Model can state diagnoses as specific behaviors with the stimuli that are most relevant or may use summary labels to convey complex concepts in abbreviated terms. During the nursing assessment of neurologic function, the nurse notes the positive functioning of this intricate system of thinking, feeling, moving, and interacting. At the same time, changes in functioning and any deficits are noted. This behavioral assessment together with data about stimuli provides a basis for nursing diagnoses in this mode component. The subtleties of behavior changes that are important suggest that Roy's first method of diagnosis is often the most appropriate. That is, the nurse makes a statement of the behavior with the relevant stimuli. For example, the nurse might note that the 13-year-old in her sixth day of coma following a car accident has flickered her eyelids when the overhead lights were turned on.

Roy has developed a typology of indicators of positive adaptation related to neurologic function (Table 12–4, column 1). Included in the typology are (a) effective processes of arousal and attention; sensation and perception; coding; concept formation, memory, and language; and planning and motor response; (b) integrated thinking and feeling processes; and (c) plasticity and functional effectiveness of developing, aging, and altered nervous system status. It is important to recognize situations of effective adaptation so that these can be maintained or enhanced. Commonly recurring adaptation problems (column 2) include decreased level of consciousness, defective cognitive processing, memory deficits, instability of behavior and mood, ineffective compensation for cognitive deficit, and potential for secondary brain damage. The NANDA diagnostic labels (NANDA International, 2007) listed in the last column include high risk of secondary brain injury; altered level of responsiveness, decreased; altered level of responsiveness, heightened; altered level of responsiveness, inappropriate behaviors and moods; and uncompensated cognitive deficit (specify type of deficit) and other diagnoses from their typology that are related to neurologic function.

In situations of neurologic disruption, it is important that the essence of the disruption be conveyed in the nursing diagnosis in such a manner as to provide direction for subsequent steps of the nursing process. This is facilitated by identification of the specific

TABLE 12–4 Nursing Diagnostic Categories for Neurologic Function

Positive Indicators of Adaptation	Common Adaptation Problems	NANDA Diagnostic Labels
• Effective processes of arousal and attention; sensation and perception; coding; concept formation, memory, language; planning and motor response • Integrated thinking and feeling processes • Plasticity and functional effectiveness of developing, aging, and altered nervous system	• Decreased level of consciousness • Defective cognitive processing • Memory deficits • Instability of behavior and mood • Ineffective compensation for cognitive deficit • Potential for secondary brain damage	• Autonomic dysreflexia • Risk for autonomic dysreflexia • Disorganized infant behavior • Risk for disorganized infant behavior • Readiness for enhanced organized infant behavior • Decreased intracranial adaptive capacity • Decisional conflict • Readiness for enhanced decision making • Unilateral neglect • Impaired environment interpretation syndrome • Deficient knowledge • Readiness for enhanced knowledge • Acute confusion • Chronic confusion • Impaired memory • Disturbed thought processes • Readiness for enhanced decision making • Risk for acute confusion

behaviors that are of concern and the relevant stimuli that are influencing them. An example of this type of nursing diagnosis could be "changes in vital signs associated with increased intracranial pressure." This diagnosis pertained to a young adult male in the emergency unit following a motor vehicle accident. Although he arrived unconscious, he regained consciousness but was disoriented. He was conversing and following commands but could not recall anything about the accident. He described severe headache, visual disturbances, dizziness, and a sense of nervousness. As time progressed, his headache worsened, he developed drowsiness and confusion, difficulty in thinking, and ultimately, he had a seizure. A medical diagnosis of subdural hematoma was made following an MRI scan and surgical intervention was initiated. Other nursing diagnoses applicable in this situation might be "decreased level of consciousness related to signs of increased intracranial pressure associated with head trauma."

Goal Setting

In using the Roy Adaptation Model, goal setting involves working with the patient and family to establish clear outcomes for nursing care. A complete goal statement includes the behavior of focus, the change expected, and the time frame in which the goal is to be achieved. Goals can be long term or short term and these time frames are relative to the situation involved. However, when working with patients with disorders of the nervous system, characteristically the goals tend to take the extremes of being very immediate, as in critical care, or very long term, as in rehabilitation and care of the elderly. For the young man with decreased level of consciousness related to increased intracranial pressure, the general goal of care is to minimize intracranial pressure and prevent secondary brain injury and complications of coma, and for the patient to progress to a higher level of responsiveness. Prevention of secondary brain injury includes the following process criteria identified by the AANN Standards (Mitchell, 1988):

1. To identify the individual's baseline level of brain function, including responsiveness, size and reaction of pupils, brain stem reflexes, respiratory rate, and behavior.
2. To institute measures to promote cerebral perfusion, including avoiding hypoxia, hypercapnia, and hypo- or hypertension.

An example of a specific goal for the young man described previously who has decreased level of consciousness related to increased intracranial pressure can be stated, "Within 30 minutes, the cause of the increased intracranial pressure will be identified and steps will be initiated to alleviate the pressure." The behavioral focus of the goal is the intracranial pressure, the change expected is that it will be alleviated, and the time frame is 30 minutes. Another example of a goal relates to a longer term situation: an individual with memory deficit. The general goals of nursing care are to provide for safety and other basic needs, to establish a sense of trust and confidence, to help the individual and family understand the individual's abilities and limitations, to improve memory function, and to develop and use methods to compensate for deficits. A specific goal for the family of an individual with Alzheimer's disease might be: "Before the nurse's home visit next week, the husband will devise two ways to remind his wife not to go outdoors alone and at that time will report on the effectiveness of their use." The focus of the goal is on the husband's development and use of effective memory devices for his wife's safety. The criteria will be whether two methods were devised that worked. The time frame is 1 week.

Nursing Intervention

Nursing interventions are carried out to meet the stated goals. According to the premises of the Roy model, altering the stimuli that make up the adaptation level is a way to promote adaptation. Managing focal stimuli is often the nursing intervention of choice when dealing with neurologic functioning, and these cover a wide range of the individual's internal and external environment. Nutritional and fluid intake can be altered according to its effect on neurologic functioning, for example, limiting fluids after cranial surgery. Another example of managing focal stimuli is providing tactile and auditory stimulation for the patient in a coma. Contextual and residual stimuli can also be the focus of nursing interventions to broaden the range of coping ability. Measures to reduce stress and fatigue are used to minimize the neuromuscular weakness of exacerbation of such conditions as multiple sclerosis and myasthenia gravis, as well as to control episodes of seizure activity in individuals with epilepsy. While teaching a mother specific exercises for her child with cerebral palsy, the nurse may also refer her to a support group for parents of children with disabilities to help her manage other contextual and residual factors affecting the situation.

Some of the key nursing interventions related to the nursing diagnoses discussed will be outlined. Basic medical-surgical textbooks and books on the neurosciences for nurses and other clinicians can be consulted for other specific nursing interventions related to neurologic functioning and all its complexities in the many situations of normal development and disruptive changes that the nurse may see. In a situation of decreased level of consciousness related to increased intracranial pressure such as that described previously, the nurse recognizes the significance of the intracranial pressure and carries out the following nursing interventions:

1. The first priority is to maintain an open airway, adequate ventilation, and circulation.
2. Observe and report slight neurologic changes, especially changes in pupils, motor response, verbalizations, and vital signs.
3. Maintain a quiet environment.
4. Elevate the head of the bed 30° with the head in alignment with the body (turning the head alone can result in constriction of vessels in the neck and decrease venous blood return from the brain).
5. Prevent sudden increases in pressure, as from vigorous coughing, isometric exercises (contraction and relaxation of a muscle without mechanical work), or straining during defecation, which can bring on the Valsalva maneuver.
6. Minimize emotional and physical trauma such as spaced visits with instructions given to maintain a quiet and encouraging environment.

Varying degrees of coma require attention to all nursing measures for physical needs, comfort, and safety. In the acute situation related to the motor vehicle accident victim, interventions with which the nurse would be involved include organizing and preparing for diagnostic assessment and ultimately emergency surgical intervention. In emergency circumstances such as that described, preoperative teaching involving the patient is not possible. Rather, conscientious neurologic assessment continues and physical preparations for surgery are made. Immediate transport is necessary and preparation of the operative site would be accomplished in the operating room. Much of the attention of the nurses will be directed toward the family members, their understanding of the situation and the required surgery, and the expected outcomes.

In any situation where family are unexpectedly called to the emergency room, and particularly when neurosurgery is involved, the nurse is mindful of the stress and emotions involved. Reinforcement of explanations provided by the surgeon will probably be necessary. Postoperatively, nursing interventions will be directed at the prevention and recognition of complications; evaluation of neurologic status; prevention, recognition, and control of increased intracranial pressure; supportive care; and, in the longer term if necessary, rehabilitation.

In situations of ongoing unconsciousness, it is the nurse's responsibility to prevent complications of the comatose state, such as decubiti, stomatitis, and atelectasis. The patient is turned and repositioned every 2 hours and given back massage. This is individualized for the older person with thinning skin. Turning alternates the pressure on different areas of the skin as well as enhances ventilation. Various devices such as gel pads, egg crate mattresses, sheepskin, alternating pressure pads, and waterbeds help prevent decubiti. An alternating pressure mattress is particularly effective because pressure in various areas is frequently altered. A rubber doughnut placed around the decubitus actually complicates matters by creating further decubiti. This is caused by the increased pressure on the skin beneath the doughnut. The nurse uses foot supports or a foot board to prevent foot drop, that is, falling of the foot related to flexor paralysis of the ankle.

If the eyes are open and blinking is absent, artificial tears can be used, but patching protects the eyes better. A usual approach is to wet eye patches in a sterile water or saline solution and gently cover the eyes with the lids closed. The nurse removes the patches to do pupil checks and allow for possible sensory input for short periods. In cases of coma, a neurologic assessment is done every 2 to 4 hours. For cranial nerves, checks are done on III (pupils), V (corneal reflex), and IX and X (swallow and gag). Any voluntary movements and responses to pain are noted. A check is made for the plantar reflex. As in all other conditions, an open airway is a priority concern. The patient's trachea is suctioned if breath sounds are congested or the airway obstructed. The nurse assesses for incontinence and abdominal or bladder distention. Mouth care is provided every 2 hours to prevent infection, such as stomatitis, respiratory tract infection, and aspiration. The nurse explains to the patient what is being done, and never discusses a negative prognosis at the patient's bedside. The sense of hearing is often present although no other neurologic faculties appear intact.

The nursing interventions for memory deficits will be tailored to the particular individual, to the deficit noted, as well as to the individual's remaining abilities. The nurse works with the family to plan care for the individual. Both family and nurse will avoid confusing the individual with details beyond the immediate. They can provide frequent reassurance when the individual shows fear of the unfamiliar. Developing a sense of trust and confidence can be enhanced by simple measures such as putting the name of the primary care nurse readily in view at the patient's bedside or attached to the individual if ambulatory. Useful, orienting information is given often, such as the time of day or how long until the next meal or bedtime. Simple routines for care in daily living are developed and used. The steps for dressing can be written out. A daily schedule is posted, put on an audio recording for those with vision problems or attached to the armrest of a wheelchair for those up in the chair. The nurse and other caregivers use a calm, matter-of-fact approach when the patient needs the same information given repeatedly or when there are signs of confabulation or lack of insight. The individual also can be guided toward productive and satisfying activity after simple self-care needs are met. For example, the list of daily activities may include watering a plant. The particular plant listed is changed according to which plant needs to be watered and the patient is not burdened with having to remember which plant was done the day before.

For some people, it may be necessary to provide protection and supportive supervision. Structures such as doors and stairwells will be checked and altered to prevent unsupervised wandering and falling. The psychological comfort of the environment can be enhanced by activities such as reminiscent groups. In the long-term care of people with memory deficits, especially those that are progressive, the nurse may recommend resources to provide relief for caregivers. The nurse can be helpful as a knowledgeable and caring individual when a family needs assistance with the issues related to long-term institutional care. Earlier in this chapter, the principles of integrated neural functioning and neural plasticity were described. Based on evidence that multiple networks in the brain can carry on the same function, and that there are possibilities for modifying central nervous system structural organization and function, in many conditions there is hope for recovering or improving memory function following brain injury, particularly in the younger person. People who suffer brain injury from stroke or head injury present difficult problems of memory deficit and levels of recovery are often uncertain. There can be continued inability to remember conversations or instructions, telephone numbers, written material, television shows, or even faces for several months after the stroke or accident. The individual may lose track of speech in mid-sentence. This is especially true if there is any distraction or interruption such as a phone ringing or someone speaking and interrupting the train of thought.

In designing nursing interventions for improving memory, two principles that have already been mentioned are used, that is, they are individualized to the individual and to the deficit. The nurse is in a good position to do this especially for the settings where these individuals will be (Sisson, 2001). Based on frequent contact with patients and their families, the nurse observes the specific deficits and reactions to them. In this way, meaningful and individualized intervention techniques and strategies can be developed. In some settings, the nurse also has available formal evaluation of memory deficits by the health care team including members with neuropsychology knowledge. In other cases, the nurse bases care primarily on the nursing assessment of the memory deficit. Nursing interventions are further individualized by the total nursing assessment, which includes the influences of the other adaptive modes. A specific factor might be tolerance to fatigue; for example, soon after head injury, a 10-minute session of memory exercises at the bedside may be the patient's limit, and when working with young adult male patients (representing nearly 80% of the head injury population), one can devise memory exercises using playing cards so that the activity is more acceptable to patient's primary role.

A final major principle in designing interventions for improving memory is that all the efforts are based on a specific theoretical approach to understanding cognitive function. This includes efforts of the nurse, family, and other health care personnel. The notion of integrated brain functioning and the model of an information processing system can be helpful here. The Das–Luria model has been used by Roy (2001) to further define a proposed cognitive information processing model. In the work of these authors (Das, Kar, & Parrila, 1996; Das, Kirby, & Jarman, 1979; Luria, 1973, 1980), the basic information-processing functions of sensory input, perception, memory, concept formation, and output have simultaneous and successive properties. Simultaneous means that the input is received all at once, such as seeing the picture of a house and synthesizing the separate parts of it into a whole. Successive processing refers to processing elements in serial order. For example, in hearing human speech, one hears one word after another and makes a sentence from the order of words. The same simultaneous and successive dimensions are present in planning functions as well. One can think of solving the task of drawing a line through a maze. If the maze formation is very simple, one can see the whole and quickly generate and execute the program for solving the task. If, however, it is a complex maze, then parts of the maze are taken in serial order while the planning functions of searching, comparing, hypothesizing, and verifying are carried out.

Based on this particular understanding of cognitive processing, the memory aids to promote retraining can be planned to activate simultaneous and successive processing. For example, capitalizing on the dimension of simultaneous processing, the individual can be taught to recall family members using a photo album. The individual is asked to repeat aloud several times the name of a given individual in a picture, seeing the entire face, speaking the name, and hearing it at the same time. The name is then used in a meaningful statement. For example, "Aunt Louise is my mother's sister." The name is further associated with a characteristic obvious in the picture, such as "Aunt Louise has red hair."

A simple method of using successive processing to improve memory is to have lists of words that the individual repeats after the nurse or family member. The list becomes increasingly long and is varied from words that are similar in some way to those that have no similarities. Another technique can be to have a deck of playing cards in which one card at a time is laid down in front of the individual. The next card is taken off the deck and placed on top of it. The individual is asked to identify the card before the last card on the stack when the caregiver stops dealing. As the individual's memory improves, the instructions can be made more difficult by having the individual name the second card back or the third card back. Simultaneous and successive processing practice (Roy, 1989) can be used with a specific deficit such as recalling place names, as in an example of an individual who cannot remember the name of the city of residence. This practice involves a set of simple exercises in which families can be involved. The simultaneous strategies are used with a map as the stimulus to learn the name of the city. Then, an additional strategy is to have the individual color the area of the city on the map. Sometimes many rehearsals of the task are required. Pictures of readily familiar landmarks of the city that contain the city's name are obtained, and then the name is placed on a card. The patient learns to match the name card with the landmark and says the name of the landmark including the name of the city each time.

There is a rapidly growing literature on memory retraining. Many different perspectives are represented. The nurse can help families evaluate any particular programs they might be considering, especially when these would add great expense to the already heavy financial burden of illness. Computer programs have not yet proven effective and most professionals in the field caution that they will never replace the human being who sits with the patient and provides support as well as feedback on performance. By increasingly understanding how the brain is operating, how memory functions, and how the individual has been affected by brain damage, the nurse can creatively help design simple and useful strategies. These strategies are aimed both at daily care of the individual with memory deficits by compensating for these and at improving memory function by stimulating simultaneous and successive processing in memory tasks.

Evaluation

Evaluation involves judging the effectiveness of the nursing interventions in relation to the individual's adaptive behavior, that is, whether the individual has attained the behavior stated in the goals. The nursing interventions would be identified as effective if the individual's behavior is in accordance with the stated goal. If the goal has not been achieved, the nurse identifies alternative interventions or approaches. This is done by reassessing the behavior and stimuli and continuing with the other steps of the nursing process. Since the goals include the behavior to be focused on, a change or level of stability expected, and a given time, these are the dimensions for judging effectiveness. Consider the goal stated earlier: "Within 30 minutes, the cause of the increased intracranial pressure will be identified and steps will be initiated to alleviate the pressure." The goal would be achieved if half an hour later a diagnosis was established and steps underway to intervene. Following the surgery to alleviate the subdural hematoma, further short- and long-term goals would be developed during postoperative care. Initially, these would be very short term in nature. For example, "Within the next hour, intracranial pressure will remain stable and within acceptable levels." The evaluation of this goal would rest with the signs of IICP and perhaps intracranial monitoring of pressure levels. As the situation stabilizes and time passes, longer term goals would be developed and continually evaluated in response to the patient's postoperative condition. Some goals related to memory deficits are particularly difficult to evaluate. The nurse again will use the notion of short-term and long-term goals. Remembering that some neurologic functions are intact or recovering and that some are functioning at a slower pace can help caregivers to be patient with the long process involved. The nurse recognizes, and helps the family to recognize, that improvement may take place only subtly, over long periods of time, and not in steady progression, but with days of better and worse functioning.

Summary

This chapter focused on the complexities of neurologic processes and how this knowledge can help one understand the thinking, feeling, moving, and interacting individual who is adapting within the changing world. Two basic life processes presented as key to neurologic function were cognition and consciousness. Compensatory strategies that act to maintain neurologic function were identified. Two examples of compromised processes, memory deficits and decreased level of consciousness, were discussed. Planning nursing care involving assessment of behaviors and stimuli related to cognition and consciousness, nursing diagnoses, goals, nursing interventions, and evaluation were described in this chapter. Particular emphasis was placed on planning nursing care related to consciousness and memory.

Exercises for Application

1. Devise a brief assessment tool for the cranial nerves. Use this tool to assess normal function of a colleague. While doing the assessment, have a mental image of the neural pathways that are operating.
2. Write down at least five different sources of information that come to you each day and think about what it might feel like to be in this environment without the ability to process it selectively.
3. Describe how an individual with severe memory deficits might be affected in each of the adaptive modes: physiologic, self-concept, role function, and interdependence.

Assessment of Understanding

QUESTIONS

1. Name the two basic life processes associated with neurologic function as identified in the Roy Adaptation Model.
   (a) _____
   (b) _____
2. Neural plasticity was provided as an example of a compensatory process associated with neurologic functioning. Describe neural plasticity.
3. Two compromised processes of neurologic function were discussed in this chapter: memory deficits and decreased level of consciousness. Label the following descriptor as associated with either memory deficits (MD) or level of consciousness (LC).
   (a) _____ deficit in restoring and retrieving information
   (b) _____ brain herniation is an associated compensatory process
   (c) _____ a critical situation that can lead to death
   (d) _____ focal stimulus may be seizure, stroke, or toxic reactions
   (e) _____ may result from increased intracranial pressure
   (f) _____ may involve degenerative brain pathology associated with alcoholism

4. Identify three behaviors associated with the assessment of cognition and consciousness.

Cognition
(a) _____
(b) _____
(c) _____

Consciousness
(a) _____
(b) _____
(c) _____

5. Identify eight stimuli that affect neurologic function, particularly of cognition or consciousness.
(a) _____
(b) _____
(c) _____
(d) _____
(e) _____
(f) _____
(g) _____
(h) _____

SITUATION

Jeffrey McClure is a 45-year-old father of two children who lives in a rural area about an hour's drive
from a major city. He has been diagnosed with
epilepsy since he was in his teens. Although multiple
treatment regimens have been attempted (control
with medications, surgical intervention), his seizures
are not under control. Intermittently he will have a
seizure at home. The nurse involved with the family
is interested in helping Jeffrey's wife and children
know what to do when Jeffrey is having a seizure.

6. Develop two nursing diagnoses related to the situation described—one focusing on Jeffrey and
the other focusing on the family members.
(a) Focused on Jeffrey: _____
(b) Focused on the family: _____
7. State goals related to the situation described
with specific focus on the nursing diagnoses
formulated.
(a) _____
(b) _____
8. List nursing interventions designed to achieve
the goals specified in item 7b.
(a) _____
(b) _____
9. Describe how evaluation of the nursing interventions would be accomplished and how further
steps of the nursing process would proceed.
(a) _____
(b) _____

FEEDBACK

1. (a) cognition
(b) consciousness
2. Neural plasticity is considered to be a fundamental property of the nervous system. It refers to
enduring modification of structures within the
nervous system to develop or preserve cognitive
and neurologic function. These modifications
occur at critical periods, can last a lifetime, and
seem to lack motivation and reinforcement for
their establishment. Plasticity is greater in early
years, with multiple new patterns of structure and
function possible. There is also increasing evidence for retaining and restoring nervous system
functional effectiveness including sprouting of
remaining nerve fibers after injury. The reservoir
of plasticity decreases over the life span.
3. (a) MD, (b) LC, (c) LC, (d) MD, (e) LC, (f) MD
4. Cognition: any three of the following: arousal
and attention, sensation and perception, coding,
concept formation, memory, language, planning,
motor response.
   Consciousness: any three of the following:
level of consciousness, motor response, response
to pain, orientation, and level of awareness.
5. Any eight of the following: pathophysiology,
immediate situation, blood gases and hemoglobin
levels, effects of treatment, knowledge about
condition, stress, nutritional status, activity and rest,
self-concept, role function, and interdependence.
6. Sample nursing diagnoses:
(a) Compromised safety related to uncontrolled
epileptic seizures and lack of success of
treatment regimens.
(b) Anxiety and uncertainty regarding appropriate
actions during seizures due to lack of knowledge.
7. Suggested goals:
(a) Within 1 week, Jeffrey will consistently employ safety precautions to enhance his personal safety in the event of a seizure.
(b) At the time of Jeffrey's next seizure when
family members are present, they will
demonstrate actions to support Jeffrey's
safety during and after the seizure.
8. Possible nursing interventions:
(a) Assess Jeffrey's knowledge level about
epilepsy and his recurring seizures; eliminate
misconceptions and provide correct information; assist in contacting agencies that can provide information and support, reassurance, and
socialization with others facing the same problem; involve him in the development of a treatment plan aimed at taking medications as prescribed, avoiding situations that precipitate
seizures, and adjusting his lifestyle (e.g., no
driving) while maintaining self-esteem.

(b) Encourage family to discuss their feelings of fear or shame, and assist them in dealing with the constant stress associated with the seizures; instruct them as to what actions to take while the seizure is in progress; point out important observations to be made both before, during, and following the seizure; explore safety precautions associated with daily lifestyle.

9. Evaluation: Nursing interventions would be judged successful if the goals were achieved. Specifically,
(a) Within 1 week, Jeffrey has instituted safety precautions to enhance his personal safety in the event of a seizure. He is no longer driving, he is taking his medications regularly and as prescribed, and he is getting lots of rest and avoiding situations that precipitate seizures. Jeffrey identified symptoms that occurred just prior to the seizure. Further

nursing care involved exploring further the significance of these and his preferred actions when they were evident.
(b) During the occasion of Jeffrey's next seizure, his family members were able to support him by staying with him, easing him to the floor, placing a padded tongue blade between his teeth before they were clenched, loosening his collar and belt, turning him on his side, not restraining him, and reassuring and reorienting him when the seizure ended. They observed carefully actions that occurred during the seizure and were able to report on his behavior, mood, and comments prior to the seizure. The nursing intervention was judged effective and further information was provided in answer to questions that were raised by family members.

References

Anthony, J. C., LeResche, L., Niaz, U., Von Korff, M. R., & Folstein, M. F. (1982). Limits of the mini-mental state, a screening test for dementia and delirium among hospital patients. *Psychological Medicine, 12,* 397.

Black, I. B. (1991). *Information in the brain: A molecular perspective.* Cambridge, MA: The MIT Press.

Das, J. P. (1984). Intelligence and information integration. In J. Kirby (Ed.), *Cognitive strategies and educational performance* (pp. 13–31). New York: Academic Press.

Das, J. P., Kar, B. C., and Parrila, R. K. (1996). *Cognitive planning: The psychological basis of intelligent behavior.* Thousand Oaks, CA: Sage Publications.

Das, J. P., Kirby, J. P., & Jarman, R. F. (1979). *Simultaneous and successive cognitive processes.* New York: Academic Press.

Eccles J., & Robinson, D. N. (1984). *The wonder of being human, our brain and our mind.* New York: Free Press.

Folstein, M. F., Folstein, S. E., & McHugh, P. R. (1975). Mini-mental state, a practical method for grading the cognitive state of patients for the clinician. *Journal of Psychiatric Research, 12,* 189.

Gazzaniga, M. S., Ivry, R. B., & Mangun, G. R. (2002). *Cognitive neuroscience: The biology of the mind* (2nd ed.). New York: W. W. Norton & Company.

Gouvier, W. D., Ryan, L. M., O'Jile, J. R., Parks-Levy, J., Webster, J. S., & Blanton, P. D. (1997). Cognitive retraining with brain-damaged patients. In A. M. Horton, Jr., D. Wedding, & J. Webster (Eds.), *The neuropsychology handbook* (2nd ed.). New York: Springer.

Hickey, J. (1992). *The clinical practice of neurological and neurosurgical nursing* (3rd ed.). Philadelphia: Lippincott.

Ignatavicius, D. D., & Workman, M. L. (2006). *Medical-surgical nursing: Critical thinking for collaborative care* (5th ed.). St. Louis, MO: Elsevier Saunders.

Jennett, B., & Teasdale, G. (1977). Aspects of coma after severe head injury. *Lancet, 1*(8017), 878–881.

Kemp, J. (1979). *The philosophy of Kant.* Oxford: Oxford University Press.

Kolb, B., & Whishaw, I. Q. (1996). *Fundamentals of human neuropsychology* (4th ed.). New York: W. H. Freeman and Company.

Lezak, M. D., Howieson, D. B., Loring, D. W., Hannay, H. J., & Fischer, J. S. (2004).

Neuropsychological assessment (4th ed.). New York: Oxford University Press.

Luria, A. R. (1973). *The working brain: An introduction to neuropsychology.* New York: Basic Books.

Luria, A. R. (1980). *Higher cortical function in man.* New York: Basic Books.

Marieb, E. N., & Hoehn, K. (2007). *Human anatomy and physiology* (7th ed.). San Francisco: Pearson Benjamin Cummings.

Mitchell, P. H. (1988). Consciousness: An overview. In P. H. Mitchell, L. C. Hodges, M. Muwaswes, & C. A. Walleck (Eds.), *American Association of Neuroscience Nurses' Neuroscience nursing: Phenomena and practice* (pp. 57–66). Norwalk, CT: Appleton & Lange.

Mitchell, P. H. (2001). Decreased behavioral arousal. In C. Stewart-Amidei, J. Kunkel, & K. Bronstein (Eds.), *American Association of Neuroscience Nursing's neuroscience nursing: Human responses to neurologic dysfunction* (2nd ed., pp. 93–118). Philadelphia: Saunders.

Mountcastle, V. B. (1997). The columnar organization of the neocortex. *Brain, 120,* 701–722.

NANDA-International. (2007). *Nursing diagnoses: Definitions and classifications, 2007–2008.* Philadelphia: NANDA-I.

Newman, M. (1994). *Help as expanding consciousness* (2nd ed.). New York: National League for Nursing Press.

Pribram, K. H. (1969). *Brain and behavior 3: Memory mechanisms* (p. 7). Baltimore: Penguin Books.

Roy, C. (1988). Altered cognition: An information processing approach. In P. H. Mitchell, L. C. Hodges, M. Muwaswes, & C. A. Walleck (Eds.), *American Association of Neuroscience Nurses' Neuroscience nursing: Phenomena and practice* (pp. 185–211). Norwalk, CT: Appleton & Lange.

Roy, C. (1989). Nursing care in theory and practice: Early interventions in brain injury. In R. Harris & R. Rees (Eds.), *Recovery from brain injury: Expectations, needs, and processes* (pp. 95–110). Northfield, South Australia: Institute for the Study of Learning Difficulties, South Australian College of Advanced Education.

Roy, C. (2001). Alterations in cognitive processing. In C. Stewart-Amidei, J. Kunkel, & K. Bronstein (Eds.), *American Association of Neuroscience Nursing's neuroscience nursing: Human responses to neurologic dysfunction* (2nd ed., pp. 275–323). Philadelphia: Saunders.

Sisson, R. (2001). Alterations in memory. In C. Stewart-Amidei, J. Kunkel, & K. Bronstein (Eds.), *American Association of Neuroscience Nursing's neuroscience nursing: Human responses to neurologic dysfunction* (2nd ed., pp. 253–273). Philadelphia: Saunders.

Wilber, K. (1997). *The eye of spirit.* Boston: Shambhala.

Additional References

Boss, B. J. (1993). The neurophysiological basis of learning: Attention and memory implication for SCI nurses. *SCI Nursing, 10,* 121–129.

Brooks, N. (1984) *Closed head injury: Psychological, social, and family consequences.* Oxford: Oxford University Press.

Brooks, N. (1992). Psychosocial assessment after traumatic brain injury. *Scandinavian Journal of Rehabilitation Medicine, 26*(Suppl.), 126–131.

Burrell, L. O., Gerlach, M. J. M., & Pless, B. S. (1997). *Adult nursing: Acute and community care* (2nd ed.). Stamford, CT: Appleton & Lange.

Pi Lambda Theta, San Jose Area Chapter. (1983). *Helping head injury and stroke patients at home: A handbook for families.* San Jose, CA: Pi Lambda Theta.

Posner, M., DiGirolamo, G., & Fernandez, D. (1997). Brain mechanisms of cognitive skills. *Consciousness and Cognition, 6,* 267–290.

Taylor, J., & Bellenger, S. (1980). *Neurological dysfunctions and nursing intervention.* New York: McGraw-Hill.

CHAPTER 13

Endocrine Function

Endocrine function is the last of the complex processes identified in the physiologic mode of the Roy Adaptation Model. The endocrine system integrates and maintains, in close association with the autonomic nervous system, the body's physiologic processes to promote normal growth, development, and maintenance of structure and function. In this dual regulatory system, nervous system actions that are acute and of short-term duration are supplemented by slower and longer hormonal actions. This sequenced action permits precise control of body functions. Even minute changes are recognized immediately and effective adaptation is accomplished. When all interrelated endocrine processes are running smoothly, adaptive behaviors are observed. However, when one component is disrupted, other parts of the endocrine system, the physiologic mode, and the individual as a whole may be affected. This chapter provides an overview of the endocrine system and includes a description of the component glands and their related functions. Emphasis is placed both on the functions as a single system and its interaction with other body processes, particularly the nervous system, in maintaining physiologic integrity. Knowledge of endocrine structure and functioning serves as a basis for understanding the life processes of this mode component. Illustrations of innate and learned adaptive responses to compensate for ineffective processes are described. Examples of compromised processes are discussed. Finally, guidelines for planning nursing care by assessing the individual's behavior and significant influencing stimuli as well as formulating diagnoses, establishing goals, selecting nursing interventions, and evaluating nursing care are described.

OBJECTIVES

After studying this chapter, the reader will be able to do the following:

1. Describe the complex processes associated with endocrine function.
2. Describe one compensatory process related to the complex processes of endocrine function.
3. Name and describe two situations of compromised processes of endocrine function.
4. Identify important first-level assessment factors for behaviors of the complex processes of endocrine function.
5. List common stimuli of second-level assessment affecting endocrine function.

6. Develop a nursing diagnosis, given a situation related to endocrine function.

7. Derive goals for an individual with ineffective endocrine function in a given situation.

8. Describe nursing interventions commonly implemented in situations of ineffective endocrine function.

9. Propose ways to determine the effectiveness of nursing interventions.

KEY CONCEPTS DEFINED

Endocrine glands: Small collections of specialized tissue located in widely separated regions of the body that release hormones into the blood for transport to the site of influence.

Exocrine glands: Specialized tissues that release hormones into a duct for transport to the site of influence.

Hormonal stimulation: The initiation of hormone secretion by another hormone.

Hormones: Secretions of endocrine glands that function as chemical messengers with regulatory effects on specific anatomical structures and physiologic processes.

Humoral stimulation: The initiation of hormone secretion by the changing composition of body fluids.

Negative feedback mechanisms: The primary means of regulating blood levels of hormones wherein hormone secretion is triggered by some stimulus; then rising hormone levels inhibit further release.

Neural stimulation: The initiation of hormone secretion by nerve fiber signals.

Target organ/tissue: The anatomical destination of a hormone wherein a physiologic response is produced.

COMPLEX PROCESSES OF ENDOCRINE FUNCTION

The endocrine system is composed of the endocrine glands, small and unimpressive collections of specialized tissue located in widely separated regions of the body. The glands of the endocrine system have specific functions in controlling body processes.

Structures and Processes

Marieb and Hoehn (2007) name the endocrine glands as pituitary, thyroid, parathyroid, adrenal, pineal, and thymus. In addition, the hypothalamus, while actually part of the nervous system, produces and releases hormones. Several organs, the pancreas and the gonads including ovaries or testes, have endocrine tissue and functions. Although other tissues and organs—for example, the heart, lungs, kidneys, stomach, and small intestine—perform minor endocrine functions, the focus of this chapter will be on the glands listed above. A distinction is made between exocrine and endocrine glands. Exocrine glands produce substances that are released into a duct for transport to the site of action. An example is the exocrine pancreas, which releases digestive enzymes into the duodenum through the pancreatic duct. The exocrine glands are not included in this consideration of endocrine function.

The endocrine glands, on the other hand, secrete one or more hormones—chemical messengers with regulatory effects on specific body parts or organs—directly into the bloodstream. The hormones are transported to and ultimately influence other anatomical structures and physiologic processes. The sites of destination for hormones are termed target organs/tissues. Figure 13–1 shows the major endocrine glands and highlights the all-important feedback loops. According to Marieb and Hoehn (2007, p. 605) the major processes controlled by hormones are "reproduction; growth and development; mobilization of body defenses; maintenance of electrolyte, water and nutrient balance of the blood; and regulation of cellular metabolism and energy balance." The major actions and source of selected hormones are outlined in Table 13–1.

Each hormone is unique, yet all hormones have some characteristics in common. In general, endocrine hormones are secreted in small amounts. They cause an alteration in cellular activity by either increasing or decreasing the rate of normal metabolic processes. Although the precise change depends on the specific hormone and the cell type, generally hormones have one or more of three actions: (1) plasma membrane permeability (electrical state) is changed, (2) enzyme function is altered (activation or inactivation), or (3) genetic material is stimulated to produce instructions for making particular enzymes. The extent of hormonal action varies among hormones. One, such as thyrocalcitonin, may have only regional effects while another, like thyroxine, exerts its effect pervasively over all metabolic processes in the body. Negative feedback mechanisms are responsible for the regulation of hormones. The sequence begins when hormone secretion is initiated by internal or external stimuli. The resulting rise in level of hormone in the body then provides feedback that inhibits further hormone release.

Most hormonal action is initiated by one of three categories of stimuli: hormonal, humoral, or neural. Hormonal stimulation involves the initiation of hormone release by another hormone. For example, the hypothalamus releases hormones that stimulate the anterior pituitary to release hormones. These, in turn, stimulate other endocrine organs to secrete hormones. Humoral stimulation refers to changing levels of certain ions and nutrients in body fluids. For example, decreasing blood calcium level prompts the release of parathyroid hormone (PTH); as calcium levels increase, the stimulus is diminished. Neural stimulation involves nerve fibers in the initiation of hormone release. An example of this is the sympathetic nervous system stimulation of the adrenal medulla to release norepinephrine and epinephrine during periods of stress. Although each endocrine gland can be viewed as a separate unit with its own independent functions, the various glands also function interdependently. As illustrated previously, the release of hormones from one gland often influences hormonal release from other glands. Similarly, a disturbance in one endocrine gland is likely to incur a disturbance in others. For example, a decrease in the release of thyroid stimulating hormone (TSH) by the anterior pituitary gland causes the thyroid gland to secrete less thyroxine and triiodothyronine.

Earlier mention was made of hormone production in locations other than the major endocrine organs. Several examples of this are provided: (1) prostaglandins—released from plasma membranes in response to local irritation; its effects range from vasoconstriction to enhancing blood clotting to increasing the digestive secretions in the stomach; (2) erythropoietin—produced in the kidney in response to hypoxia; stimulates the production of red blood cells in the bone marrow; and (3) placenta—produces hormones (human chorionic gonadotropin, estrogen, progesterone, human placental lactogen, and relaxin) that maintain pregnancy and prepare for the process of delivery. A full discussion of the complex structures and functions related to the endocrine glands and other endocrine processes is beyond the scope of this text. The reader is directed to basic anatomy and physiology and specialty nursing science textbooks for a more in-depth knowledge.

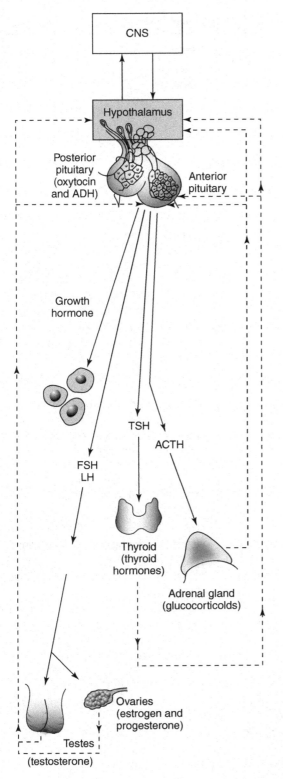

FIGURE 13–1 Control of Hormone Production by Hypothalamic-Pituitary-Target Cell Feedback Mechanism. (From Mattson-Porth, C. (2005). *Pathophysiology: Concepts of altered health states.* (7th edition). Philadelphia: Lippincott. p. 958. Used with permission).

TABLE 13–1 Major Action and Source of Selected Hormones

Source	Hormone	Major action
Hypothalamus	Releasing and inhibiting hormones 　Corticotropin-releasing hormone (CRH) 　Thyrotropin-releasing hormone (TRH) 　Growth hormone-releasing hormone (GHRH) 　Gonadotropin-releasing hormone (GnRH) Somatostatin	Controls the release of pituitary hormones Inhibits GH and TSH
Anterior pituitary	Growth hormone (GH)	Stimulates growth of bone and muscle, promotes protein synthesis and fat metabolism, decreases carbohydrate metabolism
	Adrenocorticotropic hormone (ACTH)	Stimulates synthesis and secretion of adrenal cortical hormones
	Thyroid-stimulating hormone (TSH)	Stimulates synthesis and secretion of thyroid hormone
	Follicle-stimulating hormone (FSH)	Female: stimulates growth of ovarian follicle, ovulation Male: stimulates sperm production
	Luteinizing hormone (LH)	Female: stimulates development of corpus luteum, release of oocyte, production of estrogen and progesterone Male: stimulates secretion of testosterone, development of interstitial tissue of testes
	Prolactin	Prepares female breast for breast-feeding
Posterior pituitary	Antidiuretic hormone (ADH)	Increases water reabsorption by kidney
	Oxytocin	Stimulates contraction of pregnant uterus, milk ejection from breasts after childbirth
Adrenal cortex	Mineralocorticosteroids, mainly aldosterone	Increases sodium absorption, potassium loss by kidney
	Glucocorticoids, mainly cortisol	Affects metabolism of all nutrients; regulates blood glucose levels, affects growth, has anti-inflammatory action and decreases effects of stress
	Adrenal androgens, mainly dehydroepiandrosterone (DHEA) and androstenedione	Have minimal intrinsic androgenic activity; they are converted to testosterone and dihydrotestosterone in the periphery

TABLE 13–1 (*continued*)

Source	Hormone	Major action
Adrenal medulla	Epinephrine Norepinephrine	Serve as neurotransmitters for the sympathetic nervous system
Thyroid (follicular cells)	Thyroid hormones: triiodothyronine (T_3) and thyroxine (T_4)	Increase the metabolic rate; increase protein and bone turnover; increase responsiveness to catecholamines; necessary for fetal and infant growth and development
Thyroid C cells	Calcitonin	Lowers blood calcium and phosphate levels
Parathyroid glands	Parathyroid hormone (PTH)	Regulates serum calcium
Pancreatic islet cells	Insulin	Lowers blood glucose by facilitating glucose transport across cell membranes of muscle, liver, and adipose tissue
	Glucagon	Increases blood glucose concentration by stimulation of glycogenesis
	Somatostatin	Delays intestinal absorption of glucose
Kidney	1,2 5-Dihydroxyvitamin D	Stimulates calcium absorption from the intestine
Ovaries	Estrogen	Affects development of female sex organs and secondary sex characteristics
	Progesterone	Influences menstrual cycle; stimulates growth of uterine wall; maintains pregnancy
Testes	Androgens, mainly testosterone	Affect development of male sex organs and secondary sex characteristics; aid in sperm production

Source: Mattson-Porth, C. (2005). *Pathophysiology: Concepts of altered health states* (7th ed.). Philadelphia: Lippincott. Used with permission.

COMPENSATORY ADAPTIVE RESPONSES

In viewing the person as an adaptive system, it was noted in Chapter 2 that the individual has innate and acquired ways of responding to the changing environment. Further, Roy has conceptualized these complex adaptive dynamics as the coping processes of the regulator and cognator subsystems. One particular illustration of regulator compensatory abilities associated with endocrine function relates to the neuroendocrine stress response. Both the cognator and regulator subsystems determine the body's total response to environmental stimuli. However, that part of the adaptation response associated with endocrine function is located within the regulator coping processes. The major parts of the regulator subsystem are the neural, chemical, and endocrine components; all three are activated in response to a major stimulus. The perception-psychomotor part is considered neural in nature and this overlaps with the cognator coping mechanism. It serves to connect the two mechanisms, thereby allowing physiologic response to influence cognitive responses and vice versa. The remaining two components of the regulator coping mechanisms, chemical and endocrine responses, act together to regulate the body's physiologic response to stress.

Stress was defined in early writings by Roy and McLeod (1981) as the transaction between the environmental demands requiring adaptation and the individual's cognator and regulator coping mechanisms. Later the stress response was described as the process that results from any physical or psychological stimulus disturbing the adaptive state (Andrews & Roy, 1986). The term stressor is viewed as synonymous with the notion of a focal stimulus as defined by Roy. Selye (1976) proposed that the body's physiologic response can take two forms. The first is the Local Adaptation Syndrome (LAS). This occurs when the body is confronted by a stimulus to which only one organ or part of the body reacts. One example is the inflammatory response or immune response. The neuroendocrine mechanisms are not activated during this process. The second response pattern, the general adaptation syndrome (GAS), occurs whenever a number of body systems are threatened. The syndrome also occurs when the individual undergoes prolonged periods of stress. The GAS is a neuroendocrine response involving primarily the sympathetic branch of the autonomic nervous system and the pituitary, adrenal, and thyroid glands. The body's neuroendocrine responses to stress for both long-term and short-term reactions are shown in Figure 13–2, which outlines the role of the adrenal glands and stress.

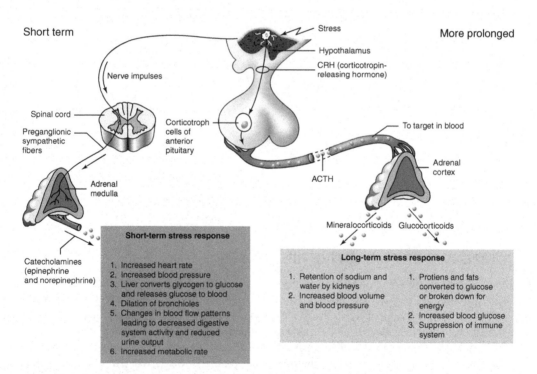

FIGURE 13–2 Stress and the adrenal gland. (From Marieb, E.N., & Hoehn, K. (2007). *Human anatomy and physiology* (7th ed.). San Francisco: Pearson Benjamin Cummings (p. 631) Used with permission).

Selye (1976) suggested that both the GAS and the LAS develop in three distinct stages. First, the alarm reaction stage occurs when the whole body's neuroendocrine defenses against the stimulus are alerted and mobilized to protect the body. The alarm occurs regardless of whether the stimulus is bacteria or verbal abuse. Second, in the stage of resistance the body attempts to cope by limiting the stimulus' affects to the smallest possible area. Lastly, the stage of exhaustion is when the body's adaptive ability to resist the stressor becomes exhausted. The phases vary in duration and intensity related to the strength of the stimuli that initiated the stress response. For example, a brief, sudden, unexpected noise may elicit only very brief immeasurable responses reflective of the alarm phase. The stress response does not continue into the resistance or exhaustion phases. On the other hand, a major surgical operation may produce more measurable, prolonged responses of the second and third phases.

In addition to regulator compensatory responses, the cognator subsystem plays an important role in adaptation relative to endocrine function. An individual with diabetes mellitus as noted in the discussion of nutrition provides an example of how an individual with a compromised process of metabolism can learn to adapt and compensate. Through education and practice, individuals learn about the important balance among diet, exercise, and insulin. They learn how to regulate each and can become very effective in maintaining an appropriate balance. They also learn about complications that occur with imbalance and what to do to intervene at an early stage to avoid more serious complications. Through cognator compensatory processes, many people with diabetes are able to adapt effectively and maintain physiologic and psychosocial integrity.

COMPROMISED PROCESSES OF ENDOCRINE FUNCTION

Ineffective endocrine behaviors are most commonly caused by compromised processes of endocrine function. The compromise is frequently associated with the interruption or dysfunction of the negative feedback mechanisms. Hancock (1997, p. 1075) identified four sources of such disruption: (1) a gland develops the ability to function autonomously; the negative feedback mechanisms are no longer influential. Hyperfunction develops. An example of this situation is hyperthyroidism. (2) A gland is absent or defective for congenital, acquired, or surgical reasons, thus, it no longer adequately responds to stimulation. Hormonal deficits occur. Surgical intervention for a glandular tumor can cause such complications. (3) Cells of target tissues/organs increase or decrease in their sensitivity to hormonal stimulation. Hypo- or hyperfunction develops. For example, diabetes mellitus is considered to be related to a loss of cell sensitivity to insulin. (4) Prolonged suppression of glandular function by administration of its hormone product, such as steroids from the adrenal cortex, may result in acute deficit upon withdrawal of the hormone product.

As with other cells of the body, those of the endocrine glands are susceptible to trauma, vascular interference, autoimmune disorders, infection, and neoplasm. The functional and structural changes in endocrine glands precipitated by these stimuli take similar forms regardless of the specific gland affected. Hormonal disturbances are characterized by either hyposecretion or hypersecretion of a hormone, or an imbalance between or among hormones. Each of these situations is characterized by particular physiologic symptoms and behaviors. Exploration of the specific consequences associated with each endocrine disorder is beyond the scope of this text. The reader is encouraged to consult a pathophysiology resource for specific descriptions of the physiologic disruptions associated with endocrine function.

NURSING PROCESS RELATED TO ENDOCRINE FUNCTION

In applying the nursing process to the complex processes of endocrine function, the nurse makes a careful assessment of behaviors and stimuli. In assessing factors influencing endocrine function, regulator and cognator effectiveness in initiating compensatory processes is considered. Based on this thorough first- and second-level assessment, the nurse formulates a nursing diagnosis, sets goals, selects interventions, and evaluates care.

Assessment of Behavior

As was the case with neurologic function, integrity of endocrine function, or lack thereof, has profound effects on physiologic integrity as a whole. Ultimately, functioning of the individual in all the other modes is affected. In addition, disruptions of the endocrine system are often long term in nature. The role of the nurse in assessment and supportive nursing interventions contributes to the promotion of integrity of the whole person over time.

Since endocrine hormones affect the functioning of all the body's needs and processes inherent in physiologic integrity, the nurse carries out an overall appraisal of the individual's physiologic integrity. A thorough nursing assessment of behaviors will show what are adaptive and ineffective behaviors related to endocrine function. The nurse uses the skills of interviewing, observation/inspection, intuition, and measurement of internal and external behaviors to gather both subjective and objective data in each of the areas of the physiologic mode. The focus is not only on the patient's current status in each area but also on any changes over time noted by the individual. Behaviors reflective of endocrine dysfunction in one or more needs or processes may be evident. The behavior manifested depends upon the characteristics of the focal stimuli. The physiologic needs and complex processes identified in the Roy Adaptation Model provide a framework for assessment of behavior in relation to endocrine functioning.

OXYGENATION In assessing oxygenation as related to endocrine functioning, the nurse considers the individual's mental status as well as respiratory and circulatory functioning. Initially, level of consciousness and mental status are noted. The individual's predominant mood, memory, degree of alertness, and thought patterns are important indicators of endocrine disruption. Depression, agitation, or psychoses are sometimes evident. Liability of mood and irritability may be associated with excessive ACTH. Blood pressure and pulses are affected by many hormones, and alterations from normal patterns may be indicative of dysfunction. Hypertension may be related to fluid retention associated with excessive ACTH. Increases or decreases in heart rate and rhythm or changes in heart sounds may result from alterations in thyroid hormone. Percussion of the chest may provide evidence of an enlarged heart, sometimes a result of alterations in growth hormone, thyroid hormone, or insulin. Respirations are assessed for increase or decrease in rate; tidal volume (affected by insulin) is measured. Changes in voice or speech are important to note. Percussion of the chest may provide evidence of pleural effusion, sometimes evident in alterations in thyroid hormone.

ACTIVITY AND REST Endocrine functioning also affects an individual's need for activity and rest. Aspects for assessment include energy level, sleep patterns, coordination and extent of body movements, and the presence of abnormal behaviors. Generalized weakness is commonly reported by people who have alterations in adrenocorticoid, thyroid, insulin, and pituitary hormonal levels.

NUTRITION   The individual's appetite, amount and type of food intake, and weight changes are all indicators of endocrine functioning as well as evidence of meeting nutrition needs. A decrease in body weight suggests the presence of underlying hormonal dysfunction in the absence of voluntary caloric restriction or a marked general increase in exercise. Obesity of the trunk may indicate altered levels of cortisol. Bowel sounds are auscultated; they are affected in disruptions of thyroid hormone or insulin. Palpation of the abdomen may indicate an enlarged liver or ascites, also influenced by the same hormones.

FLUID, ELECTROLYTE, AND ACID–BASE BALANCE   Fluid, electrolyte, and acid–base balance often is altered in endocrine dysfunction. Assessment of these complex processes addresses the individual's desire for fluid, status of the mucus membranes, and the presence of abnormalities such as diaphoresis and edema. Diabetic ketoacidosis is a serious acid–base imbalance seen when an individual with diabetes mellitus is in crisis. This metabolic problem is caused by a total or partial lack of insulin combined with counterregulatory hormones acting. Mineralocorticoids secreted by the adrenal glands play a major role in elimination or retention of body fluid through their influence on the kidney.

ELIMINATION   Elimination, in terms of the amount, characteristics, and patterns of urinary and intestinal output, are assessed related to endocrine functioning. For example, the volume, timing, and frequency of urinary output are important indicators of diabetes mellitus; the constituents of urine are important in diagnosing conditions of adrenocorticoid hormonal alteration. The report of tenderness in the kidney area may be indicative of an underlying pathophysiologic problem.

PROTECTION   In the need for protection, assessment data reflecting endocrine functioning relate to both the nonspecific and the specific defense processes—characteristics of the skin, hair, and nails and the body's ability to withstand and recover from infections. Areas of focus include skin characteristics such as color, texture, moisture, turgor, and depth; pigmentation distribution, tanning ability, tendency to bruise, presence of acne or striae, and rate of wound healing. The individual's hair is assessed for color, amount, texture, distribution over the body, and how easily it can be broken. Nail characteristics such as growth, texture, and smoothness reflect endocrine functioning. For example, abnormal behaviors resulting from an elevation of thyroxine are warm, damp, soft textured skin, silky hair, loosening of the nail from the nail bed, and absence of forehead wrinkling. In situations of excessive glucocorticoid secretion, the skin becomes very friable and capillary fragility increases dramatically. The individual bruises easily and purplish-red striae may be present on the abdomen, breasts, shoulders, and buttocks. The inflammatory response is influenced by the glucocorticoids. For example, cortisol is thought to limit both the inflammatory response and the immune response. Any evidence of changes in these body responses is important to note.

THE SENSES   Endocrine functioning can also be assessed by looking at the status of the individual's senses. The alteration of ability in the senses—hearing, touch, vision, and smell—may be indicative of endocrine problems. Hearing loss and decreased night vision may indicate thyroid dysfunction. Exophthalmus and eyelid tremor, retraction, or lag may also be evident in such situations. Retinal problems occur with insulin disruptions. Other behaviors to note are the presence of abnormal sensations such as pain and intolerance to temperature changes. Diminished sensory responses to stimuli in the lower extremities and neuropathies of the bladder and bowel are associated with decreased insulin production.

NEUROLOGIC FUNCTION Assessment of neurologic function is also involved in the first level of assessment related to endocrine function. Level of consciousness and mental function, presence of tremors, and seizures are all important indicators. As well, functioning of the central nervous system is assessed. For example, tremors of the tongue and extremities may be evident in situations of thyroid disruption. Level of consciousness is affected by thyroid hormone, aldosterone, parathyroid hormone, and insulin. In hyperthyroidism, actions of the central nervous system increase, resulting in nervousness, restlessness, decreased attention span, tiredness, and fatigue. For people with epilepsy, seizures worsen. In situations of hyperparathyroidism, changes in mental function may range from fatigue and loss of initiative to acute psychoses.

STRUCTURAL DEVELOPMENT Other assessment areas to consider involve the structural development of the body's skeletal system, soft tissues, and organs. The body's skeletal structure is affected profoundly by levels of growth hormone, thyroxine, and triiodothyronine. Therefore, assessment of endocrine functioning considers the individual's skeletal and soft tissue development in relation to age-predicted growth and body proportions. For example, decreased linear bone growth is associated with decreased thyroxine levels. An increased rate of linear bone growth, with premature closure of the epiphyseal centers and altered body proportions, can be related to decreased levels of androgen or growth hormone. Other indicators of growth hormone dysfunction are the development of a progressive underbite or space between the lower teeth. An increase and redistribution of soft tissue is associated with high levels of adrenocorticoid hormones. In cases of an increase in thyroid hormones, the thyroid gland is noted to be larger, tender, and sometimes asymmetrical in shape. Facial appearance is an important factor associated with thyroid or cortisol problems. In fact, many endocrine disorders have associated facial characteristics that are often diagnostic keys to the underlying problem.

Similarly, the growth and development of the individual's reproductive structures and their related functioning is dependent upon adequate endocrine hormones. Alterations in the size and shape of genitalia, libido, secondary sexual characteristics, onset of menarche and menopause, and penile erectile functioning are indicators of endocrine functioning. For example, reduced output of follicle-stimulating hormone (FSH) and luteinizing hormone (LH) may result in breast and uterine atrophy in females and reduced beard and testes size in males.

OTHER ADAPTIVE MODES There may be evidence of endocrine dysfunction in one or more of the other adaptive modes. Self concept is often affected by disruptions is cortisol, testosterone, thyroid hormone, and insulin levels. This situation may, in turn, have an impact on role function and interdependent relationships.

LABORATORY TESTS Because of the multiple functions of the endocrine system, various tests are used to determine whether disruption of this regulating system is present. If so, tests also help in identifying the factors influencing the individual's ineffective behaviors. These tests are of two general types. First, there are tests involving direct measurement of the concentration of various hormones or antibodies specific to chemical groups or conformations of hormones in the plasma, blood, or urine. Examples of these are bioassay of thyroid hormone and chemical assay of cortisol and PTH levels. Secondly, tests of indirect methods of measuring hormonal concentration are used, such as the urine test for 17 ketogenic steroids and the thyroid stimulation test.

A careful analysis of the individual's behavior in each of these areas is essential as the basis of a realistic, individualized nursing care plan. The nurse must determine if a particular behavior is adaptive, requiring supportive interventions, or ineffective, necessitating management of stimuli. Some behavioral changes indicate a potential emergency requiring rapid action. An example is the cognitive changes of hypoglycemia. The judgment is made by considering each behavior in light of the indicators of effective adaptation. Just as the foundation of a house determines the quality of a home, the data gathered and decisions made at this stage of assessment determine the merit and success of the subsequent nursing care plan.

Assessment of Stimuli

The second level of assessment of the complex processes associated with endocrine function is identifying focal, contextual, and residual stimuli influencing the behaviors observed in the first level of assessment. As evident in the previous discussion, the focal stimulus for the observed behaviors was primarily compromised processes of endocrine function. Other factors that exert an influence, both in situations of compromised processes and in adaptive situations, include developmental stage, family history, environmental conditions, health care interventions, the individual's knowledge level, and the integrity of other modes. As with the other needs and complex processes, compensatory processes are also important considerations.

DEVELOPMENTAL STAGE The individual's developmental stage is an important factor for consideration when assessing stimuli related to endocrine function. Certainly, there are normal developmental changes that occur in each phase of development. At puberty, there is marked development of the secondary sexual characteristics, for example. In addition, many endocrine disruptions tend to become evident at certain ages. Previously Type II diabetes mellitus most frequently had an onset after age 30. Currently there is an increasing incidence in children and adolescence as a result of obesity. Most endocrine glands show altered function with advancing age. Changes in the endocrine system related to aging include decreased antidiuretic hormone, decreased ovarian function, decreased glucose tolerance, and decreased peripheral metabolism (Ignatavicius & Workman, 2006). Anatomically, there is atrophy of glands such as the pituitary, but this may not affect hormone production. The ovaries decrease in size and weight and the target tissue is less responsive to the stimulating hormone. The nurse can help the individual understand the changes and differentiate expected changes from pathology.

FAMILY HISTORY Because of the hereditary nature of some disruptions in endocrine function (Type II diabetes mellitus, for example), it is important to inquire about the health status of other family members. In situations where endocrine disruptions have been present for other family members, it is important to explore the individual's understanding of what these situations entailed.

ENVIRONMENTAL CONDITIONS Contextual stimuli, such as external environmental conditions, frequently augment the effects of the focal stimuli. For example, the internal temperature changes noted in dysfunction of the thyroid gland may be increased by changes in environmental temperature and humidity. Similarly, the lassitude evident in hypothyroidism may be accentuated by the socially impoverished milieu.

HEALTH CARE INTERVENTIONS   Medical and nursing interventions designed to assist the individual in adapting to a disease process contribute additional contextual stimuli. For example, medications are one group of stimuli that tend to compound difficulties in adapting. It is not unusual for an individual to be receiving an antibiotic, a corticosteroid, and an analgesic all at the same time for an endocrine-related condition. Each of these drugs has a desired effect on the focal stimulus (glandular dysfunction); however, they may have associated adverse effects. Medications can affect other endocrine glands and neuroendocrine integrating mechanisms. It is important that the individual have a thorough understanding of the actions, interactions, and side effects of the medications that he or she is taking. Other nursing interventions related to treatment of ineffective behaviors in another mode can have a negative impact on endocrine function. These include diet, exercise, availability of fluids, and activity level. Surgical intervention is often an intervention selected to deal with disruption of endocrine function. Certainly, this process creates significant stimuli for the individual and this requires increased adaptive efforts. The surgical process, if utilized, is an important consideration for all steps of the nursing process and may, for a time, be the focus of a significant amount of nursing activity.

KNOWLEDGE LEVEL   In situations of endocrine disruption, the individual's knowledge level about their condition is an important stimulus. This is particularly evident in the case of diabetes mellitus. Does the individual understand the interrelationship of diet, exercise, and insulin? Does he or she know the symptoms of imbalance and the actions to take if this occurs? Is the importance of consistent and conscientious monitoring of blood glucose levels understood?

INTEGRITY OF OTHER MODES   Previously mentioned were the potential behaviors in other adaptive modes that may be observed in situations of endocrine disruption. Particularly this is noted with the individual's self concept. It is easy to understand how disruptions in the endocrine functioning could contribute to problems in role function and interdependence, as well. What is not so clear, although there is increasing evidence to indicate a linkage, is the influence that disruptions in these modes can have on physiologic functioning and on the endocrine system, in particular. For this reason, it is important to identify situations of a psychosocial nature that could be having an effect on the individual physiologically.

Nursing Diagnosis

Development of nursing diagnoses associated with endocrine regulation is accomplished in the same way as in the other areas of the physiologic mode. One method involves a statement of the individual's behaviors together with the influencing stimuli; another method makes use of summary labels. Nursing diagnoses may reflect either adaptive or ineffective behaviors. In the former case, a sample nursing diagnosis states, "Normal development of secondary sexual characteristics related to effective endocrine functioning." In the case of ineffective behaviors, a multitude of nursing diagnoses may result. The endocrine system is closely interrelated with other body systems; therefore, a disturbance in one endocrine-regulating mechanism is likely to precipitate disturbances in others. Problems commonly occur in one or several of the following areas: cardiac output, comfort, safety, nutrition, self concept, protection, activity and rest, elimination, coping abilities, compliance, fluid volume balance, knowledge level, cognitive processes, and stress tolerance. A nursing diagnosis illustrating ineffective behaviors is "Intolerance to heat, increased appetite with weight loss, frequent diarrhea, fine hand tremors, weakness, clumsiness, fatigability, and nervousness associated with thyroid hyperactivity."

It is also possible to construct a nursing diagnosis using a summary label that captures clusters of behaviors. This method is used by experienced nurses to communicate significant amounts of information in one phrase. As identified in Chapter 3, there are five indicators of positive endocrine function in the Roy Adaptation Model: (1) effective hormonal regulation of metabolic and body processes; (2) effective hormonal regulation of reproductive development; (3) stable patterns of closed-loop, negative-feedback hormone system; (4) stable patterns of cyclical hormone rhythms; and (5) effective coping strategies for stress. Likewise, five commonly recurring adaptation problems are identified: (1) ineffective hormone regulation, (2) ineffective reproductive development, (3) instability of hormone system loops, (4) instability of internal cyclical rhythms, and (5) stress. A nursing diagnosis stated with the use of a summary label reads, "Instability of menstrual cycle related to dietary restriction and excessive exercise." This situation is frequently evident in young women engaged in competitive sports. Both the behavior and the stimuli stated in this example of a nursing diagnosis communicate a wealth of information to an individual experienced in adaptation problems associated with endocrine function. However, for the inexperienced individual, the more detailed expression of behaviors and stimuli can be more meaningful.

The use of a summary label when more than one mode is affected by the same stimulus is often an effective way of communicating a cluster of behaviors. For example, the concept of "stress" might be such a diagnosis—one word captures a multitude of behaviors and stimuli. The diagnosis statement could be "stress associated with too many demanding commitments and too little time." In Table 13–2, the Roy model nursing diagnostic categories for the complex processes of endocrine functioning are shown in relation to nursing diagnosis labels approved by the North American Nursing Diagnosis Association (NANDA International, 2007).

In situations of endocrine dysfunction it may be easy for the nurse to focus on the pathophysiology involved rather than the behaviors and stimuli that are related to what is happening physiologically in the individual's body. Knowledge of pathophysiology is important to assist the nurse in the identification of behaviors and stimuli related to endocrine dysfunction. With

TABLE 13–2 Nursing Diagnostic Categories for Endocrine Function

Positive Indicators of Adaptation	Common Adaptation Problems	NANDA Diagnostic Labels
• Effective hormonal regulation of metabolic and body processes • Effective hormonal regulation of reproductive development • Stable patterns of closed-loop negative-feedback hormone system • Stable patterns of cyclical hormone rhythms • Effective coping strategies for stress	• Ineffective hormone regulation • Ineffective reproductive development • Instability of hormone system loops • Instability of internal cyclical rhythms • Stress	• Stress overload • Delayed growth and development • Risk for disproportionate growth • Adult failure to thrive • Risk for delayed development

the framework that the Roy Adaptation Model provides, behaviors and stimuli relate to the individual's behavioral manifestation of the problem and the factors that appear to be influencing it. In turn, the nursing diagnosis also focuses on behaviors and stimuli rather than on the pathophysiologic conditions(s). A well-written nursing diagnosis aids in setting priorities and establishing direction for the next step of the nursing process—goal setting.

Goal Setting

Each step of the nursing process focuses on the individual's behavior, the stimuli influencing that behavior, or both. With the nursing diagnosis, the statement developed included both the behavior and the stimuli. With the goal setting step, the focus is on the individual's behavior. Each goal identifies a behavior that is to be addressed. Many endocrine dysfunctions have a chronic as well as an acute phase. Thus, the goal setting process includes both long- and short-term goals, each of which states the behavior of focus, the change expected, and the time frame in which the goal is to be achieved. The following statements provide examples of possible goals for an individual with activity intolerance related to a decrease in metabolic rate secondary to hypothyroidism. "Throughout the next several days, the individual will develop a list of factors that increase fatigue." "Within 1 month, the individual will demonstrate an increase in activity tolerance, decreased signs of fatigue and dyspnea on exertion, and will independently perform activities of daily living." Each of these goals indicates the behavior(s) of focus, the change desired, and the associated time frame.

Consider a situation where an 11-year-old boy demonstrates the behaviors of excessive urination, excessive hunger and thirst, rapid weight loss and weakness, and is diagnosed with Type I diabetes mellitus. He requires daily injection of insulin balanced carefully with diet and exercise to control metabolic processes. Goals related to the situation could be "Within 1 week, the boy will select foods according to the guidelines recommended by the American Diabetes Association." Or "Within 2 weeks, the child will demonstrate the ability to do his own blood glucose testing." Or "Within 1 month, he will be able to calculate, prepare, and administer his own insulin." In order to be effective in guiding the progress of the individual, goals must be established in collaboration with the individual involved. As with each step of the nursing process, the individual is an active participant. Where possible, the individual's involvement helps to ensure that accurate and relevant information is obtained, that it is interpreted appropriately into nursing diagnoses, and that achievable and relevant goals are established. This is the only way that interventions to assist in achieving effective adaptation can be determined. The identification of nursing interventions is the next step of the nursing process as described in the Roy Adaptation Model.

Nursing Intervention

The nursing intervention step of the nursing process according to the Roy Adaptation Model focuses on the stimuli affecting the behavior identified in the goal setting step. The nursing intervention step is the management of stimuli, and this involves altering, increasing, decreasing, removing, or maintaining them. In the previous situation involving the boy recently diagnosed with Type I diabetes mellitus, the stimuli affecting the observed behaviors involves the balance between diet, exercise, and the action of insulin within the body. Thus, nursing interventions would be directed to these areas of influence. Dietary modifications for the diabetic person address optimum nutrition, maintenance of ideal body weight, control of the plasma glucose level, prevention of complications of the disease, and individualizing the meal pattern to the individual's lifestyle. Exercise is an important consideration that can help keep the manifestations of diabetes under control. The intricacies of insulin administration—concentration, modifications, onset/peak/duration of action, complications, administration, monitoring and control, and glucose testing—involve the development of knowledge, skills, and attitudes. This presents an educational challenge for both the individual and the nurse.

All the above nursing interventions focus on stimuli (diet, exercise, levels of insulin) that are causing the ineffective behaviors for the individual. As with many other endocrine function disturbances, the problems tend to be long-term challenges for the individual. Many nursing interventions relate to the individual's knowledge level and understanding about the problem to equip them to make the necessary adaptations on an ongoing basis. Knowledge about crisis situations associated with acute episodes is also important. The young man with diabetes requires knowledge about many serious acute complications such as hyperosmolar nonketotic coma, diabetic ketoacidosis, hypoglycemia, and infection. The same holds true for many other situations of endocrine disruption. It is not within the scope of this text to explore endocrine disorders in more depth. The reader is referred to pathophysiology resources and medical and nursing practice textbooks for further information.

Evaluation

Evaluation involves judging the effectiveness of the nursing interventions in relation to the individual's adaptive behavior. The question is whether or not the individual has attained the behavior stated in the goals. The nursing interventions are identified as effective if the individual's behavior is in accordance with the stated goal. If the goal has not been achieved, the nurse identifies alternative interventions or approaches by reassessing the behavior and stimuli and continuing with the other steps of the nursing process. In considering the previously identified goal: "Within 2 weeks, the child will demonstrate the ability to do his own blood glucose testing," the nurse, in evaluating the effectiveness of the interventions, would within 2 weeks have the boy demonstrate his ability to do glucose testing. Successful demonstration of the processes would indicate that the nursing intervention—probably an educational process—was effective. Similar evaluation could be conducted with respect to the ability to administer insulin to himself.

It is important to recognize that the nursing process and the six steps are ongoing, simultaneous, and overlapping. Although they have been separated and dealt with in an artificially linear manner for discussion purposes, often intervention can be occurring at the same time as first- and second-level assessment is proceeding. Likewise, evaluation occurs on an ongoing basis. The nurse has evaluation in mind even when nursing diagnoses are being established and as goals are being formulated.

Summary

This chapter has focused on the application of the Roy Adaptation Model to the complex physiologic processes associated with endocrine function. An overview of these basic life processes was provided along with illustration of innate and learned adaptive compensatory responses related to endocrine function and examples of compromised processes. Finally, guidelines for planning nursing care through identification of parameters of assessment behaviors and stimuli, the formulation of nursing diagnoses, goals, and nursing intervention were explored, and evaluation of nursing care was described.

The following section turns to the other adaptive modes of self concept, role function,

and interdependence of the individual. These modes are directly influenced by adaptation in the physiologic modes, and in turn, disruptions in the modes have physiologic effects.

Exercises of Application

1. Recall a recent stressful situation in your life, perhaps an examination or a car accident. Using the behavioral assessment categories in this chapter, list the behaviors you exhibited that reflect activation of your neuroendocrine mechanisms.

2. Create a table with three columns: major endocrine glands, behaviors associated with hyperactivity, and behaviors associated with hypo-activity. Use a pathophysiology or nursing textbook to complete the columns.

Example:

Endocrine Gland	Hypersecretion	Hyposecretion
Anterior Pituitary – growth hormone	giantism – proportional accelerated linear growth	midgets – very short with adult body proportions
	acromegaly – bony and soft tissue growth of extremities	dwarfism – normal trunk size with short extremities

Assessment of Understanding

1. In Column B, name the hormone(s) that stimulate(s) the process identified in Column A. In Column C, identify the endocrine gland that secretes it.

Column A: Process	Column B: Hormone	Column C: Secreting Gland
a. growth of body cells, soft tissue, and cartilage	a. _____	a. _____
b. reabsorption of water, regulator of osmolarity, blood pressure	b. _____	b. _____
c. regulates the catabolic phase of metabolism, metabolic rate of all cells, and body heat production	c. _____	c. _____
d. regulates plasma calcium and phosphorus levels	d. _____	d. _____
e. reabsorption of sodium; elimination of potassium, ammonium, and magnesium	e. _____	e. _____
f. emergency response to stressful situations similar to sympathetic nervous system	f. _____	f. _____

2. An important regulator compensatory process is termed "the stress response." The body's physiologic response takes two forms: LAS and GAS. Label the following statements according to the form (LAS or GAS) they describe.
   (a) _____ stimulus is localized
   (b) _____ neuroendocrine response
   (c) _____ collective body systems are threatened
   (d) _____ only one organ reacts
   (e) _____ periods of stress are prolonged
3. No matter what the source of endocrine disruption, the resulting structural and functional changes take similar forms; the observed behaviors are a ramification of either _____ or _____ of the particular hormone.
4. Which of the following physiologic components are important areas for assessment of behaviors related to endocrine function? (Check the ones that apply.)
   (a) _____ oxygenation
   (b) _____ activity and rest
   (c) _____ nutrition
   (d) _____ fluid, electrolyte, acid–base balance
   (e) _____ elimination
   (f) _____ protection
   (g) _____ senses
   (h) _____ neurologic function
5. Although the focal stimulus in situations of endocrine dysfunction is frequently a pathophys-

iologic problem, give an example of a situation where disruption in normal processes is caused by another factor.

SITUATION:

Mr. Jay is a 66-year-old male who has been recently diagnosed with Type II diabetes mellitus. Assessment revealed that he is experiencing excessive urination and is very thirsty. He is very weak and feels light headed. He states that he is hungry all the time. Since his diagnosis of diabetes, Mr. Jay has been following a "special diet." However, he recently has had several social events where he did not adhere to any diet. Because he has been feeling tired and weak, he has forgone his regular morning and evening walks. When asked about his blood glucose level, he commented that he has not tested it lately since he ran out of supplies. Mr. Jay has never attended an educational program for diabetics.

6. Formulate two nursing diagnoses for this situation: (a) focusing on specific behaviors and (b) using a summary label.
7. Develop a short-term and a long-term goal statement for Mr. Jay.
8. Identify two nursing interventions that will address the goals that you developed in item 7.
9. What would be the behavior that would indicate that Mr. Jay had achieved the goals developed in item 7?

FEEDBACK

1. **Column B:**
   Hormone
   a. Growth hormone
   b. Antidiuretic hormone
   c. Thyroxine and triiodothyronine
   d. Parathyroid hormone
   e. Mineralocorticoids
   f. Epinephrine

2. All of them
3. Examples:
   • Failure to ovulate caused by the administration of birth control pills.
   • Menstrual irregularity attributed to strenuous exercise and rigid weight control.
   • Unnatural strength and physical development related to the ingestion of steroids.
4. (a) LAS
   (b) GAS

Column C:
Secreting Gland
a. Anterior pituitary
b. Posterior pituitary
c. Thyroid
d. Parathyroids
e. Adrenal cortex
f. Adrenal medulla

(c) GAS
(d) LAS
(e) GAS
5. hyposecretion, hypersecretion
6. (a) Excessive urination, thirst, weakness, and light-headedness related to imbalance in diet, exercise, and insulin levels.
   (b) Hyperglycemia related to inadequate understanding of insulin regulation in relation to diet and exercise.

7. (a) Within 1 hour, Mr. Jay's blood glucose will be within acceptable levels.

   (b) Within 1 week, Mr. Jay will be regularly monitoring his blood glucose levels and recording them on a chart together with an account of his dietary intake and exercise.

8. (a) The nursing intervention would involve obtaining a blood glucose level and responding appropriately to the situation: if hyperglycemic, he may require fluid replacement and the restoration of control using diet, exercise, and medication.

   (b) The nursing intervention for goal 7(b) would involve his attendance at a diabetic instruction class to enhance his knowledge, skill, and commitment to regulating his diet and exercise.

9. (a) Evaluation for goal 7(a) involves retesting of blood glucose levels to determine whether they have responded appropriately and are now within normal parameters.

   (b) Evaluation for goal 7(b) would be a chart indicating that Mr. Jay was indeed monitoring carefully his diet, exercise, and blood glucose level.

References

Andrews, H. A., & Roy, C. (1986). *Essentials of the Roy Adaptation Model.* E. Norwalk, CT: Appleton-Century-Crofts.

Hancock, M. R. (1997). Nursing assessment and common endocrine interventions. In L. O. Burrell, M. J. M. Gerlach, & B. S. Pless (Eds.), *Adult nursing: Acute and community care* (2nd ed., pp. 1074–1084). Stamford, CT: Appleton and Lange.

Ignatavicius, D. D., & Workman, M. L. (2006). *Medical-surgical nursing: Critical thinking for collaborative care* (5th ed.). St. Louis, MO: Elsevier Saunders.

Marieb, E. N., & Hoehn, K. (2007). *Human anatomy and physiology* (7th ed.). San Francisco:Pearson Benjamin Cummings.

NANDA International. (2007). *Nursing diagnoses: Definitions and classifications, 2007–2008.* Philadelphia: NANDA-I.

Roy, C., & McLeod, D. (1981). Theory of the person as an adaptive system. In C. Roy & S. L. Roberts (Eds.), *Theory construction in nursing: An adaptation model* (pp. 49–60). Englewood Cliffs, NJ: Prentice Hall.

Selye, H. (1976). *The stress of life* (2nd ed.). New York: McGraw-Hill.

CHAPTER 14

Self-Concept Mode of the Person

The second adaptive mode is termed the self-concept mode for the individual person. The Group Identity Mode for persons in groups is described in Chapter 18. The self-concept mode for the individual is described in this chapter to guide nursing assessment and planning of care. The aim is to promote effective adaptation for people. The core self-concept is significant for the individual. Adaptation in this mode affects the other three modes because people act out of who they are. The self is involved whether making choices for promoting health or facing changes in one's health. The self-concept mode is another perspective of the holism of the person.

Self-concept is defined as the composite of beliefs and feelings that the individual holds about self at a given time. Formed from internal perceptions and perceptions of others, self-concept directs behavior. The self-concept mode is viewed in the Roy Adaptation Model as having two components: the *physical self*, including body sensation and body image; and the *personal self*, consisting of self-consistency, self-ideal, and moral-ethical-spiritual self. Some examples of these components include the statement, "I look like I haven't slept in a week"—a behavioral statement related to body image. The statement, "I know I can figure out how to get this printer to work with my new computer," illustrates self-ideal behavior.

The basic need underlying the self-concept mode has been identified as *psychic and spiritual integrity*—the need to know who one is so that one can be or exist with a sense of unity and meaning. The Roy Adaptation Model views the self and the individual's motivation to act as driven by these needs, psychic and spiritual integrity. Psychic integrity, and the related dimension of spiritual integrity, are both basic to health. Adaptation problems in this area may interfere with the person's ability to do what is necessary to maintain health or to heal when not healthy. It is important for the nurse to have knowledge about the self-concept mode to assess behaviors and stimuli influencing the person's self-concept.

This chapter provides an overview of the self-concept mode and the integrated processes of the developing self, perceiving self, and focusing self. It is through these processes that psychic and spiritual integrity is maintained. Compensatory adaptive processes related to self-concept are discussed, and examples of associated compromised processes of individuals are explored. Finally, the chapter provides guidelines for planning nursing care by outlining nursing assessment of behaviors and stimuli, formulating diagnoses, establishing goals, selecting interventions, and evaluating nursing care.

OBJECTIVES

After studying this chapter, the reader will be able to do the following:

1. Describe the self-concept mode according to the Roy Adaptation Model.

2. Describe one compensatory process related to self-concept.

3. Name and describe two situations of compromised processes of self-concept.

4. Identify important first-level assessment behaviors for the self-concept mode.

5. Identify second-level assessment factors or stimuli that influence the self-concept mode.

6. Formulate nursing diagnoses related to the self-concept mode.

7. Establish goals related to given diagnoses in the self-concept mode.

8. Select nursing interventions to promote adaptation in the self-concept mode.

9. Propose approaches to determine the effectiveness of nursing interventions for self-concept.

KEY CONCEPTS DEFINED

Anxiety: A painful uneasiness of mind due to a vague, nonspecific danger; threatens an individual's sense of self-consistency.

Body image: How one views oneself physically and one's view of personal appearance.

Body sensation: How one feels and experiences the self as a physical being.

Coping strategies: The individual's habitual responses used to maintain adaptation; the ways the individual functions to maintain integrity in everyday life and in times of stress.

Developing self: Growing self-perceptions based on physical, psychological, and cognitive development, and perceptions of others' reactions to self; these experiences are cognitively organized into self-schemas.

Focusing self: The process of being in touch with the physical and personal self in a way that surfaces hope, energy, continuity, meaning, purpose, and pride to be an individual self within the whole human community; awareness of self, consciousness, and meaning are transformed in person and environment integration, which the person focuses on by way of thinking and feeling.

Life closure: The process through which an individual resolves the issue of the meaning of one's life and accepts the reality of eventual death.

Moral-ethical-spiritual self: That aspect of the personal self which includes a belief system and an evaluation of who one is in relation to the universe.

Perceiving self: The process whereby the individual takes in what is happening in the environment and through perception defines who they are; this definition is based on how they interpret the input.

Personal self: The individual's appraisal of one's own characteristics, expectations, values, and worth, including self-consistency, self-ideal, and the moral-ethical-spiritual self.

Physical self: The individual's appraisal of one's own physical being, including physical attributes, functioning, sexuality, health and illness states, and appearance; includes the components of body sensation and body image.

Psychic and spiritual integrity: On the individual level, the basic need of the self-concept mode; the need to know who one is so that one can be or exist with a sense of unity, meaning, and purposefulness in the universe.

Schema: The structures for encoding and representing information.

Self-concept: The composite of beliefs and feelings that one holds about oneself at a given time; formed from internal perceptions and perceptions of others' reactions.

Self-consistency: The part of the personal self component which strives to maintain a consistent self-organization and to avoid disequilibrium; an organized system of ideas about self.

Self-esteem: The individual's perception of self-worth that is a pervasive aspect of the personal self.

Self-ideal: That aspect of the personal self-component that relates to what the person would like to be or is capable of doing.

Self-schema: Cognitive generalizations about the self derived from past experience that organize and guide the processing of the self-related information contained in an individual's interactions with others.

Sexual ineffectiveness: Ineffective sexual behavior related to physical or psychological factors; demonstrated by decreased sense of sexual self or aggressive sexual behavior.

SELF-CONCEPT OF THE INDIVIDUAL

From the early publications on the Roy Adaptation Model, the self-concept has been defined as the composite of beliefs and feelings that a person holds about self at a given time (Driever, 1976). This definition is consistent with the core features of the self identified today (Mischel & Morf, 2003). We develop our beliefs and feelings about self from our own internal perceptions and from feedback of how others perceive us. It is this composite self that directs behavior. The question, "Who am I?" is so central that the sense of self is a major part of everything a person does. Another author noted that the self is considered the image that the individual has of oneself as a physical, social, and spiritual or moral being (Gecas, 1982).

In the Roy Adaptation Model, the self-concept mode for the individual is viewed as having two subareas, the physical self and the personal self. Figure 14–1 is a diagram representing the self-concept with the two subareas and their components. The integrated life processes form a middle range theory basis. The physical self includes two components, body sensation and body image. The person looks at self as a physical being, including physical traits, appearance, functioning, sexuality, and health and illness states. Body sensation applies to feeling and experiencing oneself as a physical being. Statements such as, "I feel sick," "I am exhausted," or "I feel great!" are examples of body sensation behaviors. Body image applies to how one views oneself physically and one's appearance. "I need to lose some

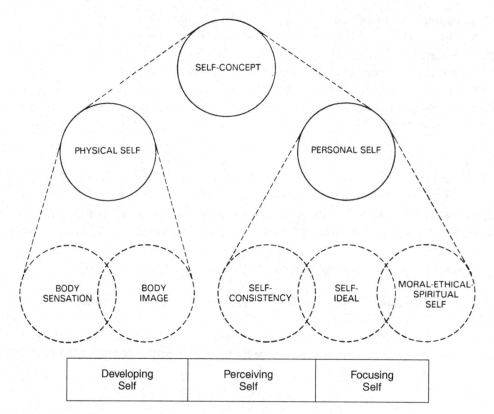

FIGURE 14–1 Self-concept mode. Theoretical basis.

weight," "I feel I really look good today," or "I'm not really physically fit," are all behavioral statements related to body image. Body sensation and body image are shown as the two component parts of the physical self.

The personal self is viewed as having three components: self-consistency, self-ideal, and moral-ethical-spiritual self. Self-consistency refers to an organized system of ideas about self. The mind works to make all the ideas in the self system seem to be consistent with, or fit together with, one another. Lecky (1961) identified that through the need for self-consistency, the person strives to maintain a coherent self-organization and avoid disequilibrium. Behavior related to self-consistency can be observed in a person's response to a situation and in verbal statements. Examples are, "I'm a person who is always on time," or "I'm really anxious about having to be in bed until the end of this pregnancy; I am usually so active." Self-ideal relates to what one would like to be or is capable of doing. "I want to be a nurse," or "I would like to be able to do better in Spanish class," are statements manifesting a person's self-ideal. The moral-ethical-spiritual self includes the belief system and an evaluation of who one is in relation to the universe. It is evidenced by such statements as, "I believe that every person deserves the same kind of health care," or "I believe that my suffering has some part to play in this world." These components will be explored further in developing an understanding of the processes related to self-concept. The underlying middle-range theoretical processes are described in the following section.

PROCESSES OF SELF-CONCEPT

The Roy Adaptation Model describes the person as having basic life processes in each adaptive mode. The nurse can evaluate the adaptation level of these processes and provide care to promote integrated processes at the highest level of adaptation possible. The basic processes of the self-concept mode include the developing self, the perceiving self, and the focusing self. These processes (see lower boxes of Figure 14–1) draw on middle-range theories to provide knowledge of the self-concept, physical and personal components, according to the Roy Adaptation Model.

Process of Developing Self

Both the physical and personal self develop throughout the person's life. For the child, the developing self is influenced by increasing physical and thinking abilities and by interactions with others. Freud (1949), Erikson (1963), Piaget (1954), and Neugarten (1969, 1979) are developmental theorists who provide understanding of the process of the developing self. Other authors provide theories about the developing self such as moral development and self-schemas. The child's physical and cognitive maturation and changing relationships are key to the development of self. At birth, humans begin to develop the self. Responses by primary caregivers enhance or inhibit the newborn's beginning attempts to make sense of the world. Bowlby (1969) is one author who emphasizes the critical nature of successful attachment between baby and parents (or surrogates). Based on his research, he proposed that the development of self-esteem is germinated within that bond. Disorganized attachments result in fragmented self. Initial relationships are with the primary caregiver, the mother or father or preferred staff person at day care. Gradually, the child interacts and adjusts as a member of a family, of a small child care group, and eventually a class at school. The work of Freud and Erikson are helpful in understanding the stages of development that include interaction with others.

Freud derived a theory of personality development from his clinical observations. His psychoanalytic model proposed two internal biological forces that drive change in the child. The first is sexual or libido. The second is aggressive energies. The five stages of development focus on a zone of pleasure or gratification. These are oral, anal, phallic, latent, and genital. There have been critiques and expansions of this work. Erikson expanded on Freud's psychoanalytic stages and included the full life span. The eight maturational crises described by Erikson (1963) are useful in understanding the influence of interactions with others on the developing self-process. It is not difficult to recognize the influences of reactions of others in the maturational crises described at each stage: trust versus mistrust, autonomy versus shame and doubt, initiative versus guilt, industry versus inferiority, identity versus role confusion, intimacy versus isolation, generativity versus self-absorption and stagnation, and ego integrity versus despair. In Erikson's maturational theory, particular emphasis is placed on identity emerging between 12 and 18 years of age. The reader is referred to the original author.

Piaget focused on cognitive development. According to Piaget, infants and young toddlers are in the sensorimotor stage. Children at this age use all their senses and motor skills to define and interpret objects and events. The major cognitive task is to experience triumph over objects. The child's thinking proceeds from directly acting as a whole on the environment to more goal-directed action. The child learns to interact with an object to make something happen. Between 6 and 12 months, self is seen as separated from objects. In Piaget's preoperational stage, toddlers and preschoolers complete the task of understanding symbols, such as classifying by color, shape, or size. Perceptually, at ages 2 to 5 years, self is the focus and purpose of the world. The child will reject another's viewpoint and be unaware that the other person can have a different viewpoint. Between ages 5 and 8, the child is less egocentric, but will have difficulty comprehending a conflicting viewpoint. The school-age child is in the concrete operational stage of cognitive development and can master classes, quantities, and relations such as time and space. Thinking is limited by relying on experience, and by the limited number and quality of past experiences. Adolescents have formal operations thought processes that include abstract and symbolic relationships. Their view of the world goes beyond the present and the concrete to include future possibilities, abstractions, and contrary-to-fact propositions. Such thinking is used in creating self-consistency, self-ideal, and a moral-ethical-spiritual self.

The developmental approach of Neugarten (1979) focuses on the second half of life. In this theory, time, age, and life cycle are significant in making a meaningful life story from a life history. The approach has been used to understand development of self in the elderly. Given the expanded life span of people today, Erikson's eighth stage of development has expanded to include three additional stages (Edelman & Mandle, 2002). The first is ego differentiation versus work roles preoccupation. The older adult achieves an identity apart from work. Body transcendence versus body preoccupation is the stage in which the physical self adjusts to normal and aging changes. Finally, ego transcendence versus ego preoccupation is the stage focused on accepting death and involves both self-ideal and the moral-ethical-spiritual self. Dobratz (1984, 2004, 2005) has studied the process of life closure from the perspective of the Roy Adaptation Model. This is discussed in the section on grieving as a compensatory process.

The development of moral thinking and moral judgment is relevant to the developing self. Kohlberg (1981) studied the reasons that people make decisions about right or wrong behaviors. In his findings he described three levels of moral judgment, and each had two stages. At the preconventional level, the child begins by keeping rules to avoid punishment. In the second stage of this level, the child believes that what is in one's own interest or what is fair is what is right. Exchange is used to meet two people's interests. The next level is the conventional in which people hold mutual expectations and feel that being good is important. The second part of this level includes being aware of social systems and one's conscience. Contributing to society is important, and the person considers self-respect as a reason for choosing right behaviors. The third level is postconventional and principled. It involves believing in a social contract to abide by laws for the good of all and using universal ethical principles. Kohlberg did not believe that all people reach this stage.

The interviews used in Kohlberg's research were of males from school age through young adulthood. Gilligan's theory of moral development (1982) showed differences between men and women. The development is parallel but differences occur in relationships and issues of dependency. Separation from the mother was important for males. Attachment within relationships was the most important factor in successful female development. Girls learn to value relationships and to be interdependent at an earlier age than boys. Care and responsibility become issues for women. Women move from the moral dilemma of how to exercise their rights without interfering in the rights of others to the more general approach of how to lead a moral life. They feel obligations to themselves, their families, and people in general.

Another theory that provides understanding of the developing self process is work on self-schema and processing information about the self (Markus, 1977). In discussing the information processing of the cognator, the Roy Adaptation Model notes that the amount of stimulation available at any time is greater than a person can process or even attend to. Tendencies to select what to notice, learn, or remember are not random. Rather Markus

(1977; Markus & Wurf, 1987) proposes that they depend on some internal cognitive structures that allow the individual to process the incoming information with some degree of efficiency. Schema is a term used for the structures for encoding and representing information. Self-schema are cognitive generalizations about the self derived from past experience that organize and guide the processing of the self-related information contained in an individual's interactions with others. Self-schemas have been documented in a variety of domains, for example, body weight (Markus, Hamill, & Sentis, 1987), exercise (Kendzierski, 1988), and sexual identity (Markus, Crane, Bernstein, & Siladi, 1982), related to physical self; and academic performance (Garcia & Pintrich, 1994), related to self-ideal.

Using several theoretical approaches, the developing self process can be summarized as stages of self growth based on physical, cognitive, and moral development, and taking in the reactions of others to self. These experiences are cognitively organized into self-schemas and involve both the physical and personal self.

Process of Perceiving Self

Another way to understand self-concept is to focus specifically on the process of perceiving self. The definition of self-concept is defined in the Roy Adaptation Model as the composite of beliefs and feelings that the individual holds about self. One's beliefs and feelings are based on perceptions. As noted in Chapter 10, perception means the person's interpretation of sensory stimuli and the conscious appreciation of it. The perceiving self means that persons take in what is happening in the environment and through perception define who they are by how they interpret the input. A number of theorists in several disciplines have examined this interactive process of the person's self-concept with the environment, particularly other persons.

In a broad self-perception theory, Coombs and Snygg (1959) see self as a constellation of self-perceptions. A number of symbolic interaction theorists (Cooley, 1964; Goffman, 1959, 1967; Mead, 1934; Sullivan, 1953) describe that the person bases self-perception on the way responses of others are perceived. Mead proposed that the concept of self refers to an individual's awareness of being a distinct entity in society. Although the sense of self is not present at birth, it arises in the process of social experience as the infant, child, and adult relate to other individuals and the wider society. Cooley expanded on this idea by maintaining that a sense of self is the result of social interactions in which one sees one's self reflected in the meanings and evaluations of others. Cooley maintained that people see in imagination the other persons' judgments of them, for example, of their appearance. If the individual is getting signals about looking good, one experiences feelings such as pride and satisfaction about self. If, however, a person interprets negative input about appearance, the result may be feelings of humiliation. Mead noted also that for the self to develop in its fullest sense, it is necessary not only to take on the attitudes of others directed toward the self, but also to acquire the attitudes of the group and society in which the person holds membership. The individual must therefore be able to comprehend the situation from the standpoint of the generalized other. For example, the teenage girl puts herself in the place of her classmates, "stands in their shoes," and perceives that in their eyes she is fashionable when she wears clothes and makeup like they wear.

The understanding that people reconfirm their self-concept through ongoing social interactions highlights the significance of interpersonal relations in health care. The nurse learns that the therapeutic use of self is important in being effective in the nursing process. Increased self awareness enhances the nurse's use of self in the therapeutic process. There are a number of approaches to learning to be more accurate in perceiving self. Luft (1969, 1984) created the

Johari window as a visual framework for understanding the extent of the individual's self-awareness. This approach is based on understanding that there are different parts to the self. Some parts are more easily known and some are unknown and even unconscious. Verklan (2007) explained that personal awareness is divided into four quadrants, like a window with four panes (Figure 14–2). The four quadrants are open, blind, hidden, and unknown. You can think of the lines between the quadrants as curtains that can be open or closed, wide or narrow. Opening the curtain occurs as interpersonal interactions grow. The open quadrant includes what everyone knows about you and that you also know. For example, people know that you are a sophomore in college, like to study hard, and will find ways to visit your family during school breaks because they mean a lot to you. This pane has a lot of facts about you, and also includes some of your likes, dislikes, goals, attitudes, and emotions. For those who know you well, the curtain is open. Others who do not know you may have a smaller view of this windowpane.

The hidden quadrant contains things that you know about yourself, but you generally keep from others. In general, people may not know the names and ages of your siblings and that one of them has a chronic illness. Your self disclosure increases with personal interactions. When one person discloses something of self, the other often responds by sharing something in the hidden category. This windowpane can get smaller and the open window gets larger as the new information moves to the top left quadrant. The blind quadrant includes what is known to others, but which is unknown to you. It takes trust and courage to tell someone what others know, but they do not know about themselves. Perhaps your friends are aware that because of your little sister's illness, you initially treat everyone as if they need your help. When someone tells you this, you can become more aware of your behavior. This growth and awareness makes it possible for you to decide how to use your natural response of being concerned about others. You may now recognize when your overconcern is not appropriate and uncomfortable for the other person. The final windowpane includes what is unknown to others and is also unknown to you. You may only learn about some of your

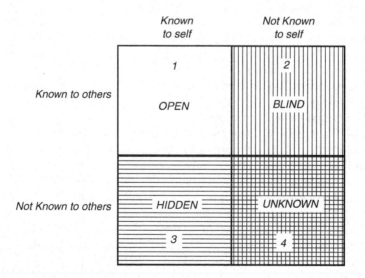

FIGURE 14–2   Johari Window. (From Luft, J. *Group processes: An introduction to group dynamics* (3rd ed.). Palo Alto, CA: Mayfield. Used with permission.)

strengths and weaknesses when you have to respond to new challenging situations. With more life situations, each person will learn more about the self. Instead of staying in a small, safe open quadrant, one can take the risk to learn more about the self in other quadrants.

Increasing self awareness involves first listening to oneself and paying attention to our thinking, feeling, and doing. Secondly, we will listen to others and learn how to incorporate their feedback. Accurate self perceptions have benefits for the nurse both personally and professionally. In addition, helping others with effective processes of the perceiving self can make nursing care more effective. Other strategies for enhancing the process of the perceiving self are values clarification and reflective practice. Values clarification was proposed by Raths and colleagues (1966). The strategy involves choosing, prizing, and action whereby the person can identify one's individual chosen values. A number of excellent publications are available to learn the strategy. As well, a number of authors have written on the process of reflective practice (see for example, Gustafsson & Fargerberg, 2003).

Process of Focusing Self

The self-concept involves both stability of the self over time and consistency, unity, and organization of self. A number of theorists discuss stability of self from varying perspectives. The term selected for the theoretical commonalities is the process of *focusing self*. Focusing implies being in touch with the physical and personal self in a particular way. One is in touch with self in a way that surfaces hope, energy, continuity, meaning, purpose, and pride. The person can focus on being an individual self within the whole human community in its struggle for peace, unity, and balance (McMahon, 1993). Focusing involves a process of awareness of who one is and of one's place as an individual among other people in society. It moves beyond individualism to perceiving self as part of the common patterns and integral relations of persons and the earth, as noted in the assumptions of the Roy Adaptation Model for the 21st century (see Chapter 2). The focusing self makes possible the executive functions of self. This means that one can set goals and make plans to achieve them. The individual directs one's own actions and can evaluate one's progress and correct behavior as needed. As noted in one discussion of self-regulation and the executive function, this ability "dramatically increases the range, complexity, and diversity of human behavior" (Baumeister &Vohs, 2003, p. 199).

In psychology in the mid-20th century, there was a focus on behaviorism. Some theorists began to see the need to focus study on the uniqueness of the person. By the 1970s there was a resurgence of focus on the self with the development of cognitive psychology. Lecky (1945, 1961) had proposed the theory of self-consistency to conceive of a person as a unique and dynamic whole whose most significant characteristic is individuality. Self-consistency, as discussed by other theorists, refers to the organization of ideas and attitudes about self that is acquired through the transaction between the person and environment (Elliott, 1986; Rogers, 1961). Lecky asserts that through the demands of self-consistency, the person strives to maintain a consistent self-organization and avoid disequilibrium. In discussing Lecky's work, Zhan (1994) noted that the most constant factor in one's experience is the self and the interpretation of one's own meaning—the kind of person one is and the place one occupies in the world.

Another theory related to self-consistency is Festinger's theory of cognitive dissonance. This theory has been elaborated by others and reflects the individual's efforts to minimize perceived discrepancies between the self-concept and other aspects of experience (Festinger, 1962; Markus & Zajonc, 1985; Rosenberg, 1968). This theory is discussed further as a compensatory adaptive process. We have noted that people reconfirm their self-concept through current social interaction. Self-consistency has been identified as the result of striving for unity or integrity during the transaction between person and environment (Beck, 1976; Lecky, 1961; Rogers, 1961). Inconsistency in self-organization results in discomfort and disturbance. The individual uses cognitive processes to reduce tension and to maintain a consistent self. Antonovsky (1986) describes the result of these processes as a sense of coherence. Coherence is described as a sense of global orientation of the extent to which one has a dynamic feeling of confidence. Erikson (1968) described identity as "a subjective sense of an invigorating sameness and continuity" (p. 19).

Both self-esteem and self-preservation are motives discussed by Rosenberg (1965, 1979). Self-esteem relates to the worth or value the person holds of self. It is a pervasive aspect of the self-concept. Rosenberg describes dimensions of self including self-attitudes of continuity, consistency, clarity, and accuracy; and structure, referring to the values or criteria used to assess different self-attributions. Other authors have described models of contingencies of self worth (Crocker & Park, 2003). In this model, the impact of events and circumstances on self-esteem depends on the perceived relevance of the events. Self-esteem is more vulnerable to and more defended in response to events that are relevant to what is important to one's self-worth. The person's interpretation of the event in relation to what is important and to reaching one's goals determines the effect on self-esteem. In summarizing related research, the authors noted that people with high general self-esteem think more positively about themselves and have more certain self-concepts. They may find it easier to not believe negative information about self or may dismiss the importance of the event to their values of self. They also are at risk for greater losses of self-esteem if they fail in areas that are important to them.

In discussing the creative self, Zohar (1990) notes the human capacity to support unity of consciousness and the construction of relational wholes. The person is capable of creative self-reflection in dialogue with the environment. Zohar adds that the concept of morality is created in response to the person's need for an integrated picture of appropriate social behavior. Whereas the middle of the 20th century advocated the view of the person as a unique individual, entering the 21st century, the unity of patterns of person and environment is noted. People share a destiny with the universe and are responsible for mutual transformations. Quoting Zohar (1990) and other authors who look at persons in relation to a purposeful universe, Roy has made the foci of assumptions for the 21st century mutual complex person and environment self-organization and a meaningful destiny of convergence of the universe, persons, and environment in what can be considered a supreme being or God (see Chapter 2).

Contemporary social changes affect the focusing self. Two trends in particular that the self deals with in creating a focusing self are the mobility of society and the information age. We have noted that the reactions of others are important to the developing self. There was a time when people may have lived in the same town or city over a lifetime. Now it is more common that people will move more frequently. With multiple changes in living situations and in jobs, the network of people that one deals with also changes. Extensive changes in human communication have occurred using digital technology. Poster (2006) noted that the digital self that participates in Internet public spheres is different from the self speaking to another person in a classroom or coffeehouse. In particular, he proposes that "Digital information machines construct subjects who are present only through their textual, aural, and visual uploads" (Poster, p. 41). Rather than a self over which the individual has some influence, Poster views the digital self as a subject, or output consequence of electronic media. Both of these changes highlight the importance of the internal value system of the focusing self. The person uses the focusing self process to maintain consistency and unity in the midst of many changes in one's environment including changing relationships and developing technology.

COMPENSATORY ADAPTIVE PROCESSES

The self-concept mode has many compensatory processes, based on the richness and flexibility of personal strengths within each individual. As defined earlier in this book, compensatory processes represent the adaptation level at which the cognator and regulator have been activated by a challenge to the integrated life processes. Two compensatory processes selected for discussion are grieving and cognitive dissonance.

Grieving

Grief recovery has been called a neglected growth process. Loss is a significant component of growth at any age. Bowlby (1969) identified the most substantial loss of childhood as separation from the mother. Birth necessitates finality to the physical oneness with mother. The way the pivotal loss of symbiosis with mother is handled by the infant and the caregiver is thought to influence the personality of the individual. Loss begins in infancy but is a common theme throughout all stages of human development. When a loss occurs, or a person considers what it means to face death, the cognator and regulator are activated. The use of coping processes provides the possibility of reaching higher levels of adaptation and person and environment transcendence. From this perspective, grieving losses and life closure are considered compensatory processes of adaptation. Common losses occur in the four adaptive modes. These include loss of physical function; loss of sense of self, including facing death; loss of role function; and loss of interpersonal relationships. Losses may be actual or potential. The series of emotional responses that occur following the perception or anticipation of a loss is grief. In the broadest sense, grieving can be applied to any situation in which loss is involved. When the compensatory process of dealing with loss is not successful, problems of compromised adaptation, such as body image disturbance, powerlessness, or unresolved loss, may result.

Life is filled with losses and grieving is a natural response. Grieving is not a pathologic process, but rather can bring healing and a higher level of personal integrity and transformation. In the literature, the process of grieving is viewed as consisting of four stages.

1. Shock and disbelief
2. Apprehending the loss
3. Attempting to deal with the loss
4. Final restitution and resolution

The nurse's role in helping the person effectively use this compensatory process is a significant part of nursing care. Table 14–1 outlines the stages of grieving a loss and lists samples of expected behaviors and common stimuli, and common nursing approaches at each stage are discussed as part of the nursing process. The nurse can be helpful to the grieving person through sensitivity to the meaning of the situation for the individual, purposeful interviewing, and validating hunches from observation and theory.

As discussed in relation to the developing self process, the work of mastering one stage of development prepares the ground for the work of the next stage. The tasks of a stage are never achieved completely. Until the end, life affords opportunities to resolve developmental

TABLE 14–1 Stages of Grieving a Loss

Expected Behaviors	Common Stimuli	Common Nursing Approaches

Stage 1: Shock and Disbelief (lasts minutes to days)
 	
Statements indicating fact of the loss has not been apprehended: "Oh, I can't believe it's true"
 	
Verbal report of stunned numb feeling
 	
Blank facial expression
 	
Sitting motionless and dazed
 	
Little or no attention to the surroundings
 	
Automatic carrying out of routine
 	
Verbal expression of intellectual acceptance and making plans for dealing with the loss
 	
Inability to look at part of the body affected by the loss
	Focal
	    Need to protect self from being overwhelmed by painful feelings
	Contextual
	    Suddenness of the news of the loss
	Residual
	    Other circumstances surrounding the loss, e.g., physical illness, need to support others affected by the loss
		Be present, use touch to communicate caring and presence
		
		Tell the person you are there to help
		
		Refrain from making judgments
		
		Provide for privacy
		
		Allow denial, don't agree or refute it
		
		Ask the person to talk about current feelings
		
		Provide for contact with significant others
		
		Provide for physiologic needs

Stage 2: Apprehending the Loss
Sighing
Verbal report of slight sense of unreality
Verbal report of intense subjective distress
Expression of anger at the circumstances and desire not to be bothered
Crying
Behaviors of fear and anxiety
Report of loss of strength
Report of emptiness in chest or epigastrium
Report of tightness in throat
Appetite changes
Weight loss
Report of inability to sleep
Inability to engage in organized activity
Report of a sense of emotional distance from others
Feeling of emptiness
Searching for lost object
	Focal
	    Mention or thought of the lost object
	Contextual
	    Presence of other people
	    Importance of the lost object
	    Degree of ambivalence toward the lost object
	    Ability to tolerate and express painful feelings
	    Response of significant others
	Residual
	    Cultural norms of how to grieve
		Be present and listen
		Gently remind person of reality
		Provide for privacy
		Tell the person the responses of this stage are normal and expected
		Reflect, paraphrase, use silence to encourage expression of feelings
		Use all the above approaches with significant others
		Notify clergy of person's choice

TABLE 14–1 (*continued*)

Expected Behaviors	Common Stimuli	Common Nursing Approaches
Beginning ability to talk about the reality of loss: "I guess it's really happening" Beginning ability to look at and touch the part of the body affected by loss		
Stage 3: Attempting to Deal With the Loss (The main work occurs intrapsychically and takes months to years.) Report of preoccupation with lost object or function Waves of sadness and crying Feelings of despair Talk about the lost object and experiences with it prior to the loss Expression of feelings of loss of intactness and wholeness of self Report of altered body sensations, e.g., itching feeling in a leg that has been amputated Development of physical illness Carrying out of self-care routine, looking at and touching the affected part of the body	Focal 　Contemplation of future without the lost object Contextual 　Importance of the lost object 　Degree of ambivalence toward the lost object 　Spiritual beliefs 　Number of and degree of resolution of past losses 　Degree of preparation for the loss 　Physical and psychological health of the person 　Ability to tolerate and express painful feelings 　Amount of guilt felt 　Age of the person Residual 　Cultural prescription of how to grieve 　Contemplation of the unexpected experience of grief itself	Be present and listen Tell person it is normal to feel sorrow, guilt, anger, helplessness Use open-ended questions to elicit expression of feelings Refrain from making judgments Ask the person to talk about the meaning of the lost object Ask person to talk about past losses—how it felt, what helped, how it was resolved Remind person it takes time to go through grieving process Use touch to communicate presence and caring Ask person about spiritual beliefs Involve clergy person as requested by person Apply above approaches to significant others
Stage 4: Final Restitution and Resolution Expression of interest in alternatives for the lost object or function Ability to talk about the loss experience without bitterness and guilt	Focal 　Level of success or completion of previous stages of grief Contextual 　All stimuli listed above Residual 　All stimuli listed above	Active listening techniques Help person problem-solve how to form new patterns of functioning and relating Refrain from judging Point out person's strengths and gains

Source: Data drawn in part from three books on nursing diagnosis: Carpenito, L. (1985). *Handbook of nursing diagnosis.* Philadelphia: J. B. Lippincott; Gordon, M. (1985). *Manual of nursing diagnosis.* New York: McGraw-Hill; Kelly, M. A. (1985). *Nursing diagnosis source book.* E. Norwalk, CT: Appleton-Century-Crofts; and from Chapter 18 "Loss" by Marjorie H. Buck In *Introduction to nursing: An adaptation model* (2nd ed.) by Sister Callista Roy. Englewood Cliffs, NJ: Prentice-Hall, Inc., 1984, pp. 337–352.

issues at yet higher levels. Related to the process of grieving is the process that Dobratz (1984, 2004, 2005) has defined as life closure. The process of life closure is the ultimate opportunity to rework previous issues in the full development of the personal self. Life closure is a normal part of the life cycle. It is the process through which a person resolves the issue of the meaning of one's life and accepts the reality of eventual death. In Erikson's (1963) developmental stages, the crisis of the last stage is ego integrity versus despair. Ego integrity involves accepting one's life as it has been. Despair includes fear of death and the feeling that time is too short and that one's life should have been lived differently.

Beginning the process of life closure is often a response to the aging and death of parents. The person is forced to confront personal feelings about aging and death when interacting with parents in the last months of their lives. Parents are a strong link to the individual's past. Death of the parents marks the end of a segment of life and leaves the individual next in line for death. Death of siblings, spouse, or peers may also stimulate facing one's own death. The physical changes of aging can serve as stimuli for the process of life closure. The relatively constant adult physical self-image is challenged by changes in appearance, function, and stamina brought on by aging. Similarly, illness raises questions of a changing self and of personal mortality. Pain, disability, and chronic health issues in late middle age and the older years cause the person to stop and rethink his or her view of life, self, and the universe. Cultural views and the person's perception of aging and death also influence dealing with life closure. Robinson (1995) used the Roy Adaptation Model to explore the grief response and the variables that have an impact on it in 65 widows. She found that social support affected coping and seemed to decrease the total grief response.

The End-of-Life Nursing Education Consortium (ELNEC, 2002) identifies America as a death-denying society. This can mean not recognizing the need to express grief and to work through the pain of loss. Kübler-Ross (1969) and many succeeding researchers (Finucane, 2002) have found that dying people are overwhelmingly grateful to have someone listen to their thoughts and feelings. With an understanding of the assumptions of the Roy Adaptation Model, the nurse is prepared to assist people to reminisce about their lives and previous experiences and to recognize the meaningfulness of the pattern of their lives. The nurse confirms the person in assurance that life has pattern and meaning, that one is united with other people in the context of a meaningful universe. Further, in a spiritual sense, all persons and creation share a common destiny. Purposeful communication using reflecting, paraphrasing, open-ended questions, and active silence will promote an effective life review. The nurse will need to be comfortable with the subject of loss, death, and dying to help others achieve greater personal integrity in the processes of grief and life closure. Reading literature, attending classes and workshops, and sharing personal feelings with family and friends helps the nurse to be prepared to assist the person with grief and life closure and with finding meaning in loss and death. The nurse respects each individual and the unique process of grieving and life closure. The nurse takes cues from the person as to when it is time to enter into, and at times to continue, the process of grieving or of life closure. The nurse continually conveys a willingness to listen and provides help and support by making eye contact, sitting down, and reflecting comments from past conversations.

Cognitive Dissonance

Cognitive balance is a concept that has been used in many theories of self-concept. Cognitive dissonance (Festinger, 1962) is the term frequently used to indicate a particular process of cognitive balancing that occurs after a difficult decision is made. Decisions, by their nature, involve alternatives, doubt, ambivalence, and conflict. Perhaps more than one alternative is attractive to the individual. Dissonance is created by considering the various choices. For example, a high school senior may be presented with acceptance letters from two equally attrractive institutions of higher learning. She vacillates between accepting the first, as it is located closer to her family, or the second, where physical distance may present increased opportunity for independence. She discusses the situation with friends, family, and her school counselor. The longer the deliberation, the more ambivalence will be created, leading to a state of cognitive dissonance. When the alternatives are under consideration, the individual feels a mixture of negative and positive emotions related to different choices. The dissonance is a continuous source of tension, and the individual attempts to reduce it in a number of ways. For example, once the decision is made, there is a tendency to begin valuing the selected choice even more than before. Persons rely on this process in order to cope with the doubts and skepticism generated during the deliberation. The student may focus on the advantages offered by the college selected. This is more satisfying than emphasizing a difference of opinion among her family members about where to attend. Living with a decision is made easier by emphasizing the positive aspects of the choice.

COMPROMISED PROCESSES OF SELF-CONCEPT

According to the Roy Adaptation Model, when ineffective compensatory processes do not restore integration, compromised processes occur. In the self-concept mode, as in other modes, compromised processes result in adaptation problems. Adaptation problems or compromised processes are the third level of adaptation. Difficulties can occur in any or all of the processes of self-concept. Two examples of compromised processes within the individual are discussed here: ineffective sexual function and anxiety.

Ineffective Sexual Function

Ineffective sexual function, an adaptation problem of the physical self, is defined as sexual behavior that does not meet the person's goals or is antisocial. It may relate to physical or psychological factors. The term sexual dysfunction has come to mean more specific sexual health issues related to desire, arousal, or orgasm. In the physical self the person may demonstrate ineffective sexual function in one of two ways—verbalization of decreased sense of sexual self or aggressive sexual behavior. Decreased sense of sexual self is revealed by the person's comments. Several factors inherent in the experience of illness contribute to this compromised adaptation process. The pathophysiology of disease, medications, and particularly chemotherapy may directly affect the physiologic sexual response. Factors during hospitalization that affect the sense of sexual self include asexual hospital gowns, hospital routines, procedures that invade and assault the person's body, lack of privacy, and the interruption of the regular routine of work, hobbies, recreation, and social interactions.

Asking for personal information about the nurse, such as address, telephone number, and/or social and sexual life is considered aggressive sexual behavior. Attempts to touch the nurse's body, seductive comments and jokes, or unnecessary exposing of the genitals are other aggressive sexual behaviors. Such behaviors by the patient may be precipitated by discomfort with lack of privacy, uncertainty about the effects of illness or surgery on sexual functioning, and feelings of helplessness to control life in the face of illness. Lack of information and clarity about sexuality may also affect ineffective sexual function, both decreased sense of sexual self and the use of aggressive sexual behaviors.

Anxiety

One of the most common compromised processes related to the personal self is anxiety. Anxiety is the result of anything that threatens a person's sense of self-consistency and is defined as a painful uneasiness of mind due to a vague, nonspecific threat. A mild or brief moderate anxiety response can activate the person to confront and cope with a threatening event in an adaptive way. At this level, anxiety is considered a compensatory process. A recurrent, prolonged, or severe anxiety response, on the other hand, may hinder the individual's attempt to adapt to the environment. Anxiety as a compromised process uses needless energy and is ineffective in integrating one's experiences into the personal self-concept. A thorough assessment of behaviors and stimuli is made before the nursing judgment of anxiety as an adaptation problem can be reached.

The behaviors indicative of anxiety are complex, individual, and diverse. They often mimic behaviors of other adaptation problems. Some of the behavioral reactions that can be associated with anxiety are identified within each of the adaptive modes. In the physiologic mode the person may manifest any of the following: constant activity, sleep disturbances, cold clammy skin, alopecia, dry mouth, dilated pupils, voice tremors and pitch changes, trembling, difficulty concentrating, amenorrhea, difficulty breathing, tachycardia, palpitations, loss of appetite or overeating, nausea and vomiting, flatus, constipation or diarrhea, polyuria, and increased perspiration. Changes specific to self-concept mode components that may occur in anxiety include changes in sex drive and performance; disgust with one's body; decreased self-care and hygiene; sadness and crying; pseudo-cheerfulness; denying of feelings; inner preoccupation; negative self-talk; rumination about problems; angry outbursts; and talking of fear, apprehension, and worry. Effects of anxiety on the role function mode include inability to make decisions, difficulty doing simple tasks, struggling to meet responsibilities, and decreased interest in usual roles. In the interdependence mode, the anxious person often expresses feeling alone and isolated. In the anxious state, individuals may seek to be with others at all times, even to the point of requiring company in order to function.

The focal stimulus for anxious behaviors is the perceived threat. Common stimuli include experiences of loss, actual or anticipated; sudden changes in lifestyle, positive or negative; assault; invasive procedures; disease; unknown or fatal prognosis in illness; rapid or extreme changes in role function; disruptive family life; history of past anxiety states; unconscious conflict; unmet needs; and transmission of another person's anxiety to the individual.

When anxiety is at a compromised level, the nurse works with the person toward three general goals.

1. The person will verbalize feeling anxiety and acknowledge its interference with the ability to effectively meet other goals and needs.
2. The person will verbalize insight into the nature and source of the anxiety.
3. The person will demonstrate the ability to cope effectively with the anxiety.

How to develop specific goals for adaptation problems is discussed later as part of the nursing process.

NURSING PROCESS RELATED TO SELF-CONCEPT

Because the self-concept is central to the person, meeting needs in this mode is important for adaptation of the person, as well as for integrity of the other adaptive modes. An understanding of self-concept processes and related compensatory and compromised processes prepares the nurse for effective use of the nursing process. The nurse will complete first- and second-level assessment for the physical and personal aspects of the self-concept. Based on judgments about adaptation levels assessed, the next step of the nursing process is the diagnosis. Goals are then set with the patient, based on assessment and diagnoses, to select interventions and to evaluate the outcomes of care.

Assessment of Self-Concept Behavior

The components of the self-concept mode form the basis for behavioral assessment of psychic and spiritual integrity. As the nurse gradually gets to know the patient, there is evidence of behaviors that indicate the self processes for both the physical and personal self. Self-concept behavior is manifest through the person's appearance such as grooming, posture, and facial expression. Further statements the person makes about self are important. For example, a person may appear pale and drawn and make the comment, "I'm not feeling very well." Both appearance and statements are behaviors related to the component of the physical self, body sensation. Similarly, a person who has brought a cross or other religious symbol into the hospital is telling something about the moral-ethical-spiritual self.

At times, the nurse makes a purposeful assessment by questioning a person relative to self-concept. To do this effectively, the nurse provides a comfortable and trusting environment for the person. In the nursing assessment of self-concept the person is asked to share some intimate feelings about self. The nurse uses sensitive awareness and observation, interviewing, interaction, and physical assessment skills to assess behaviors in each component of the self-concept mode. In considering assessment of the developing self process, assessment of the physical self is considered most relevant and will be described.

PHYSICAL SELF   Assessment of the person's physical self is of primary importance in the promotion of adaptation. Adaptation problems in the area of the self-concept mode, and specifically the physical self component, may interfere with the person's ability to heal and to do what is necessary to maintain and promote health. In addressing the physical self with the patient, it is important that the nurse understand and be comfortable with a personal physical self and related body image, body sensation, and sexuality. Not only is an adaptive physical self required by the patient in dealing with other adaptation problems, it is a personal requirement for the nurse attempting to assist the patient toward effective adaptation in the self-concept mode. After providing privacy, the nurse meets the person's immediate needs. Confidentiality is discussed. The nurse tells the person who else, if anyone, will have access to the information. The patient may wish to keep certain aspects of the interview strictly between the nurse and self. The nurse tells the patient whether that is possible in advance and honors the agreement. The nurse does not impose judgments or stereotypes on the person receiving care. Good communication skills including open-ended questions, use of silence, and reflection are used. Questions are related to the individual's need for promoting health and are placed in the realm of common concern. For example, the nurse could say, "Many people are concerned about their sexual activity following colostomy surgery." Sexuality as a human experience needs to be explored, experienced, and shared. The person receiving care, however, is often hesitant to bring up the subject. The nurse has the responsibility to show a willingness to deal with issues of sexuality.

Body Sensations   The nurse assesses the infant or nonverbal person's body sensation component by observing or obtaining a report from the nurturing person of facial expressions, body posture, physical tensions, levels of relaxation, ease of feeding and eliminating, and depth of sleep. All human beings share sexual feelings as part of body sensations. The person experiences pleasurable sexual sensations from the time of birth, or possibly before. Human sexuality involves far more than the sex act and reproduction. Sexuality involves who and what we are as male and female, how we get that way, how we feel about it, and how we deal with each other about it. Dreams, fantasies, ideals, pleasure, and laughter are involved.

Once the young person has become fairly verbal, the nurse can add questions related to the assessment of body sensations. The nurse assesses the person's knowledge, needs, preferences, losses, and any effects of a medical condition or treatment in the area of sexuality. Examples of such questions are listed in Table 14–2. The nurse puts the questions into his or her own words. The person's developmental level, personal communication style, and culture are also taken into consideration. The nurse uses accurate terminology and checks with the person receiving care for mutual understanding of terms being used. The body sensation behaviors are the observations listed, as are the individual's responses to the questions. For example, the person may state, "I feel _____ (strong, weak, sexually responsive, faint, pained)." Even when the person does not make a direct statement, the nurse can validate hunches drawn from observation. For instance the nurse might say, "I see your brow is furrowed and your jaw is clenched. What are you feeling now?"

The importance of helping people identify their body sensations is noted in an example of research-based nursing intervention. A classic program of research showed that if the nurse prepares a patient for a procedure, such as introduction of a nasogastric tube, by describing the physical sensations that will be felt, the person is better able to cope with the procedure and cooperate with what needs to be done (Johnson & Leventhal, 1974).

Body Image   Body image behaviors, how the body looks to oneself and how one feels about how the body looks and functions, is assessed next. Part of body image is identifying the self as male or female. The Roy Adaptation Model deals with gender identification in the role function mode, primary role. Sex role identification is discussed here as related to the body image component of physical self-concept. The nurse makes direct observations of the person's posture, carriage, and level of personal hygiene and grooming. A complete physical assessment including pelvic, Pap, and breast examinations for women and genitourinary examination for men is included, when relevant and appropriate. The nurse may perform this examination or obtain the information from the written record. Detailed information on how to do a physical assessment can be found in textbooks on physical assessment. During the physical exam, the nurse has the opportunity to talk with the person about any concerns and questions and to teach about self-awareness and self-care. Based on these observations and the list of questions in Table 14–2 the nurse asks open-ended questions to identify body image behaviors. Taking into consideration the person's health care situation and cues from the person, the nurse decides whether or not to carry out a detailed assessment of sexuality. The person's responses as well as the nurse's observations are noted as body image behaviors. The identified behaviors can be judged

TABLE 14–2 Assessment of Behavior of the Physical Self Component

Characteristics	How to Elicit Behavior	How Behavior is Manifested
Body sensation: how the body feels to the self.	How do you feel physically?	I feel (strong, weak, tired, rested, etc.)
Sensations allow one to experience the body.	What physical sensations are you experiencing?	I feel (cold, warm, pained, sexy, etc.)
		Facial expression
		Muscular tension
Sensations allow one to experience the self as a sexual being.	How often do you have sexual feelings?[a]	I have sexual feelings (daily, weekly, never, etc.)
	How do you usually deal with your sexual feelings?	I usually (ignore them, masturbate, make love, etc.)
	How satisfied are you with your methods of dealing with your sexual feelings?	I am (fairly satisfied, not satisfied at all, etc.)
Body image: how one feels about the body; how one's body looks to the self.	Describe how you see yourself physically.	I am (slim, fat, well-built, tall, pretty, ugly, etc.)
Level of satisfaction with appearance.	What aspects of your physical appearance do you like?	I like (my height, my hair, my smile, etc.)
	What, if anything, would you like to change about your appearance?	I would like to change (my weight, my teeth, etc.)
	How do you feel about your appearance?	I feel (pretty good, upset since this surgery, etc.)

[a] When the person does not bring up the subject of sexuality, the nurse decides if specific questions are indicated. Questions are asked in the context of the person's health situation.

Source: Content is based in part on Cho, J. M. (1998). *Nursing process manual: Assessment tools for the Roy Adaptation Model.* Glendale, CA: Polaris Press.

to be adaptive or ineffective. Adaptive behaviors contribute to the person's psychic and spiritual integrity. Ineffective behaviors detract from or prevent formation and maintenance of the person's integrity.

PERSONAL SELF   In continuing assessment of the self-concept, the nurse looks at the components of the personal self. Personal self behaviors are expressed in verbalization of thoughts and feelings as well as in actions. An individual's view of self cannot be inferred from observing only a few behaviors. A thorough assessment is done before a nursing diagnosis can be made. To obtain the assessment data, as in assessing the physical self, the nurse creates an atmosphere in which the person feels safe to express thoughts and feelings. The attitude of the nurse does much to set the tone of safety or lack thereof. Since feelings are the subjective response of the individual, there are no good, bad, right, or wrong feelings. Laughing, crying, raging, shaking, and talking are expressions of feelings. The tension of unexpressed feelings is contained within the person. It is possible to feel very angry, for example, without raging or even talking about it. Such suppression of feelings, however, ties up psychic energy and interferes with the ability to do other things, such as think clearly and heal. In terms of the Roy model, this is cognator ineffectiveness. The nurse who conveys an accepting, nonjudgmental attitude can facilitate the expression of feelings and enhance cognator effectiveness. The nurse will be able to listen to the expression of feelings by the other person without imposing personal reactions.

In addition, the nurse needs to be in touch with her or his own personal feelings and to have an appropriate outlet for feelings. One's adaptation level in all modes affects the nurse-patient interaction. Another aspect in creating a safe environment for the person is the ability to state clearly and directly the purpose of an interaction. For example, the nurse might say, "I am going to spend some time talking with you about your thoughts and feelings about yourself. Since each person is different and responds differently to (giving birth, cancer, or a new health promotion program, for example), it is important for me to understand how you are feeling now. That way I can plan with you care based on your needs and wishes." The actual wording will vary for the individual situation. The time and place of an interview and other nurse–patient interactions will be planned appropriately. The person who is in pain, for example, cannot attend to questions relating to the personal self. If the person is in a room with other people present, it may not be possible to attend to a nursing interview. As noted, the immediate physiologic needs and the need for privacy must be met prior to beginning a personal self-assessment. Table 14–3 lists the components of personal self, how to elicit behaviors, and how the behaviors may be manifested. The nurse will find the words that are appropriate to the situation and cultural background. Open-ended questions invite dialogue. The nurse pays close attention to the patient's responses, eliciting clarification when necessary to understand his or her personal meanings ascribed to particular situations and experiences. The goal of sensitive communication is to elicit the patient's perspective as they describe it, and in their own words. Given that words hold personal meaning related to the personal self, each individual will rely on different expressions to relate their reality. Nonverbal behaviors of posture, facial expression, tone of voice, and eye contact are noted. The personal self is also reflected in planning, developing moral values, and making decisions consistent with the self. Once the personal self behaviors are identified, the nurse makes an initial judgment as to whether the behavior is effective or ineffective. Adaptive behaviors promote survival, growth, reproduction, mastery, and person and environment transformations, including transcendence. Another criterion for judging behaviors as adaptive or ineffective is the extent to which the behaviors lead to the realization of the individual's goals relative to the ideal self. Assessment of stimuli is the next step in the nursing process.

Assessment of Stimuli

Identifying the influencing factors, or stimuli, related to the self-concept is important to planning nursing care. The nurse needs to know what is affecting the person as an individual self. It is the individual person with whom she will plan care. The processes of developing self, perceiving self, and focusing self, as discussed, provide the basis for factors to be included in the second level of assessment. The stimuli influencing self-concept have been grouped into 10 general categories. The order in which the categories are assessed and the type of data collected will vary according to the individual situation. For a young child,

TABLE 14–3 Assessment of Behavior of the Personal Self Component

Characteristics	How to Elicit Behavior	How Behavior is Manifested
Self-consistency: personality traits; how one views self in relation to actual performance or response to situation.	How would you describe yourself as a person? What are your personal characteristics?	I am (a smart person, a person of strong will, like a child, not worthwhile, etc.)
Self-ideal: what one would like to be or do related to what one is capable of being or doing.	What are your aspirations for yourself as a person? What would you change about yourself if you could?	I would like to be (someone who makes a difference, famous, a strong person, etc.) I would change (how I lose my temper, my inability to do math, my sense of not belonging anywhere, etc.)
Moral-ethical-spiritual self: one's sense of self in relation to one's sacred, ethical beliefs; how self is viewed in relation to one's value system, beliefs about "rightness" or "wrongness"; evaluator of "who I am."	How would you describe your spiritual beliefs? How do your spiritual beliefs affect your view of self? How do you measure up to your own standards of right living? How do you evaluate yourself?	I believe in (God, a higher being, natural order, etc.) I go to (church, AA meetings, the mountains, etc.) I like to (read certain books, meditate, practice yoga, etc.) I am (pretty consistent, a long way from doing as I believe, etc.) I tend to be (hard on myself, patient with myself, pretty happy with myself, etc.)

Source: Based on Cho, J. M. (1998). *Nursing process manual: Assessment tools for the Roy Adaptation model.* Glendale, CA: Polaris Press.

observations of interactions with the environment and consistency of behavior may be used more frequently than interview questions on one's goals or values, for example.

PHYSICAL DEVELOPMENT   Age and degree of physical development affect self-concept as abilities change and control of bodily functions change. All the normal changes of growth and development are stimuli for both the physical self and personal self behaviors. The human body is continually changing, and these changes require alterations in the sense of physical self. As the nervous system matures, the infant learns to roll over, sit, crawl, stand, and walk. Further growth leads to the physical changes of puberty. Continuing development brings on the initially subtle and then more evident changes of aging. All these events affect the person's concept of self. The nurse is aware of normal growth and development theory and applies it when identifying physical self stimuli and understanding how these stimuli affect the personal self.

In addition, physiologic behaviors are reviewed. These provide important stimuli for the physical self component of the self-concept mode. For example, the person's height, weight, color and distribution of hair, muscular strength, skin condition, ability to control bodily functions, and neurologic function all influence how the person perceives and feels about the body. Eventually these factors will also influence the person's self ideal, that is, what goals one sets for self. The nurse, using the Adaptation Model, completes the physiologic mode assessment using direct observation, physical assessment skills, and review of the written record. The information gained in assessment is useful in understanding the stimuli, or factors, affecting the self-concept.

STAGES OF COGNITIVE AND MORAL DEVELOPMENT Models of life-span development emphasize the role of the individual as a participant and partner in the developmental process throughout life. Cognitive development involves many interacting factors, for example, biologic aspects that include genetic makeup and maturation. In addition, environmental factors, including social interaction, learning, and culture are involved. All these factors interact and can affect cognitive development throughout the life span. Although Piaget's (1954) model was developed in studying children, it can be useful in describing stages of cognitive development that are relevant to understanding the developing self-concept, both physical and personal. Sensorimotor, preoperational, concrete, and abstract stages of thinking can be assessed by the nurse in both adults and children. A simple task to differentiate between concrete versus abstract reasoning is to draw a bottle that is tilted toward one side and half filled with water. To be classified as using abstract reasoning, the person must be able to explain that the water is drawn level with the floor because of gravity's pull on the water. The level of thinking greatly affects how one perceives the self in the world.

Kohlberg (1981) and Gilligan (1982) provide insights into assessing how the person makes moral judgments. The nurse can be aware of statements that show what is important to the person. The nurse can also help the person clarify the values behind a decision that is faced. Assessing what the person believes to be right in the situation and how they define what is right is significant in understanding the person.

MATURATIONAL CRISIS As noted, Erikson (1963) described eight psychosocial stages of development human beings go through from birth to death in old age. Likewise, Neugarten (1979) focused on the maturational tasks of the second half of life. Each stage challenges the individual to resolve a maturational crisis. A person moves through the stages at an individual rate. No crisis is ever completely resolved. As life events unfold, the person has the opportunity to rework each crisis. The nurse uses knowledge from theories, such as Erikson's and Neugarten's, and direct questions to assess this category of stimuli affecting the developing self.

INTERACTIONS AND TRANSACTION BETWEEN PERSON AND ENVIRONMENT Interactions of individuals with the environment is a key concept of nursing and of the Roy Adaptation Model in particular. There are several levels of interactions and transaction that are major stimuli for the self-concept mode. There is the significant interaction with primary caregivers, the reactions of others, confirmation of self from social interaction, as well as the higher levels of transactions with the broader environment.

The formation and maintenance of a sense of physical self is influenced profoundly by the *reactions of primary caregivers*. The infant gains information about self through body sensations (Montagu, 1986). Perception of touch from the nurturing person(s) as gentle, warm, and physically supportive leads to a sense of security in the infant. Consistent responses by the caregivers to the child's sensations of hunger and discomfort of position, need for touch, fatigue, and wet or dirty diapers also leads to a sense of security within the body. The nurse observes interactions between the young person and the primary caregiver when possible to gain information in this category. Questions are used to gather this earlier information from persons who are adults. For example, the nurse might ask, "What do you know about how your parents reacted to you when you were a baby?" An overweight, unemployed female adult stated, "My father never held me during my first year of life. Mother told me he was so disappointed that I wasn't a boy that he could hardly look at me. He still calls me Sam, never Samantha."

The young child's sense of self is influenced by the caregivers providing names and values to the parts, sensations, and functions of the body. Mothers play the age-old game of pointing and naming body parts with the growing infant. Comments such as "Is your nasty gut hurting you again?" or "Are you feeling pressure in your gut? Maybe you will go to the bathroom soon," help shape how the person feels about body sensations and functions. Studies have shown that physiologic arousal is the same for fear, joy, anger, and emotional attraction. It has been suggested that the interpretation of these sensations as distinct feelings of fear, joy, anger, or emotional attraction is due to input provided by others (Kleinke, 1978). The values and feelings the primary caregivers have about their own body sensations and images are communicated to the child. Some people are able to talk openly and frankly about their bodily functions. Other people talk about them indirectly using euphemisms. Some people simply never talk about physical sensations and functions. The child's developing sense of physical self is influenced by the verbal and nonverbal—what is said as well as what is not said—messages of caregivers. The nurse gathers data in this category by direct observation when possible. Questions also are used to gather these data from the person and significant others.

The person experiences *reactions of others* related to having certain physical characteristics, abilities, and sensations, as well as other characteristics of the self. These reactions strongly influence the formation of physical self behaviors. From the moment of birth and even before, parents apply societal standards to the individual. The pregnant woman might say, "I'm glad I know it's a boy, but he kicks so hard, I know he's going to be aggressive." Comments at the delivery of a newborn might include statements such as, "Too bad you had another girl," or "He's so tiny he'll never make a football player." Cultural perspectives are part of these reactions. Each society and culture values certain physical attributes. The values are communicated by others' reactions, but also by way of myths, legends, fairy tales, books, television, movies, magazines, and advertising. The individual who inherits desirable physical characteristics is rewarded while the person who does not lacks rewards and often receives negative input. The North American culture values the young, slim, firm, well-proportioned female body and the tall, muscular, male body. The ideal is infrequently the reality. It is clear that personal self is affected by reactions to the physical self.

Further, a primary view of the human body in Western societies for a long time has been that of an object, a machine which should perform to the "owner's" wishes. A level of mistrust, annoyance, and ignorance about bodily functions has pervaded the culture. Advertising promises that taking certain over-the-counter drugs will let the individual complete a full day's activities despite a cold or flu. Professional athletes take drugs to kill the pain of injury and continue playing. The message is, "Don't feel sick and you won't be sick," in fact, "Don't feel." An earlier study by Amman-Gainotti (1986) demonstrated the lack of knowledge about body structure and function. This study found that many adolescent girls do not know the source of menstrual blood. Western culture has long taught individuals to be cut off from true awareness and understanding of their own body sensations and functions (Johnson, 1983). Recently, there has been a movement in health promotion to unite body, mind, and spirit and to be aware of the physical self. In light of this mixed cultural situation, the nurse is very sensitive and patient when interviewing the person concerning physical self stimuli as well as behaviors. The person may have limited ability to discuss physical self data due to lack of information. The interview may be a beginning experience of someone truly wanting to know how the body feels and is integrated into who one is as a person.

Also from a cultural perspective, reflected by reactions of others, religious groups teach certain attitudes about body image, function, and sexuality. For example, masturbation, abortion, and homosexuality are not accepted in the religious teachings of the Orthodox Jews, Roman Catholics, and traditional Protestants. In some traditions, including Middle Eastern, intercourse is reserved only for marriage. Some liberal branches of Protestant religions may sanction any activity or behavior that is considered healthy and does not harm another person. The nurse is aware of the keen impact of reactions of others and of cultural norms, including religion, on the self and uses open-ended questions to obtain information from the individual about how such experiences have influenced that person's sense of physical self.

The self-concept is influenced by *confirmation through social interaction*. This occurs particularly as the person observes the reactions of others. As identified earlier, the work of the interactionist theorists Cooley, Mead, and Sullivan forms the basis of this stimulus. In essence, these theories state that individuals start to think of self in the ways in which they perceive that others view them. For example, the person who is repeatedly told, "You are thoughtless of others," may incorporate a sense of being a selfish person. In the same way, if the person holds this view, new situations will be interpreted in a way that confirms this concept of self. If the nurse comments that the patient in the next bed is very ill, a person with this background of social interactions may immediately believe that he or she has been disturbing the patient. Once a person reaches adulthood, the messages significant others have given regarding a person's personal value have been incorporated into the self-concept.

Interviewing the individual can provide data on all the interactions that are stimuli influencing the person's self-concept. Again, family members have a significant impact on the formation and confirmation of self-concept. The nurse assesses the family's influence on the person's self-concept in this category. Sample questions are: Who are the family members? What is the family's value of the individual? Who does the person receiving care feel particularly close to in the family? Does the person get the same message from all family members? Does the person believe that confirmations of self are realistic or sometimes could be misinterpretations? Is the person able to accept new data of positive interpretations of self? Not all of these data will be available or relevant for every patient. When possible, the nurse will also interview any significant others who are available and will observe the patient's social interactions.

Transaction with the broad environment is another stimulus influencing self-concept. Looking to the future, Roy has redefined adaptation as the process and outcome whereby the thinking and feeling person uses conscious awareness and choice to create human and environmental integration. Environment is defined as the sum total of the conditions, circumstances, and influences that surround and affect the development and functioning of the person. Therefore, the broad environment is a stimulus to the self-concept. A further feature of the complexity of the person's interaction with the environment is that there is a mutuality of influence. The person affects the environment and at the same time the environment affects the person. The particular feature of person and environment interaction as a stimulus to self-concept raises it to a new concept, that of transaction. Transaction occurs when the person and environment influence each other. Interaction means to act upon each other. Transaction adds the notion that both are changed in the process, and integration and mutual transformation are possible. Given these processes of interaction with and transaction of environment by the individual, a set of conditions and circumstances is created that is unique to that person. People are, in their essential makeup, composed of the same "stuff" and held together by the same dynamics as those that account for everything else in the universe. Swimme and Berry (1992) noted that, "To be is to be related, for relationship is the essence of existence.... Nothing is itself without everything else" (p. 77). Nurses seek to understand the particular environment in which the patient is situated, in order to develop a meaningful plan of care.

An example of how nurses include the environment in assessment is given by additions that Carnevalli and Thomas (1993) made to the definition of nursing diagnoses. The authors expand the focus from human responses to include the situation, the context surrounding the person, and the responses. In using the Roy model to assess the effect of transaction between person and environment, the nurse observes how the person and environment change each other and whether the pattern leads toward integration. On the other hand, the nurse notes whether or not the person finds the environment toxic to self and, in turn, is toxic to the environment. Data suggest that environmental stability plays an important role in self-concept stability (Demo, 1992). Newman (1994) noted that it is the pattern of our lives (transactions of person and environment) that identifies us, not the substance that goes into making up that pattern. Identifying patterns of the whole and helping people to deal with them is important developing knowledge in nursing. Both nurse-scholars, including Roy and Newman, and nurses in practice will contribute to this knowledge by insightful observations of patients in their life experiences.

SELF-SCHEMA Over time a perception of self results from the individual's interpretation of all the various interactions with others and the environment. According to Coombs and Snygg (1959), a core or inner cell of self-concept is formed of perceptions about self that are the most vital, fundamental aspects of the individual. The interactions with primary caregivers, and rewards, sanctions, and responses of others within the culture are internalized. Attempts to organize, summarize, or explain one's own behavior in a particular domain result in development of cognitive structures about the self that are called self-schema. Self-schema are cognitive generalizations about the self that organize and guide the processing of the self-related information contained in the individual's social environment. They represent the way the self has been differentiated, and as individuals have repeated experiences of a certain type, their schema become increasingly resistant to inconsistent or contradictory information. This issue is discussed later in this chapter as the tendency to self-consistency. If a person has a developed self-schema, the person can make judgments about self with relative ease. For example the person may say, "I know I can handle the diet changes needed for my health." The individual may be able to report behavioral evidence about a given domain such as to identify a body image characteristic. The person can also anticipate future behavior in a given situation. For example, she or he may say, "I am the kind of person who bounces back fairly quickly; this surgery won't keep me down." The nurse asks questions to elicit the person's perception of self and observes whether or not the data reflect a self-schema.

VALUE OF SELF ATTRIBUTES AND SELF-ESTEEM   As noted, current models of self-worth describe that the impact of events is contingent upon how the person perceives the relevance to what they value about self (Crocker & Park, 2003). The person's perception related to their self-ideal determines whether the situation will be a major stimulus or influencing factor. Contingency means that it depends on the perceived relevance of the events. If an event it highly relevant, it will have a greater impact on one's self-worth. The person's interpretation of the event in relation to what is important and to reaching one's goals determines the effect on self-esteem. Early work by Rosenberg (1979) discussed self-esteem as a motive. That is, self-esteem can be a stimulus to behavior. He noted that within the self-concept there are values or criteria used to assess different self-attributions. How one establishes the worth of personal attributes is part of the process of the focusing self. Elliott (1986) reported an empirical link between self-esteem and self-consistency among young people ages 8 to 19 years. Another study showed that how freshmen choose to spend their time was related to what was important to their self-worth before they entered college (Crocker et al., 2001). Self-evaluation generally becomes more favorable through the life span.

In earlier work on the Roy Adaptation Model, self-esteem has been defined as that pervasive aspect of the personal self component that relates to the worth or value the person holds about the self (Driever, 1976). Low self-esteem is a negative feeling of self-worth that handicaps a person's ability to adapt to the environment. The nurse may recognize many manifestations of low self-esteem including the following: withdrawal from others; decrease in spontaneous behavior; appearance of sadness, anxiety, or discouragement; feelings of isolation; inability to express or defend oneself; avoidance of situations of self-disclosure or notice; sensitivity to criticism; self-deprecation; denial of successes or accomplishments; rumination about problems; and seeing the self as a burden to others. Teaching the building of self-esteem in children is an important part of pediatric nursing. This teaching relates to the assessment done related to parent and infant attachment described above. Being aware of levels of self-esteem and their effect on the person is significant in all of clinical nursing practice.

PERCEPTUAL SELF-AWARENESS   The personal self is affected by how accurate the person is in knowing self. Thus perceptual self-awareness is a stimulus affecting the self-concept mode. As noted, the person's perceptual abilities are used to take in and interpret feedback of others. As one establishes a core sense of self and is clear about what is valued as part of the self, the perception of self can be more accurate. The nurse can use the image of the Johari window to assess her own and others' self-awareness. A self-aware person has a larger amount of information about self in the open pane of the window. There is a consistency of what one thinks about self and what others think about the person. A clear failure in perceptual self-awareness is the young woman with an eating disorder who weighs in at 88 pounds and stands 5 foot 6 inches tall and at the same time protests that her body is fat. The misperception of her physical self will affect all adaptive modes and seriously threaten her health and well-being. It is important for the person to have a hidden self, but to be aware of it and to know when and what they choose to disclose. If the person is acting out of early childhood memories without acknowledging them, then the lack of awareness may affect relationships. This can occur in a person with a history of child abuse who has difficulty establishing close relationships. The nurse can uncover issues that may be in the blind windowpane by noting discrepancies in reports from the individual and a family member's report. The patient recovering from a myocardial infarct may report that he has greatly increased his physical activity. However, the daughter may tell the nurse that her father only goes outside to pick up the newspaper in the morning. Other signs of a lack of self-awareness are lack of openness to criticism by being defensive, ambivalent, or rejecting input. The nurse examines how accurate self-awareness affects her own interactions and recognizes its affect on the behavior in the self-concept mode of patients.

COPING STRATEGIES AND CAPACITIES   Another category of stimuli the nurse will consider is the person's coping strategies. Coping strategies are defined as the person's habitual responses used to maintain adaptation. Coping strategies are the ways the person functions to maintain integrity in everyday life and in times of stress. Some of these are habitual and learned over time, and others may be developed in a new situation, based on general tendencies of the cognator and regulator. When assessing the physical self component, the nurse seeks information from the individual regarding usual practices for maintaining a positive sense of physical self. For example, many people do regular physical workouts. Some people have grooming routines such as hairdresser appointments that help maintain a positive sense of self. Eating a specific diet and taking certain nutritional supplements and vitamins may give the person a sense of well-being. Disruption of any of these and other routines might threaten the person's sense of physical self.

It is important to find out if the person has previously faced an experience similar to the current one and how that experience was dealt with. Data in this category are obtained by interviewing the person and significant others. A research instrument to measure coping strategies derived within the Roy model currently is being tested by Roy and colleagues. Research using the Roy Adaptation Model, discussed in Chapter 21, identifies some of the patterns of coping used by given patient populations. We noted the study by Robinson (1995) who used the Roy Adaptation Model to explore the grief response in 65 widows. A major finding was that stimuli and coping response explained 18% of variance in grief response. In other words, assessing stimuli and the person's coping can help the nurse predict how the widow will handle the grief of loss of husband.

STRIVING FOR UNITY OR INTEGRITY   Theorists who discuss the importance of self-consistency postulate a striving for unity or integrity (Elliott, 1986; Lecky, 1961). The striving for unity or integrity may be an innate human quality that affects adaptation in the self-concept mode as well as in the other adaptive modes. Through a consistent striving for self-organization, the person avoids imbalance and discomfort. Identifying the need for balance of the inner self as related to health is reflected in many traditions of both Eastern and Western healing.

CONSCIOUSNESS OF PERSON AND ENVIRONMENT MEANINGS   The person uses thinking and feeling to move from awareness of self to higher consciousness and meaning. Consciousness of person and environment meanings is an element of person and environment integration. Which personal characteristics are valued is determined in part by cultural and social norms. Race, sex, class, religion, and other societal discriminations affect the individual's concept of self. The nurse assesses the person's awareness of what significant people in his or her life expect, what the individual values as expected of her or him, and how these compare with social values and the current situation. The nurse may discover factors influencing changes in the person's current sense of self as different from the original ideal self. The situation of illness itself will be a stimulus for changes in both the physical and personal self, especially self-consistency and self-ideal. Helping the person find new meaning in an altered physical or personal self may be a focus for nursing care.

In considering second-level assessment, the stimuli influencing behavior, the nurse is aware that there are other factors that influence an individual's self-concept. Behaviors in the other three adaptive modes can serve as stimuli for self-concept behaviors. As the nurse interviews and interacts with the person receiving care, data may arise that do not fit in the specified 10 categories of stimuli but which do influence the person's physical or personal self. These additional data are included in the assessment as well and used to plan nursing interventions. When obtaining stimuli assessment data, the nurse refers back to the information obtained in the behavioral assessment as much as possible. For example, the nurse might say, "You mentioned earlier that you feel you are a strong and capable person (self-consistency behavior). How have people that you interact with regularly helped you feel that way about yourself?" Such a question will probably elicit stimuli assessment data under the category confirmation through social interaction. The nurse phrases the questions specifically to help keep the person focused on the current situation. In this way the nurse obtains the data needed to plan nursing interventions. Influencing factors contribute to effective adaptation or may exert an influence toward ineffective adaptation. It may be helpful to identify the effect that each stimulus has on the person. The benefit of doing so is evident in the step of planning interventions. During the intervention phase, stimuli that are making a positive contribution will be maintained and enhanced, and those that are not will be altered or eliminated when possible.

Nursing Diagnosis

Throughout the nursing process, the nurse is aware that the individual is involved whenever possible. When the person is an active participant in each step of the nursing process, then meaningful involvement with carrying out the plan is more likely. A collaborative process makes it possible for the plan to be supported by the person in need and then the plan can be effective in achieving the planned outcomes. The step of nursing diagnoses associated with the self-concept mode is done in the same way as in the other modes. One method involves the statement of behaviors together with the influencing stimuli; another method makes use of summary labels. Thus, the nurse first makes a careful assessment of behaviors and stimuli. In assessing factors influencing self-concept, regulator and cognator effectiveness in initiating compensatory processes is considered. The presence of compromised processes of adaptation becomes a nursing priority. Based on thorough first- and second-level assessment, the nurse formulates nursing diagnoses, sets goals, selects interventions, and evaluates care.

Throughout this section on planning nursing care, we will return to the case study of the Robles family from Chapter 4. The 2-year-old child who is a quadriplegic has been home from acute care and rehabilitation for 6 months. The house renovations have worked well and the maternal grandmother and two cousins are still involved in helping with home care. Mrs. Robles has for the past few weeks become concerned about her two sons. Anthony is now 7 years old and seems to be acting out at school because of his mother's time spent with Sylvia, the little sister who requires her care 8 hours a day. Luca is almost 4 years old and has become withdrawn. The extended family members are blaming Mrs. Robles for neglecting her sons. Mr. Robles wants to be supportive but knows that the family's financial status depends on him focusing on his work. Mrs. Robles finds the situation filled with challenges and conflict. She has contacted a trusted nurse to express her frustrations. In particular she feels terrible because she was sure she could make this work for her family. She highly values her role as mother. For several weeks she has not been sleeping well and has felt a general lack of energy. She is also beginning to doubt her capabilities as a caregiver and mother. She states, "Every day looks gray and gloomy," "I don't enjoy anything anymore," and "I know I am not doing a good job with any of my children." From the beginning she was fully committed to the values and goals of the plan to keep the injured child within the family. The problematic situation with Sylvia's brothers has brought her to tears. She feels she cannot do anything right. She asks the nurse, "What should I do?"

As noted, development of nursing diagnoses associated with self-concept is accomplished in the same way as in the other adaptive modes. One method involves the statement of the behaviors together with the influencing stimuli; another method makes use of summary labels. Nursing diagnoses may reflect either adaptive or ineffective behaviors. In the situation of Mrs. Robles, a sample adaptive nursing diagnosis states, "Help-seeking behaviors, that is, a coping strategy to deal with threats to self, arising from a positive relationship with the nurse." The behavior of request for help is influenced by a previous and ongoing value of her role of mother and commitment to keep the family together.

In the case of ineffective behaviors, a multitude of nursing diagnoses may result. As the self-concept mode is closely interrelated with the other modes, a disturbance in one is likely to precipitate disturbances in others. For example, for Mrs. Robles, a diagnosis might be "Feelings of insecurity and worthlessness due to behavior problems of her sons in dissonance with her value of being a good mother." The relationship between the individual and the parts of the relational environment is evident in this diagnosis.

It is also possible to construct a nursing diagnosis using a summary label that captures a cluster of behaviors. This method is used by experienced nurses to communicate significant amounts of information in one phrase. As identified in Chapter 3, there are a number of indicators of positive self-concept adaptation identified as summary labels in the Roy Adaptation Model. Indicators for the physical self include positive body image, effective sexual function, psychic integrity with physical growth, adequate compensation for bodily changes, effective coping strategies for loss, and effective process of life closure. For the personal self, the indicators are stable pattern of self-consistency, effective integration of self-ideal, effective processes of moral-ethical-spiritual growth, functional self-esteem, and effective coping strategies for threats to self. Likewise, commonly recurring adaptation problems are identified: for the physical self—body image disturbance, ineffective sexual function, rape trauma syndrome, and unresolved loss; and for the personal self—anxiety, powerlessness, guilt, and low self-esteem.

Use of a summary label when more than one mode is affected by the same stimulus is often an effective way of communicating a cluster of behaviors. For example, low self esteem might be such a diagnosis. One word captures a multitude of behaviors and stimuli. The diagnosis statement could be, "low self esteem due to inadequacy of mothering role." In Table 14–4, the Roy model nursing diagnostic categories for integrated processes of self-concept are shown in relation to nursing diagnosis labels approved by the North American Nursing Diagnosis Association (NANDA International, 2007). Once the nursing diagnoses have been stated, the nurse proceeds to the next step in the process of planning care, which is goal setting.

Goal Setting

Each step of the nursing process focuses on the individual's behavior, the stimuli influencing that behavior, or both. With the nursing diagnosis, the statement developed included the behaviors and stimuli. With the goal-setting step, the focus is on behavior. Each goal identifies a behavior

TABLE 14–4 Nursing Diagnostic Categories for Self-Concept Mode for the Individual

Indicators of Adaptation	Common Adaptation Problems	NANDA Diagnostic Labels
• Positive Body Image • Effective sexual function • Psychic integrity with physical growth • Adequate compensation for bodily changes • Effective coping strategies for loss • Effective process of life closure • Stable pattern of self-consistency • Effective integration of self ideal • Effective processes of moral-ethical-spiritual growth • Functional self-esteem • Effective coping strategies for threats to self	• Body image disturbance • Sexual ineffectiveness • Rape trauma syndrome • Unresolved loss • Anxiety • Powerlessness • Guilt • Low self-esteem	• Disturbed personal identity • Powerlessness • Risk for powerlessness • Hopelessness • Defensive coping • Ineffective denial • Grieving • Complicated grieving • Risk for complicated grieving • Post-trauma syndrome • Risk for post-trauma syndrome • Rape-trauma syndrome • Rape-trauma syndrome; compound reaction • Relocation stress syndrome • Risk for relocation stress syndrome • Self-mutilation • Risk for self-mutilation • Risk for suicide • Risk for self-directed violence • Anxiety • Death anxiety • Fear • Chronic sorrow • Readiness for enhanced hope • Disturbed body image • Chronic low self esteem • Situational low self-esteem • Readiness for enhanced self-concept • Readiness for enhanced power • Risk for compromised human dignity • Spiritual distress • Risk for spiritual distress • Readiness for enhanced spiritual well-being • Moral distress

that is to be addressed. Many self-concept problems have a chronic as well as an acute phase. Thus, the goal-setting process includes both long- and short-term goals, each of which states the behavior of focus, the change expected, and the time frame in which the goal is to be achieved.

The following statement provides an example of a possible goal for the situation of Mrs. Robles: "Within 2 weeks, Mrs. Robles will voice enhanced confidence in her capabilities and self-worth." In order to be effective in guiding the progress, goals must be established in collaboration with the person involved. As with each step of the nursing process, the individuals, where possible, must be active participants to ensure that accurate and relevant information is obtained, that it is interpreted appropriately into the diagnoses, and that achievable and relevant goals are established. This is the only way that interventions can be determined that will assist in achieving psychic and spiritual integrity for the individual. A long-term goal may be that "Within 3 months, Mrs. Robles will express pride in her ability to be a good mother to all three children."

After formulating goals, the nurse proceeds to the identification of nursing interventions. This is the next step of the nursing process as described by the Roy Adaptation Model.

Intervention

The intervention step of the nursing process according to the Roy Adaptation Model focuses on the stimuli affecting the behavior identified in the goal-setting step. Thus, the intervention step is the management of stimuli that involves altering, increasing, decreasing, removing, or maintaining the stimuli. At the same time, the nurse may help the person to use effective coping strategies to strengthen compensatory processes. A review of the stimuli affecting adaptive life processes and the discussion of compensatory processes earlier in the chapter provides insight into specific interventions aimed at psychic and spiritual integrity for individuals.

In Mrs. Robles' situation, the focal stimulus appears to be the behavior of her sons. However, given the current situation, these may be expected behaviors for both Anthony and Luca. In general, such situations will require a series of changes. The situation in which Mrs. Robles finds herself is problematic, and the interventions must be directed at changing the situation. It may be possible to alter the hours that she cares for Sylvia so that she can be with the boys from the time they come home from school and day care until their bedtime.

Evaluation

Evaluation involves judging the effectiveness of the nursing interventions in relation to the person's adaptive behavior; that is, whether the behaviors stated in the goals have been achieved. The nursing interventions are effective if the behavior is in accordance with the stated goal. If the goal has not been achieved, the nurse identifies alternative interventions or approaches by reassessing the behavior and stimuli and continuing with the other steps of the nursing process.

The previously identified goal was stated as, "Within 2 weeks, Mrs. Robles will voice enhanced confidence in her capabilities and self-worth." Indications of progress toward this goal would be Mrs. Robles talking with the nurse about her increasing confidence in her abilities and that she knows she is someone who can reach her goals. She was able to involve both Sylvia and Anthony in planning for Luca's birthday party. She stated, "Everybody had such a good time. Even my mother and the others were saying what a great idea and how good it was to see the children happy. Sylvia picked out the colors of the balloons and she was so excited when they floated to the ceiling over the bed. Anthony and Luca were shrieking with joy that she was so happy. I did not know that I could feel like a good mother again this soon." The long-term goal will be evaluated by changes in Mrs. Robles' level of satisfaction with the care of her sons. The goal that "Within 3 months, Mrs. Robles will express pride in her ability to be a good mother to all three children" may also involve some evaluation of how each child is coping with having one child in the home needing constant care.

It is important to recognize that the nursing process and the six steps are ongoing, simultaneous, and overlapping. Although they have been separated and dealt with in an artificially linear way for discussion purposes, intervention is often occurring at the same time as first- and second-level assessment is occurring. Likewise, evaluation occurs on an ongoing basis, being held in mind even when nursing diagnoses are being established and as goals are being formulated. Competency in ease in applying the adaptation model comes with increasing knowledge and experience.

Summary

This chapter focused on the application of the Roy Adaptation Model to the self-concept mode. An overview of the three processes—developing self, perceiving self, and focusing self—associated with psychic and spiritual integrity for the individual was provided. Illustration of compensatory processes related to self-concept was included and examples of two compromised processes, ineffective sexual function and anxiety, were discussed. In addition, the nursing process was outlined. The assessment of behaviors and stimuli were described. Guidelines for formulating nursing diagnoses, goals, and interventions were explored, and evaluation of nursing care was described.

Exercises for Application

1. Select one of the life processes of the self-concept mode and outline the major events of your own life story in relation to this process.

2. Select one component of the physical or personal self subareas of self-concept and create questions that would be appropriate for assessment of stimuli related to that particular component.

Assessment of Understanding

QUESTIONS

1. The basic need underlying the self-concept mode of the individual person is _____.
   The two subareas of the self-concept mode are:

(a) _____, which includes two components, (1) _____ and (2) _____.

(b) _____, which includes (1) _____, (2) _____, and (3) _____.

2. Fill in the following table for assessment of behavior in the self-concept mode.

Characteristic to Assess	How to Elicit Behavior
a. Physical self	
1. Body sensation	1.1
	1.2
	1.3
	1.4
	1.5
2. Body image	2.1
	2.2
	2.3
	2.4
b. Personal self	
1. Self-consistency	1.1
2. Self-ideal	2.1
3. Moral-ethical-spiritual self	3.1

3. Select one of the 10 stimuli affecting self-concept behavior. Describe in your own words how that stimulus affects both the physical and personal self.
  (a) Stimulus _____
  (b) Affects on physical self _____
  (c) Affects on personal self _____

4. Which of the following could be considered compensatory processes related to self-concept?
  (a) The tendency of people to select mates who have similar physical characteristics
  (b) Integrating a loss into one's physical self-concept
  (c) Prolonged ambivalence about a decision
  (d) Considering mortality when a parent dies

5. Identify one compromised process of self-concept _____

SEE BOX 14–1 CASE STUDY FOR ASSESSMENT OF UNDERSTANDING: NURSING PROCESS IN SELF-CONCEPT MODE

6. Formulate a nursing diagnosis for the person in the case study using two methods.
  (a) _____
  (b) _____

7. Construct a goal for Stella.

8. Since interventions are focused on stimuli, what interventions could be used to alleviate the situation described, considering the following stimuli?

  (a) loss of significant other (male friend)
  (b) perceptions and self-schema
  (c) coping strategies

9. How would you evaluate achievement of the goal you established in item 7?

FEEDBACK

1. Psychic and spiritual integrity
  (a) physical self, (1) body image, (2) body sensation
  (b) personal self, (1) self-consistency, (2) self-ideal, (3) moral-ethical-spiritual self

2. (a) (1.1) How do you feel physically? (1.2) What physical sensations are you experiencing? (1.3) How often do you have [physical sensation]? (1.4) How do you usually deal with [physical sensation]? (1.5) How satisfied are you with your methods of dealing with your [physical sensation]? (2.1) Describe how you see yourself physically. (2.2) What aspects of your physical appearance do you like? (2.3) What, if anything, would you like to change about yourself? (2.4) How do you feel about your appearance?
  (b) (1.1) How would you describe yourself as a person? (2.1) What are your aspirations for yourself as a person? (3.1) How would you describe your spiritual beliefs?

3. (a) Residual stimuli (b) physical illness (c) cultural norms of how to grieve

4. b, d

5. (a) ineffective sexual function

BOX 14–1

Case Study for Assessment of Understanding: Nursing Process in Self-Concept Mode

Stella Martinez is a 20-year-old Mexican-American woman who is a junior nursing student at a university in the Midwest. She has been a good student and is delighted to be in her first clinical placement. However, during her second week, she was caring for a person with a gangrenous arm. She fainted and had to be taken to the student infirmary. Stella began to confide in a trusted colleague, a graduate nursing student whose clinical placement overlaps her own. Stella indicated to her colleague that she was concerned about not feeling well and how this was affecting her work.

Physically, Stella is tiny. She is 5 feet, 1 inch tall and wears size 6 clothing. When school started in the fall, she was proud to have diminished to a size 2. She admits that she has given up her meal pass since she doesn't eat that much. Stella prefers to do heavy exercise during the meal breaks. During her younger years, Stella's closely knit family were migrant workers who moved from Texas to California to Oregon with the crops. She has an older and a younger brother who were always very protective of her when they worked in the fields. At one point, the family received an unexpected inheritance from a grandmother in Mexico. This enabled the family to purchase a small adobe house in the Imperial Valley in California and to become involved in the dried fruit industry. Stella was able to stay in one location during high school and, during this time, she did very well in her studies. Stella realized that she wanted to be a nurse when she was helping her mother care for a dying relative. A high school counselor was helpful in her successful admission to a university nursing program. During the past summer, Stella went home from the university to spend time with her family. There, she began to date the older brother of a friend, a man 10 years her senior. Her family was not in favor of this relationship and told her that he was too old for her and that he would only break her heart. The man's sister warned Stella not to trust her brother. After about 6 weeks of an intense relationship, the man suddenly broke off any association with Stella. Within the week, he announced his engagement to another woman, a tall, slim Anglo-American of his own age. She was a person that he had been involved with while Stella was away at school, but who had been out of town in the early summer. In her hurt and disappointment, Stella returned to the Midwest early stating, "It's a small town back there and I don't want everyone looking at me." She joined the university gym and began vigorous exercise morning and evening as well as running at noon when she could.

6. Examples of nursing diagnoses:
   (a) Deterioration in health and stamina due to minimal intake and severe exercise
   (b) Disconnection from support systems related to perception that significant others (family and friends) were critical of her choices
7. Example of a goal: Within 1 week, Stella will voice acknowledgment that her coping strategies of minimal intake and severe exercise are compromising her health and her career goals (self-ideal).
8. Possible interventions:
   (a) Encourage expression of feelings, thoughts, and questions about the experience.

   (b) Explore events surrounding her short-term relationship that are having a negative effect on Stella's self-concept. As details are recalled, Stella may come to realize that current thoughts and feelings about self are based on distorted self-ideal or misinterpretations of others' reactions.
   (c) Talk therapy may help Stella to understand the potential complications associated with the coping strategies she is using.
9. Stella will acknowledge that her lack of intake and severe exercise are causing her health to deteriorate and may interfere with her ability to finish her nursing education and achieve her career goals. She will initiate steps to get further help.

References

American Association of Colleges of Nursing and the City of Hope National Medical Center. (2000). *End-of-Life Nursing Education Consortium (ELNEC) Course Syllabus.* Available: http://www.aacn.nche.edu/elnec/

Amman-Gainotti, M. (1986). Sexual socialization during early adolescence: The menarche. *Adolescence, 21,* 703–710.

Andrews, J. D. W. (1990). Interpersonal self-confirmation and challenge in psychotherapy. *Psychotherapy, 27*(4), 485–504.

Antonovsky, A. (1986). The development of a sense of coherence and its impact to stress situations. *The Journal of Social Psychology, 26*(2), 213–225.

Baumeister, R. F., & Vohs, K. D. (2003). Self-regulation and the executive function of the self. In M. R. Leary & J. P. Tangney (Eds.), *Handbook of self identity* (pp. 197–217). New York: The Guilford Press.

Beck, T. (1976). *Cognitive therapy and the emotional disorder.* New York: International Psychiatry.

Bowlby, J. (1969). *Attachment and loss: Vol. 1. Attachment.* New York: Basic Books.

Carnevalli, D. L., & Thomas, M. D. (1993). *Diagnostic reasoning and treatment decision making in nursing.* Philadelphia: Lippincott.

Cooley, C. H. (1964). *Human nature and the social order.* New York: Schocken.

Coombs, A. W., & Snygg, D. (1959). *Individual behavior: A perceptual approach to behavior.* New York: Harper & Brothers.

Crocker, J., Luhtanen, R. K., & Bouvrette, S. (2001). *Contingencies of self-worth in college students: The CSW-65 scale.* Ann Arbor: The University of Michigan.

Crocker, J., & Park, L. E. (2003). Seeking self-esteem: Construction, maintenance, and protection of self-worth. In M. R. Leary & J. P. Tangney (Eds.), *Handbook of self identity* (pp. 291–313). New York: The Guilford Press.

Demo, D. H. (1992). The self-concept over time: Research issues and directions. *Annual Review of Sociology, 18,* 303–326.

Dobratz, M. (1984). Life closure. In C. Roy (Ed.), *Introduction to nursing: An adaptation model* (2nd ed., pp. 497–518). Englewood Cliffs, NJ: Prentice-Hall.

Dobratz, M. (1990). Hospice nursing. *Cancer Nursing, 13*(2), 116–122.

Dobratz, M. C. (2004). Life closing spirituality and the philosophic assumptions of the Roy adaptation model. *Nursing Science Quarterly, 17*(4), 335–338.

Dobratz, M. C. (2005). A comparative study of life-closing spirituality in home hospice patients. *Research and Theory for Nursing Practice, 19*(3), 243–256.

Driever, M. (1976). Problems of low self-esteem. In C. Roy (Ed.), *Introduction to nursing: An adaptation model* (pp. 232–242). Englewood Cliffs, NJ: Prentice-Hall.

Edelman, C., & Mandle, C. L. (Eds.) (2002). Health promotion throughout the lifespan (5th ed.) St. Louis: Mosby.

Elliott, G. (1986). Self-esteem and self-consistency: A theoretical and empirical link between two primary motivations. *Social Psychology Quarterly, 49*(3), 207–218.

Erikson, E. H. (1963). *Childhood and society* (2nd ed.). New York: Norton.

Erikson, E. H. (1968). *Identity: Youth and crisis.* New York: Norton.

Festinger, L. (1962). *A theory of cognitive dissonance.* Palo Alto, CA: Stanford University Press.

Finucane, T. E. (2002). Care of patients nearing death: Another view. *Journal of American Geriatric Society 50*(3), 551.

Freud, S. (1949). *An outline of psychoanalysis, an authorized translation* (James Strachey, Trans.). New York: W. W. Norton.

Garcia, T., & Pintrich, P. (1994). Regulating motivation and cognition in the classroom: The role of self-schemas and self-regulatory strategies. In D. Schunk & B. Zimmerman (Eds.), *Self-regulation of learning and performance: Issues and educational applications* (pp. 129–178). Hillsdale, NJ: Erlbaum.

Gecas, V. (1982). The self concept. *Annual Review of Sociology, 8,* 1–33.

Gilligan, C. (1982) In a different voice: Psychological theory and women's development. Cambridge, MA: Harvard University Press.

Goffman, E. (1959). *The presentation of self in everyday life.* New York: Anchor.

Goffman, E. (1967). *Interactional ritual.* New York: Anchor.

Gustafsson, C., & Fargerberg, I. (2003). Reflection: The way to professional development. *Journal of Clinical Nursing, 13,* 271–280.

Hanna, D. (2004). Moral distress: The state of science. *Research and Theory for Nursing Practice, 18*(1), 73–93.

Hanna, D. (2005). The lived experience of moral distress: Nurses who assisted with elective abortions. *Research and Theory for Nursing Practice 19*(1), 95–124.

Horton, A. M., Jr. (Ed.). (1990). *Neuropsychology across the life-span: Assessment and treatment.* New York: Springer Publishing.

Johnson, D. (1983). *Body.* Boston: Beacon Press.

Johnson, J. E., & Leventhal, H. (1974). Effects of accurate expectations and behavioral instructions on reactions during a noxious medical examination. *Journal of Personality and Social Psychology, 2,* 55–64.

Kendzierski, D. (1988). Self-schemata and exercise. *Basic and Applied Social Psychology, 9,* 45–59.

Kleinke, C. (1978). *Self-perception: The psychology of personal awareness.* San Francisco: Freeman.

Kohlberg, L. (1981). *The philosophy of moral development: Vol. 1.* San Francisco: Harper & Row.

Kübler-Ross, E. (1969). *On death and dying.* New York: Macmillan.

Lecky, P. (1945). *Self-consistency: A theory of personality.* New York: Island Press.

Lecky, P. (1961). In C. F. Thorne (Ed.), *Self-consistency: A theory of personality.* Hamden, CT: The Shoe String Press.

Luft, J. (1969). *Of human interaction.* Palo Alto, CA: National Press.

Luft, J. (1984). *Group processes: An introduction to group dynamics* (3rd ed.). Palo Alto, CA: Mayfield Publishing Co.

Markus, H. (1977). Self-schemata and processing information about the self. *Journal of Personality and Social Psychology, 35*(2), 63–78.

Markus, H., Crane, M., Bernstein, S., & Siladi, M. (1982). Self-schemas and gender. *Journal of Personality and Social Psychology, 42*(1), 38–50.

Markus, H., Hamill, R., & Sentis, K. (1987). Thinking fat: Self-schemas for body weight and the processing of weight relevant information. *Journal of Applied Social Psychology, 17*(1), 50–71.

Markus, H., & Wurf, E. (1987). The dynamic self-concept: A social psychological perspective. *Annual Review of Psychology, 38,* 299–337.

Markus, H., & Zajonc, R. (1985). The cognitive perspectives in sociopsychology. In G. Lindzey & E. A. Aronson (Eds.), *Handbook of social psychology* (Vol. 1., 3rd ed.). New York: Erlbaum.

McMahon, E. M. (1993). *Beyond the myth of dominance: An alternative to a violent society.* Kansas City, MO: Sheed & Ward.

Mead, G. (1934). *Mind, self and society.* Chicago: University of Chicago Press.

Mischel, W., & Morf, C. C. (2003). The self as a psycho-social dynamic processing system: A meta-perspective on a century of the self in psychology. In M. R. Leary & J. P. Tangney (Eds.), *Handbook of self identity* (pp. 15–46). New York: The Guilford Press.

Montagu, A. (1986). *Touching: The human significance of the skin* (3rd ed.). New York: Harper & Row.

NANDA International. (2007). *Nursing diagnoses: Definitions & classification, 2007–2008.* Philadelphia: NANDA-I.

Neugarten, B. (1969). Continuities and discontinuities of psychological issues in adult life. *Human Development, 12,* 121–130.

Neugarten, B. L. (1979). Time, age, and the life cycle. *The American Journal of Psychiatry, 136*(7), 887–894.

Newman, M. (1994). *Help as expanding consciousness* (2nd ed.). New York: National League for Nursing Press.

Piaget, J. (1954). *The construction of reality in the child* (M. Cook, Trans.). New York: Basic Books.

Poster, M. (2006). *Information please: Culture and politics in the age of digital machines.* Durham, NC: Duke University.

Raths, L. E., Harmin, M., & Simon, S. B. (1966). *Values and teaching: Working with values in the classroom.* Columbus, OH: Chas. E. Merrill.

Robinson, J. H. (1995). Grief responses, coping processes, and social support of widows: Research with Roy's Model. *Nursing Science Quarterly 8(4),* 158–164.

Rogers, C. (1961). *On becoming a person.* Boston: Houghton Mifflin.

Rosenberg, M. (1965). *Society and adolescent self-image.* Princeton, NJ: Princeton University Press.

Rosenberg, M. (1968). Discussion: The concept of self. In R. Ahelson, E. Aronson, W. McGuire, T. Newcomb, M. Rosenberg, & P. Tannebaum (Eds.), *Theories of cognitive consistency: A sourcebook* (pp. 384–389). Chicago: Rand McNally.

Rosenberg, M. (1979). *Conceiving the self.* New York: Basic Books.

Sullivan, H. S. (1953). *The interpersonal theory of psychiatry.* New York: Norton.

Swimme, B., & Berry, T. (1992). *The universe story.* San Francisco: Harper.

Verklan, M. T. (2007). Johari window: A model for communicating with each other. *Journal of Perinatal and Neonatal Nursing.* April–June, 173–174.

Zhan, L. (1994). Cognitive adaptation processing and self-consistency in the hearing impaired elderly (Doctoral Dissertation, Boston College, 1993). *Dissertation Abstracts International, 54,* 4086B.

Zohar, D. (1990). *The quantum self: Human nature and consciousness defined by the new physics.* New York: Quill/Morrow.

Additional References

Breakwell, G. (1986). *Coping with threatened identities.* London: Methuen.

Cathcart, R. S., Samovar, L. A., & Henman, L. D. (Eds.). (1996). *Small group communication: Theory and practice* (7th ed.). Madison, WI: Brown & Benchmark.

Hall, B. A. (1997). Spirituality in terminal illness: An alternative view of theory. *Journal of Holistic Nursing, 15*(1), 82–96.

Napier, R. W., & Gershenfeld, M. K. (1993). *Groups: Theory and experience* (5th ed.). Boston: Houghton Mifflin.

Ryan-Wenger, N. M. (1992). A taxonomy of children's coping strategies: A step toward theory development. *American Journal of Orthopsychiatry, 62*(2), 256–263.

CHAPTER 15

Role Function Mode of the Person

The role function mode focuses specifically on the roles individuals occupy in society. The basic need underlying the role function mode has been identified as social integrity, which involves the need to know who one is in relation to others so that one can act. As emphasized previously in this book, an individual is an adaptive and holistic system with life processes that are interrelated; therefore, changes in one area of the individual's functioning will affect adaptation in another. If an individual is experiencing problems in a given role such as parent, the difficulty affects the ability to heal and promote health. In turn, changes in health status affect role performance. The role function mode provides the opportunity to focus specifically on how individuals interact within society. The philosophic assumptions of the Roy model speak to the social nature of people by emphasizing common purpose and meaning for human existence within the convergence of the universe (Roy 1997; 2007). The relationships among individuals and between each individual and society are integral to the philosophic, scientific, and cultural assumptions of the Roy model. Therefore, social adaptation is as much of a concern to the nurse as is physiologic and psychological-spiritual adaptation.

This chapter provides an overview of the role function mode of the Roy Adaptation Model for individuals, including description and theoretical bases of the mode. The theoretical background of integrated life processes, compensatory and compromised adaptive processes of the role function mode are explored. Planning nursing care includes assessment of behaviors and stimuli related to the role function mode. Nursing diagnoses, goal setting, nursing interventions, and evaluation of nursing care are described.

OBJECTIVES

After studying this chapter, the reader will be able to do the following:

1. Describe the processes of the role function mode of the individual according to the Roy Adaptation Model.

2. Identify one compensatory process related to the role function mode.

3. Name and describe two situations of compromised processes of role function.

4. List important first-level assessment factors, that is, behaviors, for the role function mode.

5. Identify second-level assessment factors, stimuli, that influence the role function mode.

6. Create a nursing diagnosis, given a situation related to role function.

7. Propose goals for a given situation of ineffective role function.

8. Describe nursing interventions commonly implemented in situations of ineffective role function.

9. Derive approaches to determine the effectiveness of nursing interventions in the role function mode.

KEY CONCEPTS DEFINED

Developing roles: The process of adding new roles as one matures through life; involves learning the expectations of the roles.

Expressive behavior: The feelings and attitudes held by the individual about doing what the role requires.

Instrumental behavior: Goal-oriented behavior; activities the individual does to carry out the role.

Primary role: The role the individual holds based on age, sex, and developmental stage; it determines the majority of an individual's behaviors during a particular growth period of life.

Role: The functioning unit of society; each role exists in relation to another.

Role conflict: Inconsistent expectations held by an individual, or by other individuals, for a given role (intrarole conflict) or inconsistent expectations among the roles of the individual's role set (interrole conflict).

Role distance: Certain behaviors associated with the role that are not compatible with self-concept; emotional behaviors tend to be negative and the individual limits goal-oriented behaviors as much as possible because of dislike for the role or part of it.

Role expectations: Beliefs held by society in general, by an individual, or by those in complementary roles, about expected behavior associated with a role.

Role failure: A situation in which an individual occupying a role has an absence or ineffectiveness of expressive or instrumental behaviors.

Role mastery: Indicates that an individual demonstrates both expressive and instrumental behaviors that meet social expectations associated with a role set.

Role set: The total number of roles an individual holds at a given time.

Role-taking: A process of looking at or anticipating another individual's behavior by viewing it within a role attributed to the other; basing one's interaction on the judgment about the other's role; focuses on the meaning that the acts have for both individuals in a role interaction.

Role transition: Growth in a new role with increasing effectiveness of emotional and goal-oriented role behaviors.

Secondary role: A role that an individual assumes to complete the expectations of a developmental stage and primary role.

Social integrity: The basic need of the role function mode for individuals; the need to know who one is in relation to others so that one can act.

Tertiary role: A temporary role that is chosen by an individual and often associated with the expectations of an individual's primary and secondary roles.

PROCESSES OF INDIVIDUAL ROLE FUNCTION

A role has been defined as the functioning unit of society. Each individual's role exists in relationship to another. For example, the parent role relates to a child; the employer role, an employee; and the nurse role, a patient. Associated with each role are expectations of how an individual behaves towards an individual in the related position. Role theories, then, seek to explain behavior as acting on expectations for individuals in given positions. Individuals play roles in relation to each other. The basic need of the role function mode is social integrity. For the individual this is accomplished by knowing who one is in relation to others. The individual knows the roles occupied and the associated expectations so that one can act appropriately. Clarity for action helps meet the individual's need for social integrity.

There are many approaches to role theories that can be divided into two types: structural and interactional. Structural role theories are based on structural–functional approaches to individuals in society such as those developed by Parsons and Shils (1951). Similarly, Linton (1945) saw roles as emphasizing structural components of societies, and because they were associated with social status, they were relatively fixed. Eagly (1987) provided a view of social role theory that deals with how gender affects roles in society. Data from the U.S. Bureau of Labor Statistics (2000) demonstrated that there are still many occupations that are decidedly male while others are decidedly female. For example, the construction industry is made up of 97% men. Firefighters and police personnel also are male-dominant, with 98% and 86% of the forces being men, respectively. However, when it comes to roles associated with home, such as child care and dietician, women dominate these fields in the same proportion. It is interesting to note that while 84% of elementary school teachers are female, only 42% of college professors are female. Eagly's theory indicated that even though the real differences among these careers are the job tasks themselves, society still holds a belief about the social structure that certain occupations are more suitable for one gender over the other.

Interactional approaches to role theory draw upon symbolic interactionism based on Mead (1934) and those who followed him. This theory emphasizes socialization through an individual taking the role of the other. There is an ongoing effort by scholars to bridge the gap between these theoretical approaches and see them as complementary. Structural approaches look at the broad perspective of people within positions in society. Interactional approaches look at ways people interpret meanings within a role interaction. The theoretical bases of the role function mode are illustrated in Figure 15–1.

An example of how structural and interactional approaches work together can be seen in the situation of a student beginning the first semester of college. She is enrolled in a class taught by a professor who also happens to be her program adviser. The student is intimidated by the professor's no-nonsense way of leading discussions and is nervous about the upcoming assignments on the syllabus. She'd like to stay after class to ask some questions, but is afraid to do so. With great reluctance, the student goes to the professor's office for advisement during the registration period for the next semester. She is pleasantly surprised when the professor

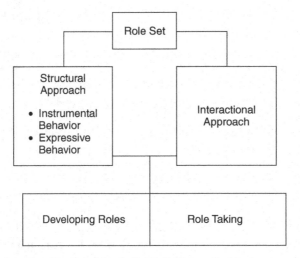

FIGURE 15–1   Role Function Mode for the individual. Theoretical basis.

greets her warmly by name. The professor seems much more relaxed in this one-on-one situation. This affects the student's behavior, and she feels comfortable asking questions about her course schedule as well as the upcoming class assignments. The student begins to understand that the professor must act in a more formal way in a classroom setting in order to successfully teach the curriculum, whereas in her own office, she is able to meet with individual students in a more informal way. The next time the student attends class, she feels more comfortable about contributing to class discussion. As she progresses through her college career, the student becomes more confident in her interaction with professors and adjusting her behavior to changing roles. She gains several mentors along the way.

Both structural and interactional approaches are useful in understanding adaptation in the role function mode. The role function mode of individuals deals specifically with the individual's place in society and how the individual interacts in reciprocal roles. The goal of the mode is social integrity. Processes used to create social integrity are developing roles and role-taking.

DEVELOPING ROLES   Developing roles refers to the process of adding new roles as one develops through life. The process involves learning the expectations of the roles. In addition, within a given stage in life, additional new roles are acquired. Role development is the assumption of a new social position by using the behaviors expected of one occupying that social role. Role expectations consist of beliefs that are held by society in general, the individual, and those in complementary roles regarding appropriate behaviors. Each time a new role is added, the individual experiences the process of developing a role. The total number of roles one has developed at a given time is defined within the role function mode as the individual's role set.

A classification of role sets as involving primary, secondary, and tertiary roles has been adopted for use in the Roy Adaptation Model (Banton, 1965; Randell, 1976). An individual will have one primary role but will also have many secondary and tertiary roles. The primary role determines the majority of behaviors that the individual engages in during a particular period of life. It is determined by age, sex, and developmental stage. Examples of primary roles are 3-year-old preschool male, 16-year-old adolescent female, and 75-year-old mature adult male. The association of age, sex, and developmental stage in labeling the primary role helps to identify many specific role expectations in relation to the developmental stage and to social expected processes.

Secondary roles are those that an individual assumes to complete the expectations of a developmental stage and primary role. For example, a 35-year-old young adult male or female may be faced with the task of being able to nurture, support, and provide for their spouse and children. Secondary roles that are assumed in relation to this expectation could be husband or wife, father or mother, and teacher or mentor. The last column of Table 15–1 identifies some general social processes expected of secondary roles for age-related developmental stages, based on classic work by Erickson (1963).

In the example given, the social process for the young adult involves becoming an independent member of society and contributing to society by having a family. Although this expectation is not as strong in society today as two decades ago, many people in society select this option. Secondary roles are normally achieved positions as opposed to primary qualities and require specific role activities. Job positions are secondary roles and are important in most societies because they affect the individual's use of time and personal resources. Secondary roles are often stable and not given up easily since they are developed and mastered over a period of time (Nuwayhid, 1984). However 21st-century society offers more mobility in job positions than ever before. Problems of role function usually occur in secondary roles and

TABLE 15–1 Developmental Stages and Social Processes Related to Developing Roles

Age (years)	Developmental Stage	Social Process
Birth–1½	Infant: trust vs. mistrust	Society contributes to the individual
1½–3½	Toddler: autonomy vs. shame	Society contributes to the individual
3½–6	Preschool: initiative vs. guilt	Society contributes to the individual
6–12	School-age: industry vs. inferiority	Individual begins to contribute to society
12–18	Adolescence: identify vs. role confusion	Individual relates to society through peer groups
18–35	Young adult: intimacy vs. isolation	Individual becomes independent member of society and begins to contribute toward the continuance of society by starting a new family
35–60	Generative adult: generativity vs. stagnation	Individual becomes involved with the survival of society through creative works and the guidance of the next generation
60 and on	Mature adult: ego integrity vs. despair	Individual becomes able to incorporate becoming a follower or a leader; sometimes in the sense of being a consultant

Source: Erickson, E. H. (1963). *Childhood and society* (2nd ed.). New York: Norton. Used with permission.

relate to whether or not the individual has what is needed to develop the role. This is discussed further in assessment of stimuli relating to developing roles.

Tertiary roles are related mainly to secondary roles and are ways that individuals meet their role expectations (Malaznik, 1976). Associated with the role of father might be that of a football or softball coach. Tertiary roles are usually temporary and chosen by the individual, and may include social or professional group activities. Figure 15–2 illustrates the role set for an individual using the classification of roles discussed. Understanding developing roles involves first identifying the primary, secondary, and tertiary roles in the individual's role set.

For an individual, there are many possible conflicting expectations within and among all the expectations of the total role set. For example, a teacher may need to meet with an administrator after school as an expectation of his developing role as teacher. At the same time, he is expected to arrive on time at a practice field in his role as football coach. This issue is discussed further as the compromised process of role conflict. Within the Roy Adaptation Model, a structural approach to roles has been useful in the assessment of developing roles. The parts of a structural approach are defined as instrumental and expressive behaviors, and apply to each role the individual occupies (Nuwayhid, 1984; Parsons & Shils, 1951).

Instrumental behaviors, or goal-oriented behaviors, are those activities individuals do to carry out their roles. The individual uses behaviors with the goal of role mastery. Role mastery is engaging in instrumental and expressive role behaviors that meet social expectations. Instrumental

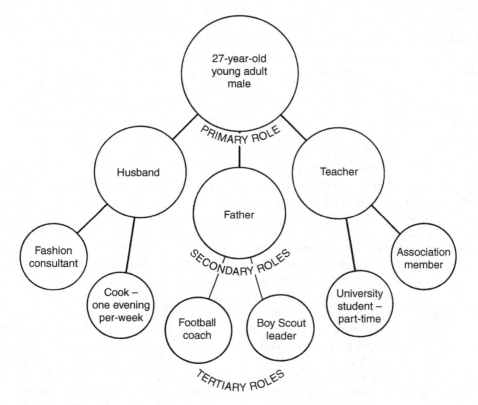

FIGURE 15–2 Illustration of a role set. Primary, secondary, and tertiary roles.

behaviors are normally physical actions that have a long-term goal. For example, maintaining a job over time meets social expectations related to the goal of supporting a family.

Expressive behaviors, or affective behaviors, involve the feelings and attitudes held by the individual about doing what the role requires. The goal of expressive behavior is direct or immediate feedback. Expressive behaviors are emotional in nature. They result from interactions in which the individual expresses these role-related feelings. For example, a mother or father might bring a child a surprise gift after returning from a business trip to experience the delight and appreciation of the child.

Similar concepts were discussed in work by Patterson (1996). He suggested that the structural–functional models tend to distinguish between relatively spontaneous affect or emotion-driven behavior and more managed or deliberate behavior. Spontaneous patterns might be rooted in emotion, but managed patterns are goal oriented or strategic; consequently, behavior patterns might be independent of affect. Instrumental (goal-oriented) and expressive (affective) behavior are thus learned in relation to developing roles of one's role set. These concepts from structural role theory are useful for nursing assessment as related to the integrated life process of developing roles.

Eagly's (1987) work on gender roles noted earlier included understanding of instrumental and expressive influences. She argued that the division of labor that emerged over time is more social-emotional based than task based. Society views men and women differently, particularly in regard to the division of labor; individuals, then, adapt their behavior to conform with their social roles. Perceived differences in men and women are based on real behaviors of people living out social role expectations that are mistakenly assumed to be based on gender differences (Brehm et al., 2002).

ROLE-TAKING   Role-taking is a process of looking at or anticipating another individual's behavior by viewing it within a role attributed to the other. The individual then shapes the interaction on a judgment about the other's role. Role-taking is based on symbolic interactionism. In Chapter 14, symbolic interactionism was introduced as a theory related to the developing self-concept. As noted, the approach also is significant in role theory. Mead (1934) and followers assert that reciprocal social relationships or interactions determine how the mind develops, and that the human individual thinks primarily in social terms. In cosmic terms, individuals are who they are by participating in the common life of the planet (Zohar & Marshall, 1994). In addition to being an influence on the developing self-concept, interactions with others involve role-taking, a key process of the role function mode. Role-taking focuses on the meaning that the acts have to both individuals in a role interaction. An individual's role behaviors emerge based on one's own meanings and interpretations of other's meanings. In early work on the theory of the adaptive modes, Roy and Roberts (1981) proposed the significance of the role-taking process of individuals in understanding the role function mode. Mead (1934) observed that individuals work out their own role by imaginatively "taking the role of the other." Turner (1979) extended this concept by specifying three standpoints from which the role-taking process occurs. First, the individual may simply adopt the standpoint of the individual in the other role, such as the individual who says, "If I were in her shoes, this is what I would do." In this case, the process directly determines behavior. One simply acts from the standpoint of the other. Second, the individual may understand the other's standpoint by adopting the standpoint of a third party, such as the individual who says, "I know what my older sister would do in relating to this person." This process shows which behavior is expected depending on inferences about the role of the other. Here, the function of role-taking is to determine how one should act toward the other. Finally, the self may take the standpoint of a purpose or objective rather than a specific directive, such as the individual who says, "I want to impress this person and although I'm not sure what would work, I'll try this approach." Here, the individual lacks a specific directive and thus shapes personal behavior according to what the individual judges to be the probable effect of the interaction between one's role and the inferred role of the other. Turner (1979) described the characteristics of the role-taking process as the following: reciprocal, with every role a way of relating to other roles in a situation; a tentative process (since role-taking occurs in interaction) continuously testing the conception one has of the role of the other; and grouping behaviors into units as a collection of possible actions that are regarded by the self or viewer as belonging together.

In applying an interactionist perspective of role, Meleis (1975) noted that through interaction and role-taking with others, the individual's roles are discovered, created, modified, and defined. This is apparent in the earlier example of the student learning to relate to various teachers in varying situations in college.

COMPENSATORY ADAPTIVE PROCESSES OF ROLE FUNCTION

The role function mode has compensatory processes, just as do the other adaptive modes. As defined earlier in this book, compensatory processes represent the adaptation level at which the cognator and regulator have been activated by a challenge to the integrated life processes. In general, to compensate means to provide a way to act or counteract as an equalizing, counterbalancing force. When a given role function process is challenged in a way that threatens to compromise adaptation, compensatory adaptive processes are activated. As compensatory processes act, the adaptation level is somewhere between the level of integrated processes and compromised processes. Effective compensatory processes increase adaptation level. Two compensatory processes selected for discussion are role transition and role distance.

Role Transition

During role development or role change, the individual goes through a process called role transition. Role transition is defined as growth in a new role with increasing effectiveness of emotional and goal-oriented role behaviors. In the case of the maternal role, for example, the new role is one of a series of secondary roles that an individual assumes to meet the developmental tasks of a primary role. It is a continuous and ongoing process. As an individual ages, the primary role changes; new developmental tasks confront the individual, and new secondary and tertiary roles are assumed to meet these developmental tasks. It is noted that the transition from one secondary role to another is much more difficult and time-consuming than moving from one tertiary role to another. Tertiary roles are usually temporary and by their nature require less emotional and physical involvement than secondary roles.

The individual does not always have a conscious choice of assuming a new role. Many secondary roles change due to environmental circumstances. For example, a man who has worked all his life as a taxi driver may have an accident that leaves him unable to drive a taxi, but he could still hold another job. This man, then, has to seek a new job that might require additional training. He did not choose to seek a new secondary role, but his ability to adapt to his new job and make an effective transition to a new secondary role is a challenge to his social integrity. Such challenges are a concern for nurses with respect to promoting integrated adaptive role function.

In assessing the role function mode adaptation of various individuals, nurses will identify many secondary and tertiary roles that are in transition. After a woman has had a heart attack, she might be able to return to work, but she might also have to give up some of her tertiary roles, like being an officer in her district nursing association. Meleis (1975) noted that role transitions require the individual to incorporate new knowledge, alter behavior, and change the definition of self in the social context. Specifically, Meleis urged that nurses be aware of developmental, situational, and health–illness role transitions. When people find their usual role set in transition, this can be a challenging time that requires nursing intervention to promote adaptation in the role function mode.

In later work, Meleis and colleagues (2000) developed a middle-range theory regarding the complexities of the transition experience. There are five essential properties of transition experiences: awareness, engagement, change and difference, time span, and critical points and events. Awareness is key to transition, because the individual must have knowledge of the fact that change is imminent. Engagement refers to the level of involvement the individual chooses to adopt in the transition. This degree of engagement will vary depending on the individual's awareness of the physical, emotional, social, or environmental changes that are a part of the transition experience. Change and difference might at first appear to be one and the same, but they are in fact separate. While all transitions are based on some degree of change, not all change is linked to transition. It is necessary to study changes in relation to their nature, temporality, importance, or severity, and the norms and expectations imposed on the individual.

Transition has a time span with a specific end point. Transition begins with the anticipation or sign of change, continues through the instable time of the actual change, and follows up with the conclusion to the transition, which is either the start of a new transition or a period of stability after the original transition. Lastly, critical points and events often play a significant role in transition. Events such as birth, death, or the diagnosis of an illness can be associated with transition, although not all events need be as obvious as these examples. Critical points are often linked to an increase in awareness or a change in the degree of engagement. There can be any number of critical points during a transition, particularly during periods of confusion and uncertainty, and so a patient requires his or her nurse to respond with care in different ways. Im and Meleis (1999) applied this middle-range theory to their study of menopausal transition of Korean immigrant women.

As nurses have used the Roy Adaptation Model, they have developed guidelines for evaluating progress in role transition. The individual is moving toward effective role transition when adaptive expressive or emotional behaviors are exhibited, with a few adaptive instrumental or goal-oriented behaviors. These behaviors partially meet with the social expectations associated with the assigned role. However, the number or quality of the behaviors is not sufficient for an integrated adaptation level relative to role transition. The adaptive behaviors, however, reflect positive movement toward the goal of role mastery. In the initial phase of effective role transition, the behaviors will primarily be expressive behaviors. However, this occurs only for a short period of time. Almost immediately, some instrumental behaviors are observable. If the transition is effective, the number and quality of instrumental behaviors will increase over time. The new role behaviors are effective in meeting goals and the individual's affect matches the role.

As noted in the literature on role theory, certain factors must be present in the environment for role transition to occur. These factors are the requirements described as stimuli influencing the developing role process. Also, the expressive and instrumental behaviors during role transition are affected by the other major stimuli described. When role transition is less successful, the individual has adaptive expressive behavior but ineffective instrumental behaviors for a particular role. Unlike the other difficulties in role function, which usually arise from some sort of conflict, difficulty with role transition usually results from a lack of knowledge, education, practice, or role models. For example, a new mother who is experiencing difficulty with transition to the maternal role has the self-concept of mother, wants to be a mother, and may even know what a mother is expected to do, but she does not know how to do the tasks as expected.

Two approaches based on role theory that nurses use to promote role transitions are introduction of role cues (Roy, 1967) and role supplementation (Clarke & Strauss, 1992; Meleis, 1975). Roy described mothers who were in role transition in adjusting their mothering roles to interacting with an ill child in the hospital for the first time. She reported the use of interactional role theory to develop and test a set of role cues that the nurse used with the mother. The pediatric staff nurse purposefully used three categories of action in interacting with the mother.

1. Congruent orientation, the focus of attention in common with the mother's focus of attention
2. Involvement, communication with the mother concerning the child's condition, treatment, or activities
3. Role reference, the nurse used words and actions to define for the mother what she might do for her child

The simple approach of role cues has been effective in pediatric nursing. For Meleis (1975), the approach of role supplementation involves any deliberative process whereby role difficulties are identified and the conditions and strategies for role clarification and role-taking are used to promote role transitions. Role supplementation can be used both as prevention, as in working with expectant mothers, or therapeutically, as when the individual fails to make progress in role transitions such as reluctance to accept rehabilitation after a major illness or injury. According to Meleis, role supplementation is useful for practice and research. The process includes role clarification, role-taking, and role modeling; role rehearsal, reference group, and communication; and interactions. To become an expert practitioner in using these approaches, the reader is referred to the original sources.

Role Distance

A second compensatory process in the role function mode is known as role distance. In role distance, certain behaviors associated with the role are not compatible with the self-concept. The individual experiencing role distance at first appears to be experiencing difficulty with role transition. However, a detailed assessment shows that the individual's goal-oriented behaviors in role distance vary greatly in number and in type from the individual in role transition. For example, the individual has the knowledge and experience to perform the instrumental behaviors associated with a role, but does so only when absolutely necessary or when there is no one else around to perform the tasks. The individual functions at a point just above role failure by performing the minimal number of expected goal-oriented behaviors for the role. In role distance, the individual exhibits both instrumental and expressive behaviors appropriate to a particular role, but these behaviors differ significantly from expected behaviors for the role (Nuwayhid, 1991; Schofield, 1976).

Perhaps the most significant difference between role distance and the other role function processes is that the role is incompatible with the individual's self-concept. The individual feels uncomfortable because he or she does not like the role, either in part or as a whole. This is important to consider because the individual may not reject an entire role, but rather certain behaviors associated with the role that the individual perceives as undesirable. The individual seeks to alleviate discomfort by exhibiting expressive behaviors that make the role seem unimportant or unnecessary. Individuals occupying complementary roles are made to feel uncomfortable in their positions. The individual makes derogatory remarks about the role and jokes, belittles, and speaks out about the role in negative terms. This behavior occurs in degrees. The more the role is disliked, the more numerous, severe, and pronounced are the exhibited expressive behaviors.

When role distance is being used as a compensatory process, the nurse focuses on decreasing the threat or discomfort to the individual's self-concept. A simple example is the patient who is joking about the hospital gown while changing for same-day surgery. The nurse can comment casually that although this is not how the individual generally appears to the world, in this setting everyone looks like this. The nurse may add that the situation is temporary and the patient will be putting their own clothes back on as soon as possible. In more involved situations of role change, the nurse recognizes that the individual basically has two choices to reintegrate their role function and reach a new level of adaptation. The nurse's approach may be to help the individual identify these choices, select the one that is best, and act on that choice.

If the individual is uncomfortable with certain role behaviors because they do not match the self-ideal, then one choice is to delete the role from the role set and focus on other roles more compatible with the self. Another choice is to reexamine the self-ideal in a way that may incorporate the role from which the self is distancing. The basis for a choice generally rests with the value and importance of the role for the individual. If this is a highly valued role such as that of new father, or one that is important because it is inevitable, such as living with a chronic illness, then the individual may need help identifying and dealing with the discrepancies felt between role behaviors and self-concept. Helping people recognize the choices they can make related to their well-being is a significant part of what nurses can do to promote adaptation. This approach is particularly relevant in actualizing the values and beliefs of the Roy model. The nurse aims to improve effectiveness in working with patients regarding choices for health since such choices are opportunities for personal growth in situations of role distance, as well as in many other patient situations.

COMPROMISED PROCESSES OF ROLE FUNCTION

Whenever an individual fails to perform the expected behaviors for a role, a compromised adaptation level exists. The focal stimulus or immediate cause for the behavior varies according to the processes involved. In some cases, it may be the absence of knowledge, lack of education, or scarcity of role models that lead to compromise. In other cases, the setting, cognator processes, or self-concept may not be adequate to achieve role mastery. A compromised adaptation level can occur related to developing structural roles or role-taking in a given situation. Two examples of compromised role function are role conflict and role failure.

Role Conflict

Role conflict refers to inconsistent expectations held by an individual, or by other people, for a given role in the role set or inconsistent expectations among the roles of the individual's role set. Role conflict, therefore, can be specified as intrarole conflict, which is conflict within a role, and interrole conflict, which is conflict between or among roles. In intrarole conflict, the individual fails in the goal-oriented and/or emotional behaviors expected for a role. This failure is a result of incompatible expectations from self or one or more individuals in the environment concerning the individual's expected behavior (Schofield, 1976). For example, Martha comes from a traditional Italian Catholic family. She maintains a very close relationship with her mother and is in mastery of her daughter role. Martha is now the mother of a 6-week-old baby girl. She has read, taken classes, and searched the Internet about baby care, and is up to date on the current trends. Martha's mother, however, is old-fashioned, and still believes in keeping the baby's head and feet covered in warm clothing in the middle of summer. Martha's mother's praise and approval are very important to Martha. In performing her role as mother, Martha finds herself performing behaviors that try to meet her own perceptions of the maternal role, while also trying to meet her mother's expectations. As she vacillates back and forth, Martha applies all of her energy trying to accommodate two opposing views of the maternal role. Given this conflict, Martha will not achieve role mastery.

Interrole conflict occurs when an individual fails in the expected goal-oriented or emotional behaviors because the role set has one or more roles with expected behaviors that are incompatible. In this situation, the individual is occupying roles that are in competition. An example of interrole conflict would be the case of Louise. Louise is an electrical engineer who was just promoted at work. She works 10 to 12 hours each day and is in role mastery. Louise delivered a baby boy 8 weeks ago, and she now considers her life to be in total chaos. She wants to be at work to maintain her position and control. At the same time, she wants to be with her baby and be involved with as much of his care as possible. As a result, she is torn between the two roles and is not experiencing mastery in either one.

Role Failure

Role failure differs from role conflict in that the individual fails to exhibit adaptive emotional behaviors. To be successful at role function, the individual must want to take on the role. In role failure, the individual does not want to assume the role, and any role behaviors that are observed are usually ineffective because they are aimed at pleasing those in complementary roles. The individual does not have emotional behaviors or has ineffective emotional behaviors. The key element in role failure is the individual's desire. If the individual exhibits any adaptive emotional behaviors concerning a role, the individual generally is not in role failure. This is important to remember because when emotional and goal-oriented behaviors are ineffective, nurses too often label the patient as being in role failure. In reality, the behavior can be indicative of role transition or role conflict. Role failure does occur and is seen in complex situations in practice such as difficulties with family roles. Role failure is a complex diagnosis in the role function mode and usually involves one or more of the other modes of the Roy Adaptation Model. In role failure, the outcome for an individual may be to choose not to fulfill the role. As in any adaptation problem, thorough first- and second-level assessment can be helpful. In the role function mode, understanding the effects of the self and interdependence modes are particularly relevant.

NURSING PROCESS RELATED TO ROLE FUNCTION MODE–INDIVIDUAL

In applying the nursing process to the role function mode, the nurse makes a careful assessment of behaviors and stimuli as in assessment of the other adaptive modes. This section identifies and describes behaviors of individuals who are developing a role or interacting in a role as well as the stimuli that affect these role behaviors.

Assessment of Behavior

The nurse begins assessment in the role function mode when first meeting the individual and is alert to behavior the individual reveals spontaneously. After creating a comfortable environment, the nurse continues with an in-depth first-level assessment. In identifying behaviors in the role function mode, the nurse is aware of the goal of social integrity. In assessing developing roles, emphasis is placed on the broad, long-term process. For example, the identification of a role set takes a broad view of the individual's life and social development. The related instrumental or goal-oriented and expressive or emotional behaviors are viewed as emerging patterns as roles develop. In assessing behaviors of the role-taking process, the perspective is narrowed somewhat to the role-taking experience in a given situation. An individual behavior is described, or a unit of behaviors is grouped. Understanding the individual within a social context requires significant knowledge and experience for both the broad and narrow views of assessment. The assessment is complex—first, because the effort is to summarize much information into a full picture, and secondly, because it requires insight into the dynamics of meaning between interacting individuals. This understanding is developed throughout the nurse's career, but basic principles are provided in this book, so that the nurse can begin to grow in this area of nursing knowledge.

Of particular relevance in assessing the role-taking process is for the nurse to understand one's own role-taking behavior in the nurse–patient interaction. A useful exercise for learning about the nurse–patient relationship is called a process recording. In a process recording, a conversation between the patient and the nurse is written down as closely to verbatim as possible in two columns. A third column is made to the right of the statements for the nurse to write down reflections about the meaning of the interaction. A sample process recording is provided in Table 15–2. In this exercise, the nurse is doing an assessment of role-taking behavior in a given situation. The purpose is to identify the role behavior of the self as it affects and is affected by the role behavior of the other.

IDENTIFICATION OF ROLES   The primary, secondary, and tertiary roles the individual occupies, and the associated goal-oriented and emotional behaviors, form the basis for behavioral assessment of social integrity of the developing roles process. In assessing behavior, the nurse begins by identifying the individual's age and related primary role. From this information, secondary roles can be projected, and by purposeful questioning, secondary and tertiary roles can be determined along with their relative importance for the individual.

GOAL-ORIENTED AND EMOTIONAL BEHAVIORS   Behavioral assessment would also include the determination of instrumental, goal-oriented, and expressive, emotional behaviors associated with each role. Direct observation of specific roles can provide further information as to the adaptive process of developing roles. Consider as an example a 19-year-old young adult female who has just entered college. In addition to the secondary role of student, one can project such roles as daughter, sister, girlfriend, and participant in sports activities. Associated with the role of student are the goal-oriented behaviors of studying, attending classes, taking exams, writing papers, and participating in laboratory sessions. Emotional behaviors include "hanging out" with peers, complaining to parents about a heavy workload, and rejoicing about exam results with the professor.

Following identification of the individual's set of roles and related goal-oriented and emotional behaviors, tentative judgments can be made relative to how adaptive the developing role processes are. Adaptive role development behaviors are those that meet role expectations;

TABLE 15–2 Sample Process Recording to Focus on Role-taking Behavior in the Nurse and Patient Interaction

Situation: The nurse enters the room where a young mother is with her child who has just been admitted to the pediatric unit of the medical center with a fever of unknown origin. The child was born with spina bifida and the mother has been caring for him at home for 5 years.

Nurse	Mother and Child	Reflection on Meaning
Good afternoon, Mrs. Fabien, and Stevie, how are you doing today? I hear you have a fever.	Oh, I am glad you are here, Ms. Moralez. Yes, Stevie's temperature started up on Friday and nothing I do has helped.	The mom is really feeling frustrated. It seems to help that she recognized me.
Sounds like you have had a hard time. What do you know so far about what is causing the elevated temperature?	Oh, the usual. Anything from urinary tract infection to meningitis.	The long haul is getting to Mrs. Fabien. I see Stevie occasionally when he needs acute care, but for her this is an everyday thing.
Yes, there have been a lot of these problems. But then I see you and Stevie only when something like this happens. For you, Stevie's care is every day. You do such a good job of meeting his needs.	Yeah. But I don't feel that I do a good job when something like this happens, and we don't know yet how serious it is.	I really can be a support to Mrs. Fabien during this time of diagnosis and treatment. (You know, my sister is expecting a baby in a few weeks; what if her baby has a serious birth defect?) Better respond to what this mother is saying now.
Well, the lab work is started and we should begin to get some answers soon. I am glad you brought Stevie in right away. Your vigilance is his best protection.	Oh, he is just such a good little guy, and a joy for the whole family. I really can't do enough for him. I know we will get through this, too, and I can't tell you how glad I am that you are here. I know you will help get information as soon as possible.	It really helps to have a relationship with the mother from the start. She is counting on me. Maybe I can help not only get through this acute episode, but show her how she can continue to grow in her mothering of little Stevie.

ineffective behaviors do not meet role expectations. Role mastery is the term used to indicate that an individual demonstrates both expressive and instrumental behaviors that meet expectations associated with one's role set. Basically, the nurse assesses whether or not instrumental behaviors are achieving expected goals, and whether expressive behaviors provide satisfaction for the individual.

Assessment of Stimuli

In second-level assessment the nurse identifies stimuli that affect developing roles and the role-taking process. The structural approach to roles provides one basis for second-level assessment. Four role requirements have been described by Nuwayhid (1984), based on the theory in sociology by Parsons and Shils (1951). These requirements are viewed as necessary within the social structure to allow an individual to develop role behavior, be it instrumental, namely, goal directed, or expressive, feeling based. Other important stimuli are derived from understanding developing roles and the role-taking process.

REQUIREMENTS   The four role function requirements are identified as major stimuli for role development. Their presence helps the individual's role development by identifying expected behaviors for each role the individual holds. The theory of roles identifies requirements for role behavior as consumer, reward, access to facilities and circumstances, and cooperation and collaboration. The following example relates to the sick role (originally described by Parsons, 1964) and to later applications by nurses to the wellness role. Illustrations are provided of the requirements to both goal-oriented and emotional behaviors.

In the sick role, a goal-oriented behavior for the patient is taking prescribed medications and one for the wellness role is the individual's self-initiated health promotion behaviors. The requirements for role behaviors are listed in Table 15–3. The four requirements of both instrumental and expressive behaviors are important to consider when assessing stimuli influencing role development behaviors. Their presence or absence may serve as focal, contextual, or residual stimuli to the observed behaviors in the role function mode.

PHYSICAL ATTRIBUTES AND CHRONOLOGIC AGE   Physical attributes and chronologic age influence which roles an individual is ready to occupy. For example, at age 18, an individual's learning abilities provide readiness for college study. Certain jobs require given physical capabilities, such as a professional athlete, yet individuals with physical disabilities may perform many roles for which their abilities qualify them. For example, it is not unusual to see an office manager or attorney who is confined to a wheelchair because of a neurologic condition that affects the spinal cord but not the brain. In addition, society is redefining age limitations on certain roles. Older individuals are allowed to adopt children and new careers are common in later years.

SELF-CONCEPT AND EMOTIONAL WELL-BEING   Self-concept, as an adaptive mode, affects developing roles. The role must fit within the individual's self-ideal, namely, it will be something that the individual expects of himself or herself. In addition, the individual must feel capable of being in the role and carrying out behaviors expected in the role. An example is a young woman who always planned to go to college and feels capable of taking and succeeding in the selected course of study she chooses. This self-motivation and confidence affect the individual's capacity or ability to develop the role successfully. The individual will also have the emotional well-being to fulfill the role. Taking on one or more new roles can be stressful, and a certain amount of emotional resilience facilitates the developing role process. The young woman in the example has no emotional concerns that would decrease her success as a student. Further, she was active in sports in high school, thus has experience in handling both winning and losing, and has developed the perspective and emotional flexibility associated with such "ups" and "downs."

TABLE 15–3 Requirements for Role Behavior. Stimuli

Goal-oriented	Description	Example
Consumer	Who or what benefits from the person's performance of role behaviors?	The patient in the sick role benefits by taking prescribed pain medication; the well person benefits by doing daily exercise.
Reward	What rewards does the individual receive for performance of role behaviors?	Pain is alleviated and physical mobilization can be increased. In the wellness role, the person who exercises feels an increased sense of well-being.
Access to facilities and set of circumstances	Are materials and time and place available to perform role behaviors?	In the sick role, medication is available, as is appropriate equipment for taking it. In the wellness role, the person is able to schedule a time and place to exercise.
Cooperation and collaboration	To what degree is the person allowed opportunities to perform role behaviors?	Medication is brought to the patient in the sick role and time is allowed to elapse before its effect is felt. The person in the wellness role has someone to stay with her child so that she can go to a group session.

Emotional	Description	Example
Consumer	The need for immediate feedback from an appropriate and receptive person.	In some situations, this person is the nurse who is available to care for the patient and assess response to medication. In the wellness role, a friend who is a nurse joins the person for her exercise session.
Reward	An established network that will provide feedback on role performance.	In both illness and wellness cases, the person receives encouragement and feedback from the nurse.
Access to facilities and set of circumstances	The need to feel confident that one has what is needed to accomplish the task.	The nurse provides time to discuss the person's concern about taking medication or doing exercise.
Collaboration and cooperation	The positive emotional tone and belief that the setting in which the role is performed provides the environment needed to fulfill the role.	Both individuals feel that they are actively involved in decisions related to care and health promotion.

KNOWLEDGE OF EXPECTED BEHAVIORS Because knowing what is expected in a role is necessary to develop the role, the individual uses cognator processes to gain knowledge of expected behaviors. In particular, perception, information processing, and learning are important in role development. The young woman beginning college is alert to formal notices such as the school catalogue and online communications from the registrar's office. She watches and listens to both faculty members and other students in the early days of classes. She is developing both formal and informal knowledge about what behaviors are expected in carrying out her new role as student. For example, she recognizes that she is expected to study, plan ahead on projects, attend and participate in classes, and maintain B average grades in order to remain in her chosen major.

OTHER ROLES Expectations of behavior in one role may interfere with behaviors in another. Likewise, skills learned in one role may facilitate developing another role. Throughout life, there are opportunities for experience in managing a variety of roles. Further, people learn how many and what kinds of roles they can accomplish successfully within the level of stress they are willing to tolerate. Thus, the developing of a new role may be dependent on the individual's assessment of their total role set, namely, all other roles. The student in college may decide that she will not compete for a position on a sports team until she has mastered other college roles and resolved expectations from the student and girlfriend roles.

ROLE MODELS The number, quality, and responses of role models influence the process of developing roles. Role modeling occurs when an individual observes a significant other with the goal of understanding and emulating the complexity of behaviors of the other's role. Imitation and trial and error are used in role modeling, without direct reinforcement for imitation. Imitating attributes of others is considered a prevalent type of social role learning. An early observation of Meleis (1975) noted that in a face-to-face society, role modeling is intensive and ensures accurate and relatively smooth role transitions. Whereas role modeling is reduced in highly developed, mobile, technical, and nontraditional societies, this observation has become even more pronounced in U.S. society in the decades since it was identified. Nurses have recognized the value of enhancing role modeling as a way of promoting healthy role behaviors (Erickson, Tomlin, & Swain, 1988). In the example of the college student, she can look to her parents, older siblings, and other students as role models for student behaviors. She might begin professional role development by observing which journals her teacher reads.

SOCIAL NORMS General rules of conduct for role behavior established by society are referred to as norms. Norms represent standards of socially approved and disapproved behavior. Norms can provide an important mechanism for social control of an individual's behavior in society. The tendency to change perceptions, opinions, or behavior in ways that are consistent with society norms is referred to as conformity. Norms usually include sanctions, such as reward or punishment, for those who do or do not behave within the social or group norm. Norms vary greatly in different situations and in different cultures. The individual role behavior is affected by changing norms. The effect of social norms and how solidified they can be is illustrated in Eagly's (1987) social role theory relating gender and occupations.

SOCIAL SETTING The setting or environment is important in promoting or limiting the learning of roles and role-taking interaction. In this case, setting means the environment of learning a role and the conditions under which two individuals interact. You can ask yourself what kind of settings allow the nurse to enter the role-taking process as a partner in health care with the patient. The close interaction for role taking requires an environment with at least the basics for interaction. The setting, whether a hospital room, clinic, or home, will provide privacy for interaction, at least at times. The nurse needs to manage the setting with the patient in such a way so as to not feel rushed by other commitments. Further, planning of assignments will include continuity of care by the nurse with the patient over time. To develop a role similarly requires basics such as the access to facilities described earlier as a role function requirement.

COGNATOR PROCESSES   For the processes of both developing roles and role-taking, the cognator activities of perceptual and informational processing and judgment are key. In developing roles, the cognitive and emotional abilities of the cognator are maturing along with the opportunities to develop new roles. This was noted in the example of the new college student who takes in her environment and shapes her role within the local norms and her goals. Likewise, in role-taking, all of one's perceptual awareness and ability to process informational cues are used. In addition, an immediate judgment is made about the information to alter one's behavior within the interaction. An example of the nurse interacting with the mother of a child with fever of unknown origin demonstrates the use of the cognator processes in the role-taking process. The nurse perceives the mother, where she sits, her facial expression, body posture, and the words she uses. The nurse processes the perceptions and makes the judgment that the mother is both frustrated and welcoming of the nurse. Thus, the nurse acknowledges the mother's feelings and engages her in discussion of possibilities for this episode of illness and provides support for her as caring for a child with a chronic condition. Note that the setting, and likely the gender and age, of the nurse and the mother also may be influencing factors for the behavior.

COGNITIVE RESOURCES   Cognitive resources refer to cognitive capacity available for attending to, processing, and managing concept formation and judgment while in a role development or role-taking situation. Each part of cognator processing requires energy, and regardless of total cognator effectiveness, one must have energy to use this capacity or it is not available for learning roles or role interactions. Further, when cognitive resources are concentrated on the immediate situation, they can be distributed among monitoring self, interpreting the role partner, or awareness of the setting or the topic of conversation. An individual can be highly motivated to participate in role-taking; however, over time the amount of energy required by the interaction may be draining for either or both individuals. Caregiver burden and nurse burnout are two examples described in the nursing literature that illustrate how cognitive resources drained by intense interactions contribute to energy depletion in given roles. Factors that help an individual use cognitive resources to promote adaptation in learning roles or role-taking include focus of attention and cognitive effort. Emotions and goals help to increase energy that is needed to focus the attention of cognitive resources developing a role or on a role-taking interaction. For example, positive attitude, or liking of the other individual, helps to maintain the focus on the other. Similarly, if an important goal is at stake, as in a job interview, then attentional focus is more easily maintained. Similarly, there are many reasons for the individual to put more cognitive effort into an interaction. A nurse may be very committed to developing a role as health partner with a particular patient, both because of strong professional commitments as a nurse and also because of acute awareness of the health consequences for the patient depending on this interaction.

SOCIAL PERCEPTION   Social perception is a general term for the processes by which people come to understand one another. It is clear that some individuals are better at understanding others, and this is a major influence particularly on role-taking. Again, skill at social perception is a complex nursing ability, and the reader is referred to additional sources for further understanding. In a basic sense, social perception is described as a three-step process (Brehm et al., 2002). Observation of individuals, situations, and behavior is the first step. These are the raw data of social perception. Second, there is a process whereby people explain and analyze behavior. To interact effectively with others, it is useful to know how they are feeling and to identify dispositions, namely, more stable characteristics. Attributing certain personality traits, attitudes, and abilities helps an individual to predict another's behavior. Basically, we want to infer that an individual is friendly and can be trusted. Since people cannot observe these attributes, they must infer them from what an individual says and does. The last step of social perception is for the individual to integrate observations into a coherent impression of the other person.

There are many overt and subtle ways in which impressions create a distorted picture of reality. On early observations, an individual may make immediate judgments based on initial cues and these are referred to as "snap judgments." The inferring of attributes about an individual may be correct or incorrect. A study of integrated impressions about people was done by showing different groups brief videotapes of 10 women telling the truth or lying about their feelings (Ekman & O'Sullivan, 1991). Among the following observer groups of college students, police investigators, trial judges, and psychiatrists, all scored only slightly better than chance, making the correct judgment between 53% and 58% of the time. Only the U.S. Secret Service agents scored better than chance, making correct judgments 64% of the time.

Despite the fact that social perception is imperfect, there are ways in which people are more competent as social perceivers. The more experience people have with each other, the more accurate they are; for example, they are more accurate in judgments about friends and acquaintances. Although people are not good at making global judgments, such as knowing what people are like across a range of settings, they can make predictions in given situations. For example, one can predict a coworker's action on the job, which is more important than being mistaken about the other's personality. Social perception skills can be enhanced in people who learn the rules of probability and logic; for example, taking a statistics course can improve ability to reason about social events. That is, the individual uses the information that probabilities of .80 help one anticipate that a behavior is likely to occur in 8 out of 10 cases. At the same time one knows the behavior likely would be different in 2 out of 10 times. Further, the .80 prediction has possibility for error included.

Finally, people can form more accurate impressions of others when motivated by a concern for accuracy and open-mindedness. Nurses can benefit from knowing that understanding of people can be enhanced and the problems of bias can be minimized to the extent that we observe others with whom we interact, make judgments that are reasonably specific, have some knowledge of rules of logic, and are sufficiently motivated to form an accurate impression. Social perception is a potent factor particularly influencing effective role-taking.

GENERAL DETERMINANTS   Just as age, gender, and developmental stage help to determine the role set in a structural approach to developing roles, so, too, have biology, gender, culture, and personality been noted to be primary influences in the choice of social environments (Patterson, 1996). Choosing a college in a small town or a large city may be based on personal factors, but it will determine some of the dimensions of the social environment. The social environment in turn influences the role-taking interactions that are available. For example, going to college with a twin in a small town may influence the amount and type of one-to-one social interactions with others. As to cultural factors, members of international student organizations often notice the rich experience of differences as they begin to know each other and learn to interact.

Stimuli other than those discussed above may be relevant in an individual's role situation. These should be considered as additional influencing factors in the second-level assessment. The context and meaning of the situation is taken into account using an interactionist perspective discussed earlier. Once the stimuli influencing the individual's developing roles have been identified, the behaviors, in light of the theoretical bases, are evaluated as adaptive or ineffective in maintaining social integrity. The individual's own goals for role behavior are key to this judgment. Stimuli are identified as focal, contextual, or residual and are labeled as to whether they are exerting a positive or negative influence on the developing role process.

CASE STUDY FOR PLANNING NURSING CARE   In this section a case study is used to illustrate application of the role function mode of the Roy Adaptation Model in patient care. The case involves a 25-year-old young woman, Lin, who recently emigrated to the United States from Korea with her husband. Although she was qualified as a pharmacist in her homeland, her qualifications are not recognized in the United States and she cannot work in her profession. She is currently working in a fabric warehouse as a laborer. She has made some acquaintances in the Korean community; however, she does not yet feel as though she has developed close friends. Lin is 6 months pregnant. She is hoping that her mother can come for an extended period to help with her new baby, but those arrangements have not been completed.

Although other elements of the Roy Adaptation Model are useful in this situation, the focus of the case examples will be on the role function mode. First, the nurse identifies the primary, secondary, and tertiary roles occupied by the individual with particular attention to the integrated processes of developing roles and role-taking. The nurse will assess instrumental, goal-directed, and expressive or emotional behaviors. As stimuli are assessed in second-level assessment, analysis of role requirements points to focal, contextual, or residual stimuli that are of importance in planning nursing care. Other important stimuli to be considered were identified earlier in this chapter. The nurse also is aware continually of evidence of compensatory or compromised processes with respect to role function. Based on a thorough first- and second-level assessment, the nurse proceeds to plan nursing care by initially formulating nursing diagnoses.

Nursing Diagnosis

It is important to note, once again, that the individual receiving care will be involved, where possible, as an active participant in each step of the nursing process. It is only through meaningful involvement of the patient with the nurse that the plan of care will be realistic. Using this collaborative process, the plan will be supported by the individual whose needs it addresses, and it can be effective in achieving the planned outcomes. Development of nursing diagnoses associated with role function is accomplished in the same way as in the other modes. One method involves the statement of the behaviors together with the influencing stimuli; another method makes use of summary labels. Nursing diagnoses may reflect either adaptive or ineffective behaviors. Consider the situation of the young immigrant woman. In preparation for the baby's arrival, she and her husband have begun to assemble equipment and supplies for the baby. At the warehouse where she is employed, there are remnants of fabric that are available at a substantially reduced price. Lin has purchased some of this fabric and is making clothes for the baby. She has also been able to obtain enough fabric for bedding. She and her husband have discovered that baby furniture can be purchased at garage sales at a reasonable price, and they have been spending recent Saturdays searching for what they need. Lin is demonstrating behaviors appropriate to her developing role of mother. A nursing diagnosis capturing these adaptive behaviors could be "Effective goal-directed behaviors preparing for the baby's birth related to anticipating the baby's needs." Each day at work, Lin enthusiastically reports to her coworkers regarding recent accomplishments or finds at the yard sales. This constitutes expressive behavior and can be captured in a nursing diagnosis stating, "Appropriate expressive behaviors related to the presence of the four role performance requirements: consumer—coworkers; reward—their interest and enthusiasm; facilities and circumstances—opportunity to socialize at work; and collaboration and cooperation—supportive work environment."

One factor that is causing Lin some concern is the physical distance from her mother. She would really like to be able to speak with her mother for advice and support, yet the distance between them prohibits long telephone conversations and Lin does not have access to an Internet connection. A diagnosis statement that captures this concern is "Absence of mother's advice and support during pregnancy related to mother living in Korea and Lin living in the United States."

There are six indicators of positive role adaptation identified as summary labels in the Roy Adaptation Model.

1. Role clarity
2. Effective processes of role transition
3. Integration of goal-oriented and emotional role behaviors
4. Integration of primary, secondary, and tertiary roles
5. Effective pattern of role activities
6. Effective processes for coping with role changes

These summary labels can be applied to individual situations in a way that provides useful information. For example, in the case study, a diagnosis using a summary label could be, "Effective processes for coping with role change related to evidence of the role requirements." Likewise, four commonly recurring adaptation problems are identified. They are ineffective role transition, prolonged role distance, role conflict, and role failure. The use of a summary label when more than one mode is affected by the same stimulus is often an effective way of communicating a cluster of behaviors. For example, "role failure" is a complex diagnosis that usually involves more than one mode. For the experienced nurse, this label would convey the absence of expressive behaviors related to the role and the lack of the individual's desire to assume the role. It would point to the need to look further into the situation for ineffective role transition or role conflict.

In Table 15–4, the Roy model nursing diagnostic categories for the integrated processes of role function are shown in relation to nursing diagnosis labels approved by the North

TABLE 15–4 Nursing Diagnostic Categories for Role Function Mode for the Individual

Positive Indicators of Adaptation	Common Adaptation Problems	NANDA Diagnostic Labels
• Role clarity • Effective processes of role transition • Integration of goal-oriented and emotional role behaviors • Integration of primary, secondary, and tertiary roles • Effective pattern of role activities • Effective processes for coping with role changes	• Ineffective role transition • Prolonged role distance • Role conflict—intrarole and interrole • Role failure	• Parental role conflict • Improved parenting • Risk for impaired parenting • Ineffective role performance • Readiness for enhanced parenting

American Nursing Diagnosis Association (NANDA International, 2007). Once the nursing diagnoses have been stated, the nurse proceeds to the next step in the process of planning care, which is goal setting.

Goal Setting

Each step of the nursing process focuses on the individual's behavior, the stimuli influencing that behavior, or both. With the nursing diagnosis, the statement developed included both behaviors and stimuli. With goal setting, the focus is on behavior. Each goal identifies a behavior that is to be addressed, the change expected, and the time frame in which the goal is to be met. In the case of the young immigrant woman, Lin, a goal might focus on her continued transition into the role of mother. An example is, "Before the due date for the baby's arrival, Lin will have acquired all the necessary supplies and equipment to care for her new baby." The behavior in this goal relates to the readiness for the baby's arrival in terms of supplies and equipment, the change is that "all" is obtained, and the time frame is "before the due date for the baby's arrival." Another goal for Lin will focus on a support system in case her mother is unable to arrange her visit by the time the baby arrives. It may be stated as follows: "Within 1 month, Lin will be developing relationships with other expectant and new mothers in her community." Here the behavior relates to supportive relationships, the change relates to developing these, and the time frame is "within 1 month."

Nursing Intervention

The nursing intervention step of the nursing process according to the Roy Adaptation Model focuses on the stimuli affecting the behavior identified in the goal-setting step. The nursing intervention step is thus the management of stimuli, and this involves altering, increasing, decreasing, removing, or maintaining given stimuli. In the case of Lin, one of the goals relates to her developing a support system with other expectant and new mothers in her community. The stimulus is presence of role requirements, a common stimulus needed for effective role development. For example, it is important that this new mother have an established network that will provide support and feedback on her transition into the role of mother. The nurse can involve Lin in prenatal classes where she will not only receive knowledge regarding childbirth and child rearing, but also get to know other women who are expecting babies around the same time. As it happened, there was a Korean nurse involved in presenting the prenatal instruction to the class of expectant parents. This individual was able to put Lin in touch with several other Korean immigrants who had just delivered new babies. The above nursing interventions focused on stimuli, that is, role performance requirements and knowledge of expected behaviors that were contributing to the potential for problems of role function. The next step of the nursing process returns to focus on the behaviors evident in the situations following the nursing interventions.

Evaluation of Outcomes

Evaluation involves looking at the outcome of the nursing intervention to judge whether it was effective in relation to the individual's adaptive behaviors, that is, whether the behaviors stated in the goals have been achieved. The nursing interventions are effective if the behavior meets the stated goal. If the outcome is that the goal is not achieved, the nurse identifies alternative interventions or approaches by reassessing the behavior and stimuli and continuing with the other steps of the nursing process. In considering the previously identified goal for Lin, "Within 1 month, Lin will be developing relationships with other expectant and new mothers in her community," if the nursing interventions were effective, as an outcome Lin would report friendships with other new mothers who are in close proximity to her home. If at the time of evaluation Lin had made no new friends, other approaches would have to be considered to develop a support system for Lin as she develops her new role as a mother.

It is important to recognize that the six steps of the nursing process are ongoing, simultaneous, and overlapping. Although they have been separated and dealt with in a linear manner for discussion purposes, often nursing intervention is occurring at the same time that the nurse is assessing behavior and stimuli. Likewise, evaluation of outcomes occurs on an ongoing basis, being held in mind even when nursing diagnoses are being established and as goals are being formulated.

Summary

This chapter focused on the application of the Roy Adaptation Model to the role function mode. An overview of the two integrated processes—developing roles and role-taking—associated with social integrity was provided. Illustrations of innate and learned compensatory responses related to role function were described, and examples of the compromised processes of role conflict and role failure were provided. Finally, guidelines for planning nursing care included a discussion of assessment of behaviors and stimuli, and a case study showing nursing diagnoses, goals, nursing interventions, and evaluation of outcomes of nursing care was described.

Exercises for Application

1. Identify the primary, secondary, and tertiary roles in which you are currently involved.
2. Select one of your secondary roles and list the associated instrumental and expressive behaviors. Assess the requirements for role function of one instrumental and one expressive behavior.
3. Imagine a 45-year-old generative adult male. Project secondary roles for him and formulate appropriate questions or comments that would elicit information about these roles. Speculate about specific behavior related to the role requirements.

Assessment of Understanding

QUESTIONS

1. The two integrated processes associated with the role function mode for the individual and as defined by the Roy Adaptation Model are developing roles (DR) and role-taking (RT). Label each of the following statements according to the process to which they apply.
   (a) _____ based on symbolic interactionism
   (b) _____ role set
   (c) _____ imaginatively, taking another's role
   (d) _____ anticipating another individual's behavior
   (e) _____ adding new roles as one matures
2. Which of the following behaviors would an individual exhibit with a nursing diagnosis of ineffective role transition?
   (a) ineffective expressive behaviors
   (b) effective instrumental behaviors
   (c) ineffective instrumental behaviors
   (d) none of the above
3. The Roy Adaptation Model describes two compensatory processes associated with the role function mode: role transition (RT) and role distance (RD). Label the following descriptive phrases according to the compensatory process to which they pertain.
   (a) _____ performance of the minimal number of prescribed instrumental behaviors for a role
   (b) _____ closely related to self-concept
   (c) _____ instrumental behaviors increase over time
   (d) _____ initially, primarily expressive behaviors
   (e) _____ role is viewed as undesirable, in part or in whole
   (f) _____ related to developmental tasks
   (g) _____ role is spoken of in derogatory terms

4. Name the four compromised processes associated with the role function mode for the individual as identified in the Roy Adaptation Model.
   (a) _____
   (b) _____
   (c) _____
   (d) _____

SITUATION

Consider an example of an 18-year-old young adult female who has just entered college. In addition to the secondary role of student, one can project such roles as daughter, sister, girlfriend, and participant in sports activities. Associated with the role of student are the instrumental behaviors of studying, attending classes, writing exams and papers, and participating in laboratory sessions. Expressive behaviors include "sounding off" with peers, complaining to parents about the heavy workload, and rejoicing about exam results with the teacher.

Analysis of the role performance requirements (second-level assessment) is as follows:

Instrumental behavior—studying
   A. Consumer: self, significant others, teacher
   B. Reward: gets good grades, passes courses, receives scholarship
   C. Access to facilities and set of circumstances: library is available, evenings are reserved for study time
   D. Cooperation and collaboration: teachers identify important material, boyfriend calls after 9 p.m., classmates study at the same time

Expressive behavior—"sounding off" with peers
   A. Consumer: peers
   B. Reward: understanding of peers

C. Access to facilities and set of circumstances: peers have opportunity to get together after class and in residence situation

D. Cooperation and collaboration: peers are supportive of each other and all are in the same circumstances

5. Develop a nursing diagnosis that identifies effective adaptation related to the data provided:

During her second semester at school, the student experiences a fractured femur as a result of an accident during her sports activities. For a period of time, she is required to assume the "sick role." Derive a goal related to this circumstance interfering with her student role. The nursing diagnosis on which to base this goal is role conflict related to immobilization and treatment of injury and need to keep up with study requirements at school. Note the goal components of behavior, change expected, and time frame.

6. Suggest nursing interventions that would help her accomplish the previously stated goal.

7. Identify behavior that would indicate that the nursing interventions have been successful and the goals have been achieved.

FEEDBACK

1. (a) RT, (b) DR, (c) RT, (d) RT, (e) DR
2. (c) Ineffective instrumental behaviors

3. (a) RD, (b) RD, (c) RT, (d) RT, (e) RT, (f) RD, (g) RT
4. (a) ineffective role transition
   (b) prolonged role distance
   (c) role conflict
   (d) role failure
5. Nursing diagnosis example: Effective pattern of student role performance associated with presence of all role performance requirements. Example of a goal: During her time of immobilization (time frame), the student will continue (change expected) to work on assignments (behavior) as she feels physically able.
6. Suggested nursing interventions: friends could be asked to take notes for her during class, teachers could be contacted for assignment information, requests could be made to have exams deferred, a laptop computer could be accessed to enable work on assignments.
7. Possible evaluation indicators: assignments would be completed on schedule, exam would be rescheduled for a realistic date in the future, courses would be completed in an appropriate time frame, no courses would have been dropped.

References

Banton, M. (1965). *Roles: An introduction to the study of social relations.* New York: Basic Books.

Biddle, B. J., & Thomas, E. J. (Eds.). (1979). *Role theory: Concepts and research.* Huntington, NY: Kreiger Publishing.

Brehm, S. S., Kassin, S. M., & Fein, S. (2002). Social psychology. (4th ed.). Boston: Houghton Mifflin Company.

Clarke, B. A., & Strauss, S. S. (1992). Nursing role supplementation for adolescent parents: Prescriptive nursing practice. *Journal of Pediatric Nursing, 7*(5), 312–318.

Eagly, A. H. (1987). *Sex differences in social behavior: A social-role interpretation.* Hillsdale, NJ: Erlbaum.

Ekman, P., & O'Sullivan, M. (1991). Who can catch a liar? *American Psychologist, 46,* 913–920.

Erickson, E. H. (1963). *Childhood and society* (2nd ed.). New York: Norton.

Erickson, H., Tomlin, E., & Swain, M. A. (1988). *Modeling and role modeling: A theory and paradigm for nursing.* Lexington, SC: Press of Lexington.

Goode, W. J. (1960). A theory of role strain. *American Psychological Review, 25,* 483–496.

Handel, W. (1979). Normative expectations and the emergence of meaning as solutions to problems: Convergence of structural and interactionist views. *American Journal of Sociology, 84*(4), 855–881.

Im, E. O., & Meleis, A. I. (1999). A situation specific theory of menopausal transition of Korean immigrant women. Image: *Journal of Nursing Scholarship, 31,* 333–338.

Linton, R. (1945). *Cultural background of personality.* New York: Appleton-Century.

Malaznik, N. (1976). Theory of role function. In C. Roy (Ed.), *Introduction to nursing: An adaptation model* (pp. 245–264). Englewood Cliffs, NJ: Prentice-Hall.

McMahon, E. M. (1993). *Beyond the myth of dominance: An alternative to a violent society.* Kansas City, MO: Sheed & Ward.

Mead, G. H. (1934). *Mind, self, and society.* Chicago: University of Chicago Press.

Meleis, A. I. (1975). Role insufficiency and role supplementation: A conceptual framework. *Nursing Research, 24*(4), 264–271.

Meleis, A. I., Sawyer, L. M., Im, E., Hilfinger Messias, D. K., & Schumacher, K. (2000). Experiencing transitions: An emerging middle-range theory. *Advances in Nursing Science, 23*(1), 12–28.

NANDA International. (2007). *Nursing diagnoses: Definitions and classifications, 2007–2008.* Philadelphia: NANDA-I.

Nuwayhid, K. A. (1984). Role function: Theory and development. In C. Roy (Ed.), *Introduction to nursing: An adaptation model* (2nd ed., pp. 284–305). Englewood Cliffs, NJ: Prentice-Hall.

Nuwayhid, K. A. (1991). Role transition, distance, and conflict. In C. Roy & H. Andrews (Eds.), *The Roy Adaptation Model: The definitive statement.* Norwalk, CT: Appleton & Lange.

Parsons, T. (1964). *The social system.* New York: The Free Press.

Parsons, T., & Shils, E. (Eds.). (1951). *Toward a general theory of action.* Cambridge, MA: Harvard University Press.

Patterson, M. L. (1996). Social behavior and social cognition: A parallel process approach. In J. I. Nye & A. M. Brower (Eds.), *What's social about social cognition? Research on socially shared cognition in small groups* (pp. 87–105). Thousand Oaks, CA: Sage Publications.

Randell, B. (1976). Development of role function. In C. Roy (Ed.), *Introduction to nursing: An adaptation model* (pp. 256–264). Englewood Cliffs, NJ: Prentice-Hall.

Roy, C. (1967). Role cues and mothers of hospitalized children. *Nursing Research, 16,* 178–182.

Roy, C. (1988). An explication of the philosophical assumptions of the Roy Adaptation Model. *Nursing Science Quarterly, 1*(1), 26–34.

Roy, C. (1997). Future of the Roy model: Challenge to redefine adaptation. *Nursing Science Quarterly, 10*(1), 42–48.

Roy, C. (2007). Knowledge as universal cosmic imperative. In C. Roy & D. A. Jones (Eds.), *Nursing knowledge development and clinical practice* (pp. 145–161). New York: Springer.

Roy, C., & Roberts, S. L. (Eds.). (1981). *Theory construction in nursing: An adaptation model.* Englewood Cliffs, NJ: Prentice Hall.

Schofield, A. (1976). Problems of role function. In C. Roy (Ed.), *Introduction to nursing: An adaptation model* (pp. 265–287). Englewood Cliffs, NJ: Prentice-Hall.

Turner, R. H. (1979). Role-taking, role standpoint and reference group behavior. In B. J. Biddle & E. J. Thomas (Eds.), *Role theory: Concepts and research* (pp. 151–159). Huntington, NY: Kreiger Publishing.

US Bureau of Labor Statistics (2000). US Department of Labor, Washington, DC.

Zohar, D., & Marshall, I. (1994). *The quantum society: Mind, physics, and a new social vision.* New York: Quill/Morrow.

CHAPTER 16

Interdependence Mode of the Person

The final adaptive mode to be introduced is the interdependence mode. This mode, like the role function mode, involves interaction with others. Interdependence, however, focuses on close relationships of people rather than roles in society. The interdependence mode for the individual person is introduced in this chapter. The interdependence mode for people relating in groups is described in Chapter 20. The basic underlying need of the interdependence mode is relational integrity. Relational integrity means the feeling of security in relationships. A sense of security is experienced through mutual and satisfying relationships with others and with the environment. For people, this need is often met through interaction with significant others and support systems. Two basic life processes of the interdependence mode of the individual are affectional adequacy and developmental adequacy. The Roy Adaptation Model notes that each individual strives for relational integrity by adequacy and mastery in these processes. This chapter provides an overview of the interdependence mode with a focus on integrated processes of affectional adequacy and developmental adequacy. Illustrations of compensatory adaptive processes related to interdependence for the individual are provided, and examples of compromised processes of interdependence are explored. Finally, guidelines for planning nursing care by assessing behaviors and stimuli, formulating diagnoses, establishing goals, selecting interventions, and evaluating nursing care are described.

OBJECTIVES

After studying this chapter, the reader will be able to do the following:

1. Describe the interdependence mode according to the Roy Adaptation Model.
2. Describe one compensatory process related to the interdependence mode.
3. Name and describe two situations of compromised processes of interdependence.
4. Identify important behaviors for first-level assessment of the interdependence mode.
5. Identify second-level assessment factors or stimuli that influence the interdependence mode.

6. Develop a nursing diagnosis, given a situation related to interdependence for the individual.

7. Derive goals for a given situation illustrating ineffective interdependence in a given situation.

8. Describe nursing interventions commonly implemented in situations of ineffective interdependence.

9. Propose approaches to determine the effectiveness of nursing interventions.

KEY CONCEPTS DEFINED

Affectional adequacy: One of two processes associated with the basic need of relational integrity for the individual; the need to give and receive love, respect, and value satisfied through effective relations and communication.

Alienation: A condition or feeling of being estranged or separated from self and others; feelings develop when significant others are not meeting what is expected as givers of affection and relationship.

Developmental adequacy: One of two processes associated with the basic need of relational integrity for the individual; learning and maturation in relationships achieved through developmental processes.

Interdependence: For the individual is defined as the close relationships of people aimed at satisfying needs for affection and development of relationships.

Nurturing ability: Involves providing growth-producing care and attention.

Relational integrity: The basic need of the interdependence mode; the feeling of security in relationships.

Significant others: The individuals to whom the most meaning or importance is given.

Support systems: Persons, groups, and organizations with whom one associates in order to achieve affectional and developmental adequacy.

PROCESSES OF INTERDEPENDENCE FOR INDIVIDUALS

Interdependence for the individual is defined as the close relationships of people aimed at satisfying needs for affection and development of relationships. The purpose is to achieve relational integrity—the basic need of the interdependence mode. In Chapter 14 the significance of feedback from others for the developing self was noted. It is through affectional and developmental processes that one continues to grow as an individual and as a contributing member of society. The quest for adequacy in relationships is part of today's culture. Intact families try to spend time together, divorced people seek new relationships, social groups for young and old proliferate. There is a preponderance of self-help books on "satisfying relationships." Movies and novels focus on the struggles of intimate and loving relationships. However, the times reflect that fewer people are married and more are living alone. Relationships are affected by demographic and societal changes. These include the aging population, family separations, and frequent job changes. These and many other demands challenge people to find new ways to achieve relational integrity. For example, immigrant groups alone in a foreign country tend to form groups to fulfill their need for relational adequacy and security when their families are absent and they are isolated in a culturally strange environment.

The literature on relationships discusses their influence on quality and length of life. Some authors tie length of life and the good life to relationships with others or social support (see, for example, Cohen, 1985; Dimond & Jones, 1983; Gottlieb, 1981; Greenblatt, Beccera, & Serafetinides, 1982; Roy, 1981). House, Landis, and Umberson (1988) reviewed the literature noting a relationship between social interaction and health. The classic study of Spitz (1945) showed that infants who were deprived of touch or affection simply wasted away and died. For years, it has been known that married people live longer and are healthier, and often happier, than unmarried people. The "social contact index" (Berkman, 1978) often used in these studies takes into account whether the individual is married, has close contacts with friends and relatives, belongs to a religious group, or has organizational links. People who have contacts in only one of these categories appear to have a greater risk of dying than those who have contacts in more than one category.

Interdependent relationships involve the willingness and ability to give and accept from others aspects of all that one has to offer: love, respect, value, nurturing, knowledge, skills, commitments, material possessions, time, and talents. People who demonstrate adaptive interdependence have a comfortable balance between their needs for affiliation or dependence and achievement or independence. They have learned to live successfully in a world of other people, animals, objects, the environment, and a God figure. Interdependence needs are met through social interaction on many levels. For the individual, relationships are developed primarily with significant others and support systems. Productive and rewarding relationship processes meet needs related to affection, that is, love, respect, value, nurturance, care, attention, affirmation, belonging, approval, and understanding. Secondly, the individual meets developmental needs associated with learning and maturation in relationships.

Interdependent relationships are divided into two categories, significant others and support systems. Significant others are the individuals to whom the most meaning or importance is given. The significant others for a person may be parents, spouse, friends, family members, God, or even an animal. These significant others are loved, respected, and valued, and in turn, they love, respect, and value to a degree greater than in other relationships. Significant others can be identified by answering the question of who are the most important people in my life. For most people, the significant others are relatively stable and remain for periods of time. Individuals usually can identify at least one person who is a significant other. In some situations, material possessions or money become more significant than other people. However, in these instances, the love, respect, and value is not reciprocal and ineffective interdependence results.

Support systems include people, groups, and organizations with which one associates in order to accomplish goals or to achieve some purpose. The meanings of relationships with support systems do not usually carry the same intensity as those of relationships with significant others. Consider the example of an adult woman who might identify her spouse and children as significant others and a friend at work and her book club as support systems. A place of work, itself, becomes part of a person's support system. At times of illness, the nurse can occupy a position in a support system for an individual who requires health care. Thus, interrelationships, whether they are with significant others or support systems, become an important consideration in providing nursing care.

A central notion of interdependent relationships is the giving to and receiving from others. As noted, this includes giving and receiving aspects of that which we have to offer as persons, such as love, respect, value, nurturing, knowledge, skills, commitment, time, talents, and material possessions. This giving and receiving is evident in friendships, family relationships, and interactions in groups. Such relationships involve both giving and receiving of something, love and nurturing in parent–child relationships, work in return for pay in employment relationships, participation in return for security and belonging in cultural groups, as simple examples. Figure 16–1 shows the theoretical basis for the interdependence mode for the individual. Giving and receiving with significant others, such as the family, and with support systems, such as relations, friends, clubs, associations, work groups, or components of larger social service systems, are viewed as based on the underlying middle range theories of affectional and developmental processes.

An important consideration when evaluating the effectiveness of interacting components in achieving the goals of the relationship is the congruence and alignment of the interrelated components. Disruption occurs if any one component is not compatible with or does not complement the other. Ineffective adaptation is the outcome. For example, if a young person begins to see support systems as more important than family members, the interrelations of the entire family are affected. If the example set by parents differs from the developing child's support system, new ways of balancing relationships are sought. Kane (1988) reported beginning work toward a conceptual model of family social support and presented three interaction factors: reciprocity, advice and feedback, and emotional involvement. This work on reciprocity is based on the earlier work of Cobb (1976) that described an individual as involved in a network of mutual obligation. This belonging is noted by the sharing of resources with others and the giving and receiving of help. Advice and feedback relates to the quality and quantity of communication between the family and its network. Kane also drew on the work of Caplan (1974), who emphasized the importance of relationships with significant others to work through the issues of living. Kane (1988) noted that communication is done through a process of giving advice and feedback. Emotional involvement includes the concepts of intimacy and trust. This final factor includes emotional bonds such as love, caring, warmth, and compassion.

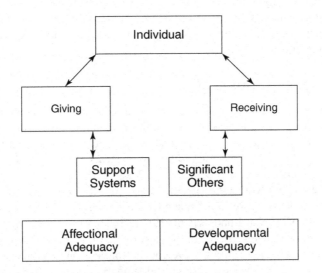

FIGURE 16–1 Interdependence Mode for the individual. Theoretical basis.

The importance of communication in the achievement of effective relationships was also described by others. Koch and Haugk (1992, p. 18) observed that, "Without communication in a personal relationship, you risk collapse of that relationship." Selman and Andrews (1994) claimed that relationship issues are inseparable from communication issues, and in most cases are the same thing. Since relationships exist for a purpose, there must be a way of accomplishing the goals and plans associated with that purpose. Communication is that vehicle. As Selman and Andrews (1994) observed:

> Success in realizing intentions is accomplished through relationships with others. The future is continually being created through conversations with others—by asking for or making commitments, by making requests and promises. Any potential future exists only as a possibility unless and until it is realized through action. From this perspective, commitments are actions. Successful coordination in relationships is the coordination of commitments.
>
> As the vision and commitments [in interrelationships] grow, so do the relationship breakdowns. This is both inevitable and healthy—an indication that the real underlying patterns and negative behavioral mechanisms are beginning to surface. These mechanisms normally are concealed, buried...; they often thwart the best intentions to change. When they are uncovered, breakdowns in relationship are no longer taken for granted or covered over with platitudes. Rather, practices for getting to the bedrock question of what constitutes a "good relationship" begin to develop—that is, what are an individual's commitments, and how can one learn to develop and continuously improve effective relationships? (p. 54)

Selman and Andrews (1994) presented seven principles of effective relationships that have proven valuable, both in relationships with significant others and in interaction with support systems. These are identified and defined in Table 16–1. As they are applied, the effectiveness of relationships is markedly enhanced. The basic need of the interdependence mode is relational integrity—the feeling of security in relationships. As previously noted, two processes are involved in achievement of relational integrity: affectional adequacy, that is, the giving and receiving of love, value, and respect; and developmental adequacy, that is, learning and maturing of relationships.

Process of Affectional Adequacy

Affectional adequacy involves the willingness and ability to give to and receive from others aspects of all one has to offer as a person: love, respect, value, nurturance, knowledge, skills, commitments, talents, possessions, time, and loyalty, for example. Affectional adequacy incorporates the need to be nurtured and to nurture in terms of care, attention, affection, affirmation, belonging, approval, and understanding. These needs are met primarily by establishing in-depth relationships with other people. Behaviors that demonstrate this exchange of personal attributes and assets are called receptive (receiving) and contributive (giving) behaviors (Randell, Tedrow, & Van Landingham, 1982). Receiving behaviors are those that indicate that a person is receiving, taking in, or assimilating that offered by another. Receiving behaviors include allowing another to care for and protect oneself, accepting a thoughtful gesture, and receiving physical or psychological support. Giving behaviors are those of giving or supplying nurturance to another person. Examples include caring for another, touching, providing physical and psychological support, and performing thoughtful gestures.

TABLE 16–1 Principles of Effective Relationships

Listen Generously

Listen for the contribution and commitment of the other person, suspending assessments, judgments, and opinions about what he or she is saying. This does not mean that we agree or disagree with what is being said, but that we are committed to the legitimacy and value of the other's view.

Talk Straight

Speak honestly in a way that forwards the action as opposed to reacting or attacking what is being said. This includes learning to make clear and direct requests.

Be for Each Other

Believe and commit to the premise that we are all in this together and that no one individual can win at the expense of another. This is the basis for trust and for making it safe for each other to take risks without fear of censure or being undermined by one's colleagues.

Honor Each Other's Commitments

Respect each other's commitments including one's own.

Appreciate and Acknowledge Each Other

Each member in the relationship commits to continuously acknowledge and appreciate the contributions of others and the team itself, even when things do not work out. It also means requesting and receiving acknowledgement from others if it is missing.

Be Concerned for Inclusion

Ask the question "Who else should be included or has a stake in what we are talking about?"

Be Concerned for Alignment

Participate in every conversation with a commitment to build alignment. Alignment does not mean consensus or universal agreement. It means that everyone is either "committed to" or "able to support" the commitments of others. No one is committed against the direction in which we are moving.

Source: Selman, J. C., & Andrews, H. A. (1994). Effective relationships: Rethinking the fundamentals. In H. A. Andrews, L. M. Cook, J. M. Davidson, D. P. Schurman, E. W. Taylor, & R. H. Wensel(Eds.), *Organizational transformation in health care: A work in progress* (pp. 55). San Francisco: Jossey–Bass. Used with permission.

These giving and receiving behaviors reflect the mutual relationship between an individual and others in the environment. People who successfully maintain relationships have developed the ability to recognize and deal with their own love and support needs, as well as those of other people. The process of achieving affectional adequacy includes many components of interaction such as language skills, nonverbal communication skills, and the ability to recognize the feelings and attitudes of others. The development of sympathy and caring, as well as sharing, is inherent in this process. This development begins early and continues throughout a person's life. Focus on learning and maturation in relationships is further addressed in the section on developmental adequacy.

Process of Developmental Adequacy

Developmental adequacy refers to the processes associated with learning and maturation in interrelationships. These relationships often involve two people relating and also extend to the groups to which they belong. Each relationship undergoes development and transition in terms of dependency and independency throughout the span of the relationship. The appropriateness of this balance as learning and maturation proceed influences adaptation and the ability to achieve relational integrity. In early interpretations of the adaptive modes, Randell, Tedrow, and Van Landingham (1982) proposed the belief that when a baby is born, two adaptive modes are operational, the physiologic mode and the interdependence mode. Many studies document the infant's need for touch, physical contact, the bonding process, and love. Out of the interactions that are primarily affectional and nurturing arises the beginning of self-concept; finally, roles are learned. These authors further suggested that, with the living out of one's life, the modes are given up in reverse sequence. For example, people who are admitted to convalescent centers in their final years give up many of their previously held roles. Sometimes even the identity of their self-concept becomes less apparent if the individual moves to dementia or a state of coma. The expression of self is diminished by decreased meaningful social interaction. A form of the interdependence mode, the receiving part of interaction, and the physiologic mode remain operational.

According to this view, a person begins and ends life as a physiologic and interdependent being. There are exceptions to this continuum, such as sudden death or a long productive life with minimal deterioration of functioning. This general picture of the development and relinquishing of the four adaptive modes is illustrated in Figure 16–2. Many sociological and psychological theorists have studied the development of relationships in terms of dependence and independence. The works of Erikson (1963), Selman (1980), Fromm (1956), Havighurst (1953), and Maslow (1954) provide an understanding of the development and maintenance of relational integrity. Selman (1980) provided a description of five stages of friendship that are similar to Erikson's work but apply more specifically to the development of affectional needs. The stages and their characteristics are listed in Table 16–2.

A friendship builds out of some commonly held beliefs, values, and interests. Some people experience the growth of a friendship from which an adult love relationship can develop. Fromm (1956) talked about love being a feeling and an action. Love has the characteristics of knowing, caring about, respecting, and feeling responsibility toward the receiver of love. Each of us has a need to be loved and supported and to love and support. The love relationship is an intense interaction with close identification with the loved one. As such, the joy and pain, as well as stresses and happiness, of the other, are experienced by both people in the relationship. The love relationship includes a friendship with the other person. Havighurst (1953) described developmental tasks for the infant to the mature adult. Each stage of life includes tasks related to establishing and maintaining relational integrity.

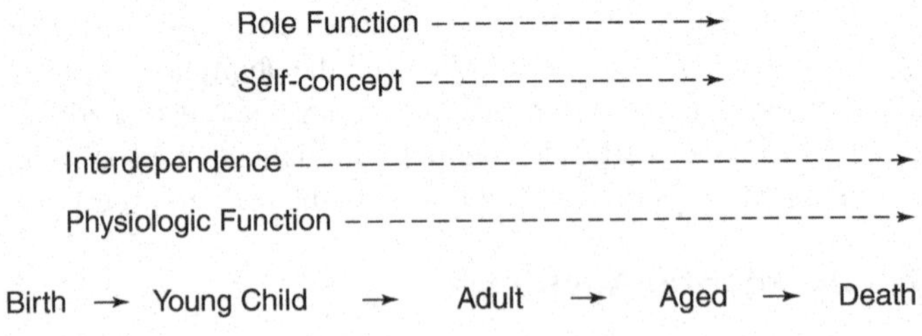

Role Function – – – – – – – – – –➤

Self-concept – – – – – – – – – – – –➤

Interdependence –➤

Physiologic Function –➤

Birth → Young Child → Adult → Aged → Death

FIGURE 16–2 Four adaptive modes for the individual from birth to death.

TABLE 16–2 The Five Stages of Friendship

Stage	Age (Years)	Characteristics
0	3–7	*Monetary Playmate*: The child has difficulty distinguishing between a physical action, such as grabbing a toy, and the psychological intention behind this action. Friends are valued for their material and physical attributes and defined by proximity.
1	4–9	*One-way Assistance*: At this stage, the child can differentiate between his or her own perspective and those of others. However, the child does not yet understand that dealing with others involves give-and-take between people. In a "good" friendship, one party does what the other party wants to do.
2	6–12	*Two-way Fair Weather Cooperation*: The child has the ability to see that interpersonal perspectives are reciprocal, each person taking into account the other's perspective. Conceptions of friendship include a concern for what each person thinks about the other. It is much more a two-way street. The limitation of this stage is that the child still sees the basic purpose of friendship as serving many separate self-interests rather than mutual interests.
3	9–15	*Intimate, Mutually Shared Relationships*: Not only can the child take the other's point of view, but by now he or she can also step outside the friendship and take a generalized third-person perspective on it. With the ability to take a third-person perspective, the child can move from viewing friendships as reciprocal cooperation for each person's self-interests to seeing it as a collaboration with others for mutual and common interests. That is, friends share feelings, help each other resolve personal and interpersonal conflicts, and help each other solve personal problems.
4	15 on	*Autonomous Interdependent Friendships*: The individual sees relationships as complex and often overlapping systems. In a friendship, the adolescent or adult is aware that people have many needs and that in a good friendship, each partner gives strong emotional and psychological support to the other, but also allows the friend to develop independent relationships. Respecting needs for both dependency and autonomy is seen as being essential to friendship.

Source: Selman, R. C. (1980). *The growth of interpersonal understanding: Development and clinical analysis.* New York: Academic Press. Used with permission.

COMPENSATORY ADAPTIVE PROCESSES

Viewed as an adaptive system, individuals have innate and acquired ways of responding to the changing environment (see Chapter 2). Further, Roy conceptualizes these complex adaptive dynamics as the coping processes of the regulator and cognator subsystems for the individual. Compensatory processes represent the adaptation level at which the cognator–regulator have been activated by a challenge to the integrated life processes. Compensatory processes associated with interdependence for the individual often involve support systems. Individuals often call on these for assistance when affectional or developmental challenges occur. Two illustrations of interdependence compensatory adaptive responses are provided: a mentorship program for disadvantaged young people and programs to assist those affected by alcohol abuse.

Many social service programs have arisen in response to a need to provide assistance to individuals in the achievement of relational integrity, that is, affectional and developmental adequacy. Agencies participating in and supporting such initiatives often include the business community, labor associations, school districts, and civic councils. One such program is a mentorship program for disadvantaged young people. This program provides an opportunity for employed adults to mentor students at their workplace. The mentor functions as a positive role model for the student and encourages that individual to develop his or her fullest potential and to develop a vision for the future. Mentorship is an attempt to encourage young people in disadvantaged situations to stay in school and to be successful in life. The impact of such a program is reflected in the following quotation from a high school principal: "Today schools and educators are asked to take on so many responsibilities in nurturing and developing young people, but we cannot do it by ourselves. We are grateful for the support provided by all the partners in [the program] as we challenge our students to seek their greatest potential."

Another example of a support system that is assisting families in compensatory processes is focused on a major interdependence problem, alcohol abuse. The Al-Anon Family Group Headquarters, Inc. is an organization designed to support those whose lives and relationships have been affected by someone else's drinking problems. There is also an arm of the organization directed at the needs of teens in such a situation. For the individual who has the desire to overcome alcohol dependency, Alcoholics Anonymous is an agency with branches throughout North America. Through interdependent relationships with individuals experiencing the same dependency problem, mutual support and encouragement have helped many individuals to gain control of their situation.

COMPROMISED PROCESSES OF INTERDEPENDENCE

When integrated and compensatory life processes are inadequate, the third adaptation level of compromised processes results. Adaptation problems are compromised processes of adaptation. They can be caused by difficulties in one or both of the processes of interdependence since affectional adequacy and developmental adequacy are interrelated. Four examples of compromised processes of interdependence for individuals are discussed in this section. They are separation anxiety, loneliness, substance abuse, and aggression.

Separation Anxiety

Separation anxiety is the painful uneasiness of mind related to separation from a significant other. The focal stimulus for this condition is the actual or threatened separation from a significant other; it is discussed as a compromised process of the interdependence mode.

Separation anxiety is first experienced in infancy. The individual has the potential for experiencing separation anxiety throughout the life span. There are developmental crises in the individual's life that create a vulnerable period for anxiety related to separation. These developmental crises are addressed in the works of Mahler (1979), Bowlby (1969, 1973), Robertson (1953), and Erikson (1963).

The infant is separated physiologically at birth from the mother with the cutting of the umbilical cord. The beginning of emotional separation occurs during later stages of development. Before emotional separation can occur, emotional bonding or attachment with the significant other must occur (Klaus & Kennel, 1981). Bonding is a term that describes a reciprocal joining or unity. It begins for the woman as she experiences pregnancy and proceeds through the tasks of pregnancy. Bonding probably begins for the fetus during this time, but is accelerated during and immediately following birth. By the time the child is ready to enter school, a process of bonding and attachment, followed by a stage of separation and becoming a distinct separate individual, has occurred. It is after that attachment phase, and during the separation–individuation phase, that separation anxiety first occurs and is most intense.

Mahler (1979) described three phases of the attachment–separation process that are experienced in sequence. The first phase, autism, occurs during the first few weeks of life. The infant does not differentiate the self from the environment, but does learn to differentiate between pain and pleasure. The second phase, the symbiotic phase, refers to the attachment to the mother. At this time, about 1 month of age, the infant does not differentiate the self from the nonself but does attach to the mother. Mahler's third phase, the separation–individuation process, begins soon after the symbiotic or attachment phase. There is a four-part progression that occurs during the separation–individuation process. Separation refers to separation from the constant caregiver, usually the mother. Individuation refers to clearly becoming a self. The first subphase is termed differentiation and emerges as the infant becomes mobile by creeping, walking, climbing, and exploring self and the environment. The infant stays near the mother and enjoys playing games with objects and people that repeatedly disappear and reappear, such as "where did it go?" and "peek-a-boo." The next subphase is termed practicing, during which the child explores the environment near the mother and develops motor skills. The child in this stage accepts strangers readily as long as the mother is near and the stranger does not approach.

Rapprochement is the next subphase during which the child actively resists separation. It is manifested by the toddler using negative behavior, such as repeatedly saying "no" or self-identity behavior such as saying "me" and "mine." There is an intense period of growth in the formation of the self-concept mode during the rapprochement phase. The separation from the mother is for longer periods, but the toddler continues to return to her frequently. The self-concept and interdependence modes are interconnected closely at this point of the toddler's life. The final subphase, object constancy, occurs from 18 to 36 months of age. The child develops intrapsychic symbols for the significant other. This development enables the child to begin separating without the overwhelming fear of abandonment.

Early work in separation anxiety was done by Robertson (1953) and Bowlby (1969). These authors described the infant between 3 and 6 months of age as recognizing the mother as an individual. They defined the period of 18 to 24 months as a time of peak dependency on the caregiver. The child at this time is possessively and passionately attached to the mother. The child is overwhelmed when separated from the mother. Bowlby and Robertson documented on film the behavior of children who were separated at the time of hospitalization. They defined three stages of separation anxiety through which children proceed if their significant other is separated from them. They are protest, despair, and denial or detachment. In the protest stage, children are acutely aware of their need for their mothers. They will do anything and do it vigorously to recapture their mothers. They do believe that their energetic protesting behaviors will, in fact, return their mothers to their sides.

The next state of separation occurs in a few hours or days, the stage of despair. During this stage, children are actively mourning the loss of the significant other, and they withdraw. While mourning, each child remains preoccupied with the loss of the mother and remains vigilant for her return. It is the quiet phase of separation anxiety. The child is passive and will perform self-comforting activities such as thumb-sucking or clinging to a favorite toy. The final phase of denial (detachment) is moved into slowly. At this point, children repress the need for their mothers and begin to be interested in the environment. Children begin to seek comfort in food and support from anyone who will give it to them. A stranger viewing a child at this stage would tend to remark on how well-adjusted the child has become. When parents return, the child who has gone only as far as the stage of despair will usually reject the parents initially and then respond to them slowly. The attachment is reestablished slowly as the child and significant other are reunited. Passing through these stages to a resolution hopefully will lead to a more comfortable separation another time.

Although separation experiences are essential to the development of the individual, they should be minimized during periods of increased stress, such as hospitalization. These early works of Robertson and Bowlby were helpful in the movement of extending visiting hours in pediatric hospitals and instituting policies of rooming-in for parents and families so that they can stay with their ill child. Erikson (1963) identified eight developmental crises, or stages, that are to be mastered sequentially through the life span. These were identified in Chapter 14. The tasks of infancy and early childhood relevant here are building trust and achieving autonomy. This stage is relevant to the issue of attachment and separation through which the child proceeds to attain a separate identity. Ainsworth (1964) and Mead (1971) explored child behavior in other cultures. Ainsworth studied children and parents in Uganda, and Mead, in Samoa. Both cultures have extended family units with many adults in the child's environment. Both researchers documented that the infant did not attach as intensely to the mother and therefore did not experience the degree of separation anxiety that children do who are reared in a society without extended families.

Another crisis period for separation anxiety occurs for the school-aged child with the beginning and the end of the school year. Phenomena identified as school phobias are frequently separation anxiety. Ezor (1980) studied the separation anxiety related to school. The adolescent experiences separation anxiety with high frequency. This chaotic period is not unlike the toddler period, with an emphasis on clarifying one's identity and again separating from one's parents. Separation from the peer group also causes anxiety. The adult can experience separation anxiety. An example of adult separation anxiety is the couple who is separated for a long period for a business or a military deployment. During the process of saying good-bye, the stages of protest, despair, and denial (detachment) can be experienced. Protest is manifested by such statements as "I'd like to be going with you" "I wish you didn't have to go." Feelings related to the protest stage are feelings of anxiety surrounding the actual separation and the projected time alone. The despair state can be manifested by behaviors of listlessness and lack of interest in the environment or anger behaviors. Many couples experience feelings and behaviors of anger that are unexpected and disturbing to them as they separate. Most adults move into detachment quickly, maintain the relationship in whatever way is possible, and look forward to being reunited and the resolution stage.

When living in a highly mobile society, adults and children terminate from their support systems with some frequency. Stanford's (1977) work with groups, especially cohesive groups, reported on separation anxiety as a group comes to a closure. If the individual has given importance to the group, many of the behaviors identified by Stanford will be evident. Although Stanford's work was with students, his observations can relate to individuals in the general population who are terminating with a support group. Stanford's behaviors of termination anxiety are as follows.

1. Increased conflict: Students may start bickering with one another for no apparent reason, or at least no significant reason. It is almost as though they were trying to prove to themselves that "I don't really like these people, or else I wouldn't be fighting with them. And since I don't like them, it won't be painful for me to leave them."

2. Breakdown of group skills: Working together on a task, the group may suddenly exhibit what appears to be a complete lack of skills, and they may violate all the norms that were established previously. It is almost as though they were saying to themselves and the teachers, "You see we really didn't change much this year. We're still like every other class. And since this is like every other class, it won't be so hard to leave."

3. Lethargy: Some students begin to show less and less interest in their work, as if to say, "What does it matter any more? If we're going to have to break up, what's the use of continuing to work?" Their lethargy may also be a symptom of depression indicating feelings of sadness about the imminent breakup of the group.

4. Frantic attempts to work well: Conversely, some groups may actually increase their productivity, taking on more and more projects and rushing to do everything they can before the term ends. They may display impeccable group skills, working far more effectively than ever before. Implicit in this behavior may be the message, "If we're a model class, maybe the teacher will like us so much we won't have to leave. Maybe our group can continue forever." Thus separation anxiety can be demonstrated throughout the life span often caused by a temporary separation from the significant other and more often by a permanent separation from a support system.

Loneliness

From the aged individual to the infant, from the economically privileged person to the more deprived, loneliness exists as a common adaptation problem. No one is immunized against loneliness. It is a lifelong struggle for everyone to maintain relational integrity. Even the individual who has mutually satisfying relationships experiences periods of loneliness and alienation. The individual who does not attain affectional adequacy and who, for the greater part, may have no or very few satisfying relationships suffers great emotional pain. Alienation is a condition or feeling of being estranged or separated from self and others. Alienation feelings develop when significant others are not meeting what is expected as givers of affiliation. This deprivation of presence or contact leads to a feeling of not being needed, valued, or appreciated by others, and therein lies the root of loneliness.

Alienation is a serious problem in contemporary society. Many social theorists have written on its pervasiveness in North American life and on the contextual factors that affect this pattern. Among these are the diminishing of the family as the basic unit of society, mobility, urbanization, and computerization. Early childhood experiences of affectional adequacy or inadequacy can further contribute to interdependence adaptation. Socially, friends seem to be transient, families are physically separated, and after all, "Who does care what happens to me?" Many more individuals end up living in the streets because they have no human ties that can be of help in a housing crisis. That alienation exists is undeniable. Particularly because of the contemporary situation, people in our society have a good to excellent chance of developing one of the variants of alienation.

The classic types of alienation were described by Seeman (1959) as powerlessness, meaninglessness, normlessness, isolation, and self-estrangement. Any of these types of alienation can cause the individual to feel further separated from others. Some individuals can handle these alienated feelings by innovative ways of building relationships. An example of this is the young adult who appraises the situation and says that things are not good, not the way one would like to have them. But the individual recognizes that things do not have to remain as they are. The individual proceeds to become involved in changing things and building relationships. People can use less positive means to deal with alienated feelings. These avenues involve a dependency on things or others to ward off feelings of alienation. There is a pattern of using "something" to act as a bridge to relationships. These patterns include the following.

1. Dependency on a lifestyle that emphasizes withdrawal and retreatism to feel secure.
2. Dependency on performing ritualistic behaviors to deal with anxieties of alienation, such as chain-smoking, overeating, psychosomatic illness, or any activity that is done to excess to stay busy.
3. Rebelling against society by joining an alternate cultural group with subsequent dependency on it such as the drug culture, alcoholic state, or sexual variancy groups.
4. Dependency on situations retaining the status quo. This individual sees no possibility for change and considers turning against the world as the only way to deal with alienation.

Some of these alternatives can be so ineffective as to stimulate self-concept disruption. An example of this would be the individual who chooses to withdraw from the real world and stay in a fantasy existence. This condition is referred to as self-alienation and can involve a total collapse of the self-concept. Too often, alienated schoolchildren or young adults have been involved in planning shootings of students and faculty on school campuses.

Substance Abuse

Substance abuse, as it relates to the individual, is a pressing concern associated with dependency behaviors and ineffective relational integrity. Contemporary society is highly drug oriented with increasing numbers of individuals becoming involved in various forms of substance abuse. The roots, dynamics, and effects of these problems are complex. However, literature in the field cites connections between these problems and what the Roy Adaptation Model calls unmet interdependence needs. The complexities of modern society in industrially developed countries have brought about high levels of stress at the same time that close relationships with others are less available to help individuals cope. The breathtaking rate of change, the erosion of family life, and the threat of internal and external hostile political forces are but a few of the factors causing stress. In these situations, the basic need for relating to others in mutual love, respect, and valuing is intensified. When this need goes unmet through a lack of meaningful significant others and support systems, the individual can develop a condition known as insatiable longing.

Insatiable longing is a vague yearning or gnawing sensation that keeps a person in a constant state of anticipation, which is never fulfilled and cannot be fulfilled in an ordinary way. The individual with insatiable longing is vulnerable to addiction or being taken over by some substance or activity. People can become dependent on almost anything; legal drugs or illegal drugs are common, such as, morphine, OxyContin, phenobarbital, heroin, cocaine, crack cocaine, marijuana, alcohol, food, or even work or hobbies (Brown & Fowler, 1969). Once people are in the condition of insatiable longing, they are also prone to frustration, anxiety, and depression. Life's experiences for these individuals easily become exhausting and unmanageable, and dependence on drugs results when more effective coping mechanisms are not available within the person's cognitive-emotional domain.

Aggression—Individual

When an individual does not have an effective pattern of control over aggression, a generalized pattern of behavior develops that indicates a need to control others. The problem of aggression stems from an unmet need for balance in dependency and independency. Where an overemphasis on dependency exists, passive behavior tends to predominate. If independency is overbalanced, aggression becomes evident. In understanding aggression, it is helpful to first explore the notion of passive behavior. Koch and Haugk (1992, p. 16) described passive behavior as "behavior that moves against the self." This includes physical passivity, personal withdrawal from the situation, or verbal passivity. The tendency of the individual is to keep quiet or to withhold feedback. "Passive performers frequently give up important parts of their own personalities to avoid disapproval or criticism so others will like them" (Koch & Haugk, 1992, p. 17).

Aggressive behavior, on the other hand, moves against others. Aggressive people have few internal restraints and few external limits. The expression of aggression can be physical, nonverbal, verbal, or in a pattern labeled passive aggression and are described as follows.

1. Physical aggression. Koch and Haugk (1992) pointed out, "You are all too familiar with physical acts of aggression as you read the daily news reports of abused spouses, abused children, and abused older persons. You hear of murders, assaults, drive-by shootings and gang warfare. You doubtless know more than you want to know about physical aggression" (p. 19).

2. Nonverbal aggression. Aggressive patterns in interrelationships can also develop nonverbally. "Individuals move against others simply by the expression on their faces, by the gestures they use, or their tone of voice" (Koch & Haugk, 1992, p. 20). Has a decision you made while driving ever irritated another driver? Other instances of nonverbal aggression include sneers, looks of scorn, rolling the eyes, or an exasperated sigh. All of these are an effort to move against another individual by trying to establish superiority over them.

3. Verbal aggression. Verbal aggression constitutes moving against others with words as weapons. It can take the form of insults, put-downs, profanity, blaming, or sarcasm. Each of these is an attempt to humiliate or demean another individual in an attempt to manipulate or dominate an encounter.

4. Passive aggression. Koch and Haugk (1992, p. 22) described passive aggression as subtle, "an underhanded way of moving against another individual or manipulating others to get one's own way." Passive aggression can take the form of procrastinating, forgetting, dawdling, pouting, silent treatment, or manipulative tears. For example, the individual who uses the "silent treatment" is trying to punish the other individual by withholding the love and affection associated with relational integrity. All of this is contrasted with assertive behavior in interrelationships. Assertive behavior is defined

by Koch and Haugk as "a constructive way of living and relating to other people...
that reflects concern about being honest, direct, open, and natural in relations with
others" (1992, p. 23).

NURSING PROCESS RELATED TO INDIVIDUAL INTERDEPENDENCE

The interdependent relationships of individuals are an important part of the person's total
adaptation. In applying the nursing process, the nurse will make a careful assessment of the
behaviors and stimuli related to the basic processes of affectional and developmental adequacy. In assessing stimuli influencing interdependence needs, a number of common influencing factors, including regulator and cognator effectiveness in initiating compensatory
processes, will be considered. Based on these thorough first- and second-level assessments,
the nurse makes a nursing diagnosis, sets goals, selects interventions, and evaluates care.

Assessment of Behavior

The nurse begins assessment in the interdependence mode when first meeting the person and
is keenly attuned to behaviors that the person might reveal spontaneously. After creating a
comfortable setting, the nurse proceeds with an in-depth assessment of behaviors related to
affectional adequacy. These focus on the identification of significant others and support systems and the giving and receiving behaviors evident in these relationships.

SIGNIFICANT OTHERS AND SUPPORT SYSTEMS   The nurse first addresses the two major
categories of interdependent relationships, significant others and support systems. Who does
the individual name as significant others? Who or what are his or her support systems and to
what extent does he or she depend on them? With what groups, associations, or organizations
is the individual involved? What significance do they hold in terms of time commitments and
associated responsibilities? Does the individual work? All of this information is significant in
terms of interdependence and affectional adequacy.

GIVING AND RECEIVING   What giving behaviors are evident? What receiving behaviors are
evident? Some questions that can be helpful in the identification of giving and receiving
behaviors are as follows. How do you express your caring to the significant other? How does
the significant other express caring and affection to you? It is important to observe nonverbal
behaviors when others are present with the individual. Do they touch each other, look at each
other, give gifts, share jokes or stories? An example of giving behaviors on the part of a wife
could be the statement, "I tell him often that I love him," or "I always make his lunch."
Receiving behaviors could include statements such as, "I love the way he rubs my back," or
"Look at the beautiful roses he brought me," or "He calls me from work several times a day."

Assessment of Stimuli

Stimuli that are important when assessing affectional and developmental adequacy for individuals include the following.

1. Expectations of relationships and awareness of needs
2. Nurturing ability of both parties
3. Levels of self-esteem

4. Levels and kinds of interaction skills

5. Presence of others in the physical environment

6. Knowledge about relationships and the behaviors that enhance them

7. Developmental age and tasks

8. Significant life changes

EXPECTATIONS   The expectations of the individuals who are involved in a relationship affect the quality of the relationship. If one individual expects that affection is expressed by physical proximity, spending time together, physical contact, and remembering birthdays, it is important that the other individual in the relationship be aware of these expectations and responds to them. When two people in a relationship can define their expectations clearly and communicate them, the relationship is enhanced. Once each individual is aware of expectations and needs of self and the other, it is essential that they all act on this information in a consistent way.

NURTURING ABILITY   The nurturing ability of each individual in the relationship also contributes to the quality of the relationship. Nurturing involves providing growth-producing care and attention. A person who experienced early bonding as an infant and tactile and verbal loving as a child will usually be able to move into adult love relationships with ease. They have experienced a high-quality love relationship and know what it feels like and what the characteristics are. An adult who experienced delayed bonding or minimal bonding in a parent–child relationship that was characterized by distance, separation, and verbal negating will probably need help in learning how to build a friendship or love relationship. Likewise, traumatic experiences in the early years, for example, loss of a parent or abuse by a trusted adult, can interfere with later effective nurturing ability.

LEVEL OF SELF-ESTEEM   The level of self-esteem, as related to the self-concept mode, is an influencing factor for interdependent relationships. People tend to choose friendships and love relationships with individuals who have a similar level of self-esteem, that is, people who have low self-esteem choose friends with low self-esteem. They then are reinforced in the feelings of negative self-worth and the circular process continues. Similarly when two people who experience high self-esteem develop a caring relationship, the reinforcement for the other serves to enhance the already high level of self-esteem. An individual's level of self-esteem influences the degree to which the person feels that he or she can go out to others. Likewise, self-esteem is a basic contextual factor when interdependent circumstances in life change, for example, the permanent separation from one who has been a significant other. Level of self-esteem influences the person's ability to adapt in such situations.

COMMUNICATION SKILLS   The level and type of communication skills are closely related to affectional adequacy and relational integrity. Similarly, knowledge and skills about how to build and maintain relationships are important. If the individual has open communication, is flexible, can articulate clearly, and is sensitive to other people's verbal and nonverbal behavior, the relationship is facilitated. If one of the partners does not have interaction skills at the level desired, those skills can be learned with help. Learning begins with recognition that one needs to communicate more effectively. Many self-help books are available on this subject. Feedback from a knowledgeable person as changes are initiated is an important factor. Specific knowledge about friendship and how to build and maintain a relationship is part of this relevant stimulus. There are many theoretical discussions of friendship available. McGinnis (1980) described five activities that can deepen a friendship.

1. To put friendships or relationships first or give them top priority
2. To talk about and express affection for the other individual
3. To create space in the friendship so that both people can maintain their identity and autonomy
4. To cultivate the art of affirmation, making sure that the other person knows what is valued about them
5. To accept own and the other person's anger on a temporary basis. When an individual has developed nurturing ability and has significant knowledge regarding the dynamics of friendship, there is a greater possibility of an in-depth, long-lasting relationship.

PRESENCE   Presence in the physical environment influences interdependent relationships. If friends or a couple are separated often and for long periods, it is more difficult to maintain the relationship. The impact of presence on bonding between a mother and child has been mentioned previously. It is evident that attachment occurs more readily when the mother and baby have frequent and early access to each other. Any relationship is maintained more effectively when proximity is possible.

DEVELOPMENTAL STAGE   In the case of developmental adequacy in particular, developmental stage is considered to be both a behavior and a stimulus. Erikson's (1963) eight developmental crises are often manifested in terms of interdependent relationships and the development and maturation of these relationships. For example, in the stage of identity versus identity diffusion, the peer group and models of leadership are important. The development of trust versus mistrust is a stimulus to the receiving behaviors of the interdependence mode. Two other theories that are particularly relevant to understanding how interdependence behavior develops are those described by Havighurst (1953) and Selman (1980) as noted above. The reader is encouraged to consult the primary sources for further information about these perspectives.

SIGNIFICANT CHANGES   There are times in each person's development that radical life changes occur. These include events such as divorce, serious illness, death of a significant other, and change in support system. Their impact on the individual's interdependence and adaptation as a whole is great. The individual's ability to cope with changes results in either effective or ineffective adaptation.

In applying the nursing process to the integrated processes of interdependence, the nurse makes a careful assessment of behaviors and stimuli. Based on this thorough first- and second-level assessment, the nurse formulates nursing diagnoses, sets goals, selects interventions, and evaluates care. For the remaining discussion of planning nursing care, the situation of Mr. and Mrs. Edwards is used for illustrative purposes. This is an older couple living in the community. Although Mr. Edwards is showing signs of decreasing cognitive capacity, his wife is dedicated to being is caregiver. Although many perspectives could be taken with this case, the focus will be on the two processes associated with interdependence and the achievement of relational integrity.

Nursing Diagnosis

Development of nursing diagnoses associated with interdependence is accomplished in the same way as in the other adaptive modes. One method involves the statement of the behaviors together with the influencing stimuli. The second approach is to use summary labels. Nursing diagnoses can reflect either adaptive or ineffective behaviors. For Mrs. Edwards, a sample adaptive nursing diagnosis states, "Commitment to at-home care for mentally impaired husband related to deep affection for him, confidence in own capabilities, and assistance provided by significant others and support systems." In the case of ineffective behaviors, a number of nursing diagnoses may result. The interdependence mode is closely interrelated with the other modes. A disturbance in one is likely to precipitate disturbances in others. For example, for Mr. Edwards, a diagnosis might be, "Increased agitation, restlessness, and risk of injury due to environment that does not provide the required freedom or security." The interdependent relationship between the individual and the environment is evident in this diagnosis.

Two additional diagnoses that focus on Mrs. Edwards are (1) Fatigue and exhaustion due to sleep disturbances of Mr. Edwards and (2) Concern about ability to cope with husband's decreasing functional abilities related to lack of knowledge about effective approaches and actions to support a mentally impaired individual. It is also possible to construct a nursing diagnosis using a summary label that captures clusters of behaviors. This method is used by experienced nurses to communicate significant amounts of information in one phrase. As identified in Chapter 3, there are five indicators of positive interdependence adaptation for individuals identified as summary labels in the Roy Adaptation Model. They are affectional adequacy, stable pattern of giving and receiving, effective pattern of dependency and independency, effective coping strategies for separation and loneliness, and developmental adequacy. Likewise, five commonly recurring adaptation problems are identified: ineffective pattern of giving and receiving, ineffective pattern of dependency and independency, inadequate support systems, separation anxiety, loneliness, and ineffective development of relationships. A nursing diagnosis using a summary label reads, "Inadequate support systems and resources in home environment to ensure adaptive interrelationship between environment and its affect on Mr. Edwards." Both the behavior and the stimuli stated in this example of a nursing diagnosis communicate a wealth of information to an individual experienced in adaptation problems associated with interdependence. However, for the inexperienced person, the more detailed expression of behaviors and stimuli is more meaningful. In Table 16–3, the Roy model nursing diagnostic categories for the integrated and compromised processes of interdependence are shown in relation to nursing diagnosis labels approved by the North American Nursing Diagnosis Association (NANDA International, 2007).

Goal Setting

Each step of the nursing process focuses on the individual's behavior, the stimuli influencing that behavior, or both. With the nursing diagnosis, the statement developed included both behaviors and stimuli. With the goal-setting step, the focus is on behavior. Each goal identifies a behavior that is to be addressed. Many interdependence problems have a chronic as well as an acute phase. Thus, the goal-setting process includes both long- and short-term goals, each of which states the behavior of focus, the change expected, and the time frame in which the goal is to be achieved.

TABLE 16–3 Nursing Diagnostic Categories for Interdependence Mode for Individuals

Positive Indicators of Adaptation	Common Adaptation Problems	NANDA Diagnostic Labels
• Affectional adequacy • Stable pattern of giving and receiving love, respect, and value • Effective pattern of dependency and independency • Effective coping strategies for separation and loneliness • Developmental adequacy of learning and maturing in relationships • Effective relations and communication • Nurturing ability to provide growth-producing care and attention • Security in relationships • Adequate significant others and support systems to achieve affectional and developmental adequacy	• Ineffective pattern of giving and receiving • Ineffective pattern of dependency and independency • Ineffective communication • Lack of security in relationships • Insufficient significant others and support systems for affection and relationship needs • Separation anxiety • Alienation • Loneliness • Ineffective development of relationships	• Risk for impaired parent/child attachment • Impaired religiosity • Risk for impaired religiosity • Readiness for enhanced religiosity • Impaired verbal communication • Readiness for enhanced communication • Impaired social interaction • Social isolation • Risk for loneliness

The following statements provide examples of possible goals for the situation described previously: (1) Within 1 week, Mr. Edwards will demonstrate fewer episodes of aggression, (2) Within 1 month, Mrs. Edwards and her family will express an increased sense of security and support as they care for Mr. Edwards, or (3) Following enhancement of their home environment to provide for appropriate environmental influences, Mr. and Mrs. Edwards will confirm through their statements and behavior an enhanced quality of life. In order to be effective in guiding the nursing progress, goals are established in collaboration with the people involved. As with each step of the nursing process, the individuals, where possible, are active participants. This participation helps to ensure that accurate and relevant information is obtained, that it is interpreted appropriately into nursing diagnoses, and that achievable and relevant goals are established. This is the only way that interventions can be determined that will assist in achieving relational integrity. After formulating goals, the nurse proceeds to the identification of nursing interventions, the next step of the nursing process as described in the Roy Adaptation Model.

Intervention

The intervention step of the nursing process according to the Roy Adaptation Model focuses on the stimuli affecting the behavior identified in the goal-setting step. The intervention step is thus the management of stimuli, and this involves altering, increasing, decreasing, removing, or maintaining them. In the previous situation involving Mr. and Mrs. Edwards, the problem of Mr. Edwards' aggressive behavior was addressed in the first goal. As Fabiano (1993) described, aggressive outbursts in mentally impaired individuals are often circumstantial in origin. The key to controlling aggressive behavior is in discovering the underlying problem and determining what can be done to prevent its recurrence. The manner in which the individual is approached is often to blame. Four factors of an approach that tends to produce agitation and subsequent aggression are interrogation, forced eye contact, intimidating posture, and restraint. Fabiano (1993) recommended that the caregiver sit at a right angle to the individual so that eye contact is optional and the individual does not feel trapped; communicate at eye level so as to avoid intimidation; touch the individual (holding the individual on their dominant side will avoid injury in the event of aggression); and use a soft level of speech. Above all, the caregiver must read the individual's behavior. If the individual shrugs when his or her shoulder is touched, do not persist; aggressive behavior will result. By informing caregivers of these points related to approach, much aggressive behavior can be prevented. The same analysis can be conducted for other factors that seem to be initiating the aggression.

A second goal pertained to Mrs. Edwards' stress and fatigue related to Mr. Edwards' sleep disturbances. In this situation, a suitable intervention may be to enroll Mr. Edwards in a night care program where he could go for the night to receive care and monitoring in a safe environment while Mrs. Edwards sleeps at home. By enhancing her support systems, Mrs. Edwards can continue to provide the majority of the care for Mr. Edwards at home and still have adequate rest. Yet another goal identified enhancement of the home environment to provide increased security and support. Zeisel, Hyde, and Levkoff (1994) described eight parameters of environment design that promote safety, security, and quality of life for people with Alzheimer's disease: exit control, wandering paths, individual private and personal places, common space structured to accommodate a variety of activities, outdoor freedom, residential scale, autonomy support, and sensory comprehension, that is, noise management and meaningfulness. Attention to these parameters provides for greater safety and security both for the individual and the caregivers, improved quality of life for the individual, less stress for the caregivers, and greater control for the individual over his or her life.

Through some minor renovations to their home, many of these objectives were accomplished for Mr. and Mrs. Edwards. Three sides of their yard were fenced. Installing a fence with a locked gate on the front of their yard allowed Mr. Edwards to spend time out of doors.

The home was located in a quiet neighborhood, so the environment was relatively free of traffic noise and other chaos. Mrs. Edwards developed visual cues throughout the house to assist Mr. Edwards with orientation. When she understood the impact of change, she avoided moving furniture or otherwise altering the surroundings in the home. At the suggestion of the nurse, Mrs. Edwards made contact with the Alzheimer's society in her area as a further support in helping her care for her husband. She found that the information and advice from others involved with the disease was of great assistance in helping her understand what further steps could be taken to enhance her husband's quality of life. All the above interventions focus on stimuli (approach, disturbances of sleep, environmental influences, and knowledge levels) that are contributing to interdependence problems for Mr. Edwards or his family. The next step of the nursing process returns to focus on the behaviors evident in the situation.

Evaluation

Evaluation involves judging the effectiveness of the nursing interventions in relation to the individual's adaptive behavior, that is, whether the behaviors stated in the goals have been achieved. The nursing interventions are effective if the behavior is as stated in the goal. If the goal has not been achieved, the nurse identifies alternative interventions or approaches by reassessing the behavior and stimuli and continuing with the other steps of the nursing process. In considering the previously identified goal: Within 1 week, Mr. Edwards will demonstrate fewer episodes of aggression, the intervention of informing caregivers about the factors that contribute to aggressive episodes was successful if their revised approach to him produces less agitation and subsequent aggression. If Mrs. Edwards reported that her husband was aggressive three times as opposed to 10 times within the same time period, the intervention would be judged successful.

The second goal stated: Within 1 month, Mrs. Edwards and her family will express an increased sense of security and support as they care for Mr. Edwards. The interventions related to this goal focused on some enhancements around their home. Mrs. Edwards reported "Now that my husband can go outside whenever he feels he wants to, he is not as restless and agitated. He appears to have an increased level of orientation and increased awareness of others." Another goal focused on Mrs. Edwards' level of fatigue and stress. The proposed intervention involved a night care program at a nearby care center. Unfortunately, that arrangement did not work well for Mrs. Edwards. The night program began at 8 p.m. and often Mr. Edwards was asleep before that. It was also inconvenient for Mrs. Edwards to get him to the program's location at that time, and he could not be accommodated at an earlier hour. Thus, the problem of stress and fatigue was not resolved. In reassessment of the situation, it was decided to try a rotation of home care personnel during the night so that Mrs. Edwards could sleep. This is provided through their health insurance for five nights a week. The son and daughter will provide the coverage for the other two nights. This approach will be assessed after a period of implementation in about 2 weeks.

The final goal stated: Following enhancement of their home environment to provide for appropriate environmental influences, Mr. and Mrs. Edwards will confirm enhanced quality of life through their statements and behavior. It may be possible to evaluate this goal for Mrs. Edwards through the use of a quality of life assessment tool. Mr. Edwards may demonstrate outcomes such as decreased restlessness, decreased socially inappropriate behavior, decreased use of psychotropic medication, maintenance or increase in weight, regained sense of humor, or increased awareness, for example. It is important to recognize that the nursing process and the six steps are ongoing, simultaneous, and overlapping. Although they have been separated and dealt with in an artificially linear manner for discussion purposes, often intervention is occurring at the same time as the nurse proceeds with first- and second-level assessment. Likewise, evaluation occurs on an ongoing basis, being held in mind even when nursing diagnoses are being established and as goals are being formulated.

Summary

This chapter has focused on the application of the Roy Adaptation Model to the interdependence mode for the individual. An overview of the processes of affectional adequacy and developmental adequacy associated with relational integrity was provided. Illustrations of compensatory responses related to interdependence were described and examples of four compromised processes, that is, separation anxiety, loneliness, substance abuse, and aggression, were discussed. Finally, guidelines for planning nursing care through identification of parameters for assessment of behaviors and stimuli, the formulation of nursing diagnoses, goals, and interventions were explored, and evaluation of nursing care was described.

Exercises for Application

1. Identify who you would describe as significant others and support systems in your life at this time.
2. Provide an example of giving and receiving behaviors in one relationship.
3. Think of an interrelationship situation that was ineffective. Which of the principles of effective relationship would have helped to improve the situation?

Assessment of Understanding

QUESTIONS

1. The basic need of the interdependence mode is _____, which is viewed as consisting of _____ and _____ adequacy.
2. Classify the following behaviors as being related to affectional adequacy (A) or developmental adequacy (D).
   (a) _____ giving and receiving behaviors
   (b) _____ significant others and support systems
   (c) _____ developmental stage
   (d) _____ dependency and independency
3. List three stimuli associated with affectional and relational adequacy.
   (1) _____
   (2) _____
   (3) _____
4. Which of the following could be considered compensatory processes related to interdependence?
   (a) volunteer work in a hospital
   (b) joining a book club
   (c) applying for social assistance
   (d) being part of a lay caregiver ministry at a local church
5. Name three compromised processes of interdependence.
   (a) _____
   (b) _____
   (c) _____

SITUATION:

Upon transferring to a new school, a child in second grade bursts into tears after being left in her new classroom by her mother.

6. Formulate a nursing diagnosis for the above situation using two methods.
   (a) _____
   (b) _____
7. Construct a goal for the child described in the above situation.
8. Since interventions are focused on stimuli, what interventions could be used to alleviate the situation described above, considering the following stimuli?
   (a) departure of the mother
   (b) classroom of unknown children
   (c) unfamiliar teacher
9. How would you evaluate achievement of the goal you established in item 7?

FEEDBACK

1. relational integrity; affectional and developmental adequacy
2. (a) A, (b) A, (c) D, (d) D
3. Any three of the following: Expectations of relationships and awareness of needs; Nurturing ability of both parties; Levels of self-esteem; Levels and kinds of interaction skills; Presence of others in the physical environment; Knowledge about relationships and the behaviors that enhance them; Developmental age and tasks; and Significant changes.
4. All the items could be considered compensatory processes related to interdependence.
5. Any three of the following: separation anxiety, loneliness, substance abuse, and aggression.

6. Examples of nursing diagnoses:
   (a) Crying related to strange environment and departure of significant other.
   (b) Separation anxiety related to being left by mother in a strange setting and absence of support system in new class.
7. Examples of goals:
   (a) Within 15 minutes, the child will have settled and will be calm in classroom environment.
   (b) During lunch hour, the child will make friends with two girls from her class.
8. Examples of interventions related to the stimuli identified could include:
   (a) Departure of the mother: Invite the mother to accompany the child into the classroom for a time (perhaps 15 minutes) to establish familiarity and comfort.
   (b) Classroom of unknown children: Assign another student who will act as a buddy for the child for the first week.
   (c) Unfamiliar teacher: Introduce the child to the teacher on another occasion, preferably before the actual classroom encounter. This is an anticipatory goal. It would not work in a situation such as that described but it might help avoid a similar situation in the future.
9. The goals would have been achieved if the following behaviors were evident.
   (a) Within 15 minutes, the child was composed and the crying had ceased.
   (b) After the lunch break, the child reported meeting two new children.

References

Ainsworth, M. D. (1964). Patterns of attachment shown by the infant in interaction with his mother. *Merrill Palmer Quarterly, 10*(1), 51–58.

Andrews, H. A., Cook, L. M., Davidson, J. M., Schurman, D. P., Taylor, E. W., & Wensel, R. H. (Eds.). (1994). *Organizational transformation in health care: A work in progress.* San Francisco: Jossey-Bass.

Berkman, B. (1978). Mental health and the aging: A review of the literature for clinical social workers. *Clinical Social Work Journal, 6,* 230–245.

Bowlby, J. (1969). *Attachment and loss: Attachment* (Vol. 1). New York: Basic Books.

Bowlby, J. (1973). *Attachment and loss: Separation: Anxiety and anger* (Vol. 2). New York: Basic Books.

Brown, M. M., & Fowler, G. R. (1969). *Psychodynamic nursing: A biosocial orientation.* Philadelphia: Saunders.

Caplan, G. (Ed.). (1974). *Support systems and community mental health.* New York: Behavioral Publications.

Cobb, S. (1976). Social support as a moderator of life stress. *Psychosomatic Medicine, 38,* 300–312.

Cohen, S. S. L. (1985). *Social support and health.* New York: Academic Press.

Dimond, M., & Jones, S. L. (1983). Social support: A review and theoretical integration. In P. L. Chinn (Ed.), *Advances in nursing theory development* (pp. 235–249). Rockville, MD: Aspen.

Erikson, E. H. (1963). *Childhood and society* (2nd ed.). New York: Norton.

Ezor, P. R. (1980). *Student teacher: Separation anxiety.* Unpublished manuscript, Mount St. Mary's College, Los Angeles.

Fabiano, L. (1993). *Dealing with aggression. Caring for the Alzheimer's victim* [Video series]. Seagrave, Ontario, Canada: FCS Media Production.

Fromm, E. (1956). *The art of loving.* New York: Harper & Row.

Gottlieb, B. H. (Ed.). (1981). *Social networks and social support.* Beverly Hills, CA: Sage.

Grant MacEwan Community College, Siberian Branch of the Russian Medical Academy of Medical Science, Siberian Business Development Corporation, & The University of Calgary—Gorbachev Foundation Joint Trust Fund. (1997). *Reform of the Novosibirsk Health Care System.* Edmonton, Alberta: Grant MacEwan Community College.

Greenblatt, M., Beccera, R., & Serafetinides, E. A. (1982). Social networks and mental health: An overview. *American Journal of Psychiatry, 8,* 977–984.

Havighurst, R. J. (1953). *Human development and education.* New York: Longman.

House, J., Landis, K., & Umberson, D. (1988). Social relationship and health. *Science, 241,* 540–545.

Kane, C. R. (1988). Family social support: Toward a conceptual model. *Advances in Nursing Science, 10*(2), 188–225.

Klaus, M. H., & Kennel, J. H. (1981). *Parent–infant bonding* (2nd ed.). St. Louis, MO: Mosby.

Koch, R. N., & Haugk, K. C. (1992). *Speaking the truth in love.* St. Louis, MO: Stephen Ministries.

Mahler, M. S. (1979). *The selected papers of Margaret Mahler: Separation–individuation* (Vol. 2). New York: Jason Aronson.

Maslow, A. H. (1954). *Motivation and personality.* New York: Harper & Row.

McGinnis, L. (1980). *The friendship factor: How to get close to the people you care for.* Minneapolis, MN: Augsburg Publishing.

Mead, M. (1971). *Coming of age in Samoa.* New York: Morrow.

NANDA International. (2007). *Nursing diagnoses: Definitions and classifications, 2007–2008.* Philadelphia: NANDA-I.

Randell, B., Tedrow, M., & Van Landingham, J. (1982). *Adaptation nursing: The Roy conceptual model applied.* St. Louis, MO: Mosby.

Robertson, H. (1953). Some responses of young children to loss of maternal care. *Nursing Times, 49.*

Roy, C. (1981). A systems model of nursing care and its effect on quality of human life. In G. E. Lakser (Ed.), *Applied systems and cybernetics* (Vol. IV, pp. 1705–1714). New York: Pergamon Press.

Roy, C., & Roberts, S. L. (1981). Interdependence. In C. Roy & S. L. Roberts (Eds.), *Theory construction in nursing: An adaptation model* (pp. 272–282). Englewood Cliffs, NJ: Prentice Hall.

Seeman, M. (1959). On the meaning of alienation. *American Sociological Review, 24*(6), 783–791.

Selman, J. C., & Andrews, H. A. (1994). Effective relationships: Rethinking the fundamentals. In H. A. Andrews, L. M. Cook, J. M. Davidson, D. P. Schurman, E. W. Taylor, & R. H. Wensel (Eds.), *Organizational transformation in health care: A work in progress* (pp. 53–69). San Francisco: Jossey-Bass.

Selman, R. C. (1980). *The growth of interpersonal understanding: Development and clinical analyses.* New York: Academic Press.

Spitz, R. A. (1945). Hospitalism: An inquiry into the genesis of psychiatric conditions in early childhood. In O. Fenechel, P. Greenacre, H. Hartmann, E. B. Jackson, E. Kris, L. S. Kubie, B. D. Lewin, M. C. Putnam, & R. A. Spitz (Eds.), *The psychoanalytic study of the child* (pp. 53–74). New York: International Universities Press.

Stanford, G. (1977). *Developing effective classroom groups.* New York: Hart.

Zeisel, J., Hyde, J., & Levkoff, S. (1994). Best practices: An environment–behavior (E–B) model for Alzheimer special care units. *The American Journal of Alzheimer's Care and Related Disorders & Research,* March/April, 4–21.

PART THREE

Adaptive Modes of Relating Persons

From the early development of the model, nurses used the four adaptive modes of the Roy Adaptation Model in their care of groups as adaptive systems. However, it was soon recognized that some additional theoretical development was needed for these more complex applications. A number of publications developed the content of the model to apply to families (Hanna & Roy, 2001; Roy, 1983), to communities (Roy, 1984), and to nursing administrative systems (Roy & Anway, 1988). Chapters on the family and the nursing care group were included in the 1984 edition of the textbook on the model. More extended theory development of the adaptive modes for groups was introduced in the last edition of this text (Roy & Andrews, 1999). However, the complexity of the content called for devoting separate chapters to each adaptive mode at the group level. Figure 1 shows the expansion of view from the individual to groups including the family, organization, community, and global society.

Part 3 of this book includes chapters that develop new content for each adaptive mode at the group level. Chapter 17 focuses on the physical mode of the group. Chapter 18 discusses group identity and Chapters 19 and 20 deal with the role function mode and interdependence mode on the group level. The chapters move from an understanding of the theoretical basis of the adaptive modes to the use of the nursing process to plan care for groups. Each discussion of an adaptive mode at the group level is based on understanding the parallel mode on the individual level. The examples provided purposefully use different levels of groups to apply the basic concepts. The reader will note that the adaptive modes are all interrelated in presenting a holistic perspective of the group as an adaptive system.

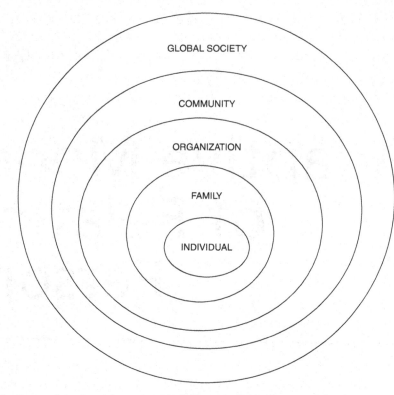

FIGURE 1   Focus of the Roy Adaptation Model from individual to group levels.

For example, a family has a group identity, which greatly affects the socialization for role expectations in the role function mode. The holism of groups is reflected in each view of the kaleidoscope.

References

Hanna, D. R., & Roy, C. (2001). Roy Adaptation Model perspectives on family. *Nursing Science Quarterly, 14*(1), 9–13.

Roy, C. (1983). Roy Adaptation Model and application to the expectant family and the family in primary care. In J. Clements & F. Roberts (Eds.), *Family health: A theoretical approach to nursing care* (pp. 255–278, 298–303, 375–378). New York: Wiley.

Roy, C. (1984). The Roy adaptation model: Applications in community health nursing. In M. K. Assoy & C. C. Ossler (Eds.), *Conceptual Models of Nursing. Applications in Community Health Nursing* (pp. 51–73). Proceedings of the eighth annual community health nursing conference. Chapel Hill, NC: University of North Carolina.

Roy, C., & Andrews, H. (1999). *The Roy Adaptation Model* (2nd ed.). Stamford, CT: Appleton & Lange.

Roy, C., & Anway, J. (1988). Roy's Adaptation Model: Theories and propositions for administration. In B. Henry, C. Arndt, M. DeVincenti, & A. Marriner-Tomey (Eds.), *Dimensions and issues of nursing administration*. St. Louis, MO: Mosby.

CHAPTER 17

Physical Mode of Relating People

Groups are basically relating persons. The classic definition of a group is two or more people who interact and influence each other. The Roy Adaptation Model expands this definition and proposes that groups include larger systems that influence each other even if people do not directly interact. Families, communities, organizations, societies, and the globalized world are all groups. In describing the four adaptive modes for groups, we begin with the physical mode. This approach is similar to discussion of the physiologic mode of the individual before describing self-concept, role function, and interdependence. According to the Roy Adaptation Model, the adaptive modes together form an integrated whole of people and of groups. The physical mode of groups is related to the group identity, role, and interdependent modes in groups. However, understanding the physical adaptive mode of groups provides a foundation for understanding holistic groups. This chapter will focus on the physical mode of people in groups according to the Roy Adaptation Model. The following three chapters deal with the other three adaptive modes for groups. The relationship among the modes is noted in several ways in this chapter. For example, the participants for the physical mode are the same people who form a group identity and who have reciprocal roles. Further, the factors or stimuli that affect groups will affect all four adaptive modes.

The definition of the physical mode was introduced in the overview of the adaptive modes in Chapter 4. The physical mode is defined as the way the group adaptive system manifests adaptation relative to needs associated with basic operating resources. In short, the physical mode provides whatever is required for the group system to survive and to enable it to adapt to changes. The underlying need of the physical adaptive mode is operating integrity. Operating integrity means that wholeness is achieved by adapting to changes in operating resource requirements. Such integrity is based on integrated processes involving the participants, physical facilities, and fiscal resources.

Examples of processes by which groups reach operating integrity and the integrated level of adaptation of the physical mode are described. These processes include strategic planning and resource management. Compensatory adaptive processes related to the physical mode of the group also are explored. Of the many possible compromised processes for the physical mode of groups, two examples are discussed, that is, ineffective response to disaster and health disparities. The nursing care planning section outlines examples of nursing assessment of behaviors and stimuli for the physical mode of groups and provides guidelines for formulating diagnoses, establishing goals, selecting interventions, and evaluating care in this adaptive mode.

OBJECTIVES

After studying this chapter, the reader will be able to do the following:

1. Describe the integrated processes of the physical mode for groups according to the Roy Adaptation Model.

2. Describe one compensatory process related to the physical mode for groups.

3. Name and describe two situations of compromised processes in the physical mode for groups.

4. Identify important first-level assessment behaviors for the physical mode for groups.

5. Identify second-level assessment factors or stimuli that influence the physical mode for groups.

6. Formulate nursing diagnoses related to the physical mode for groups.

7. Establish goals related to given diagnoses in the physical mode for groups.

8. Select nursing interventions to promote adaptation in the physical mode for groups.

9. Propose approaches to determine the effectiveness of nursing interventions in the physical mode for groups.

KEY CONCEPTS DEFINED

Community: From a geopolitical perspective, a group of people living in the same place such as a town or neighborhood; from a phenomenological perspective, an organized group of individuals with common interests or beliefs, for example, a patient support group or an ethnic group.

Contamination: Exposure to an environmental agent in quantities sufficient to cause adverse health effects.

Family: Commonly called the basic unit of society; evolving descriptions are two or more people who are joined together by bonds of sharing and emotional closeness and who identify themselves as being part of the family.

Health disparities: Racial or ethnic differences in the quality of health care that are not due to access-related factors or clinical needs, preferences, and appropriateness of intervention.

Mission statement: Brief written descriptions of the purpose of the group; increasingly important to include vision and values statements in the mission statement.

Resource management: The efficient and effective deployment of resources when they are needed.

Resources: Include participants and their skills, the physical resources needed to accomplish the strategic plans of the group, the funding, and also the information technology (IT) resources.

Strategic planning: Also called long-range planning; provides philosophy, mission, vision, and values statements; uses strategic analysis to review the internal environment and outside changes; sets goals, strategies, objectives, responsibilities, and timelines.

Support individuals: People that families can depend upon for material and emotional help; includes emotional support in times of crisis.

PROCESSES OF THE PHYSICAL MODE FOR RELATING PERSONS

Operating integrity is the underlying need of the physical adaptive mode for groups. The key components of the mode include participants, physical facilities, and fiscal resources. To begin examining the theoretical basis of the physical mode, we can look first at the participants, physical facilities, and fiscal resources of the most common groups in society, the family and communities (Figure 17–1).

Family Participants, Physical and Fiscal Resources

In nursing practice the family is the group consistently encountered. The family is discussed throughout Part 3 as the primary example of a group and described from the perspective of four adaptive modes at the group level. In the past, sociologists described the family as the basic unit of society. This concept, in its broadest sense, holds true, although the definition of family has evolved considerably from the traditional definition. A definition that reflects the range of *participants* of families in 21st-century American society describes a family as "two or more people who are joined together by bonds of sharing and emotional closeness... who identify themselves as being part of the family" (Friedman, Bowden, & Jones, 2003, p. 10). This definition is sufficiently broad to include both blood relatives and significant others as well as illustrate formation of close ties and relationships between individuals.

In the past, roles within the family were more or less predetermined. Adult males assumed primary responsibility to be the head of the household and provided for the family. The adult female managed home responsibilities. Although this notion of family participants persists, as we see in later chapters, many forms of participants functioning as families are the

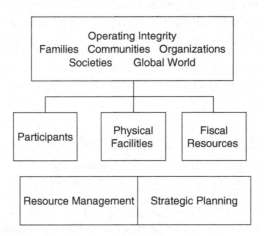

FIGURE 17–1 Physical Mode for groups. Theoretical basis.

norm today. The family network includes one or more individuals who assume leadership roles or coordinate functions within the family. This individual might assign specific roles or responsibilities to other family members or make decisions for the family. Particular roles might shift over time, for example, adult children caring for their elderly parents or a relative who had previously cared for them. More importantly, setting and achieving goals within the family is typically a shared responsibility.

Every family regardless of its size or composition has *physical resources* that contribute to the operating integrity of the group. A description of physical resources is not limited to material possessions but includes attributes that support the group integrity. The most important resource for a family is the number of individuals in close proximity who comprise a family's support system. These support individuals include close friends or extended family members. They are the people that families can depend upon not only for social relationships, but also for material and emotional help. This assistance takes forms such as child care or providing transportation. It also includes emotional support in times of crisis.

Another physical resource is living space. The space in which a family lives can affect greatly physical and emotional health. Tight, overcrowded living space or squalid conditions will affect individuals' personal health and social interactions. Homelessness is devastating for families and creates despair and embarrassment. Without a personal dwelling or personal and private space, families face an uncertain future. An available supply of nutritious foods and of adequate clothing that is climate appropriate also contributes to family operating integrity. Safety is a primary concern, and community infrastructure supports family operating integrity by protecting all its residents from problematic events. This includes fully functioning police and fire departments. Communities provide educational and recreational facilities with schools, libraries, public art, parks, and recreational facilities that are the physical resources for families.

Fiscal resources are dependent on different contributory factors. Employment is typically the primary source of income for operating household expenses. Ideally, one or more family members have stable employment that will ensure that the family can cover expenses for housing, food, clothing, recreation, and health care. Families, too, depend on the earners' benefit packages that offset costs of preventative health and dental care. Employers' and union benefit packages also help earners plan for a secure financial future with tax-deferred annuity plans for retirement and disability insurance in the event of catastrophic illness. Unemployment threatens family operating integrity and can deplete available resources. The social and emotional toll can be enormous. Families whose income source is either unstable or can barely cover the minimal expenses often rely on state or federal assistance for food, housing, or health care. Hardship can also arise when spending exceeds the family budget. Increased dependence on loans and credit card debt can deplete a family's savings and create long-term financial instability.

Community Participants, Physical and Fiscal Resources

Communities are examples of a more complex operating system within society. The individuals and groups living within specific borders provide operating integrity on several levels. In order to understand participants, physical and fiscal resources, different types of communities are described. A community refers to a "group of people living in the same place" (The Oxford Dictionary, 2004), for example, a town or neighborhood. Specific attributes of a group or locale such as size, location, or characteristic also define communities. Certain connotations or images come to mind with terms like "small town" or "rough neighborhood." A community also can refer to an organized group of individuals with common interests or beliefs. Frequently, groups whose organization either has loose bonds or no organization are also considered to be communities by virtue of their shared interest or attributes.

Identifying a community as either geopolitical or phenomenological helps to understand the infrastructure of how each functions. Regardless of its size, a geopolitical community has circumscribed borders and an established system of governance. Examples include municipalities, states, and countries. *Participants* of that community include individuals who live within its borders and those who work there. In the United States, citizens can participate in local, state, and national decisions in a number of ways, most commonly in the elective processes. Citizens in other global communities, however, might have more restricted access to participation. A phenomenological community is based on interpersonal connections between its participants who share common interests, beliefs, or goals (Smith & Maurer, 2004). A primary distinction between phenomenological communities and geopolitical communities is that their borders are frequently less well defined. Groups such as the homeless or people with disabilities are examples of a phenomenological community. The term community of solution is another type of phenomenological community (Smith & Maurer, 2004). These communities organize groups of participants, for example, to respond specifically to health concerns within a given area. They function similarly to *ad hoc* committees or a task force to respond to a community health threat, for example, a source of pollution or outbreak of an infectious disease. Often, individuals or groups from neighboring geopolitical communities will become participants of a community of solution.

Physical resources in communities are varied and dependent on many factors. Individuals and groups that comprise the aggregate largely influence the types and availability of resources. Generally, the larger the infrastructure in a community, the more varied and developed its resources. A typical example is a municipality. Larger towns and cities with a well-developed infrastructure depend on subsidies from their local, state, and federal tax bases to support vital services like police and fire departments, schools and libraries, and recreational facilities. Communities with high revenues from their tax base usually offer a wider range of services, such as state of the art public recreational centers and well-kept parks. The number of local commercial and manufacturing enterprises is regulated through local zoning ordinances. Furthermore, communities depend on commercial outlets and businesses to provide revenues to support its budget. Compared to larger towns and cities, rural communities typically have fewer resources. Although they might have independent police and fire departments, vital services, for example, schools, libraries, hospitals, and social centers, are often shared with neighboring communities. Probably the greatest resource communities provide are the individuals and groups that comprise it. Participation in local government through voting or attending public meetings is one important avenue to become involved in community affairs. Celebrating the community at local events, whether attending July 4th parades or volunteering at a school event, is vital to building a strong, cohesive working group.

Resources encompass a range of attributes. *Fiscal resources* are a key consideration for community resources. Large organizations or foundations, such as the American Heart Association, have a national base and can engage in year-round fund-raising activities to support it. Additionally, larger organizations receive additional federal, state, or local funds, which enable the organization to provide some services at cost or free of charge. Special interest organizations, however, have more difficulty raising funds and frequently make appeals through individuals and groups who have a personal connection to the agency. Examples of this type of group might include Mothers Against Drunk Drivers or The Samaritans, a suicide prevention group. Communities with individuals belonging to particular ethnic or linguistic groups often have local agencies to meet the needs and interests of these groups. For example, a community with a growing number of Chinese immigrants might offer English as a second language classes at local social or senior centers.

The actual usefulness of resources for the community integrity depends on a number of factors. Two major factors that have been identified are endorsement and accessibility of the resources. Use of resources is dependent on previous experiences with agencies as well as how easy it is to access services (Hunt, 2001). Individuals rely on word of mouth reputation as well as the support of others. Accounts of positive experiences from friends, family, and health providers will encourage others to pursue contact with the agency. Easy access will affect use. A well-organized system of public transportation in a community can be a valuable resource for local residents. Yet, as much as residents can benefit from access using public transportation, the system can present some drawbacks. Travel time can be longer, especially covering longer distances in larger cities that require transfers. Systems in smaller communities often provide limited services and riders might have to pay extra for taxis to get them to their destinations. Dependence on public transportation can be especially challenging for individuals with impaired mobility, mothers with young children, and the elderly.

Discussion in this section has focused primarily on communities at a local level, yet, in the 21st century, community has more far-reaching connotations. The national community is a collection of towns and cities across the United States. International air travel and communication networks among nations have made the world smaller and created a global community. This changing perspective has led to understanding and appreciation for others and their lives outside local communities. Current discussions related to global warming and energy use in emerging nations, for example, are of concern to the global community. Affecting change in matters like climate change cannot be isolated within a country and require cooperation among nations. Organizations like the World Health Organization (WHO) consider global health as a shared responsibility and have called for equitable access to essential care and collective defense against transnational health threats (WHO, 2008). Box 17–1 provides an insightful allegory about the relationship between ecology and health on a global level. Awareness and action will lead toward solutions that benefit the common good across world communities.

INTEGRATED PROCESSES OF THE PHYSICAL MODE

As groups meet the need for operating integrity, many processes are used. These processes are focused on the participants, physical facilities, and fiscal resources of families, communities, organizations, societies, and the global world. The processes aim to maintain and enhance the numbers and skills of participants and to maintain stable participants in the group. Groups have processes in place to ensure adequate physical and fiscal resources. In addition, to maintain operating integrity, groups from families to the global community have processes to plan for future participants and resources in meet changing physical needs. Planning becomes a focus of maintaining integrity of the physical mode. Of the many possible processes, two that relate to planning are highlighted here, strategic planning and resource management (see bottom line of Figure 17–1).

BOX 17–1

Example Relating Ecology and Health

Case Report

The patient is an elderly woman, beloved in her community, who comes to your office with a list of serious problems. She has night sweats and fevers that have been getting worse for the last few years. She has difficulty breathing and on examination seems to have suffered from aspiration pneumonia. She has alopecia, having lost her hair in a patchy distribution. Her normal gastrointestinal flora has been invaded by a few noxious species, and she has persistent diarrhea. Her skin is marked by an extensive dermatitis: It is fissured, inflamed, gouged, scraped, denuded, and cracking in many places. These excoriations are caused by a small but extremely industrious organism whose numbers have grown exponentially during the last few years, displacing and even eliminating other organisms that used to be widely distributed on the skin of our patient.

Interpretation: The Patient is the Earth; Symptoms Night Sweats and Fevers = Global Warming; Respiratory Disease = Poor Air Quality; Alopecia = Deforestation; Diarrhea = Loss of Biodiversity; Dermatitis = Overpopulation

Differential Diagnosis: Global Environmental Change

Rosenblatt, Roger A. Ecological change and the future of the human species: Can physicians make a difference? (REFLECTIONS). *Annals of Family Medicine 3.2*(March–April 2005): 173. Adapted with permission.

Strategic Planning

Groups use many approaches to planning for meeting operating integrity. A common process used by many groups is called strategic planning. The process involves determining where an organization is going for a given time period and how it's going to get there. The process has also been referred to as long range planning, but adding the connotation of strategic to planning has focused the process. The group defines its strategy, or direction. Decisions of resource management discussed below depend upon this broader process. A basic principle is to involve all group participants in the process. For example, in conducting a strategic plan a patient care service will involve all units involved in the service and all participants within those units. Likewise a university or school of nursing undertaking a strategic planning process will involve all departments and levels of personnel. Similarly a geographic community will include many participants from the various governing bodies to the citizen constituents who are involved. Setting up the structure for involvement of the total group is an important part of the process. For small groups with a given project such as planning an annual budget for a family, the structure may be relatively simple but is no less important. For a larger group such as a university making a 10-year plan or a town looking at issues related to adequacy of health care, setting up an effective planning structure will take more time and effort.

There are many various approaches to strategic planning provided in basic management books. However, the literature reflects some common steps. The steps may not be done in the same order or the same way and will always be adjusted to the needs of the group. In keeping with the assumptions of the Roy Adaptation Model, it seems that setting the strategic direction is the logical first step. Planners begin by identifying or updating the philosophy of the group. The group or organization's mission, vision, and values statements are clarified. Mission statements are brief written descriptions of the purpose of the organization. Such statements vary in length and depth from very brief to more comprehensive. The overall mission statement includes a specific statement of purpose for the group. It is increasingly important in the world of the 21st century to include vision and values statements. In writing a vision statement, the group prepares a compelling description of how the group or organization will operate at some point in the future. Secondly, the vision statement shows the contributions the group will make for the benefit of those they serve. Mission relates to current purposes, and vision shows where the group wants to go.

Values statements list priorities for the group and include moral values. Moral values are values that suggest overall priorities in how people ought to act in the world. For example, groups using the Roy Adaptation Model will include values such as those included in the philosophical, scientific, and cultural assumptions of the model. These include that people find meaning in mutual relations with each other, the world, and a God-figure; the commonality that includes the unity and diversity of people; the common purposefulness destiny; respect for the dignity and individuality of people; systems theory expanded to view the universe as progressing in structure, organization, and complexity; and encouragement of making ideas culturally relevant. Many groups with which nurses are involved share the value of providing quality care to enhance the health of all people.

Another step in strategic or long-range planning has been called the strategic analysis. This stage of the process includes a review of the group or organization and its environment including, for example, the political, social, economic, and technical environment. Outside changes may be occurring such as demographic shifts, funding uncertainties, or other groups developing similar programs. One common technique used by many groups at this stage is the SWOT analysis. Factors internal to the group are classified as strengths (S) or weaknesses (W). Factors that are external are listed as opportunities (O) or threats (T). The SWOT analysis provides information that is helpful in matching the group's participants and resources to the mission and vision statement and environment in which the group operates. The formulation and selection of specific strategies for action depend on SWOT assessment. The assessment is followed by looking at the mission and vision in the context of the current environment and SWOT assessment. Goals are set to carry out the mission with the new vision. The focus is on maximizing the strengths of the group and minimizing weaknesses. At the same time, the opportunities and threats in the environment are taken into account. Actions are formulated and implemented to reach the goals. Finally, monitoring of the implementation process is put in place to see that goals are accomplished. The reader will note the similarity of this process to the nursing process.

To set goals, the members of the group draw conclusions about what the group or organization will do as a result of the major issues and opportunities they face. These conclusions include what overall accomplishments, or strategic goals, the group plans to achieve. Secondly, they outline the overall approaches or strategies to achieve the accomplishments. As in the nursing process, goals have a specific focus, the change expected, and the time frame in which to be accomplished. One author of organizational theory notes that the goals are worded as much as possible to be specific, measurable, acceptable to those working to achieve the goals, realistic, timely, extending the capabilities of those working to achieve the goals, and rewarding to them, as well (Wilson, 1991).

In setting up approaches to meet the goals, sometimes a series of objectives, or specific results, are stated for each strategic goal. Accomplishing a strategic goal involves meeting a set of smaller objectives over the time frame. The action plan includes specifying participant responsibilities and timelines for each objective. The plan describes who needs to do what and by when. The group puts in the plan methods for monitoring the implementation process so they will know who has done what and by when to meet the objectives. One group of authors suggests the development of an annual plan that is sometimes called the operational plan or management plan (Bradford et al., 1999). This includes the strategic goals, strategies, objectives, responsibilities, and timelines that should be done in the coming year. The group or organization develops plans for each major function, division, or department and calls these work plans.

Resource Management

Another major process that groups use to meet the need for operating integrity is resource management. Many readings in organizational studies describe resource management as the efficient and effective deployment of an organization's resources when they are needed. As noted earlier, resources encompass a range of attributes, and those for families and communities were discussed. Resources include the participants and their skills, the physical resources needed to accomplish the strategic plans of the group, the funding, and also the information technology (IT) resources. The values, priorities, and goals that the group has identified in planning processes will indicate what participants and resources are needed.

Budgeting is a major part of the process of resource management. Budgets are included in the strategic and annual plan, and with work plans. The budget specifies the money needed for the resources to implement the strategic plan. The categories of the budget depend on the group. Basically, a budget depicts how the money will be spent. For organizations or communities, for example, budgets include the human resources, equipment, and materials for system maintenance and growth. The term operating budget usually means the budget associated with major activities over the coming year. Capital budgets relate to operating some major asset, for example, a building, automobiles, furniture, and computers. Project budgets relate to major projects, for example, construction of space for a clinic or implementing a nonsmoking health promotion program in a community.

A major issue of resources related to participants is the need to have adequate numbers of nurses at clinical agencies prepared to give the levels of care needed. Many agencies in the United States and elsewhere have been impacted by a shortage of prepared practicing nurses. In addressing this issue, in 1983 the American Academy of Nursing's Task Force on Nursing Practice in Hospitals conducted a study of 163 hospitals. The purpose was to identify and describe what created an environment that attracted and retained well-qualified nurses. These were institutions that promoted quality patient, resident, or client care. The report (McClure et al., 1983) noted that 41 of the 163 institutions were described as "magnet" hospitals because of their ability to attract and retain professional nurses. Today the program has developed into a certification program developed by the American Nurses Credentialing Center (ANCC) (http://www.nursecredentialing.org/magnet/index.html). The Magnet Recognition Program® aims to recognize health care organizations that provide nursing excellence. Successful nursing practices and strategies are disseminated through the program. The nursing shortage is one example of a resource management issue that is being addressed in a number of ways including the Magnet Recognition Program.

In considering the two processes identified in the physical mode, we can note also that family function is dependent on setting mutual goals and allocating available resources.

Sources of income, the family home, health insurance, supportive others, and community resources support operating integrity in families. Fiscal resources help determine how the family lives. Available resources can help to sustain the family during a period of crisis. For example, the availability of 3 months' salary can help to keep up with monthly expenses if a family member becomes unemployed. Setting mutual goals is one way that family leadership can prepare for problematic events and ensure operating integrity within an entire family system.

COMPENSATORY PROCESSES

As in each adaptive mode on both the individual and group levels, there are many compensatory processes. The Roy Adaptation Model defines compensatory processes for groups as representing the adaptation level when the stabilizer and innovator are activated by a challenge to the integrated processes. The group looks for ways to maintain stability and to grow as the situation changes. The number of possible compensatory processes for groups is great because of the variety of types of groups and the many possible challenges they face. In the physical mode for groups, the compensatory processes include all the possible responses to changes or threats to the group participants, physical facilities, and fiscal resources. A compensatory process that is common in groups is risk preparedness.

As noted above, families participate in risk preparedness by having resources available to sustain the family during a period of crisis. This includes the availability of 3 months' salary, which can help to keep up with monthly expenses if a family member becomes unemployed. Part of the planning is for the family participants to set mutual goals to prepare for challenging events and ensure operating integrity within an entire family system. This is particularly challenging when the national economic scene is uncertain. Another common example occurs in school health nursing. The increasing number of food allergies in children is the changing situation that requires the school system to initiate anticipatory planning.

The following is an example of a specific situation of risk preparedness. The number of children with documented severe peanut allergies who are enrolled in a mid-sized town's public school system has risen from 4 to 13 in the past year. Parents have expressed concern about inadvertent exposure to peanuts or food products that have been exposed to peanuts during production. To date none of the children has had an anaphylactic reaction. The school nurse initiates a process of anticipatory planning. First, she creates a documented history of peanut allergy and a treatment plan for each child who is affected. The nurse is aware that parents expressed concern about school meals and snacks. She requests a "nut free" table in the school cafeteria. At this table not only the school staff and children abide by never having any kind of nuts at the table, but in addition, no group that visits the school may use the table. This is an added anticipatory protection in the event that another group, for example, having a bake sale, might inadvertently leave the peanut antigen on surfaces.

The school nurse also develops a written policy to manage anaphylactic reactions. All participants in the school system, teachers, cafeteria staff, and school bus drivers are instructed in how to use EpiPens in an emergency. Given participants of the school community are at risk for exposure to a life-threatening allergen. The purpose of risk preparedness is to maintain the operating integrity of the group by minimizing the threat of the risk as much as possible. Box 17–2 summarizes a list of the risk preparedness planning in place.

Not all compensatory processes will be successful. The current economic climate in the United States has shown that even with meticulous anticipatory planning the expected resources

BOX 17–2

Risk Preparedness for Students With Allergies to Peanuts

- Teachers have a list of children with allergies in the classroom.
- An EpiPen is in a central location in the cafeteria and on the child's person on school buses.
- No foods with peanuts or that are processed with peanuts are served in the cafeteria.
- School administration sends a letter to parents with a request to avoid sending baked goods or snacks for distribution in classrooms.
- EpiPen training for all classroom teachers and cafeteria personnel is conducted.
- Teachers keep a supply of peanut-free treats to distribute when children have a special classroom event.

are not always on hand. Housing foreclosures, unemployment with loss of benefits, and catastrophic illness or death occur within families. These can tax family resources and functioning and lead to compromised adaptation.

COMPROMISED PROCESSES

According to the Roy Adaptation Model, compromised processes occur when ineffective compensatory processes do not restore integration. In all the adaptive modes for both individuals and groups, compromised processes result in adaptation problems. This is the case for the physical mode of groups. Adaptation problems or compromised processes are the third level of adaptation. Ineffective efforts can occur in any of the processes for maintaining operating integrity of the group. There are two examples of compromised processes in the physical mode discussed here: ineffective response to disaster and health disparities. As mentioned above, within the planning process, a system of feedback and reporting looks at progress towards goals. Similarly there are feedback systems for evaluating the effectiveness of how a group functions when faced with a crisis to the health and integrity of a community. Natural disasters and catastrophic accidents require a coordinated response team that can alleviate the threat to physical, psychological, and social health of communities. Often, the effort to stem the effects of untoward events requires assistance from surrounding communities.

In the recent past, events like the attack on the New York World Trade Center in 2001 and the outbreaks of anthrax that immediately followed underscore the need for emergency preparedness in communities. After Hurricane Katrina hit New Orleans in 2005, surviving residents struggled for years to regain stability. National agencies, including the Centers for Disease Control and the Department of Homeland Security with its Federal Emergency Management Agency (Table 17–1), set standards for states, cities, and towns to create plans to handle emergencies and mass casualties to suit individual topography and climate.

Ineffective Response to Disaster

As an example of a compromised adaptation process, we can discuss an example of the contamination of a community water supply after a natural disaster. Consider the situation in which the water supply for household use in an agricultural community is contaminated with raw sewage during a major storm. Initiation of the public health response system is an important first step in

TABLE 17–1 Government Agencies That Set Standards for Emergency Preparedness and Disaster Planning

Centers for Disease Control (CDC)	www.emergency.cdc.gov	Supports the nation's ability to prepare and respond to public health emergencies.
Department of Homeland Security	www.dhs.gov/xprepresp	Has the primary responsibility to ensure that emergency response professionals are prepared to handle any type of emergency.
		Leads a coordinated, comprehensive federal response to disasters and leads recovery efforts.
Federal Emergency Management Agency (FEMA)	www.fema.gov	Plans, responds, and carries out recovery to disasters.

the event of a contamination. First responders to contamination include local and state health departments, fire and rescue personnel, police, engineers who manage water filtration and safety, toxicologists, and the media. Efforts to avert panic are critical to prevent serious illness and potential mortality. The media in particular can present area residents with information related to water contamination and provide concise information from the health department. Additionally, providing the public with hotline numbers can also help to allay fears. This planning is in place and is considered that it will be effective in meeting such an emergency.

As we look at the specific situation, we will see what might influence the effective use of participants and resources. In this community both the state and local departments of health are actively part of the investigation. The affected area includes small farming operations that grow vegetables sold in city farmers' markets. Sections of the community are severely flooded and the local fire departments are evacuating people from these areas. The local health department is organizing volunteers to check on the most vulnerable residents, that is, the infirm, disabled, elderly, and those with small children, to make sure they have a supply of bottled water. A major concern is contamination. Contamination is defined as exposure to an environmental agent in quantities sufficient to cause adverse health effects (Polk & Green, 2007). In this case the contamination brings a high risk for gastrointestinal illness within the community.

Initial actions included the local water authorities inspecting storm drains and removing waste. The public health department issues announcements for local television and radio stations about the contamination and gives instructions about how to boil water before use and where to get bottled water. Public health nurses organize a telephone hotline to answer residents' questions related to flooding and how to get potable water. The state public health department orders shipments of bottled water to meet the needs of the communities affected. The health department also is tracking outbreaks of illnesses that result from the contamination. Plans are in progress to notify local agricultural agencies to send produce samples for testing for contamination. Although the initial actions were appropriate, major parts of the response system did not work as intended because of the loss of a major resource, the electrical system. With the downed trees and electrical wires, many of the needed rapid communication systems were not in use. In addition some of the resources were reallocated to deal with serious accidents like drowning or electrocution. As the reports about outbreaks of gastrointestinal illness began to come in, they were incomplete. However, it was clear that there was significant contamination and resulting illness. The resulting situation is an example of an ineffective response to disaster.

Health Disparities

A second example of a compromised adaptation process is the existence of health disparities in the use of the resources of health care services and resulting differences in health outcomes. The Institute of Medicine (IOM) began a study in 1999 with the following aims: (1) to assess the extent of disparities in the types and quality of health services for racial and ethnic minorities and nonminorities; (2) to explore factors that may contribute to inequities in care; and (3) to recommend policies and practices to eliminate these inequities. The report *Unequal Treatment: Confronting Racial and Ethnic Disparities in Healthcare* was published in 2002. The report found that a consistent body of research demonstrated significant variation in the rates of medical procedures by race, even when insurance status, income, age, and severity of conditions are comparable. In the United States, racial and ethnic minorities were reported less likely to receive even routine medical procedures and more likely to experience a lower quality of health services. Some examples provided are that minorities are less likely to be given appropriate cardiac medications or to undergo bypass surgery, and are less likely to receive kidney dialysis or transplants. On the other hand, they are more likely to receive some less desirable procedures such as leg amputations for diabetes or other conditions.

The IOM report defined disparities in healthcare as "racial or ethnic differences in the quality of healthcare that are not due to access-related factors or clinical needs, preferences, and appropriateness of intervention" (p. 32). In a review of the nursing literature, Flaskerud and colleagues (2002) used the operational definition that disparities are "differential patterns of morbidity and mortality in vulnerable versus advantaged social groups." Since the IOM report, the issue of health disparities has been studied increasingly. Multiple causes for disparities have been postulated and studied. Some of the possible factors include socioeconomic realities, flawed systems, or inadequate training in cultural competence. Race or ethnicity, English proficiency, socioeconomic status, gender, sexual orientation, cognitive or physical ability, and religious or spiritual belief systems are characteristics that have been demonstrated to minimize the quality of care provided to an individual. An open question still being studied is the possibility that health outcomes for ethnic groups are impaired by bias in clinical decision making. Unfortunately it is possible that deep cultural stereotypes can be part of the schema that health professionals unconsciously use in making decisions about care of minority patients.

Regardless of increased awareness of disparities among the general public, health care providers, insurance companies, and policy makers, the reports of disparities in quality of care persist long after the original report. Efforts to increase consistency and equity of care through the use of evidence-based guidelines continue. A more recent report by the IOM (2004) focused on ensuring diversity in the health care workforce. The report noted that increasing racial and ethnic groups is important because the evidence shows that diversity is associated with improved access to care for racial and minority patients, greater patient choice and satisfaction, and better educational experiences for health professions students, among other benefits. The report examined institutional and policy-level strategies to increase diversity among health professions. In responding to this need, the National League for Nursing (2008) has convened a think tank on expanding diversity in the nursing educator workforce. The issue of health disparities provides an example on the national system level of compromised processes related to the physical adaptive system of groups and the inadequate distribution of resources for all participants.

NURSING PROCESS RELATED TO PHYSICAL MODE

The physical mode focuses on basic operating resources of groups including families, communities, organizations, societies, and the global society. The use of the nursing process based on the Roy Adaptation Model in groups is similar to the process described for the nursing care of individuals. In this section the six steps of the nursing process are described. The examples provided show how to use the model-based nursing process with a variety of groups.

Assessment of Behavior

First-level assessment of the physical mode for the group includes assessing behaviors related to a set of group characteristics. Assessment for groups includes direct observation and interviewing individuals in the group. In addition, in this mode public records and written reports also are sources of assessment data. The focus of the assessment is patterns of behavior. Particular areas to assess are patterns in the characteristics of structure, functions, relationships, and consistency. The nurse assesses patterns of behaviors related to the ability of the group to maintain and enhance operating resources to accomplish group goals. Table 17–2 outlines the characteristics of groups and lists the focus of assessment. To understand the structure of the group, the nurse focuses on who the participants are, how membership is organized, and the special relations among the participants. As noted earlier, families have differing membership patterns and organization. The group functions are part of the assessment and can include the major purposes of the group as well as more specific issues related to safety and resources to

---

TABLE 17–2 Assessment of the Physical Mode in Groups

Characteristics	Focus to Assess the Physical Mode in Groups
Structure	Who are the group members? Is there a formal infrastructure or loosely organized membership? What type of space does the group occupy?
Functions	How does the group take care of its members? What safety mechanisms are available? What parts of the physical space can change? Which cannot? What resources are available to maintain space?
Relationships	What are the group boundaries? What proximity is the space to other spaces? Are any spaces shared? How is information about the physical space for the group communicated to others in the group? What threats, if any, are there to the group's physical space? Do any regulations exist to control threats?
Consistency	What heritage and traditions exist? Does the group have a shared mission? Are there shared goals and a vision for the group? What values does the group have in common with other groups?

maintain space. A geopolitical community has many functions related to safety, yet usually does not alter its space. Relationships will include such patterns as group boundaries, shared spaces, and any threats to the group's space as well as regulations to control such threats. Communities located on shorelines have risks of flooding. Regulations about how far a family can build from the ocean, lake, or river can help to control the threat. The characteristic of consistency includes the shared mission, goals, vision, and values of the group, as well as heritage and traditions. This characteristic is discussed further when group identity is discussed in Chapter 18. It is relevant in the physical mode as the basis for allocating operating resources.

Assessment of Stimuli

Using the nursing process according to the Roy Adaptation Model, the second level of assessment identifies the influencing factors, also called the internal and external stimuli. The behaviors identified in the first level of assessment are used to focus assessment of stimuli. Behaviors of compromised adaptation, or the ineffective responses, are of initial concern, since the goal of nursing is to promote adaptation. Adaptive behaviors also are important because they are to be maintained or enhanced. Some of the key stimuli that impact the behavior in the physical mode are similar to stimuli that affect groups in the other adaptive modes: self identity, role function, and interdependence. The stimuli identified for the interdependence mode of groups are particularly relevant. These include context, infrastructure, and member capability. We will discuss these as they apply to the physical mode and add the innovator and stabilizer processes as major stimuli of the physical mode.

In general, context includes the internal and external environment that affects people and groups as adaptive systems at both the individual and group level in situations of health. In Chapter 20 context is more specifically defined as a component of the interdependence mode for groups. External context includes systems such as economic, social, political, cultural, belief, and family. As we have noted, the financial stability of a family or nation is an important stimulus in the physical mode. Similarly, how the local government system makes fiscal decisions is important assessment data in understanding resource adequacy. The local zoning codes will affect what health care agencies can be located in given sections of the community. In the physical mode, as our clinical examples have shown, climate and weather of a given geopolitical community is an important consideration when looking at context. It affects the resources needed related to heating and cooling living and work places; the family budget for clothing is affected as well.

In the physical mode, as in the interdependence mode, the internal context relates to mission, vision, values, principles, goals, and plans that influence the group. The discussions above of the adaptive processes of strategic planning and resource management illustrated the role that these factors play in promoting adaptation. A clear mission, vision, and values statement has a positive effect on the group setting goals and making plans. It is the plan that is a major stimulus in effective outcomes related to the goals. One example is the planning for a hospital to gain Magnet Status recognition. The group has the internal context to prepare them for a successful site visit because all participants share the vision and goals. When considering what is affecting a group in meeting their operating needs, a nursing assessment will look at the context as one major category of possible stimuli.

Infrastructure is another stimulus that clearly affects the physical mode. In Chapter 20, infrastructure is referred to as another component of the interdependence mode of groups and refers to the procedures, processes, and systems that exist within a group through which the goals of the group are accomplished. The level of each of these affects behaviors related to the structure of the group, functions, and particularly the relationships of the group. The risk preparedness planning in schools to address the increasing number of food allergies in children is an example of creating an infrastructure within an established system. The procedures, processes, and new systems established will be an influencing factor in how well the system meets the particular needs of those children. At the same time, the infrastructure of the school district resources will affect this or any other plans at the school level. The next stimulus that is common to the physical and interdependence modes of groups is member capability. In the physical mode, we assess the knowledge, skills, and commitments of participants within the group. Consider the description of the participants for families and communities earlier in this chapter. It shows the relevance of member capability for operating integrity. A key influencing factor in health facilities and schools of nursing currently in the United States is the shortage of nurses with the knowledge, skills, and commitments needed to operate major systems of care and education.

Resource adequacy is another stimulus that affects all adaptive modes, but the physical mode in particular. A basic need of the physical mode is to maintain basic operating resources. Again, the discussion of physical facilities and fiscal resources as part of the theoretical background for this mode makes clear how the availability of adequate resources is a major influencing factor. As noted, resources include physical space, funding, supplies, communication, and security. In the example of an ineffective response to a disaster, the allocation of resources initially seemed adequate. However, when the key resource of electricity was lost, the situation quickly changed and strategies to protect the community from illness were ineffective.

As with the other adaptive modes, the stabilizer and innovator processes are other major stimuli of the physical mode. We noted in the overview of the adaptive modes in Chapter 4 that just as the goals of the individual human adaptive system are identified in the Roy Adaptation Model, so are the goals of adaptation for systems that are groups of people. Adaptive responses of groups such as families, organizations, communities, or society relate to goals. Ongoing existence of the group and its continuing growth are the basic goals of groups. The stabilizer and innovator adaptive systems are the processes to maintain and enhance adaptation. We see these broad coping processes acting in the integrated adaptive processes of the physical mode. A group with good processes of resource management will be able to survive. Secondly, a group that does periodic strategic planning and leaves itself open and flexible to respond to new opportunities has strong innovator strategies that lead to growth. The earlier example of an ineffective response to disaster can become a stimulus for innovative programs of alternative systems for communication that do not require electricity. The innovator system of this community can further build into their planning backup participants to handle additional emergencies such as injuries.

Nursing Diagnosis

Nurses who work with groups involve the group participants throughout the nursing process. When the participants are active in the nursing process from the beginning of assessment, then they are more likely to be involved in a meaningful way in carrying out the plan. Nurses who work with families, communities, and other groups use collaborative processes to obtain and maintain the support of the group in need. This joint involvement will increase collaboration so the plan for achieving outcomes can be effective.

As learned in this text, nursing diagnoses according to the Roy Adaptation Model uses two basic approaches. The first method involves the statement of the behaviors together with the influencing stimuli. The second approach is to state a diagnosis by using a summary label with the relevant stimuli. The careful assessment of behaviors and stimuli is basic to both approaches. The summary labels for diagnostic categories for the physical mode of the group according to the Roy Adaptation Model are shown in Table 17–3 in relation to nursing diagnosis labels approved by the North American Nursing Diagnosis Association (NANDA International, 2007). Indicators of positive adaptation identified are adequate number of participants, adequate knowledge and skills of participants, stable membership, satisfactory physical facilities, effective structure and processes to meet changing physical needs, adequate fiscal resources, effective planning for future adequacy of participants, physical facilities, and fiscal resources. Commonly recurring adaptation problems for the physical mode of groups include shortage of personnel; debt for family,

TABLE 17–3 Nursing Diagnostic Categories for the Physical Mode for Groups

Positive Indicators of Adaptation	Common Adaptation Problems	NANDA Diagnostic Labels
• Adequate number of participants • Adequate knowledge and skills of participants • Stable membership • Satisfactory physical facilities • Effective structure and processes to meet changing physical needs • Adequate fiscal resources • Effective planning for future adequacy of participants, physical facilities, and fiscal resources	• Shortage of personnel • Debt for family, organization, community, nation • Homelessness • Health disparities • Global hunger • Inadequate potable water • Ineffective response to disaster	• Readiness for enhanced community coping • Readiness for enhanced immunization • Readiness for enhanced therapeutic regimen management • Risk for sudden infant death • Risk for contamination • Relocation stress syndrome • Impaired home maintenance • Ineffective protection • Ineffective family therapeutic regimen management • Ineffective community therapeutic regimen management • Contamination

organization, community, or nation; homelessness; health disparities; global hunger; inadequate potable water; and ineffective response to disaster.

To continue the discussion of the nursing process, we will introduce a situation of women who are pregnant living in the area of a nuclear power plant. A recent article (O'Connor & Roy, 2008) addressed the critical role that nurses can play in preventive strategies related to harmful pollution from energy production. In addition, nurses can be part of the national debate on issues of energy related to health. In the situation used here, a community health nurse has recently become aware that 40 pregnant women live within 5 miles of the nuclear power plant. Over 70% of these women state that they do not know what risk the location of their home involves. They are concerned about how they would handle an announcement of immediate danger. When asked specifically, at least half the women said that they had family or friends living out of the area where they could stay in an emergency. The nurse collaborates with the nurse midwife and a few of the women who are pregnant to assess the situation further and identifies the following:

- Unknown to women of area the risk to fetal development from radiation
- Lack of rapid channels of public communication in the event of an accident
- Lack of public awareness of need for information and plan for evacuation
- Little or no political participation and control by local residents
- A former midwife lives nearby and is concerned about the danger

In stating the diagnosis as significant behavior and stimuli, the nurse would write: A large number of pregnant women living near nuclear power plant generally do not know about risk and how to handle immediate danger related to lack of processes for public communication with plant officials and of awareness of health needs and related political processes. For this situation a diagnosis stated by a summary label with relevant stimuli is: High level health risk for pregnant women related to lack of processes for public communication with plant officials and of awareness of health needs and related political processes.

Goal Setting

In using the nursing process, the nurse focuses on behavior, the stimuli influencing that behavior, or both. With the nursing diagnosis, the statements developed included a summary of behaviors and stimuli. For the step of goal setting, the focus is on the behavior. Each goal identifies behavior that is to be addressed. In the physical mode of the group, the focus is on patterns of behavior. For this situation the first pattern of behavior is the lack of knowledge about the risk and about how to respond to immediate danger by the pregnant women. An appropriate goal will include the behavior, change expected, and a time frame. This can be stated: All women in the area will express adequate knowledge of risk and appropriate response to announcement of immediate danger within 2 months.

Intervention

According to the Roy Adaptation Model, in the intervention step of the nursing process the nurse focuses on the stimuli affecting the behavior that is the focus of the goals. The management of stimuli is the focus of intervention. This involves altering, increasing, decreasing, removing, or maintaining the stimuli. At the same time, the nurse may help the group to use effective coping strategies to strengthen compensatory processes. A review of the stimuli affecting adaptive group processes for both adaptive diagnosis and adaptation problems helps to identify specific interventions to reach the goals. In the case situation outlined above, interventions aimed at knowledge of risk and how to respond in an emergency include

- Collaborate with local leaders, former midwife, and interested women in publicizing the health needs involved.
- Mobilize local resources for more effective ongoing information and processes for emergency communication.
- Provide for community development of evacuation plan in an emergency, giving priority to pregnant women.

Evaluation

The final step of the nursing process is evaluation. According to the Roy Adaptation Model nursing process, this means looking at the effectiveness of the nursing interventions in relation to the group's adaptive behavior. The nurse judges whether the behaviors stated in the goals have been achieved. If the behavior is in agreement with the stated goal, then the nursing interventions are effective. However, if the goal has not been achieved, the nurse identifies alternative interventions or approaches. There may be a need to repeat the assessment of the behavior and stimuli. Based on new data, the other steps of the nursing process are continued.

In the situation described, the community health nurse would survey the pregnant women in the area in 2 months and ask about their knowledge of risks to fetal development from radiation and about their knowledge and comfort with plans for evacuation in the event of an emergency. If some of the women do not meet the goal, the nurse would reassess for other possible influencing factors not taken into account in the interventions. Perhaps there is a non–English-speaking woman in the group or one who is not in touch with the routine public education approaches used. Modified interventions are used for those who have not reached the goal.

Summary

The physical mode of the group was described in this chapter. Two major processes to meet the need for operating integrity were identified and described, strategic planning and resource management. Risk preparedness was explored as an example of a compensatory adaptive process. The examples of compromised processes that were described included ineffective response to disaster and racial disparities in health care. Many more integrated, compensatory, and compromised processes are involved in the physical adaptive mode. However, some initial examples within this mode were examined. The nursing process was described beginning with the behaviors and stimuli relevant to assessment of the physical mode of groups. The remaining steps of nursing diagnosis, goal setting, interventions, and evaluation were illustrated using a particular community health situation.

Exercises for Application

1. Identify a potential disaster in a local community. Go to the Citizen Corps Web site and determine what mechanisms are already in place for an emergency. Evaluate whether there are any gaps in the system.

2. Select one group to which you belong and list the major resources for the group. Considering the resources as a whole, list one change that might provide a threat to adequate management of these resources.

Assessment of Understanding

QUESTIONS

1. Name two integrated processes of the physical mode. _____, _____.

2. Name one compensatory process and give an example different from the one described in the chapter. _____

3. List two compromised processes in the physical mode for groups. _____, _____

   For one of these processes, identify one way that the compromised adaptation affects health. _____

4. List the major characteristics of groups that are assessed in first-level assessment and give an example of one behavior to assess for each characteristic.
   (a) _____, example: _____
   (b) _____, example: _____
   (c) _____, example: _____
   (d) _____, example: _____

5. Discuss one of the second-level assessment factors or stimuli and give an example of what you would assess in a group with which you are familiar.

   _____
   _____

   Example: _____

6. Situation:

   A community bordering a midsize city has discovered that household water supply has been contaminated with toxic chemical waste from nearby industry. Residents are largely elderly citizens whose goals are limited to personal survival. A private community health nursing service has a substation office within the geographic boundary of the community. Other factors relevant in this situation: Federal investigation of previous complaints related to industrial waste has been delayed by administrative policy changes. There is little social interaction and integration among the citizens of the community. People within the community obtain their goods and services within the community and are not socialized into the ecological problems of the larger society. A young activist group has recently established a storefront community relations center.

7. State a nursing diagnosis for this situation:
   _____.

8. Write one goal that relates to the nursing diagnosis given above. _____
   _____

9. List nursing interventions to accomplish the goal above. _____, _____,
   _____, _____,
   _____

10. Describe how you would evaluate the effectiveness of the nursing interventions named. _____.

FEEDBACK

1. Strategic planning and resource management.

2. Risk preparedness. Examples will vary. Emergency evacuation routes marked on city streets.

3. Ineffective disaster planning and health care disparities.

   Answers will vary. Ineffective disaster planning can lead to outbreaks of illness and multiple injuries not being treated in a timely way so that people suffer both physical harm and personal distress.

4. Structure, examples will vary; e.g., Is there a formal infrastructure or loosely organized membership?
   Functions, e.g., What safety mechanisms are available?
   Relationships, e.g., Are any spaces shared?
   Consistency, e.g., Does the group have a shared mission?

5. Answers vary. Context is a major stimulus and includes both the internal and external environment. Some important aspects of the external context are economic, social, political, cultural, belief, and family. Example: The context for the softball team I play on includes the talent of the team members and the availability and upkeep of the field we play on, as well as the equipment we use.

6. Local community faces serious health risk with limited view of the problem and related lack of processes for responding effectively.

7. Within 6 months the members of the community will be involved in becoming more informed and in mobilizing resources to lower the health risk.

8. Interventions
   • Community health nurse provides leadership for mobilizing the resources of the young activist group to assist with the community problem-solving process.
   • Use the nursing service substation office as a "safe" place for all community meetings.

- At community meetings relate the current health risk to the personal survival goals of the citizens.
- Use professional staff to search out and provide data on the history of the problem.
- Bring in politically active senior citizens from bordering city to socialize with local citizens.

9. The effectiveness of the interventions will be evaluated in 6 months by judging whether or not the goal was reached, that is, have the members of the community been involved in becoming informed and mobilizing resources to lower the health risk?

References

Bradford, R. W., Duncan, P. J., & Tarcy, B. (1999). *Simplified strategic planning: A no-nonsense guide for busy people who want results fast!* Worcester, MA: Chandler House Press.

Flaskerud, J. H., Lesser, J., Dixon, E., Anderson, N., Conde, F., Kim, S., Koniak-Griffin, D., Strehlow, A., Tullmann, D., & Verzemnieks, I. (2002). Health disparities among vulnerable populations. *Nursing Research, 51*(2): 74–85.

Friedman, M. M., Bowden, V. R., & Jones, E. G. (2003). *Family nursing: Research, theory and practice* (5th ed.). Upper Saddle River, NJ: Prentice Hall.

Hunt, R. (2001). *Community-based nursing.* Philadelphia: Lippincott.

Institute of Medicine. (2004). In the nation's compelling interest: Ensuring diversity in health care workforce. Washington D.C.: National Academic Press.

Magnet Recognition Program. In American Nurses Credentialing Center. Retrieved March 12, 2008, from http://www.nursecredentialing.org/magnet/index.html

McClure, M. M., Poulin, M., Sovie, M., & Wandelt, M. (1983). *Magnet hospitals: Attraction and retention of professional nurses.* American Academy of Nursing Task Force on Nursing Practice in Hospitals. Kansas City, MO: American Nurses Association.

NANDA International. (2007). *Nursing diagnoses: Definitions & classification, 2007–2008.* Philadelphia: NANDA-I.

National League for Nursing. (2008, February 4). National League for Nursing Convenes Innovative Think Tank on Expanding Diversity in Nurse Educator Workforce [Press Release]. Retrieved from http://www.nln.org/newsreleases/divthinktank_02042008.htm

O'Connor, A., & Roy, C. (2008). Electric power plant emissions and public health. *American Journal of Nursing, 108*(2), 62–70.

Polk, L. V., & Green, P. M. (2007). Contamination: Nursing diagnoses with outcome and intervention linkages. *International Journal of Nursing Terminologies and Classifications, 18*(2), 37–44.

Smedley, B. D., Butler, A. S., & Bristow, L. R. (Eds.). (2004). *In the nation's compelling interest: Ensuring diversity in the health care workforce.* Committee on Institutional and Policy-Level Strategies for Increasing the Diversity of the U.S. Healthcare Workforce. Washington, DC: The National Academies Press.

Smith, C. S., & Maurer, F. A. (2004). *Community health nursing: Theory and practice* (3rd ed.). Philadelphia: W. B. Saunders Co.

Soanes, C., & Stevenson, A. (Eds.). *The Concise Oxford English Dictionary.* Retrieved August 26, 2005, from http://www.oxfordreference.com/views/ENTRY.html?subview=Main&entry=t23.e16054

Wilson, C. K. (1991). *Building new nursing organizations: Visions and realities.* Boston: Jones & Bartlett.

World Health Organization. (2008). Retrieved March 4, 2008, from http://www.who.int/about/en/

Wright, L., & Leahey, M. (2000). *Nurses and families: A guide to family assessment and intervention* (3rd ed.). Philadelphia: F. A. Davis Co.

CHAPTER 18

Group Identity Mode of Relating Persons

This chapter focuses specifically on the second adaptive mode for relating persons which is called group identity. Like self-concept for the person, it involves perceptions based on feedback. Further group identity affects how the group acts. Groups are relating persons in systems such as families, people committed to a certain cause, local communities, networks with given goals, and organizations. This view of groups includes, for example, a nursing care group in a given practice area. Through group identity, nurses can identify their group as all those assigned to a certain hospital unit caring for patients assigned to that unit. Another way to identify the group of nurses is to include only those who work on a given shift. Group identity depends on various perceptions and will affect how the group works.

The group identity mode includes the self-image and shared responsibility of the group. The basic need underlying the group identity mode is termed identity integrity. This means the ability of group members to relate to each other in ways that indicate awareness of group identity. This awareness includes such things as shared goals and values. If awareness of a shared identity is effective and efficient, it maintains and enhances the identity of the group and moves it toward achieving common goals.

This chapter provides an overview of the group identity mode and how people in groups meet the basic underlying need for identity integrity. We will describe the integrated processes of shared identity and family coherence that are associated with identity integrity for groups or systems of relating persons. Compensatory adaptive processes related to group identity are discussed. Low morale and out-group stereotyping are the examples of compromised processes for groups that are explored. Finally, guidelines for planning nursing care are provided. The nursing process includes outlining nursing assessment of behaviors and stimuli, formulating diagnoses, establishing goals, selecting interventions, and evaluating nursing care.

OBJECTIVES

After studying this chapter, the reader will be able to do the following:

1. Describe the group identity mode according to the Roy Adaptation Model.
2. Describe one compensatory process related to group identity.

3. Name and describe two situations of compromised processes of group identity.

4. Identify important first-level assessment behaviors for the group identity mode.

5. Identify second-level assessment factors or stimuli that influence the group identity mode.

6. Formulate nursing diagnoses related to the group identity mode.

7. Establish goals related to given diagnoses in the group identity mode.

8. Select nursing interventions to promote adaptation in the group identity mode.

9. Propose approaches to determine the effectiveness of nursing interventions for group identity.

KEY CONCEPTS DEFINED

Community: A group of persons with some common bond, whether living near one another; having the same religious beliefs; or perhaps coming from the same country of origin, but not necessarily living in close proximity in the country of immigration.

Community cohesion: The link that connects members of a community through support, trust, and affection.

Family coherence: A state of unity or a consistent sequence of thought that connects family members.

Group culture: The group's agreed upon expectations, including values, goals, and norms for relating.

Group identity: Shared relations, goals, and values, which create a social milieu and culture, a group self-image, and co-responsibility for goal achievement.

Identity integrity: Implies the honesty, soundness, and completeness of the group members' identification with the group

Low morale: The state in a group that results from the challenges to the usual tendency toward cohesiveness and failure of the processes for shared identity; it is evident in low energy for activities related to group goals or relationships.

Out-group stereotyping: Beliefs that associate groups of people other than one's own group with certain types of characteristics; these beliefs then influence judgments of individuals.

Shared identity: The process whereby the members of the group come to common perceptions of the environment, common cognitive and feeling orientations, and shared goals and values.

Social culture: A specific part of the milieu or environment of the group made up of socioeconomic status and ethnicity in particular.

Social milieu: Refers to the total human-made environment that surrounds the group in which it is embedded.

GROUP IDENTITY OF RELATING PERSONS

The group identity mode for relating persons is like the self-concept mode for the individual. It reflects how people in groups perceive themselves based on environmental feedback about the group. The perceptions of persons in a group can be about their shared relations, goals, and values. The feedback the group receives comes from the social milieu and the culture. Milieu is another word for environment. Social relates to human societies. Social milieu refers to the total human-made environment that surrounds the group and in which it is embedded. This includes the economic, political, religious, family, and other structures. Each of these has established beliefs. Social culture is a specific part of the milieu or environment of the group. Socioeconomic status and ethnicity in particular make up the social culture. The belief systems held within the milieu and social culture are particularly significant for a group. The social milieu and social culture act as stimuli for the group. In turn the group sets up its own social milieu and culture. The group milieu and culture affects the other groups with which the group interacts. As noted, the group self-image and shared responsibility for goal achievement is central to group identity. The basic need underlying the group identity mode is termed identity integrity. Identity integrity implies the honesty, soundness, and completeness of the group members' identification with the group at large.

In summary, group identity refers to shared relations, goals, and values, which act within and create a social milieu and culture, a group self-image, and co-responsibility for goal achievement. Understanding each concept of the definition contributes to knowledge of the components of the group identity mode. Understanding the components leads to understanding of the integrated processes of group identity. Figure 18–1 depicts the interrelated subareas and components of the group identity adaptive mode. These concepts, then, are the basis for understanding the integrated processes of shared identity.

According to the Roy Adaptation Model, groups have basic life processes in each adaptive mode. Nursing care uses the understanding of these processes to evaluate the adaptation level and to provide care to promote integrated processes at the highest level of adaptation possible. There are many basic processes for the shared identity mode. To date, two processes have been identified and the related theoretical knowledge developed. These are the group's shared identity process and family coherence. Topics related to shared identity, such as interpersonal relations and the importance of communication, are found in Chapter 16 in discussion of the interdependence adaptive mode. The consideration here is on the shared identity of voluntary personal and professional groups and the family. The family most often is the first group with which a person identifies. The group identity processes are described by synthesizing middle-range theories to provide knowledge of the group identity mode for the Roy Adaptation Model.

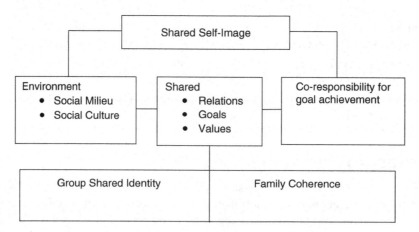

FIGURE 18–1 Group Identity mode. Theoretical basis.

Process of Shared Identity

In the group identity mode, a major process of adaptation is shared identity. Studying shared identity involves studying more than individual self-concepts and people relating to one another as members of groups. Some authors build upon ideas of Lewin (1948), who was an early theorist on small-group interaction. They noted that goal-directed behavior of individuals, groups, organizations, nation-states, or any other large-scale social system is a function of the perceived external environment and of shared understandings. These shared understandings are cognitive, emotional, motivational, and normative orientations of members of these social systems (Rabbie & Lodewijkx, 1996). Shared identity, then, is the process whereby the members of the group come to common perceptions of the environment, common cognitive and feeling orientations, and shared goals and values.

Another approach to group identity is social identity theory that was developed from studying how different groups relate to each other. This theory proposes that each person has both a personal identity, or self-concept, and social identity, or group identity. The person moves back and forth between the dominance of self or group identity depending on the demands of the situation (Brown & Capozza, 2000; Tajfel, 1979). Often the person creates a positive value of the self based on being included in a group. For example, a student nurse who is doing well in her studies welcomes the opportunity to be inducted into the nursing honor society. This group membership allows her to interact with other professionals who are committed to the goals and values she believes in. However, the premises of the theory also allow for negative identifications that can marginalize some groups.

According to social identity theory, individuals are categorized by using labels. Cognitively, it is easier to sort single objects into groups, rather than to think of each as unique. Biologists classify species; nurses classify nursing diagnoses. In some ways, categorizations are useful and adaptive. However, when people are categorized, there is a tendency to misinterpret likenesses and differences (Stangor & Lange, 1994). The second step in the theory is identification. Groups that the individual identifies with—country, ethnic region, working unit—are called *in-groups* whereas groups other than one's own are called *out-groups*. The third part of the process is social comparison. Added to the tendency of social categorization is a common bias called *out-group* homogeneity. Put simply, this means that people in the *in-group* feel that "we" have interesting and subtle differences between "us," but "they" are all alike. Beliefs about groups that are built on these categorizations tend to be overgeneralized. Much of the work on race relations uses social identity theories of *in-group* and *out-group* awareness. These natural tendencies among groups can lead to stereotyping, discussed later as an adaptation problem.

The term group culture is used to describe the group's agreed-upon expectations that include values, goals, and norms for relating (Kimberly, 1997). The expectations are shared and result in patterned behavior relevant to the group's relation to its environment and to interaction of its members among themselves and with outsiders. Communal sharing is another term related to the process of shared identity. Communal sharing is a relationship of equality in which people are merged for the purposes of the group, so that individual selves are not distinct (Fiske, 1991). People attend to being a member of the group and have a common sense of identity in which individuality is not marked. Emphasis is placed on the common characteristics that brought the group together. What is important to individuals is membership in the group and the boundaries that contrast the group members with outsiders. The group members have a sense of solidarity, unity, and belonging. Fiske noted that they identify with the collectivity and think of themselves as being all the same in some significant respect, not as individuals but as "we." This principle is demonstrated in the example of a recent national basketball championship series. Commentators noted that the team that had a strong group identity won over the team built around an individual star player.

Relevant theory and practice in nursing moves beyond the concept of communal sharing by describing a particular kind of group culture based on women's experiences. The culture described by Chinn (2008) emphasizes that recognizing the individuality of each group member enables the shared identity of the group. The individual identity is not secondary to group identity but they grow together. The author uses the acronym, PEACE, to discuss effective ways of relating in all kinds of groups and communities. Chinn sees PEACE as intent, process, and outcome. Peace is both the means and the end. It is the process and the product. Carefully chosen values are made real in action. The process is rooted in women's ancient wisdom of peacemaking. However, the skills required were often limited to home and family life. Chinn noted that the values and skills can be articulated and applied to overcoming all types of imbalances of power in both private and public relationships. The close link between values and action is referred to as "doing what we know, and knowing what we do."

The process Chinn outlined is an effort to describe the values of women's ways of making peace in groups, and the skills, actions, and abilities that go with those values. The author draws from the experiences of women's groups dedicated to transformation to present a process represented by five words. Use of the process requires conscious awareness of the group interaction and commitment to particular values, and the congruent actions, of the ways in which individuals can choose to relate to one another. The PEACE intent, process, and outcome described by Chinn (2008) articulated the values reflected in the assumptions of the Roy Adaptation Model and can be viewed as a process for shared identity. The words chosen to describe the process are praxis, empowerment, awareness, consensus, and evolvement.

Praxis refers to thoughtful reflection and action that occur in synchrony, in the direction of transforming the world. In praxis, values are made visible through deliberate action. Empowerment includes growth of personal strength, power, and ability to enact one's own will and love for self in the context of love and respect for others. It requires inward listening to the senses as well as listening intently and actively to others. One consciously takes in and forms strength by active engagement with others whose values you share. It is possible when people express respect and reverence for all other forms of life. All are one with the ground of energy and with the earth. Chinn described awareness as an active, growing knowledge of self and others, and the world in which one lives. It means a heightened awareness of the present moment and valuing one's own experience. With this awareness one sees beyond the present to integrate the past and the future. This awareness makes one conscious of the contradictions in the world. One example might be that what is defined as peace is often war. Being silent at a meeting only to rant and rave afterwards does not add to peace. Cooperation is an active commitment to group solidarity and group integrity. It grows out of mutually defined values. Each individual's viewpoint and abilities are honored equally. Everyone is encouraged to use their abilities, ideas, and energy to create a coordinated and cohesive whole. In the process described by Chinn, evolvement means a commitment to growth in which change and transformation are conscious and deliberate. Growth and transformations of the group happen in cycles and are valued and celebrated by the group.

Process of Family Coherence

The family is often the first group identity the person has and the related integrated process in this mode is identified as family coherence. In Chapter 3 the family is identified as a common stimulus affecting all of adaptation. In the group identity adaptive mode, we can understand further shared identity by understanding family coherence. Family systems theory since the early eighties presented much in the area of "dysfunction" in families. However, Tolstoy (1961) noted "Happy families are all alike; every unhappy family is unhappy in its own way." In describing the integrated adaptive process, the focus is on the working of families who share a group identity.

One of the early texts on the Roy Adaptation Model defined family as a group of two or more persons united by ties of marriage, blood, or adoption, or a group of persons who relate to one another through specified patterns or roles, regardless of ties, and thereby create and maintain a common culture (Hanson, 1984). As noted in Chapter 17, families also include a variety of living groups and structures which may or may not have biological or legal ties. The family of orientation is the one in which persons have grown up and in which they learned interactional skills. Childbearing families are one or two parents and a young child or children. Other examples are relationships such as cohabitating partners and homosexual couples, with or without children, as well as communal groups. There are blended families when one or more divorced parent remarries and takes on stepchildren and may have additional children with the new partner. Increasingly, families may include an older adult. The significant numbers of teen pregnancies, and sometimes parent illnesses, often means that a grandparent may be caring for a grandchild. Basically, families exist to nurture the growth and development of the members. In discussing the family as the unit for health promotion, Pender and colleagues (Pender, Murdaugh, & Parsons, 2002) noted that one responsibility of the family is to promote healthy development of distinct individuals while maintaining family cohesion. The common saying that blood is thicker than water emphasizes the family cohesion that is a particular kind of group identity.

Coherence refers to a state of unity. The word can also refer to a consistent sequence of thought. The family is considered as a whole rather than the sum of the members. It is an integrated system with interdependent structures, functions, and relationships. Structure includes the members and the responsibilities they have within the group. Function includes ongoing activities as well as change within the system as the environment changes. Relationships include the close interactions of give and take and strengthening unity when needed. The family unit has a concept of itself as a unit. There is consistency among the members in this view. The consistent thought about who the family is includes history, traditions, meanings, and moral-ethical values. Satir (1991) was an early theorist who emphasized how people are made up of patterns of behavior that are transmitted through family generations.

Family coherence is evidenced by certain observable characteristics (Bowen, 1978). The solidarity of the family is noted by an atmosphere of love, respect, and loyalty. The members provide understanding and companionship. They will defend each other and stand up for each other when conflicts occur with those outside the family. Members acknowledge and honor their own needs as well as those of each other. While individuals strive for competence and independence, there is a strong sense of the family commonality. Boundaries of the family from other groups are important, as noted below. In addition clear boundaries between family members create an atmosphere of mutual respect and a sense of personal integrity. A cohesive sense of boundaries within the family provides an individual with the trust and creativity necessary to be in relationships outside the family. Individuals with a strong history of family coherence tend to relate well in groups. They show the values that are intrinsic to the family of origin. Such individuals are more inclined to take risks and to exhibit honesty and freedom of expression. They use appropriate humor, ask for what they need, and respect the needs and limits of other members. The group members of coherent families know the balance of power created by the process of working through fear to intimacy.

Culture can be part of the family coherence. This is particularly evident in the Native American culture. While Native Americans believe in an individual's autonomy, the individual is always part of the tribe and the family clan. One of their beliefs is that everything has spirit and is inner-connected. The connections of the family group are part of the circle of energy from birth to death and rebirth. The nurse always considers culture, but notes in particular how it relates to family coherence. Knowledge about what groups are important to a person and who they define as family are useful in planning individual nursing care. In addition, the knowledge of shared identity can help nurses contribute to the effectiveness of groups in which they participate, such as communities, families, hierarchical institutions, committees, and self-help groups. Insights from the theories related to the shared identity processes are useful in understanding the integrated adaptation level.

COMPENSATORY ADAPTIVE PROCESSES

As with the self-concept mode of the individual, the self identity mode for groups has many compensatory processes. These processes are expanded because of the variety of types and purposes of groups and the richness of personal strengths of group members. As defined earlier by the Roy Adaptation Model, compensatory processes for groups represent the adaptation level at which the stabilizer and innovator are activated by a challenge to the integrated life processes. In this chapter we discuss two compensatory processes: community cohesion and transcending crisis.

Community Cohesion

As noted, people form groups for a variety of reasons, both personal and professional. A community is a group of persons with some common bond, whether living near one another, having the same religious beliefs, or perhaps coming from the same country of origin. The term has different meanings depending on the context. Healthy People 2010 as well as the WHO use the following definition: "A specific group of people, often living in a defined geographic area, who share a common culture, values, and norms and who are arranged in a social structure according to relationships that community had developed over a period of time" (USDHHS, 2000, p. 7). Members of a community may not necessarily be in close proximity to each other. An example is an immigrant group with even stronger ties to each other in the United States than they had in their own country. They find it important to cohere as a community even though they live in different areas. Their coherence becomes a compensatory process to help stabilize their culture within the new environment. In addition, together they seek innovative ways to be part of the larger culture. The new demands call upon stabilizer and innovator adaptive processes. Most major cities in the United States have community centers for recent immigrant populations that draw people from throughout the geographic area. For example, community centers in metropolitan Boston include Brazilian, Chinese, and Islamic. Also, there are many Jewish, Irish, and Italian centers that date back many years.

Chinn (2008) talked about communities of women with common goals, some of whom interact mainly by email. Most of her writing relates to groups of people within communities that interact on personal levels. Their explicit values, concerns, and purposes bring them together. The author emphasized both the importance of cohesiveness and diversity. It is these two values that create the solidarity of the group. The solidarity allows the focus of energies and resources so that the group can accomplish goals and promote growth. Chinn broadens the perspective by noting that we refer to global community to encompass all who live on the planet earth. The concept implies a shared concern about the global environment, economies, and politics. Derber (2004) noted that globalization promises economic stability, cultural cooperation, international solidarity, and universal human rights. However, too often it has been seen as having the goal of spreading consumerism at the expense of workers. To date, globalization has not realized the possibilities it offers.

Singer (2002) argued that the complexities of globalization should lead us to reconsider the moral significance we currently place on national boundaries. It may be better if we begin to consider ourselves as members of a community of the world. The author provides a dramatic example of facts to consider. UNICEF (2001) released a report *The State of the World's Children* on September 13, 2001. This was two days after the September 11 terrorist attacks on the United States. From the UNICEF report it can be figured that likely on the day of the attack close to 30,000 children under the age of five died from preventable causes. These include malnutrition, unsafe water, and the lack of even the most basic health care. This number of child deaths is about 10 times the number of victims of the attacks. Yet UNICEF did not receive an "avalanche" of money following the report, whereas the public appeals for victims of the terrorist attacks totaled $1.3 billion in the 3 months after the disaster. These facts provide pause for comparing national and global communities. Still, the example of the public outpouring after the terrorist attack also provides an example of extraordinary cohesion in response to violence aimed at the United States community.

In considering global issues requiring effective group action, Perry and Gregory (2007) began by quoting Roy's belief that nursing as a profession carries a social mandate to contribute to the common good. The authors introduced two major approaches. The first was transcendent pluralism as a foundation for global understanding. The aim was to create a peaceful evolution of an increasingly globalized society. Transcendent pluralism is an ethical framework to build understanding between people of diverse backgrounds. The approach creates transcultural understanding and social justice. Going beyond any single tradition to a higher spiritual realm can serve as a foundation for relationships with any group of people that are other than one's group. The second approach was for nurses to develop a broader knowledge of the environment. In keeping with the philosophical assumptions of the Roy Adaptation Model, environment can be defined as the global ecosystem. Persons are responsible for physiologic integrity and sustainability of our planet. The authors noted that advances in communications and technology make it possible to think and act globally as well as locally.

When people form a specific community, there is a natural tendency toward cohesion. This is a predictable outcome of the group identity and, if not taken to excess, can lead to positive effects for the individual and the group. Cohesiveness has been defined as the extent to which the features of the group bind the members to it. It was noted that, within a family, coherence is based simply on being a family member. The bases of cohesiveness for a group, however, includes the liking or attraction among members, similar norms and values, the effective pursuit of goals, and maintaining good working relations (Kimberly, 1997).

Individual members of a community enjoy the link that exists between them and the group. The support, trust, and affection among the community contribute to personal growth. This exists even if there is an occasional expression of hostility, dissatisfaction, or frustration. Cohesion has been called the "glue" that causes the members to remain in the community even when there are pressures or influences to leave it. For the community, the benefit is that cohesive groups usually enjoy low turnover and high participation because members desire continuation of the group and its commitment to common goals. Cohesion enhances group norms, and norms contribute to cohesion. The immigrant centers noted are voluntary that use community cohesion to enhance the group adaptation. In the group they find structure, identity, camaraderie, recognition, and positive role models. In return, the immigrant community can also contribute more to the larger society.

Transcending Crisis

A second compensatory process for groups that activates the stabilizer and innovator in response to a challenge to the integrated group identity processes is transcending crisis. Groups face crisis just as individuals do, and some of the same theoretical understanding is helpful. Crises occur when the usual coping strategies are not working. In early work to understand the phenomenon of crisis on the individual level, Caplan and Caplan (1993) distinguished between developmental and situational crisis. The same approach is useful in looking at crisis in groups. How the crisis is managed determines the outcome. Transcending a crisis can be an adaptive compensatory process leading to growth.

The development stages and situations that a group faces vary widely with the type and purpose of the group. Worchel (1996) developed one model of group development from observations of ongoing groups. The author regarded these stages as important in any group-based analysis. This model's Stage I was named the stage of discontent, because this period often creates the foundation for group formation. Although groups may be created by other factors, such as a work team, group formation issues need to be examined. Group members may feel alienated at first, and helpless to influence the group; hence, participation may be low and dominated by a few. Stage II may be initiated by a precipitating event. The incident may be relatively minor and unplanned, such as the rumor of pay inequities among the workgroup, or an emotional outburst by a single group member. The event often surfaces common dissatisfactions and initiates meaningful contact between members. Stage III of group development occurs when the members focus on defining the group and determining its membership. Members become concerned with demonstrating that they are the "in-group." The period of identification incorporates features of group activities referred to for a long time as forming, storming, and norming activities (Tuckman, 1965). Stage IV involves group productivity in which identity issues are less apparent and the group sets goals and initiates planning for how to achieve those goals. Processing information revolves around productivity issues. Differentiating members by skills, motivation, and leadership are issues. This leads to Stage V, the individual stage. The members begin to demand recognition for their contributions and request resources on the basis of equity rather than equality. The group takes a more cooperative stand toward out-groups because members may be exploring opportunities for themselves in the out-groups. The author describes Stage VI as that of decay. As increasing attention is paid to personal needs, the group becomes less important to each person. Subgroups may form and compete for power. The group drifts into a new period of discontent, Stage I. These generalizations about stages of group development present possibilities for developmental crisis with opportunities to transcend the crisis.

One example of transcending a crisis can occur in Stage III, defining the group and determining its membership. The group can take the time to clarify its values and goals. You may be a member of a Research Committee at your hospital. The group may find itself meeting without any real purpose or direction. The question of whether of not to dissolve the group has been raised. The group can take a session to clarify why the committee exists, what is important to the members, and what it wants to accomplish. This can lead to greater commitment of members to the group identity. Furthermore, the group may decide that it is time to recruit new members. The clarity needed for recruitment is helpful to both the current and new members. You may decide you need nurses from different units and perhaps one or two people with more experience in research. The new members bring additional viewpoints, energy, skills, and commitment. This infusion will be contagious to the commitment of the whole group. In this way a developmental crisis about identity is transcended as a source of growth. Note that stabilizing processes are used in clarifying the values and goals. Innovative processes are used in seeking new members.

In Chinn's (2008) approach to building community in groups, she discussed the issue of conflict transformation. This is one example of transcending situational crisis. Chinn emphasized that conflict transformation can be anticipated before there is conflict in a group. She suggested that the group build a strong foundation of three traditions when things are calm. These traditions build a strong foundation for transforming conflict when it occurs. In a group that consistently rotates leadership, each individual already feels supported in a leadership role. When conflict occurs, anyone can move into the leader role while those at the center can step aside to listen and focus on their own responses and actions. Secondly, practicing critical reflection promotes communication skills that focus on the group's responsibility for what happens in the group. The clarity developed over time about the group's principles of solidarity is a resource for addressing conflict. Lastly, the group that has worked on valuing individual differences has a strong basis for transforming the crisis of conflict in the group.

Chinn (2008) went on to point out that when the group or individuals become aware of conflict, they need to address it. Conflict cannot be ignored or handled by individuals. If it occurs in the group, it requires a group response for it to be transformative for the group. Each person addresses the points of a framework for critical reflection. These are: "I feel... when (or about)...I want...because." The exchange of all individual perspectives leads to understanding of the group. The exchange using this process brings out many possibilities and provides insight for common ground to emerge. The same principles apply to conflict in online groups. It may be easy to miss early signals of a conflict, but if not handled, conflict will have a negative influence on the group. If the group has built a strong foundation as described above, Chinn suggested that the online form of communication becomes an ideal way to address conflict. One can think about a response before pushing the send button. Also each person can respond and not reply again until each has sent the first response. The group may decide to close the discussion of the conflict or shift into a decision-building process to begin anew. Each person acknowledges what was learned and how the group grew in transforming the conflict.

COMPROMISED PROCESSES OF GROUP IDENTITY

Compromised processes occur, according to the Roy Adaptation Model, when ineffective compensatory processes do not restore integration. For groups in the group identity mode, compromised processes result in adaptation problems, as it does in other modes for both individuals and groups. Adaptation problems or compromised processes are the third level of adaptation. Difficulties can occur in any or all of the processes of group identity. The two examples of compromised processes within the group for the group identity mode that are discussed here are low morale and out-group stereotyping.

Low Morale

Morale is defined simply as the state of mind of a person or group as exhibited by confidence, cheerfulness, and productivity. Low morale in a group is a state resulting from challenges to the usual tendency toward cohesiveness and failure of the processes for shared identity and cohesion. Manifestations of low morale are evident in low energy of the group for activities related to the goals of the group or to maintaining group relationships. Complaints about small issues multiply and individuals retreat to self-interests. The members of the group are no longer interested in putting energy into sharing cognitive and emotional orientations. Commitment to values and goals of the group become less active and intense. There are many factors that can precipitate low morale in a group, or lead to its insidious development. Changes in any of the stimuli considered relevant to shared identity may be responsible for changes in morale. If demands on a group increase without the resources to meet the demands, frustrations can evolve quickly into low morale. If ways to communicate over distance are altered, there may be a gradual erosion of morale in the group. When a group that has met annually about common research interests loses funding to travel, they may find that alternate ways of sharing do not create the same joy and productivity.

In the discussion of the group's perception of changes in behavior of other people or groups, it was noted that this can lead to efforts to strengthen shared identity. The example was given of a department perceiving that they are being targeted for budget cuts by the administration. In this situation, if the perceptions turn out to be validated by layoff notices to one third of the staff, and if all efforts to deal as a group with the issue are ineffective, then low morale is a likely consequence. The cycle of low morale continues downward as changes are implemented and the demands of greater workloads are placed on fewer staff.

Leadership and how responsibility and accountability are distributed are key factors in enhancing or lowering morale. One of the most devastating blows to group morale is a leader's inequitable distribution of responsibility and accountability for group goals. If even one nurse on a given unit consistently receives lighter patient loads and never attends unit meetings, resentment and the powerlessness to explain or change the situation leads to low morale in the whole group. Perhaps equally distressing for the group is the situation in which goals are altered by the leader without consulting the group. Many nurses have experienced the low morale resulting when a health care agency is purchased by a larger corporation and new leadership changes the philosophy and mission of the institution by announcement in a newsletter. The problems resulting from low morale provide a real threat to any group, and certainly affect the type of patient care nurses can provide when it occurs in a health care setting. Nurses may also meet many patients whose health issues are exacerbated by low morale resulting from the many changes occurring in contemporary work settings.

Out-Group Stereotyping

A particular adaptation problem in the group identity mode that interferes with group functioning has been termed stereotyping. Stereotypes are beliefs that associate certain groups of people with certain types of characteristics and these beliefs then influence judgments of individuals. Stereotyping represents ineffectiveness in processes of group identity. In particular it is a violation of the need for groups to value diversity. Diverity is noted as a value in the assumptions of the Roy Adaptation Model. The expectation is also included in Chinn's work (2008) discussed in relation to the process of group identity and the compensatory process of transcending crisis. Illustrations of stereotyping in society, and resulting discrimination and prejudice, are related to gender and race.

The formation of stereotypes begins with the tendency for people to group themselves and others into social categories. While stereotypes can offer convenient summaries of social groups, their harmful effects are that they cause people to overlook diversity within categories and lead to inaccurate judgments about particular individuals. Furthermore, stereotypes provide the basis for discrimination and prejudice. Discrimination refers to any behavior directed against persons, often unfairly, based on out-group membership. Prejudice refers to negative feelings toward others based on group membership. There are mutual links among the three concepts. Stereotypes may cause people to become prejudiced; discriminatory practices may stem from and support stereotypes and prejudice; and prejudiced people may use stereotypes to justify their feelings (Brehm & Kassin, 1996). Group functioning is extremely difficult in a situation of out-group stereotyping. In this situation, groups fail to appreciate individuals with their own abilities and talents that can contribute to the group.

As discussed in Chapter 15, stereotypes of men as dominant and women as subordinate persist because men occupy higher status positions in society (Eagly, 1987). This division of labor may be the product of many factors (biologic, social, economic, and political). Men and women then act in ways that fit their assigned place in the workforce. Rather than attribute the differences to assigned roles, people attribute the differences to the group, that is, gender. Similarly, there are many classic studies of ethnic and racial stereotypes, particularly of African Americans in the United States. Surveys given over the years from the 1950s to the 1980s note that negative images of blacks have decreased (Dovidio & Gaertner, 1986). However, contemporary authors describe modern racism as a form of prejudice that surfaces in subtle ways when it is safe, socially acceptable, and easy to rationalize. According to these theories, many people are racially ambivalent. Generally, people want to see themselves as fair, but they still have deep feelings of anxiety and discomfort in the presence of other racial groups (Hass, Katz, Rizzo, Bailey, & Moore, 1992). Evidence of this ambivalence lies in the fact that many white Americans may speak about principles of racial equality, but in practice they oppose mixed marriages, black political candidates, and racially symbolic policies.

Desegregation of schools was anticipated to be a significant force against out-group stereotyping. This hope was based on the contact hypothesis, which proposes that direct contact between hostile groups will reduce prejudice under certain conditions. Desegregation has not cured problems of racism because it was also the case that the key conditions of intergroup contact—equal status, personal interactions, the need to achieve a common goal, and social norms that favor intergroup contact—have not been present (Brehm & Kassin, 1996).

Since out-group stereotyping is socially pervasive and distorts perceptions of individuals, for nurses to interact with people as individuals, they will find ways to deal with stereotyping.

Second, nurses can make a difference in promoting group effectiveness in others by making efforts to decrease stereotyping. Some authors describe stereotypes as being implicit and automatic, or stereotypes as being explicit and controlled. Brehm and Kassin (1996) noted that the individual does not need to be trapped into evaluating specific persons in terms of social categories, that is, to use implicit and automatic stereotypes. They quoted research that identifies three factors to enable a person to overcome stereotypes and judge others on a more individualized basis (Fiske & Neuberg, 1990). The first factor relates to the amount of personal information one person has about the other. The nurse is in a position to listen to the person's own story and to help others to do the same. Second, the person must have the cognitive resources to focus on the individual member of a stereotyped group. People are more likely to form an impression based on existing stereotypes when they are busy or pressed for time and unable to think clearly about the unique attributes of a single person. Although nurses are often busy, they can strive to maintain their value of the need to focus on the individual within every interaction. The researchers identify motivation as the third factor to alleviate stereotyping. When the person is highly motivated to form an accurate impression of someone, he or she often manages to set aside preexisting beliefs. Common examples are when the person is in an interdependent relationship or needs to compete against the other person. However, by the choice of nursing as a profession, the nurse has the highest motivation possible to overcome stereotyping.

NURSING PROCESS RELATED TO GROUP IDENTITY

In the group identity mode, the focus of nursing practice is on relational systems such as families, communities, and society. The Roy Adaptation Model framework for systematic nursing practice is parallel to that described for the nursing care of individuals. In this section the six steps of the nursing process are presented according to the Roy Adaptation Model. Examples are given for a variety of groups. It is understood that each illustration is one simple part of what is a complex process for nurses working with various groups over time.

Assessment of Behavior

First-level assessment of the group identity mode includes assessing behaviors of shared identity in groups and cohesion in families. Assessment can be made by direct observation and by reports from persons in the group. The nurse assesses the patterns of behavior in the group. Areas to assess are the group's common perceptions of the group boundaries, common thinking and feeling orientations, and shared goals and values. Since patterns are being assessed, the assessment is done over time, not as a single observation or report. Each group has its own particular structure and purpose that gives rise to the group. Particular applications will be made to assessing the shared identity in groups built on the group culture described by Chinn (2008). For the assessment of family coherence, the most relevant behaviors from broader family assessments are described. Again the focus is on patterns of family behavior.

PERCEPTIONS OF GROUP BOUNDARIES An important consideration in assessing patterns of shared identity is to understand how the group defines the boundaries between members of the group and nonmembers. In a school, does the workgroup include faculty and staff of a department? Are the tenure-track faculty and clinical faculty considered the same group? On the hospital administrative team, are vice presidents for all services included in a group, or is the vice president for nursing included in a separate group with other nurse administrations in the institution? Behaviors of shared identity include the group's common understanding of who are internal and who are external.

Chinn (2008) identified that usually all groups based on PEACE processes seek to be open to all who wish to join them. Being completely open may become a dilemma. The group wants to include new thinking and integrate diversity within the group. On the other hand, they also need to remain effective in accomplishing the work of the group. Chinn suggests that the group consider openness as relative and changing. Rather than making an opposing choice between open or closed, membership can change as demands of tasks change. This will encourage a natural flow of movement with people both leaving and joining the group, possibly on a temporary basis. A group responsible for a given task can set up times when membership is open and new volunteers can be oriented and introduced as members of the group. A research group may be a closed group until the project is completed. In contrast a research committee may decide to accept new members twice a year.

THINKING AND FEELING ORIENTATIONS Whether the group members share common thinking and feeling orientations is important evidence of shared identity. The group identifies which orientations are important to the group. For example, a group working on repealing death penalty laws may welcome people who have differing reasons for their support of the group. Some members may come from a humanitarian perspective and others from their religious background. Still, belief in the need to repeal the laws and the emotional energy to work toward this goal are the relevant common orientations.

Chinn (2008) provided a list of questions about the congruence of intent and actions that are the most relevant cognitive and emotional orientations in the culture of groups based on PEACE processes. These can be used, and modified, for assessing groups, and oneself, when a group is built on similar principles. They include the following questions.

- Do I know what I do, and do I do what I know? (Praxis)
- Am I expressing my own will in the context of love and respect for others? (Empowerment)
- Am I fully aware of others and myself, and do I bring such awareness to our discussions? (Awareness)
- Do I honor and encourage everyone's opinions, skills, and contributions? (Cooperation)
- Do I welcome practices that encourage growth and change for others, the group, and myself? (Evolvement) (Chinn, 2008, p. 13)

GOALS AND VALUES The process of group identity can also be assessed by observing, directly or indirectly, the patterns of behavior related to goals and values. Group goals are simply defined as goals upon which the members agree. Kimberly (1997) related goals to values. She noted that individuals accept a group goal when they can relate it to one or more of their values. A group goal can express an individual goal at a more concrete level. The group defines the goals and values that are relevant to its shared identity. These are based on what defines the group as a group and on the shared cognitive and emotional orientations. Goals and values prescribe behavior related to attaining goals. For example, a group working on repeal of death penalty laws may decide that group members will be involved in activities related to collecting studies of the effects of the death penalty, lobbying efforts, media contacts, and public education. Shared identity is strong when group actions focus mainly on commitment to common values and attainment of group goals.

In an analysis of group action, Chinn (2008) introduced the concept of power. She noted that power is the energy from which action arises. Chinn distinguished clearly, however, that the power within PEACE groups is different from power as it is usually understood. The world at large sees power as reflecting hierarchical ideal. In a hierarchical culture, power refers to the capacity to impose one's will on others. Too often people who are being manipulated or controlled do not realize the dynamic taking place. Chinn clarified that the kind of power required to create and live within PEACE comes from the power of love. What is valued in groups established on PEACE principles is the capacity to be in harmony with others and with the earth. The group strives to join others in directing collective energies toward a future that the group seeks together. Strategies for use of this kind of power are familiar to nurses. However, often they are not recognized as power because they contrast sharply with hierarchical power. They are not yet common modes of action in many groups. Chinn provided a contrast between the power of hierarchy and the power of solidarity. The power of hierarchy depends on a linear chain of command where multiple layers of responsibilities are subdivided into separate and discreet areas of responsibility. The power of solidarity shares the responsibility for decision making and for acting on those decisions in a lateral network of equals. It values deliberation and emphasizes the integration of differences in the group. Such power calls forth the fundamental values held by the whole group. Understanding these distinctions, nurses can assess behaviors related to shared identity processes in groups based on PEACE principles by evaluating group actions indicating values related to the use of power. These insights can be helpful in assessing behavior of any group.

BEHAVIORS OF FAMILY COHERENCE   The behavioral categories for assessing group identity can also be used for family coherence. In addition there is a rich literature on assessing families. Here we are focusing specifically on family coherence. Assessment of family coherence includes observations over time related to family unity. Table 18–1 lists some characteristics of family coherence and how to focus assessment of behavior about each one. It is important to note that the order and depth of assessment depends on the situation. How the nurse asks specific questions depends on the relationship to the family. The list provides a general guideline.

Assessment of Stimuli

The second level of assessment is identifying the influencing factors, or stimuli, related to group identity and family coherence. Knowing the factors influencing group identity is important in planning nursing care. When the nurse knows what is affecting the group, then she will be able to plan with the group to handle challenges. Based on a behavioral interaction model for studying groups (Rabbie & Lodewijkx, 1996), particular stimuli that affect shared identity of groups are selected for discussion. These include demands and distance, external social environment, and leadership and responsibility. As with assessment of the individual, the order in which the factors are assessed and the type of data collected will vary according to the type of group.

DEMANDS AND DISTANCE   Demands refer to the problems posed for a group to solve. Distance indicates whether or not the group has face-to-face interaction. Often a situation stimulates a group to form based on common interests in the situation. The intrusion of the profit motive in health care systems in the United States has led to creation of ad hoc groups of physicians and nurses concerned about the quality of care. The civil rights movement and the many groups working on this issue in the United States in the 1960s was a reaction to the

TABLE 18–1 Assessment of Family Coherence

Characteristics	Focus to Assess Family Behavior
Structure	Who are the family members? Who does chores such as housekeeping, shopping, repairs? How are child-rearing responsibilities divided? Which family members work outside the home? How is space allocated for being together and being alone?
Functions	How are day-to-day and larger decisions such as health care made by the family? What are the family short-term and long-term goals, for example, related to children, health care, and retirement? Is there flexibility in changing functions?
Relationships	How are love, respect, and loyalty shown? Do members find understanding, support, and companionship within the family group? Are the boundaries of the family as a group and boundaries between members clear? Are both individual needs and family needs honored? Does the family unite under stress?
Consistency	What history and traditions are important? What moral-ethical values do they share? What cultural beliefs are important?

reality of segregation, and the less apparent effects of pervasive racial prejudice and intolerance. The family constantly faces demands such as providing for basic needs for food, clothing, shelter, safety, and health care. Because of the nature of the family group, a challenge faced by one member is a demand upon all members. This can be as simple as a child having a history test the next day or as devastating as one person losing a job or receiving a medical diagnosis with uncertain outcomes.

Group action is often dependent on face-to-face interaction. For example, the PEACE groups described by Chinn (2008) are based generally on members being physically present with each other, at least some of the time. However, today video conferences and Internet communications are changing the definitions of group interactions. The distance between members of a group and how the group bridges that distance are important stimuli for shared identity. Chinn also has discussed the increasing effectiveness of groups who interact on the Internet. Other authors have shown that individuals in the same social category can coordinate their actions with one another in responding to external demands (Rabbie & Lodewijkx, 1996). The North American Jewish community acted as a group to support, financially and morally, the new country of Israel more than 50 years ago. Today many families in the United States face repeated deployments of one or more members in military service away from home and too often in harm's way. This is an unusual stress upon the family coherence.

EXTERNAL SOCIAL ENVIRONMENT The external social environment refers to the group's perception of changes in the behavior of other people or groups with whom the group interacts.

If a given department in the health care agency perceives that it is being targeted for budget cuts by the administration, this becomes a powerful external stimulus for the members of the department to strengthen their shared identity. The staff of the department will develop strategies to attain common perceptions of the situation and will share beliefs and feelings. Based on this interaction, they will develop shared goals and values.

In relation to the external social environment, Chinn (2008) addressed the challenges faced when introducing PEACE processes into existing groups within hierarchical institutions. The possibilities for transformation are great. Overcoming expectations for groups to function as usual can make the transition a challenge. Chinn suggested that a beginning can be made by the group introducing the change making a conscious commitment to a value that they freely choose. The group then chooses one PEACE process to focus on as a starting point. For example, the power of unity, referred to earlier, can be a constant focus whereby the group actively seeks to understand differing perspectives that each person brings. Allowing time for each person to speak often is in conflict with tightly scheduled agendas of meetings. However, gradually, members of the group can ask to hear what others think. Chinn noted that change may be slow and invisible and suggested that forming a group outside of the institution may be helpful in sustaining the efforts to create institutional change. Nurses are accustomed to working with opposing value structures, but sometimes are not as skilled at how to make changes. Chinn's work offers some alternatives.

Families are constantly interpreting changes in the reactions of others toward them. In a family with two parents of the same sex, a debate about gay marriage or child adoption will be an important influencing factor. The public discussion can stimulate changes in the reactions from people who know the family. This is an important time for family coherence.

LEADERSHIP AND RESPONSIBILITY   In the literature on group processes and structures, there is much discussion about how authority structures develop in groups. The effect these structures have on group behaviors also is explored. In assessing factors influencing group identity, then, the issue of authority is an important consideration. As noted, the goals and values determine the actions of the group. Attaining goals requires creating some division of labor. Even in the simple group action of holding a meeting, someone may secure the place to meet, another may send out notices, and someone else may volunteer to take minutes of the meeting. Some theorists of group processes note that, based on what people do in the group, positions emerge. Some positions relate directly to reaching goals. Other positions relate to coordinating the goal-directed activities of the others and thus become authority positions (Kimberly, 1997). The group sets limits on how much discretion the authority person has with respect to such activities as redefining the group goal, establishing norms, changing positions of people in the group, or allocating new members to positions. Authority operates differently based on the goals and values of the group, but the pattern of leadership and responsibility that emerges in a group clearly has an affect on the shared identity and family coherence.

In working with PEACE groups, as noted Chinn (2008) recommended rotating leadership and responsibility. The process of rotating leadership means more than having a different leader for each meeting. Chinn noted that the rotation process turns over to each member of the group the rights and responsibilities for leadership, tasks, and decisions. A convener may begin a meeting, but after that, whoever is speaking is the leader. The person who is speaking passes leadership simply by calling the name of the next person who indicates readiness to speak. During the discussion, each person makes notes of personal thoughts and ideas about what others are saying. The group listens carefully and allows people to complete their thoughts before indicating a desire to speak. The notes taken by each person facilitate the process of rotating leadership and are a personal tool to remain in touch with one's own thoughts while others are speaking. They can be a personal journal of experiences in the group. Based on the goals of the group, it may also be necessary to have at least one person record minutes of the meeting. A PEACE group at times rotates responsibilities to a task group. The group determines the responsibilities of the task group and provides direction that helps the task group accomplish its work in concert with the goals and values of the total group. The task group is then accountable to bring its work back to the larger group.

Families generally cohere over time and through different stages. The development of authority likely follows the pattern of the structure, functions, and relationships that have developed. However, sometimes there is an overt and a covert authority structure. As noted in the first-level assessment, it is important to know how decisions are made in the family. This process is likely influenced by how leadership and particularly authority are distributed. Assessing behavior and stimuli in groups is a skill that will increase as the nurse's knowledge and experience in understanding group process grows. There is significant literature in nursing and in related fields, particularly social psychology, organizational behavior, and family studies to facilitate this growth.

Nursing Diagnosis

When the nurse is working with a group, the members of the group are involved throughout the nursing process. With each member an active participant in each step of the nursing process, then meaningful involvement in carrying out the plan is more likely. A collaborative process makes it possible for the plan to be supported by the group in need. In this way the plan for achieving outcomes can be effective. Nursing diagnoses, according to the Roy Adaptation Model, uses two basic approaches. One method involves the statement of the behaviors together with the influencing stimuli. The second way to state a diagnosis is to use summary labels with the relevant stimuli. With both approaches, the diagnosis is based on a careful assessment of behaviors and stimuli. In assessing adaptation level in the group identity mode, stabilizer and innovator effectiveness are important. If the group system faces a challenge, are compensatory processes initiated that need to be strengthened? If compromised processes are present, this is the priority focus for nursing.

The summary labels for diagnostic categories for the group identity mode according to the Roy Adaptation Model are shown in Table 18–2 in relation to nursing diagnosis labels approved by the North American Nursing Diagnosis Association (NANDA International, 2007). Indicators of positive adaptation identified are effective interpersonal relationships, supportive milieu and culture, shared goals and values, shared expectations, expressing self in the context of others, values in action, understanding and support, shared leadership, positive morale, flexibility in functions, and unity in crisis. Commonly recurring adaptation problems for group identity include ineffective interpersonal relationships, values conflict, oppressive culture, low morale, out-group stereotyping, and abusive relationships.

We will return to the case study of Robles family first introduced in Chapter 4, and addressed in Chapter 14, to continue this discussion of the nursing process. Box 18–1 provides a brief history and update on the Robles family. This family has highly developed processes of family coherence based on their strong shared values and relationships as well as flexibility in meeting changing demands. However, recently the school nurse was asked by Sylvia's home teacher to visit the Robles family. The teacher reported to the nurse that Sylvia's grades are dropping and that she finds the child uncooperative when different

TABLE 18–2 Nursing Diagnostic Categories for Group Identity Mode

Indicators of Adaptation	Common Adaptation Problems	NANDA Diagnostic Labels
• Effective interpersonal relationships • Supportive milieu and culture • Shared goals and values • Shared expectations • Expressing self in the context of others • Values in action • Understanding and support • Shared leadership • Positive morale • Flexibility in functions • Unity in crisis	• Ineffective interpersonal relationships • Values conflict • Oppressive culture • Low morale • Out-group stereotyping • Abusive relationships	• Compromised family coping • Disabled family coping • Readiness for enhanced family coping • Risk for other-directed violence

BOX 18–1

History of the Robles Family

The family includes the parents, Mr. and Mrs. Robles, and their three children. The extended family closely involved includes the children's maternal grandmother and two cousins. The 2-year-old daughter, Sylvia, had a serious spinal cord injury in a motor vehicle accident and after a lengthy hospitalization was taken home on a ventilator. Anthony was 6 and Luca was 3 years old at that time. This Mexican American family has strong cultural commitment to the value of family. Mr. Robles earned a good income, and the family was able to handle the renovations on the house to accommodate the needs of the child with quadriplegia. About 6 months after Silvia came home, Mrs. Robles was feeling depressed because she did not feel that she was being a good mother to her sons. Changes were made in her hours of providing care for Sylvia so that she could give more attention to each child. This worked well and the extended family members were once again supportive rather than critical.

We rejoin the Robles family just before Sylvia's 12th birthday. Her brothers are now ages 16 and 13. The maternal grandmother has since died and one of the cousins was divorced and became less involved with the family. Physically Sylvia has done well, having only one hospitalization for pneumonia. She has learned the use of the computer controlled by eye movements and been able to keep up with her grades in school. Mrs. Robles is happy that she has been able to keep the family together though she still grieves the loss of her own mother. Mr. Robles still earns a good living, but turned down an opportunity for a higher paying position with another company. This was a family decision made primarily because a change in health insurance would be devastating since it would not cover the preexisting condition of Sylvia's neurologic condition.

teaching approaches are tried. On her visit to the home, the school nurse quickly notices that the family is facing another set of challenges. These are similar to those any family would face at this stage of development. However, the circumstances make the responses more difficult.

Mrs. Robles reports that she has difficulty getting Sylvia to focus on her homework; she just wants to play video games. Mrs. Robles is ambivalent about using firm discipline with Sylvia. She wants her to be as much like any other child as possible, yet sometimes she feels it may be better to let the child who is disabled do what she enjoys. Anthony is on the high school football team and Luca has just joined the marching band. They want their parents to attend more of their school events. The nurse talks with Sylvia for a few minutes and confirms her hunch that the preteen child is trying to assert her independence in the only way she can—by not doing her schoolwork. Mrs. Robles reports that in general everyone is feeling a little down. Her husband and the boys know that the teacher and Mrs. Robles are struggling with Sylvia, but they don't want to talk about it. The nurse suggests a family meeting. It takes some effort to coordinate everyone's schedule, but finally a time is set.

The nurse comes to the meeting with two tentative diagnoses for the family. The first is "shared values and goals based on strong ethnic heritage and group responsibility to maintain values and goals." The second is "low morale related to current conflicts in the children's developmental needs and a lessening of external support." As noted earlier, a major stimuli for groups is the demands they face, that is, the problems posed for them to solve. The current situation presents a problem to be addressed. In addition, the loss of the grandmother to the family is being felt by all and the withdrawal of the cousin lessens the total family support. The resulting lack of energy has inhibited the family's usual effective group decision-making. At the family meeting the nurse planned to confirm with the family her observations in the form of the nursing diagnoses. She hoped to move on to goal setting. However, she finds that the family really needs time for each one to express their thoughts and feelings. The nurse gives everyone the opportunity to talk and everyone contributes, including Sylvia. Luca is the least forthcoming and speaks only once and mutters a couple of times. By the end of the meeting the nurse has confirmed the first diagnosis but notes the need for restatement of shared goals and values. Everyone quickly confirmed her second diagnosis. After time for hearing from each person, the nurse feels she knows the family better as individuals and as a group. She sets up another family meeting to work on the next step in the process of planning care, which is goal setting.

Goal Setting

Throughout the nursing process the nurse focuses on behavior, the stimuli influencing that behavior, or both. With the nursing diagnosis, the statements developed included summaries of the behaviors and stimuli. With the goal-setting step, the focus is on the behavior. Each goal identifies behavior that is to be addressed. In the group identity mode the focus is on patterns of behavior. For the Robles family the first major pattern of behavior is the shared goals and values. They decide it would be important to restate their goals and values in the current situation and to expand these to shared expectations. The nurse helps them to state the behavior of focus, the change expected, and the time frame in which the goal is to be achieved. They set the goal "to have a written statement of goals, values, and expectations that takes into account the individual and family needs by the next meeting with the nurse in 2 weeks." Sylvia volunteers to be the secretary to type up the goals on her computer and Luca says he will be the editor. The second goal focuses on the low morale in the group. The Robles family sets the goal that they will use the project of restating their values, goals, and expectations to help each other feel better about working together to continue to grow as a group. The goal is stated as: family members will report that they feel encouraged about group efforts after 2 weeks. Before the nurse leaves, Mr. Robles volunteers the statement, "I feel better already now that you have helped us get back on track." The outcome of the first goal will be a written document, and for the second, a change in morale evidenced by statements of encouragement and particularly by sharing positive feelings.

Intervention

In the intervention step of the nursing process according to the Roy Adaptation Model, the nurse focuses on the stimuli affecting the behavior that is the focus of the goals. The management of stimuli is the focus of intervention. This involves altering, increasing, decreasing, removing, or maintaining the stimuli. At the same time, the nurse may help the group to use effective coping strategies to strengthen compensatory processes. A review of the stimuli affecting adaptive group processes for both adaptive diagnosis and adaptation problems helps to identify specific interventions to reach the goals. In the case of the Robles family it can help to achieve and maintain identity integrity for the family. Although she uses somewhat different words, the nurse frequently points out how good this family is at transcending crisis, a compensatory process. She is very authentic as she lets her own feelings of admiration and hope for the family show.

The goal of having a written statement of goals, values, and expectations has its own intervention and makes use of the family strengths. Each person puts out expectations for themselves and for the family. By having Sylvia as the secretary, then the focus of interaction is in one room of the house. This helps to keep everyone accountable and involved. Luca is constantly checking that only changes agreed upon are on the final list. For the second goal, the stimuli relate partly to the children's developmental needs. These are being clarified in the interventions for the first goal. The nurse pointed out the lessening of external support and encouraged the family to explore additional resources. Mrs. Robles decided to call her cousin whom she had not seen for awhile. Mr. Robles began to check on some long-term plans related to his job.

Evaluation

Evaluation is the final step of the nursing process and means looking at the effectiveness of the nursing interventions in relation to the group's adaptive behavior. The nurse judges whether the behaviors stated in the goals have been achieved. The nursing interventions are effective if the behavior is in agreement with the stated goal. If the goal has not been achieved, the nurse identifies alternative interventions or approaches. This involves repeating the assessment of the behavior and stimuli. Based on new data the other steps of the nursing process are continued.

When the nurse attends the next Robles family meeting, she finds that short-term goals have been met and that the family is now also thinking about long-term goals. They agree that it was fun to work on the revised list of goals, values, and expectations. They had trouble reaching consensus on expectations because some were in conflict. However, they agreed to leave all expectations on the list and to work toward finding ways to take two contradictory expectations into account. One such contradiction was that the boys expect that both parents attend the homecoming football game. At the same time, Sylvia expects that one parent would help her with her homework every night. The only problem Sylvia had with her homework in the past 2 weeks was having her leave the list alone and having quiet in her room when she needed to study. She had completely forgotten about the video games.

In regard to additional resources, there were two major developments. Mrs. Robles found out that her cousin's oldest daughter was preparing to get a second degree in nursing. She has a baccalaureate degree in sociology, but decided not to get a graduate degree in that field. Her mother talking a lot about Sylvia made her think about nursing, and she found a program for second-degree students. Currently she is taking prerequisite sciences courses at the community college. She is eager to learn about Sylvia's care and can provide respite care for Mrs. Robles. She also is excited to get to know her younger "girl cousin."

In addition, Mr. Robles had been in dialogue with his superiors at work for some time. He was cautious in raising the hopes of the family too soon. However, he checked in with them again and it seemed more certain that he would be getting a promotion. The promotion would involve an increasing amount of higher level administration and decrease his daily hands-on supervisory work. This offers the possibility for a more flexible schedule. Also, the new position involves stock options. He had been "running the numbers" and felt that the stock would mature at about the same rate as Sylvia. The whole family was excited about the possibility of a long-term plan for when Sylvia is an adult. Mr. Robles proposed that they will build Sylvia her own house on the same property where she could have her own hired caregiver. This is a way for her to be an independent adult. The nurse left with further admiration for the Robles family. Although they still had a great deal to face, they remained strong as a cohesive family system.

Summary

In this chapter we discussed the group identity mode. Two major processes for identity integrity of groups were identified and described, shared identity and family coherence. The compensatory processes of community cohesion and transcending crisis were explored. The examples of compromised processes that were described included low morale and out-group stereotyping. Although many more integrated, compensatory, and compromised processes are involved in group identity, the theoretical work completed at this time was explained. The nursing process was described beginning with outlining behaviors and stimuli relevant to assessment of group identity. The remaining steps of nursing diagnosis, goal setting, interventions, and evaluation, were illustrated by using the case study introduced earlier in the text.

Exercises for Application

1. Choose a group to which you belong and identify it in terms of shared relations, goals, and values; its social milieu and culture; group self-image; and co-responsibility for goal achievement.

2. Select one of the areas you described and identify the most relevant behaviors and stimuli you note for your group in that area.

Assessment of Understanding

1. The basic need underlying the group identity mode is _____. The subareas of the group identity mode are:
   (a) _____ and
   (b) _____ ,
   which exist within and create their own
   (1) _____ and (2) _____ .

2. Fill in the following table for assessment of behavior of group identity.

Areas of patterns to assess	Possible examples of group behavior
a. _____	a. 1. _____
	a. 2. _____
b. _____	b. 1. _____
	b. 2. _____
c. _____	c. 1. _____
	c. 2. _____

3. Fill in the following table for assessment of behavior of family coherence.

Characteristic	Two samples of focus for assessment
a. _____	a. 1. _____
	a. 2. _____
b. _____	b. 1. _____
	b. 2. _____
c. _____	c. 1. _____
	c. 2. _____
d. _____	d. 1. _____
	d. 2. _____

4. For each of the following stimuli for shared group identity, provide an example based on your understanding of each for any one group you select.
   (a) Demands and distance _____
   (b) External social environment _____
   (c) Leadership and responsibility _____

5. Which of the following could be considered compensatory processes related to group identity?
   (a) the tendency of people to select mates who have similar physical characteristics
   (b) coherence of immigrant groups
   (c) prolonged ambivalence about a decision
   (d) public outpouring during disasters
   (e) redefining the group and its membership

6. Identify one compromised process of group integrity related to each of the following components.
   (a) group self image _____
   (b) shared goals and values _____

FEEDBACK

1. identity integrity
   (a) group self image (b) shared goals, values, and responsibility (1) social milieu (2) culture
2. a. Common perceptions of group boundaries
   a. 1. Deciding to allow open group membership
   a. 2. Stratification of a workplace
2. b. Common thinking and feeling orientations
   b. 1. Identifying which orientations are important to the group
   b. 2. Cooperation among members
2. c. Shared goals and values
   c. 1. Shared identity   c. 2. Attaining goals
3. a. Solidarity
   a. 1. Loyal to other members
   a. 2. Sense of community
3. b. Boundaries
   b. 1. Ability to be in a relationship outside of the family
   b. 2. Respect for/from other family members

3. c.   History of coherence
c. 1. Exhibit honesty and freedom of expression
c. 2. Mutual respect between members
3. d.   Culture
d. 1. Worldview specific to group
d. 2. Reverence for beliefs of group
4. a.   Loss of funding for travel
b.   Budget cuts within a department

c.   A leader's inequitable distribution of responsibility and accountability
5. b, d, e
6. a.   ineffective interpersonal relations
b.   value conflict

References

Bowen, M. (1978). *Family therapy in clinical practice.* New York: Aronson.

Brehm, S. S., & Kassin, S. M. (1996). *Social psychology* (3rd ed.). Boston: Houghton Mifflin.

Brown, R., & Capozza, D. (Eds.). (2000). *Social identity processes: Trends in theory and research.* Thousand Oaks, CA: Sage Publications.

Caplan, G., & Caplan, R. (1993). *Mental health consultation and collaboration.* San Francisco: Jossey-Bass.

Chinn, P. L. (2008). *Peace and power: Creative leadership for building community* (7th ed.). Sudbury, MA: Jones and Bartlett.

Derber, C. (2004). *The wilding of America: Money, mayhem, and the new American dream* (3rd ed.). New York: Worth.

Dovidio, J. F., & Gaertner, S. L. (Eds.). (1986). *Prejudice, discrimination, and racism: Theory and research.* Orlando, FL: Academic Press.

Eagly, A. H. (1987). *Sex differences in social behavior: A social-role interpretation.* Hillsdale, NJ: Erlbaum.

Fiske, A. P. (1991). *The structures of social life.* New York: Free Press.

Fiske, S. T., & Neuberg, S. L. (1990). A continuum of impression formation from category-based to individuating processes: Influences of information and motivation on attention and interpretation. In M. P. Zanna (Ed.), *Advances in experimental social psychology* (pp. 1–74). New York: Academic Press.

Hanson, J. (1984). The family. In C. Roy (Ed.). *Introduction to nursing: An adaptation model* (pp. 519–533). Englewood Cliffs, NJ: Prentice-Hall.

Hass, R. G., Katz, I., Rizzo, N., Bailey, J., & Moore, L. (1992). When racial ambivalence evokes negative affect, using a disguised measure of mood. *Personality and Social Psychology Bulletin, 18,* 786–797.

Kimberly, J. C. (1997). *Group processes and structures: A theoretical integration.* Lanham, MD: University Press of America.

Lewin, K. (1948). *Resolving social conflicts.* New York: Harper & Row.

NANDA International. (2007). *Nursing diagnoses: Definitions & classification, 2007–2008.* Philadelphia: NANDA I.

Pender, N. J., Murdaugh, C. L., & Parsons, M. A. (2002). *Health promotion in nursing practice* (4th ed.). Upper Saddle River, NJ: Prentice-Hall.

Perry, D. J., & Gregory, K. E. (2007). Global applications of the cosmic imperative for nursing knowledge development. In C. A. Roy & D. A. Jones (Eds.), *Nursing knowledge development and clinical practice* (pp. 315–326). New York: Springer.

Rabbie, J. M., & Lodewijkx, H. F. M. (1996). A behavioral interaction model: Toward an integrative theoretical framework for studying intra- and intergroups dynamics. In E. Witte & J. H. Davis (Eds.), *Understanding group behavior: Small group processes and interpersonal relations* (Vol. 2, pp. 255–294). Mahwah, NJ: Erlbaum.

Roy, C. (1983). Roy Adaptation Model and application to the expectant family and the family in primary care. In J. Clements & F. Roberts (Eds), *Family health: A theoretical approach to nursing care* (pp. 255–278, 298–304, 375–378). New York: John Wiley and Sons.

Roy, C. (1984). The Roy Adaptation Model in nursing: Applications in community health nursing. In M. K. Asay & C. C. Assler (Eds.), *Proceedings of the eighth annual community nursing conference.* Chapel Hill, NC: University of North Carolina.

Roy, C., & Anway, J. (1989). Roy's Adaptation Model: Theories and propositions for administration. In B. Henry, C. Arndt, M. DiVicenti, & G. Marriner-Tomey (Eds.), *Dimensions and issues of nursing administration*. St. Louis, MO: The C. V. Mosby Co.

Satir, V. (1991). *The Satir model: Family therapy and beyond*. Palo Alto, CA: Science and Behavior Books.

Singer, P. (2002). *One world: The ethics of globalization* (2nd ed.). New Haven, CT: Yale University Press.

Stangor, C., & Lange, J. (1994). Mental representations of social groups: Advances in understanding stereotypes and stereotyping. *Advances in Experimental Social Psychology, 26*, 357–416.

Tajfel, H., & Turner, J. (1979). An integrative theory of intergroup conflict. In W. G. Austin & S. Worchel (Eds.), *The social psychology of intergroup relations* (pp. 33–47). Monterey, CA: Brooks/Cole.

Tolstoy, L. (1961). Anna Karenina. (D. Margarshack, Trans.) New York: New American Library. (Original work published between 1873–1877.)

Tuckman, B. W. (1965). Developmental sequences in small groups. *Psychological Bulletin, 63*, 384–399.

UNICEF's The State of the World's Children. (2001). Retrieved January 22, 2008, from http://www.unicef.org/sowc02/

U.S. Department of Health and Human Services (USDHHS). (2000). *Healthy people 2010* (2nd ed.). Washington, DC: U.S. Government Printing Office.

Worchel, S. (1996). Emphasizing the social nature of groups in a developmental framework. In J. L. Nye & A. M. Brower (Eds.), *What's social about social cognition? Research on socially shared cognition in small groups* (pp. 261–281). Thousand Oaks, CA: Sage Publishing.

CHAPTER 19

Role Function Mode
of Relating Persons

The third adaptive mode on the group level is referred to as the role function mode of relating persons. Individuals hold roles, but at the same time within any group, people relate through the various roles they hold. These roles are reciprocal, that is, there is mutual exchange between and among individuals in joint roles. It is the integrating of all of the roles in the group that determines the adaptation level of the group. This chapter focuses specifically on the third adaptive mode for groups, the role function mode for relating individuals. We understand groups as relating individuals in systems such as families, people who form a group for a particular purpose, local communities, networks of people with common goals, structured workgroups, organizations, nations and the global community. This view includes, for example, a health care agency in which many people hold differing, but mutually interacting, roles.

As noted in Chapter 15, roles are considered the functioning units of society and each role exists in relation to another. In groups, roles may be assigned or they may be assumed by an individual group member. Role clarity is the basic need of the role function adaptive mode on the group level. When the nurse is dealing with groups it is particularly important to be aware of the formal role structure and the informal role structure as well. Role function for groups, as for individuals, is learned through socialization and affected by factors such as gender, age, and social status.

This chapter describes an overview of the role function mode for interacting individuals. For the group the basic role function processes include clarifying expectations, reciprocating roles, and integrating roles. These are the processes by which role clarity is reached and the group reaches an integrated level of adaptation. Compensatory adaptive processes related to group role function also are explored. The examples of compromised processes for group role function that are discussed include interrole conflict and caregiver role strain. The section on planning of nursing care includes guidelines and examples of nursing assessment of behaviors and stimuli, formulating diagnoses, establishing goals, selecting nursing interventions, and evaluating care.

OBJECTIVES

After studying this chapter, the reader will be able to do the following:

1. Describe the processes of the role function mode for the group according to the Roy Adaptation Model.

2. Describe one compensatory process related to group role function.

3. Identify and describe two situations of compromised processes of group role function.

4. List important first-level assessment behaviors for group role function.

5. Identify second-level assessment factors or stimuli that influence the group role function.

6. Formulate nursing diagnoses related to group role function.

7. Establish goals related to given diagnoses in group role function.

8. Select nursing interventions to promote adaptation for the role function mode of groups.

9. Propose approaches to determine the effectiveness of nursing interventions for group role function.

KEY CONCEPTS DEFINED

Role clarity: The basic need for role function at the group level that depends on socialization to clarify role expectations.

Role expectations: Beliefs held by society in general, by an individual, or by those in complementary roles, about what is appropriate behavior associated with a role.

Role function for groups: Focuses on the series of actions of how the goals of the group system are accomplished; a structure of expectations developed formally or informally for what members will do to accomplish the functions of the group.

Role integration: The process of handling different roles of all of the members so that the functions of the group can be carried out; provides for regulating responsibilities and expectations between individuals in complementary roles and among all members of the group.

Role reciprocity: Involves individuals in different roles in mutual exchange, with give and take that influences the other; there is a high mutual dependence in the division of labor; helps to maintain the coherence or unity of the group.

Role set: The total number of roles an individual holds at a given time.

Role-taking: A process of looking at or anticipating one individual's behavior by viewing it within a role attributed to another; basing one's interaction on the judgment about the other's role; focuses on the meaning that the acts have for both individuals in a role interaction.

Socialization: In a broad sense, the process by which children are transformed into members of society; in particular, the process of learning role expectations in any group.

PROCESSES OF ROLE FUNCTION FOR RELATING PERSONS

An understanding of the role function adaptive mode at the group level is based on knowledge of role function on the individual level. Roles are positions in society that have certain expectations for behavior towards individuals in complementary roles. The example commonly given is that the parents are expected to love and to provide for children. Children respond by appreciating what the parents do and loving them in return. As adaptive systems, individuals strive to know who they are in relation to others so that they can act accordingly. The role function mode for individuals and for groups provides knowledge of how people interact within society. The philosophical assumptions of the Roy Adaptation Model described in Chapter 2 emphasize the common purpose and meaning for human existence within the universe. Relationships of people are integral to adaptation and to health. Role relationships in groups are a particular way of understanding how people relate and how groups of people can be effective as adaptive systems. Group identity was discussed in Chapter 18 and includes the group's self-image and shared responsibility. However, it is through the roles occupied in the groups that the work of accomplishing the purposes of the group takes place. Figure 19–1 identifies the theoretical basis for the role function mode of groups.

As the multiple roles in any group are played out by all the group members, many processes are involved. Processes involve series of activities that proceed from one to the next. The role function mode for the group focuses on the series of actions of how the goals of the group system are actually accomplished. The group either formally or informally sets up a structure of expectations for what the various members will do to accomplish the functions of the group. Some general functions relate to how the work is divided up, how information is managed, how decisions are made and how order is maintained. For example, in a health care agency, different people have responsibility for the many tasks involved in delivering patient care. Within the nursing group certain people are responsible for management activities such as hiring and performance evaluation. We noted that families have structures and relationships. In the last chapter the focus was on family coherence as an example of the integrated adaptive process of group identity. This coherence is manifested by a state of unity and connection among family members. When we move from group identity to group role function, for the family we are more focused on the structure of how tasks are accomplished.

For the family these tasks include earning a living, child care, communication, decision making, and promoting growth, as well as limit setting. We can also consider the roles that nations play in the global community. Tasks will involve challenges such as interrelating and

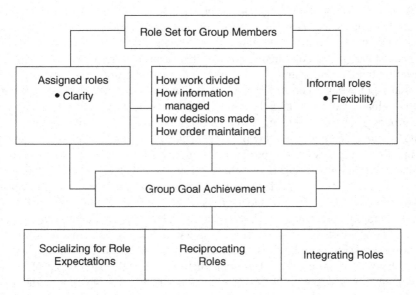

FIGURE 19–1   Role Function Mode for groups. Theoretical basis.

sustaining economies, languages, and cultures; structures for communicating and assuring shared needs such as the global environment and nation-specific needs such as given health issues; and forums for settling differences and ensuring global human rights. Regardless of the group, its size, and purpose, important processes are socialization for role expectations, reciprocating roles, and integrating roles.

Basic Process of Socializing for Role Expectations

In a broad sense socialization begins with the process by which children are transformed into members of society. This includes learning the values, standards, habits, skills, and roles appropriate to sex, social class, and ethnic group of the particular society where they are expected to be a responsible and productive member (Murray & Zentner, 2001). Socialization continues throughout one's lifetime. As social settings change, the individual gains the knowledge, skills, attitudes, values, needs, motivations, and thinking and feeling patterns that relate to that setting. The socialization process is successful if the individual can perform the roles he or she attempts. This involves being able to respond to rapid social change and many different life tasks as one grows older. Socialization in particular, then, is the process of learning role expectations in any group.

In looking at theories of roles in Chapter 15, the structural approach and the interactional approach were discussed. These are illustrated in Figure 15–1 and reviewed here briefly. Structural role theories are based on structural–functional approaches to society, look at the broad perspective of people within positions in society, and are associated with social status. For this reason, they are relatively fixed. People use learning processes to know what is expected for a given role. This learning may involve such approaches as instruction, observation, imitation, and trial and error. Interactional approaches to role theory are based upon symbolic interaction. In this case socialization takes place through an individual taking the role of the other. That is, the individual "stands in the shoes" of the other to figure out how to act. Interactional approaches look at ways people interpret what is happening in a role interaction.

The introductory section on group adaptive modes noted that groups include relating individuals who influence each other by direct interaction. However, the Roy Adaptation Model advances the notion that at the same time groups include the larger structures of society such as nations and global communities. It may be easier to learn about role function on the group level by thinking of groups of people that interact with each other. We can then show how the same processes relate to larger systems. The reader is asked to consider groups to which you belong. This may include family, and for students and faculty, there are many campus groups such as clubs and organizations, sports teams, and given committees. Similarly, for nurses in various nursing positions, you will belong to some of the same types of groups and also to other work and professional groups. By the roles you hold in the groups, you influence each individual and they influence you.

Role clarity, the basic need for role function at the group level, is dependent upon the socialization process. The basic element of socialization is clarifying role expectations. As noted, expectations are learned through approaches such as instruction, observation, imitation, and trial and error. Most roles involve some instruction. For example, instruction in the skills of new baby care such as bathing, feeding, and safety are included in nursing care for new mothers. Other roles require a great deal of instruction. This is the case with professional roles such as nursing or law. A period of formal education is required along with guided practice of the role. Many professionals in senior and teaching positions provide the role models for new members of the profession. Their behavior is observed and then imitated by the individual taking on the role behavior of a professional in that field. To take on her role, the developing nurse learns knowledge and skills. At the same time she also learns attitudes, values, needs, motivations, and thinking and feeling patterns expected for the role of nurse.

ROLE MODELS   Three approaches for clarifying role expectations for either new nurses or nurses changing positions include role models, preceptors, and mentors (Marquis & Huston, 2006). Anyone can be a role model. The role model serves as an example of someone who is experienced and competent in performing the role. For many nurses, their first significant role models are their clinical instructors. Others have had family members who are nurses that they admire and want to imitate. Marquis and Huston pointed out that the role model is a passive position for the expert individual. Beginning nurses see the role model's skilled behavior and attempt to make their behavior like what they see. However, the role model generally is not appointed to carry out this function and does not seek the emulation. Other authors noted that on the part of the individual learning the role, the process is more active (Markman et al., 2007). Besides general attempts to imitate, comparisons are being made by using mental simulation with thoughts such as "Could I ever be as good as her?" or "What would it be like to be a nurse like her?" Marquis and Huston also noted that role models have a cumulative effect. The greater the number of excellent role models available for the developing nurse to observe, the greater the possibilities for new nurses to perform well. Some significant research on excellence in hospitals has demonstrated this effect (Kramer & Schmalenberg, 1988).

PRECEPTORS   Preceptors are those who socialize into role expectations from an assigned complementary role that is active and purposeful. Assigning preceptors for student nurses in their advanced clinical placements has increased in nursing education over the past 30 years. This experience allows students to work with clinical experts in specific settings while still being guided by a faculty member. The main focus of an assigned clinical preceptor is to provide socialization into the role of the professional nurse, including the independent clinical judgment required. The preceptor combines the educator and role model functions. The preceptor is a resource individual and is immediately available to the student in the clinical setting. Lambert and Lambert (2001) noted in particular that "working alongside a preceptor allows the student to (1) observe and acquire knowledge about the role, (2) work in an environment where the demands of the role can be carried out, and (3) be in a climate that fosters motivation to meet the demands of the role" (p. 243). The careful selection of preceptors is of utmost importance. Likewise, a successful experience depends on the clarification of role expectations for each individual in this situation, the preceptor, the student, and the faculty.

Similarly, new nurses in their first positions after graduation, or nurses who are changing positions, often are assigned a preceptor. Through teaching and role modeling, the preceptor in practice has an important function to socialize the new nurse by clarifying role expectations. In addition, the experienced nurse provides emotional support. Sometimes the learning is complex and the new nurse may not succeed in first attempts. The preceptor provides support and reinforcement once the skill or approach is learned. Marquis and Huston (2006) pointed out that a preceptor can influence the maintenance of new learning through rewards and benefits on the job. Through the process of continual reinforcement of the new behaviors, attitudes and values are internalized. One research study of the transition from student to qualified nurse recommended that both preceptors and managers who work with new nurses acknowledge the stressful transition and support nurses through the process (Gerrish, 2000).

MENTORS Mentors are a third approach to socializing for role expectation. The origin of the term mentor comes from Homer's (1999) *Odyssey.* The story tells how Odysseus, the king of a small Greek island, had one son, Telemachus. When his son was an infant, Odysseus left to fight in the Trojan War. Before he left, Odysseus appointed Mentor, an old and trusted friend, to tutor Telemachus. Even though in 1978, Shapiro and colleagues called for clarification of concepts related to mentoring, multiple meanings have prevailed. The term varies in definition based on the scope and setting for which it applies. Snelson and colleagues (2002) stated that "the use of mentoring in many areas of nursing has been documented in the nursing literature such as the development of clinical practitioners, researchers and educators" (p. 655).

As early as 1977 Vance identified the classic mentor-protégé relationship as one in which an older, more experienced individual guides and supports a younger, less experienced individual. In her study of nurse leaders, Vance found that the mentoring relationship can include a combination of behaviors and roles that enhance both the professional and personal development of the protégé. Role modeling is used as it is by preceptor or faculty so that the mentor enhances the learning of the protégé. The difference is that this is done within the context of an ongoing relationship. Vance (1982) noted that a mentor serves many roles including model, guide, teacher, tutor, coach, confidant, and visionary-idealist. Roy, Murphy, and Eisenhauer (2003) noted that the role of mentoring is a complex process and requires multiple skills and abilities. It is a key process in the development and socialization, particularly of nursing scholars. Mentors can acquire the skills needed by understanding the process, and these skills and abilities can be improved with practice and patience.

In addition to being older with more experience and skill, the mentor is an individual with innate qualities of wisdom and faithfulness (Fields, 1991). A definition of a mentor synthesized from the literature is "Mentoring is viewed as a long term adult developmental process with active involvement in a close personal relationship. Mentors can serve as counselors, teachers, sponsors, and guides for neophytes learning about their professions and how to cope with dynamic workplace realities" (Prestholdt, 1990, p. 26). Within different contexts and the roles held by the mentor and the protégé, what is important is that mentoring is as effective and transformative as possible for socializing into role expectations, particularly in a profession such as nursing. Finding a mentor is important to developing professionals. However, this is a mutual relationship that develops over time and not a role relationship that can be assigned.

Socialization into role expectations takes place in broader level groups. When we consider the roles that nations play in the global community, we can also note that this happens in ways that are similar in face-to-face groups. In the time of the great monarchies, kings and queens certainly learned from each other about how to play their regal roles. Members of one generation were role models for the next. In Europe in particular, close relationships among royal families were part of transnational role development for royal leaders. In the current global society of established and developing democracies, clarifying expectations take place by public statements that nations can agree upon. One example is The Universal Declaration of Human Rights (United Nations Department of Public Information, 2007). This agreement includes the basic assertion that all human beings are born free and equal regardless of race, color, sex, religion, politics, or status. The World Health Organization also sets out expectations for action across the globe (WHO Europe, 2005).

However, it is what countries do, rather than what they say, that leads to clarifying expectations. A country models human rights by actions to provide rights to their citizens. The members of the government make obvious to other nations the specific approaches they use consistently to fulfill the expectations of securing and protecting the human rights of all people. One scholar has described the phenomenon of globalization creating a new politics (Derber, 2003). In the United States dissent movements have helped to realize the expectations for human rights. Three waves of change started with the landmark civil rights and antiwar movements in the 1960s. The universal values of peace and justice were taken seriously and the consciousness of a whole generation was transformed. This helped to end legal segregation in the Southern states and the Vietnam War. The second wave in the 1970s involved women, minorities, and gays. These people developed what Derber described as an acute consciousness of their own separate identities. Being victimized in the first wave provided the energy for these communities to build their own freedom movements. These groups remained relatively isolated from each other in the efforts to establish their own identity. The attaining of equal human rights of these groups was limited. This seemed to be related to the politics of globalization of the 1980s in which corporate power over the country and world at large was consolidated.

Derber (2003) wrote that the third wave was the first movement to explicitly organize a challenge to how globalization was emerging. It envisioned an alternative to a corporate-dominated world system. People involved in this wave think globally about markets, democracy, and social justice. Also they are linking global and local politics. They are organized in ways that have not been used before but are necessary to sustain cooperation among thousands of different groups and communities both in the United States and around the globe. Because of members worldwide, there is a need to take into account many issues and points of view. To quote the author, "They all believe that human need should trump money and that we need new rules putting jobs, health, and human rights over property rights" (p. 106). The organizational model described is called "the network." Groups all over the world communicate on a continuing basis, and as Derber pointed out, they are not just planning trade-summit protests. People from labor, environmental groups, and Third World countries are logging on to each other's listservs. They learn about each other's issues and build dialogue. This type of process is another way that socialization of role expectations within society, that is, across nations, takes place.

Basic Process of Reciprocating Roles

In describing roles in Chapter 15, we noted that each role of the individual exists in relationship to another role. One role corresponds to another; the role of one individual is complementary to the role of another. Common examples are the parent role relates to a child; the teacher role relates to a student; and the employer role, to an employee. When we describe role function in groups, we consider how all of the interrelated roles of people in a group act to establish group role clarity. This clarity makes possible the activities to accomplish the goals of the group. Role reciprocity, then, is the second basic process of integrated adaptation for the role function adaptive mode for groups.

Reciprocating roles involves individuals in different roles in mutual exchange. There is give and take; one influences the other. The sharing from one role to the other affects decision making in the group. In addition, the group maintains coherence or unity by way of reciprocating roles. When roles are reciprocated, the needs of the group and of individuals are met. Groups with reciprocating roles have a high mutual dependence in the division of labor. Further, reciprocating roles result in potential for growth for individuals and for the group. With each individual in a given role acting in relation to the other, common commitments develop and are maintained. It is also through the mutuality of roles that conflict is reduced.

A good example to understand the process of reciprocating roles is to consider a nurse accepting a management position. One author describes that the new nurse manager position will have at least three roles. The roles include leader, manager, and follower (Gray, 2003). Each of these roles is complex because they reciprocate with many other roles held by unique individuals all acting in a rapidly changing environment. Gray created a table to show this complex of interactions and the processes involved (Table 19–1). In her leader role, the new nurse manager has reciprocal roles with all the individuals whom she leads as well as her peers in other management positions. As you look at the processes involved, you can see the reciprocity involved with other roles. When the leader is listening, there is someone talking. Perhaps a nurse from her unit is explaining a family situation that provides a rationale for why she needs a given day off. If the leader is motivating the staff members with whom she works, she is constantly checking to see how each one and the group as a whole are reacting. The interaction is mutual and reciprocal. The nurse manager is also interacting with her peers to check on strategies they have found useful in motivating staff.

In the assigned role of manager, the number of individuals with whom the nurse interacts and the complexity of the reciprocal roles increases. The manager may have a large number of staff on assigned units whom she is responsible to supervise. The group includes staff in varying roles with different backgrounds, including education and experience. For example, a patient care unit may include a number of clerical staff, some of whom learned on the job and others who had a short course following high school. There may be nursing assistants who received certification in 6-month programs. Perhaps other nursing assistants

TABLE 19–1 Leader, Manager, and Follower Roles: People With Whom You Interact and Processes Involved in Each Role

Role	People with Whom Interactions Occur	Processes Involved in the Role
• Leader	• Persons being led • Peers	• Listening • Encouraging • Motivating • Organizing • Problem solving • Developing • Supporting
• Manager	• Persons being supervised • Administrators • Supervisors • Regulating agencies	• Organizing • Budgeting • Hiring • Evaluating • Reporting • Disseminating
• Follower	• Supervisor • Peers	• Conforming • Implementing • Contributing • Complementing assignments

Source: Gray, J. J. (2003). Role transition. In P. S. Yoder-Wise (Ed.), *Leading and managing in nursing* (3rd ed.). St. Louis, MO: Mosby. (p. 401) Used with permission.

have higher degrees in nursing or other fields from other countries, but do not hold RN licensure. The unit will likely include RNs with associate, diploma, baccalaureate, and masters' preparation. The experience of RNs on a unit can vary as much as 2 months to 40 years. One can see that the nurse manager will be mutually interacting with people in all these roles in her role responsibilities such as organizing and evaluating.

Since the unit or units that the nurse manager is responsible for are a group embedded in the larger group of the agency, the manager has several other groups with whom she interacts. As she is interacting with all those on her units, the manager also interacts with administrators and supervisors above her in the organizational structure. Each individual in these reciprocal roles will affect all of her responsibilities, but one can think particularly of budgeting and reporting processes. The health care agency exists within the larger society. Representatives of regulating agencies play reciprocal roles with the nurse manager. In particular these include evaluating and reporting.

Gray (2003) pointed out that the manager also is in a follower role and relates from this position to a supervisor and to peers in parallel positions. Perhaps she knows other nurses who are now in management positions in other agencies who also provide a peer group for her. The nurse manager is reciprocating when she is conforming to supervisor expectations and implementing policies. She may also use the process of negotiating to mutually set expectations. The new nurse manager plays a reciprocating role with her peers when she contributes to a project that the nurse manager group undertakes. They work mutually to complete the assignment.

This one example of a given nurse in one position, describing three particular roles, clearly demonstrates the process of reciprocating roles. At the same time it shows how complex the network of reciprocating roles can be in any group. This is true of the reciprocating roles of families, communities, and societies on national and global levels. You can also see how the effectiveness of the group is closely tied to the reciprocity of roles. The success of the group in meeting goals depends on each individual carrying out responsibilities attached to each role. A highly successful professional football coach is known to have continuously told each team member, "Just do your job." Each job was reciprocal with others. When the quarterback threw the football, a receiver had to catch it. This was only possible if both the quarterback and receiver were protected by their players blocking the opposing team efforts to stop the play. With each player carrying out the responsibilities of his assigned position, the team accomplished the group goal of a winning season.

Considering role reciprocity of nations in the global community, one organization is promoting that the reciprocal interaction be based on cooperation [Global Cooperation for a Better World (GCBW) Global Vision Statement, 2008]. One effort of the group was to redefine human progress. For the latter years of the last century, human progress meant progress for some at the expense of others (de Carteret, 1992). Examples included progress in the fields of science, technology, and industry at the expense of the environment and the human spirit. The group identified that one urgent task for the global community was to create a new goal or vision for human progress. The new goal is beneficial to the whole world and can ensure the full development of all individuals. The group implemented a process of change based on an ethic of cooperation to stimulate and strengthen the appropriate social, human, moral, and spiritual values to underscore the vision and make it a reality. With the belief that human progress such as this requires a collective will, they focused on the method to create the vision as much as the need to do it.

The approach was developed to stimulate change from the bottom up. Global cooperation was sought to provide a framework for learning in which positive attitudes and values were rediscovered. To generate cooperation is an ideal, it requires understanding of the dynamics and skill of cooperation. The group coordinator (de Carteret, 1992) noted that the first principle of cooperation is to work towards an aim that is common to all and for the benefit of all. The values required include respect, tolerance, understanding, responsibility, honesty, integrity, and generosity. de Carteret stated that, "The biggest hurdle facing the world in coming together as a global community is a lack of ability to respect our differences while perceiving our commonalities." What the author identifies as needed is similar to th philosophical assumptions of the Roy Adaptation Model. The assumptions speak of a common purposefulness of all people as well as the belief that the development of the Roy Adaptation Model takes place within given cultural perspectives. The process of cooperation helps us to see the reality of our interdependent world. Using principles of cooperation, everyone participates; the approach is multidisciplinary. Current problems are set aside and participants are asked to share their visions of the ideal. The author noted that cooperative approaches can be used in all levels of reciprocal groups—in schools, universities, businesses, community groups, among nongovernmental organizations, and at government levels.

The Global Cooperation for a Better World group carried out a project to create the document *Visions of a Better World* (GCBW, 2008). The project was supported by 400 companies worldwide and involved tens of thousands of people. The visions, hopes, and aspirations of a vast cross section of individuals from 129 countries were collected. People were asked to respond in words or pictures to the question: "What is your vision of a better world?" The only rule was that responses could be made in positive terms only. A team of project coordinators from all regions of the world synthesized the material collected. They found that despite the uniqueness of personal values and statements, there was a commonality of ideals and values that provided unity across boundaries of nationality, race, and creed. A summary of the 12 main points of the vision statement is provided in Box 19–1. This example of reciprocating roles on a global level shows how this action can enhance health and adaptation for all.

Basic Process of Integrating Roles

As noted in Chapter 15, each individual has many roles that create a role set for the individual. Each role within the set has given expectations coming from self, others, and society. As we saw in the example of a new nurse manager, in her work role alone she has at least three separate roles and each role has sets of interactions. The individual is often confronted with the need to articulate roles and expectations from many groups. Similarly, all of the roles within a group as a whole will be integrated for the group to reach goals and be at an integrated level of adaptation. For groups the differentiation of roles requires that members of the group clarify and articulate their role expectations and behaviors. The differing roles are integrated to meet group goals. At the group level, integrating roles is the process of handling different roles of all of the members so that the functions of the group can be carried out. Integrating roles provides for regulating responsibilities and expectations between individuals in complementary roles and among all members of the group.

Roy and Roberts (1981) noted the early work by Merton that described six social processes for integrating role sets for the individual. These approaches can be reinterpreted to apply to the process of integrating roles for the group. First, the individual evaluates the relative importance of various statuses. For example, an individual knows that family and job obligations have priority over voluntary organizations. In most groups there are some roles that are more crucial than others. In the process of integrating roles, the group will clarify the crucial functions. The group members will adjust to carrying out all crucial functions. A simple example is that if a committee is to meet and the chair who has the agenda is absent, the group functioning is definitely slowed down. On the other hand, if the secretary is absent

BOX 19–1

Vision Points of the Global Cooperation for a Better World

In a better world:

1. All people celebrate the joy of life.
2. Human rights are respected and upheld and the dignity and integrity of all people is assured.
3. People live in ways that preserve nature's ecological balance in an environment that is beautiful and clean.
4. The planet's natural and abundant resources are shared equitably and the basic human needs of all people are provided for.
5. All people have equal opportunities to realize their potential through an educational process that has human, moral, and spiritual values at its heart.
6. Life within the immediate family is loving, caring, and fulfilling and is the foundation for harmony within the broader human family.
7. There is respect, understanding, and tolerance in all human relations.
8. People communicate openly and in a spirit of equality and goodwill.
9. Social, economic, and political justice is ensured through honesty, responsibility, and respect for the rule of the law.
10. Governments, as representatives of their people, are committed to their well-being. People participate cooperatively in efforts for a secure and peaceful world.
11. Science serves humanity and appropriate technology is applied to ensure sustainable development and enhance the quality of life.
12. All people enjoy freedom of expression, movement, and belief while respecting the liberties and rights of others.

Brahma Kumaris World Spiritual University. As seen on http://www.bkun.org/socdev/wit7.html. Used with permission.

the group may feel that the reading of the minutes of the last meeting can wait until the next meeting. In a family with integrated roles, all crucial functions are being fulfilled. One parent is willing to limit professional goals and work less to be the major child caregiver for a time. Since the goals of the family include individual and group growth, the family members may then switch roles. The other parent will limit work and provide more child care for a given period of time.

Second, Merton noted that the power differences of those in the role set gives the individual a larger measure of autonomy. For example, if two members of the role set have competing power to impose their will, the individual may choose to whom he or she will respond. Power issues in groups can be centered in the formal and informal structures or in the changing of leadership. Chinn's (2008) approach to power in groups to build communities was discussed in Chapter 16 in relation to group identity. Chinn recommended that groups rotate leadership and responsibility. In this approach the formal structures are minimized while all group members are given the equal opportunity to participate regardless of any informal structures that develop. The purpose is to reverse the familiar structure with a linear chain of command. In the old structure a single individual or elite group manages the group and assumes leadership and control. The author described instead a group convener who facilitates announcements, focuses the discussion, and provides leadership for the process. However, whoever is speaking is considered the chair; others listen and do not interrupt.

When someone indicates a desire to speak and has not already spoken, or not recently, then the chair is passed to that individual. This is done by using the individual's name as a way of honoring the individuality of group members. One of the benefits of rotating leadership is that everyone acquires skills of leadership and critical reflection.

The third approach Merton discussed is the situation of the insulation of role activities from being observed by members of the role set. If one's activities in another role are not known to a member of one's role set, then the individual is less subject to competing pressures. Mothers may not discuss at work the time they spend helping a child work on homework or a weekend volunteering for a church function with family. For a group it may be possible to insulate their activities from other groups in the role tree of the members. Rules about conflicts of interest come into play here. For example, if a group of researchers is seeking investors for products that may emerge from their research, it is prudent to have the two groups function separately without overlapping members. If a member of the research group wants to be an investor, professional ethics requires that the exact nature of the investment be disclosed. In this way it is possible for the public to judge whether or not the roles within the two groups have been properly integrated. Improper influence in either direction is to be avoided. Investors cannot bring pressure on the researchers to make findings favorable to the business. At the same time the researchers will not provide information links to the investors that affect their behavior in ways that are unethical or illegal.

Fourth, being able to observe conflicting demands by members of the role set may serve to integrate the roles. When contradictions are plain, it becomes the task of members of the role set to resolve the contradictions. Compromise is usually the result. The same approach can be used in groups. A simple example is that the nurse manager may be asking the staff to have a problem-solving session on the unit. However, the administrative group has already scheduled a mandatory continuing education program at that time. When both groups observe the conflicting schedules, a compromise can be reached. Merton's next consideration is that there is mutual social support among status occupants. Individuals in certain statuses form supportive associations, for example, parents of teenagers who are in drug rehabilitation programs. This is the way that the individual receives support for integrating role demands. At the same time, different groups provide support for each other. Women's groups have supported gay groups in efforts for equal rights. In situations of chronic understaffing, nurses as a group may seek both social support and collaboration with patient groups and groups of other health professionals.

Lastly, Merton said that one may delete roles from one's role set. This was discussed earlier in considering the compromised process of role failure for the individual. The individual can drop a role that is not succeeding and also may choose to break off a given role relation. This can be to leave greater consensus among role expectations of the remaining role set. Similarly a group may decide that it can better integrate its roles and expectations if it deletes some of its goals. As an example, a group that has served primarily as a patient advocate group may have become more involved in political action. The multiplying of varying role activities can lead to problems of integration. The group may decide that both the patient and political foci are important. However, specific goals can be accomplished more effectively with two groups. The larger group can become two groups that work collaboratively. The members with interest more aligned with each function can join the group where they want to put their energies. In the end both groups are more effective and the shared goals can be met.

In addition to these social processes, in a system of integrated role sets there is feedback for control of output, or integrated behavior. When one perceives one's own behavior and the behavior of the other in an interaction, this perception acts as feedback to control further role behavior, as noted in the discussion of the interactional approach to roles. Turner (1962) referred to internal validation of the interaction itself. Internal validation lies in the successful anticipation of the behavior of others within the range necessary for carrying on one's own role. External validation derives from the generalized other. It is based on the individual's perception of whether the behavior is judged to constitute a role by others whose judgments have a claim to correctness or legitimacy. If role behavior is not validated, internally or externally, there will be corrections in behavior or the output of role performance. This is another part of the process of integrating roles for groups.

Handel (1979) saw a convergence of structural and interactional views in providing answers to problems of integrating roles. From the structural view, social stability and patterned conduct are explained by structures that lessen the intensity of adverse consequences of conflicting expectations. However, the author noted that there has not been much middle-range structural theory developed to explain how the individual copes with conflicting expectations. Interactional theories have addressed the negotiation of meaning in interaction as the individual's practical solution to the problems generated through conflicts of expectations in role sets. Negotiated meanings do not replace conflicting expectations. They coexist as a working consensus among the interacting individuals or groups about how to resolve conflicts in given situations. The combined structural and interactional approaches are useful to understanding the process of integrated roles. The processes of clarifying role expectations, reciprocating roles, and integrating roles lead to an integrated level of group adaptation in the role function mode.

COMPENSATORY ADAPTIVE PROCESSES

Each adaptive mode has compensatory processes as well as integrated processes. In the role function mode, groups will have many compensatory processes just as individuals do. Because we are dealing with adaptation of groups, the possibilities grow with the complexities of role function in groups. The complexity of meeting the need for role clarity in groups was noted in the discussion of the integrated processes. The Roy Adaptation Model defines compensatory processes for groups as the adaptation level at which the stabilizer and innovator are activated by a challenge to the integrated processes. Goode (1960) noted that role strain occurs in role systems. Role strain in functioning groups is associated with activating ways for reducing it. The author further describes that two basic techniques are used. First, the individual or group manages the role set in the following ways: compartmentalization, delegation, elimination of role relationships, extension, and barriers against intrusion. Secondly, the individual or group responds by setting or carrying out the terms of the role relationships. Setting the terms leads to role clarity and thus increases accountability for role performance within the group. Of all possible compensatory processes, two are described here, that is, role playing and role negotiation.

Role Playing

One description of role playing comes from seeing it described as an innovative teaching strategy for nursing. When the process is understood it will be clear that it can be used in many groups as a way of activating the stabilizer and the innovator. The stabilizer acts to maintain the group through the established structures, values, and daily activities to accomplish the group purposes. The innovator goes farther and uses structures and processes for change and growth. Either the stabilizer or the innovator can be activated by role playing for the group purposes.

One author describes role playing as a technique that encourages group members to improvise behaviors that show the expected actions of individuals involved in defined situations (Lowenstein, 2001). Role playing is a type of simulation that uses the adult learning principles of involvement and immediate feedback. A situation is described and characters assigned to be the major players. For example, a group of students, either in a basic nursing program or in a continuing education session, can take on a given clinical situation. The situation may be that they are involved in the care of a patient the day the patient and family are told that medical treatments have been exhausted and hospice care at home is recommended. The assigned roles can include primary care nurse, physician, clinical nurse specialist in oncology, chaplain, the patient, the patient's husband, and the patient's adult daughter. The situation calls upon the health care provider group and the family group to use resources to bring stability and to enhance growth of both groups.

The main advantage of using role playing processes is that participants can test behaviors and decisions in an environment without real risk. The role play situation is generally not scripted. There is spontaneous interplay among characters so that the actions and reactions of the various character roles provide material for analysis after the presentation. The participants have the opportunity to interact with others in certain roles. They experience other people's reactions to what they say and do. The process also allows participants to explore why people do and say what they do. In the analysis part of role playing, Lowenstein pointed out that the scenario and behaviors of the actors are discussed to clarify feelings, provide rationale for potential behaviors, and anticipate reactions to decisions as well as to increase observational skills and suggest new behaviors that might be tried.

In setting up the role playing situation, the challenging situation is described with some background. The parts are assigned and important characteristics of the major players are described. Enough information is given to provide a framework for role expectations and to elicit behaviors and actions. The other members of the class have the role of observing how the characters interact and analyzing the dynamics occurring. The instructor's role is more passive as a facilitator, clarifying and guiding the discussion. In describing the use of the method, Lowenstein suggested that allowing the students in the character roles a few minutes to warm up and relate to the roles they will be playing is often helpful. The three parts of the exercise are the briefing, the role playing, and the analysis. The timing suggested is about 10 to 20 minutes for the actual play and likely twice that for the analysis.

Another example of using the process of role playing might be in preparation for an accreditation visit. The nurse manager might mix the roles assigned to her staff. The nurse assistant may play a staff nurse; a nurse might play the desk clerk; some nurses may represent nurses from other shifts, and some can be given the roles of the different members of the interdisciplinary visiting team. It can be anticipated that this compensatory process will be helpful in handling the real life roles of the unit staff during the accreditation visit. At the same time the exercise might have a secondary gain of better understanding among the unit staff in differing roles.

Role Negotiation

In a general sense we can see role negotiation as an extension of socialization for role development at the individual level and socialization for role expectations at the group level. Socialization, or roles based on understanding of structured positions and on role interactions, develops over time. The formal and informal socialization processes are expected occurrences and generally contribute to a certain amount of role clarity. This makes it possible for the individual or group to interact effectively in the role function mode. However, at times an increased need for role clarity calls for an adjustment of role relationships. For groups this may happen at specified times such as when an organization or country elects new leaders. At other times the activities of the group may result in issues of role clarity that increase awareness of the need for role adjustments. The process entered into is called role negotiation. For the group the goal is to enhance group stability and growth. Role negotiation can be described as the compensatory process whereby increased need for role clarity stimulates role adjustments.

Role negotiation focuses on influencing the expectations and behaviors of reciprocal role participants in significant ways with the result that behavior is altered to some degree (Goshlin, 1969). The related approach of role bargaining is described in classical sociology (Goode, 1960). This is a process of negotiation on acceptable role behaviors for two or more individuals. There is a wide range for how explicit the bargaining process becomes. Sometimes role bargaining is an open communication process to reach agreement. In other situations, the process is less explicit. In this case one role occupant becomes the primary decision-maker and the individual in the reciprocal role indicates acceptance or rejection of the solution. In the less explicit situation, the results of the bargaining are known only by the resulting behavior. Role relationships are considered as dynamic where actors with varying degrees of awareness use role bargaining.

Different role situations are more or less open to role negotiation. Some roles have highly institutionalized expectations that offer little opportunity for role negotiations. The rights and duties are specified clearly in advance and do not allow for a new contract. An example is an organization with bylaws that describe the expectations for the various members. In other situations, or at other times, role expectations are more general and unspecified or more open. This provides the opportunity for role negotiation. The role participants who are able to accurately access the negotiability of a situation have an advantage. Hurley (1978) described how awareness of negotiation of roles is learned in childhood. Parents who are not authoritarian encourage children to express their own feelings and recognize their rights. As a result children see the possibility of negotiation. Also they develop specific skills in handling self in role-bargaining situations. The child who experienced freedom to bargain, however, may be at a disadvantage when in situations in which negotiating is not possible. The situation may be viewed as frustrating and intolerable. The author noted that this is particularly the case when the child has not learned to distinguish between the two types of situations.

Bargaining is more likely to be successful when one recognizes appropriate situations for role negotiation, has learned the necessary skills, and can be flexible. Effective role negotiation depends on good verbal skills, the ability to take the position of the other, and a strong sense of self. Sometimes freedom to negotiate a role may be restricted by internalized values and standards of conduct that inhibit exercise of abilities when situations are negotiable. The resources of those in varying roles are significant in the exchange. Resources include education, experience, and skill of each role occupant. We may consider a nurse researcher who is involving the community in a project. The nurse may have more education; however, the community members clearly have more experience and skill in knowing and working with the community. The recognition of what each brings to the situation can lead to successful role negotiations. The challenge to negotiate roles can lead to higher levels of adaptation for groups.

COMPROMISED PROCESSES OF ROLE FUNCTION

Within groups, compensatory processes at times are not effective in bringing role clarity and adaptive group role functioning. When role function within the group fails, a compromised adaptation level exists. The focal stimulus or immediate trigger for the difficulty varies widely according to the multiple roles and processes involved. A change in group membership can lead to issues of inadequate socialization for specific role expectations. In other groups the reciprocity of roles may be lacking in that not all members are fulfilling expectations, which interferes with the effectiveness of the group. There are many possible influencing factors for difficulties with integrating all the roles of all the members of a group. There may be differences of values, goals, or power relations that lead to ineffective role function for the group. A compromised adaptation level can be manifested by many patterns of ineffective adaptive behaviors. We describe two examples of compromised role function in groups: interrole conflict and caregiver role strain.

Interrole Conflict

In discussing roles for individuals, interrole conflict referred to role failure resulting from expectations of different roles for the same individual not being compatible. At the group level interrole conflicts exist when there are contradictions between two or more people in a group regarding expectations for differing roles in the group. The conflicts compromise the effectiveness of the group in reaching goals. The example of competing expectations for an individual was the woman who is an electrical engineer and was just promoted at work. As the mother of an 8-week-old baby boy, she finds herself in great conflict between two important roles. She wants to be at work to maintain her position and new role in the group. At the same time, she wants to be with her baby and be involved with as much of his care as possible. The role function problem for the individual creates role function problems for at least two groups to which the woman belongs. At work her project team needs for her to carry out her reciprocal role responsibilities for them to reach project goals. It is possible that the peer pressure is increased because she is the first woman to be the electrical engineer for the team. At the same time the mother's family is greatly affected because immediate and extended family members both want her to fulfill a traditional mothering role and want her to be happy in her role choices. This family situation may be more intense because the mother delayed having her first child until she completed her higher education and established a career. Conflicts will be acknowledged and dealt with so that role function for the group is effective.

The list of early studies of role conflict that Hardy (1978) identified showed a number of group situations of role conflict and types of role conflict. Some examples included: directors of nursing service had conflicting role demands; hospital nurses found disparity between role norms and behavior and in another study, disagreement over role demands; family members experienced disparity in attitudes; families and community had competing values; union members felt incompatible role demands and discrepancy in norms; military and civilian personnel had disagreement over role expectations; and head nurses and educators held discrepancies in role expectations. In discussion of the history of research on intergroup relations, other authors pointed out the classic work whereby researchers studied groups in teenage boys' summer camps. After two groups had developed significant rivalries, they were given a cooperative project to work on. The result was diminished hostilities and less name-calling. Perceptions of likeness of the other group increased. The intergroup cooperation actually changed the perceptions of the rival group members and they were seen as being more like the self (Wedell et al., 2007).

Chinn (2008) described conflict transformation in her discussion of creative leadership for building community. The process draws upon powers of diversity, solidarity, and creative responsibility, all of which are compatible with the assumptions of the Roy Adaptation Model. Chinn recommended recognizing the limits of adversarial definitions of conflict and knowing that the group has a choice in dealing with conflict and can learn ways to transform conflict. Important traditions in the group that can be a foundation for transforming conflict are nurturing a strong sense of rotation leadership, practicing critical reflection, and practicing ways to value diversity. The author emphasized that conflict is the responsibility of everyone in the group. To transform the conflict, someone in the group summarizes the conflict using what Chinn identifies as elements of reflection. Each member of the group shares from this reflective process to lend individual perspectives to the process of creating a complete understanding for the group. Important steps are being specific about responsibilities, each member acknowledging feelings and observations, group members stating what they want, and responding positively to the critical reflection. When conflicts are transformed, it leads to the kinds of group decisions that "represent deep commitments, insights, shifts in ways of being together, and shifts in attitude" (Chinn, 2008, p. 125).

Caregiver Role Strain

Role strain has been described as the subjective state of distress experienced by an individual in a role when role stress is encountered. Role stress is the social structural condition in which role obligations are vague, irritating, difficult, conflicting, or impossible to meet (Hardy, 1978). Using an engineering analogy and general systems theory, Hardy defined stress as an external force that disturbs the internal stability or steady state of the system. The resulting disturbance is called strain. Strain is recognized as a temporary or permanent alteration in the structure subjected to stress. Early work by Gross and colleagues (1957) identified factors to be considered before resolving conflicts that create role strain: "(1) the relative legitimacy of the expectations, (2) the sanctions incumbent upon the non-fulfillment of each of the expectations, and (3) the moral orientation of the actor."

Gray (2003) illustrated that role stress and strain affects the organization's outcomes. In health care this means that quality of patient care and patient satisfaction are decreased when there is role strain. The greatest strain seems to be among those who span the organization's boundary. A particular situation that nurses will find in practice is the common issue of caregiver role strain. This affects families greatly and is a focus for nursing efforts to promote adaptation. Many publications discuss what is described as the *sandwich generation.* Adults in their middle years are in the middle of the generation older than them and those younger. Their parents are living longer and may develop complex health care needs as they age. In addition the middle age adults may be involved with others of the older generation such as aunts and uncles, and even grandparents. Their child care responsibilities generally are decreasing. However, there usually remains considerable care or involvement with their own children. Often it is the case that the middle-aged woman is in close relationships with elder relatives more than the middle-aged man.

Caregiver strain is discussed in basic nursing textbooks and has been the subject of significant nursing research. We will review some of the basic issues for families as a group. Caregiving to parents is the most frequent topic. The same issues, however, apply to situations of providing care for a disabled or chronically ill spouse or child. Murray and Zentner (2001) noted that the family roles in our society focus on the dynamics of the marriage bond and socialization of young children. There is an emphasis on affection, compatibility, and personal growth of each individual in the nuclear family as the most important aspects of family life. In addition the emphasis on personal independence and social mobility of middle-aged and young adults sometimes creates generational households that are separated by distance. Families develop new patterns of intimacy across time and space. These cultural trends contribute to the dilemma of caring for older dependent relatives.

In addition, Murray and Zentner raised the issue of strain caused by difficulty with role reversal. The family's traditional protective function has been *filial responsibility*. Filial responsibility is "an attitude of personal responsibility towards parents that emphasizes duty, protection, care and financial support" (p. 693). However, some parts of the culture believe that good relationships between parents and adult children depend upon the parents keeping their autonomy. For the child to become the caregiver is not a sanctioned role. It is assumed that both children and parents resent it. Other cultural groups within the larger society have developed structures of extended family systems that provide support and assistance across generations. Murray and Zentner (2001) pointed out that a middle-aged person can be seen as having energy, free time, and money. The older relatives can become more demanding at a time the middle-aged adult would like some time for self, such as a vacation, additional education, or a social cause.

The caregiver role of older parents has become more common and often this is a mutually satisfying relationship. However, it can be a stressful experience. The stress causes strain, the subjective state of distress. The factors or stimuli that influence the caregiving role and the diversity of outcomes for the family are listed in Box 19–2. The identification of these factors and their outcomes are a major contribution of nursing research to understanding the occurrence of caregiver stress. It is clear that the family as a group is affected. Each person is affected individually. In addition, however, the role relationships among the members are affected. The observation made earlier that the greatest strain seems to be among those who span the group's boundary is relevant. The definitions of family boundaries may differ. An adult daughter may consider her mother to be within the boundary of her family. But other family members who are competing for the time, attention, and resources of the caregiving woman may feel that the mother-in-law or grandmother is on the outside of their definition of their family. We have also discussed that roles in groups are reciprocal and integrated. Another source of strain is that one caregiver may resent other siblings who do not participate in the caregiver role.

Because the caregiver role is meaningful on many levels, the adult child continues to care for the parent beyond physical or psychological abilities to do so. Murray and Zentner (2001) listed some indicators that the caregiver needs assistance. These included the relative's condition worsens regardless of continued efforts; the individual may feel that what they do is never enough or that there is no one else enduring what they are; there is not time to be alone or have any respite; family relations are breaking down because of the caregiving strain; the interference of caregiving with work, family, and social life are at an unacceptable level; the caregiver continues in a no-win situation to avoid feeling failure; coping mechanisms become destructive such as over- or undereating, abusing alcohol, or drugs; or being harsh with the parent. The most important danger signal is when the caregiver's loving and caring gives way to exhaustion and resentment and the individual no longer feels good about self.

Families experiencing caregiver role strain will benefit from the nurse's involvement in helping them to recognize the strain and the effects on the family system. The nurse is in a key position to help family members work through the conflicts, feelings of frustration, guilt, and anger generated by the role demands and past conflicts with parents or siblings. The caregiver

BOX 19–2

Caregiving Role and the Family

Factors or Stimuli That Influence the Caregiver Role

- Seriousness of the elder's health status
- The caregiver–care recipient relationship and living arrangement
- Duration of the caregiving experience
- Other roles and responsibilities of the caregiver
- Overall coping effectiveness of the caregiver
- Caregiver sex and age
- Number of generations needing care
- Help and support from others—family or social agencies
- Information needed to carry out tasks related to physical care of parent

Possible Outcomes of Caregiver Role for the Family

- Financial hardship
- Physical symptoms such as sleeplessness and decline in physical health, especially in the primary caregiver
- Emotional changes and symptoms in the caregiver and other family members, including frustration, inadequacy, anxiety, helplessness, depression, guilt, resentment, lowered morale, and emotional distance
- Emotional exhaustion related to restrictions on time and freedom and increasing responsibility
- A sense of isolation from social activities
- Conflict because of competing demands, with diversion from care of other family members
- Difficulty in setting priorities
- Reduced family privacy
- Inability to project future plans
- Sense of losing control over life events
- Interference with job responsibilities through late arrival, absenteeism, or early departure needed to take care of emergencies or even routine tasks
- Interference with lifestyle and social and recreational activities

Murray, R. B., & Zentner, J. P. (2001). *Health promotion strategies through the life span.* (7th ed.). Upper Saddle River, NJ: Prentice-Hall. (p. 694). Used with permission.

can be encouraged to maintain other roles. Helping the family to find community resources for care for elders is important. The family may need counseling to deal with complex emotional reactions raised by caregiver stress. In this situation as in other compensatory and compromised processes, the role function for the group requires careful planning with the group.

NURSING PROCESS RELATED TO GROUP ROLE FUNCTION

For the role function mode of groups, nursing practice focuses on systems of relating people such as families, organizations, communities, and society. The Roy Adaptation Model framework for nursing practice in groups is parallel to that described for the nursing care of individuals. The six steps of the nursing process are presented in this section as described by the Roy Adaptation

Model. The examples given consider a variety of groups. Each example is one part of what we know are complex processes that nurses work with over time for various groups.

Assessment of Behavior

First-level assessment of the role function mode for the group includes assessing behaviors that relate to socializing for role expectations in groups, reciprocating roles, and integrating roles. As explained throughout this text, assessment can be made by direct observation and by reports from individuals in the group. Patterns of behavior are the focus of the nursing assessment. Particular areas to assess are patterns of role performance within the group, comfort level of role adjustments, and problem-solving strategies for interrole conflict and role strain.

Major methods of assessment are observations of role behaviors and listening to group members' perceptions of how well the roles are performed and role sets integrated. The nurse assesses patterns of behaviors related to successful role performance, that is, the members of the group carry out activities that accomplish group goals. Patterns related to satisfaction with integrating and adjusting roles are also assessed. Are the reciprocal roles working for the group? Is the division of labor adequate and are the members doing their jobs? Are the strategies the group uses for role integration working to their satisfaction? Given the multiple role sets within the groups, do the members adequately integrate expectations for roles inside and outside the group? Does the group use flexibility in meeting expectations of multiple others and of multiple groups? Does the group feel comfortable adjusting role expectations frequently? Does the group identify role conflicts or strains when they occur? Can they problem solve strategies to decrease role conflict or strain? When negotiations of meanings of roles or clarification of expectations are needed, are all those involved included in the negotiation? Do the negotiated meanings lead to better role integration and role performance? Are new roles incorporated without undue stress on existing roles? Is the group able to feel comfortable with terminating roles?

The nurse is aware that it is not conformity to role expectations that is the focus of assessment of integrating roles at the group level. Rather the nurse assesses behaviors related to success and satisfaction with integrating roles. Successful integration of roles is observed in effective patterns of role performance. This means noting roles performed in a way that the purposes of the group are carried out. Satisfaction with integration of roles is shown in the joy of achieving goals and minimizing the strain of competing expectations.

Assessment of Stimuli

Many factors influence the role processes of groups as indicated by theoretical understanding of the processes. For example, in some situations, socialization for role expectations depends on adequate role models. Among all possible influencing factors, some specific and commonly occurring ones can be identified and described briefly. Socialization for expectations, reciprocity, and integrating roles are particularly affected by stimuli such as size and complexity of role sets, the developmental stage of the group, and group stabilizer and innovator processes. The strategies the nurse uses in assessment of stimuli of group role function are similar to those used for assessment of behaviors. Assessment begins with observation and reports from group members. Further approaches are also used. For example, observation of the group in specific situations and detailed interviews sometimes are needed to identify underlying factors influencing the group role performance. The nurse can help to bring these influencing factors to the awareness of the group as a significant part of planning for promoting adaptation in the role function mode for groups.

SIZE AND COMPLEXITY OF ROLE SET   In discussing the process of reciprocating roles we considered a nurse accepting a management position. Table 19–1 showed three reciprocal roles and some of the complexity of the new role set for this one role position. When we think of the family, there are multiple other individuals in reciprocal roles, for example, a father may relate to several sons and daughters, and to stepchildren, as well. A teacher who is part of one workgroup at school has many students, and also many groups associated with the teacher role. These include administrators, other faculty, and staff responsible for the goals of the school, and to parent-teacher groups. Each of these other groups often has a broad range of concerns. The examples of the extensiveness of role interactions relate only to a few of the roles of group members. Actually the number becomes extensive when the entire role set of each group member is mapped out.

In addition to the number of roles, a role set has another characteristic referred to as complexity. Merton (1968) used the notion of patterns of role sets to illustrate the fact that even a seemingly simple social structure is extremely complex. Complexity in regard to role sets stems from the fact that any individual occupying a particular role set interacts with complementary roles that are differently located in the social structure. Values and moral expectations of those in other statuses may in some measure differ from those of the individual in the role. Merton noted, for example, that members of a school board are often in social and economic strata quite different from the public school teacher. A salesperson for an international firm has a highly complex role set, considering the different views of client statuses in different cultures.

The rapid social changes are creating a global society among the people of the earth. Thus the number and complexity of roles is almost infinite. We need to see ourselves as part of a global and interacting community. Cultural norms still will vary, but there is increasing emphasis on creating ways that norms and values can be inclusive of the good of the individual and the group worldwide. Zohar and Marshall (1994) noted that both individualism and collectivism are mechanistic social models. The authors spoke to the social need for commitment to higher common values. Further, a community is held together neither by complex calculations of self-interest nor by sets of bureaucratic roles and rules. Rather, it draws on its common culture of collective patterns of thinking, feeling, and acting. The search for meaningful social norms, according to these authors, involves the creative use of both freedom and ambiguity. McMahon (1993) spoke of finding the common ground for a global spirituality and community in the human bodily experience. Roy (1997) has noted that human participation in transformation is the key to future human development and that nurses are an important part of society's redefining of norms. Chinn's (2008) approach to PEACE groups, described in Chapter 18 and discussed in relation to leadership roles in groups, is a way of creating social norms based on unity, diversity, commitment, and consensus, rather than culturally established hierarchies. Creating global norms is a challenge, but remains a significant goal for the survival of people and the planet.

DEVELOPMENTAL STAGE OF THE GROUP   In assessing role function for groups, an influencing factor to consider is the developmental stage of the group. The model Worchel (1996) developed for stages of group development was described in Chapter 18. Just as stage of development is significant for group identity, it also affects group role function. Stage I is named the stage of discontent. As a group forms, issues related to formation are examined. Group members may feel uncertain about their role in the group and how they can contribute to group goals. The informal role development may be taking shape at the same time that the members are learning the formal roles. A precipitating event may initiate Stage II of group development. As noted earlier even a relatively minor incident can trigger this stage. A rumor of someone leaving the group can surface common dissatisfactions. The result is to initiate meaningful contact among members. During Stage III the group members focus on defining the group. With this definition they are clear about roles within the group. Members become concerned about participating in the group. Productivity increases in Stage IV. The group sets goals and plans how to achieve those goals. Information shared among members is focused on productivity issues. The members' skills in carrying out differing roles are important as are the leadership roles. Stage V is referred to as the individual stage. It was noted earlier that in this stage the members want recognition for their contributions and resources on the basis of equity rather than equality. The group relates in a cooperative way toward other groups. Members may be exploring opportunities to play a role in the goals of another group. According to the author, Stage VI is described as decay. Personal needs may get more attention, especially if individuals feel conflict about roles in other groups. The forming of subgroups leads to competition for power. A new period of discontent, the beginning of a new Stage I may follow. There are many descriptions of the stages of group development. However stages are described, it is clear that the stage of group development affects role performance of the group.

STABILIZER AND INNOVATOR PROCESSES Strong influencing factors for effective role function in groups is their use of stabilizer and innovator processes. The stabilizer acts to maintain the system. The group uses established structures, values, and daily activities to make it possible to accomplish the purpose of the group. In some groups, written bylaws are consulted to reach role clarity. In another group, members may have a discussion of their values to bring their purpose into focus. This can act as a stabilizing force for all members of the group to fulfill their reciprocal role responsibilities. When daily activities aim towards the goals of the group, it is a stabilizing strength. For example, the family may have a specific routine of who carries out what family chores. The daily routine helps to maintain the family as a system. When assessing factors influencing the group's role function, the nurse will look to how the group uses the established structures, values, and daily activities. These stabilizer strategies are essential to using any of the social processes identified for socialization for role expectations, reciprocating roles, and integrating roles.

The innovator subsystem involves processes for change and growth. These processes lie within the group members and how the group stimulates the human potential of the members. The problem-solving of the cognator is significant for the individual in handling roles. In a similar way as people interact in groups, the role function effectiveness of the group depends on group problem-solving and decision-making skills. For example, a new task may be identified by a group involved in lobbying for better health care when they receive notice of a special legislative hearing on the issue. To respond to the challenge, roles will be adjusted and integrated to accommodate the new task while maintaining focus on their ongoing goal-oriented projects. How the group works together to define and solve the problem of adjusting tasks and role expectations, and how they work together quickly and effectively to make group decisions, has a significant impact on their role integration at this time.

Nursing Diagnosis

Using the nursing process for the role function mode for groups, the nurse makes a careful assessment of behaviors and stimuli. Based on thorough first- and second-level assessment, the nurse formulates nursing diagnoses, sets goals, selects interventions, and evaluates care. Table 19–2 lists the positive indicators for adaptation and common adaptation problems for the role function mode for groups according to the Roy Adaptation Model, along with the list of NANDA diagnostic labels (NANDA International, 2007). In discussing the latter steps, we

TABLE 19–2 Nursing Diagnostic Categories for Role Function for Groups

Positive indicators of Adaptation	Common Adaptation Problems	NANDA Diagnostic Labels
• Role clarity • Effective processes of socialization for role expectations • Structuring of expectations to accomplish goals of group • Effective processes for reciprocating roles • High mutual dependence in division of labor • Effective processes for integrating roles • Regulating responsibilities and expectations between individuals in complementary and relating roles • Flexibility in carrying out all roles to meet group demands • Sufficient mentoring for role development	• Role confusion • Inadequate socialization for role expectations • Failure of some roles in group • Ineffective give and take in role responsibilities • Uneven distribution of responsibilities to detriment of goals of the group • Interrole conflict • Caregiver or other role strain • Inadequate role development to meet growing needs of group	• Compromised family coping • Disabled family coping • Readiness for enhanced family coping • Caregiver role strain

will focus on a nurse who has significant roles in a number of related groups. Jackie Trotier has been a nurse practitioner in central Maine for about 5 years. She enjoys working with the underserved rural population with complex health problems. Her group practice provides a family medicine residency and placements for nurse practitioner students. Ms. Trotier has collaborated with a group of social workers and psychologists to hold group sessions for patients with substance abuse problems. In addition, all staff of the agency are working together to enhance their communication through the use of patient electronic health care records. Ms. Trotier's family has lived in the community for generations, and this helps her to make contacts to support projects her groups initiate. Ms. Trotier has kept in touch with her faculty advisor from her master's program and often calls upon her as a mentor.

Describing nursing diagnoses in the role function mode for groups is carried out in the same way as in the other adaptive modes. One method involves the statement of the behaviors together with the influencing stimuli. The second approach is to use summary labels. Nursing diagnoses can reflect either adaptive or ineffective behaviors. When Ms. Trotier last visited with her mentor, the mentor noted a number of positive diagnoses in the role function of her mentee. One can be stated: Reports feeling comfortable in the role of leader with the group providing special programs for substance abuse patients related to her collaborative and reciprocal relations with other professionals and their shared goal for patients. Another positive diagnosis is the summary: Integrated role set.

However, in their discussion, Ms. Trotier talks with her mentor about an organizational change that may affect her role performance in her larger workgroup. She notes that she already carries heavy teaching responsibilities both for medical residents and nurse practitioner students, as well as her practice responsibilities. She anticipates being asked to be the nursing representative to the electronic health care record committee. Ms. Trotier recognizes the importance of this role and that she is the logical choice. However, she has concerns about intrarole conflict as she tries to manage all her role commitments, and she knows that this is not an area of her greatest expertise. A nursing diagnosis may be stated as follows: Potential for interrole conflict related to adding new role expectations of committee assignment.

Goal Setting

As noted throughout this text, each step of the nursing process focuses on behavior, the stimuli influencing that behavior, or both. In stating nursing diagnoses, the statement developed includes both behaviors and stimuli. The focus is on behavior in the goal-setting step. The goal identifies a behavior that is to be addressed. Each goal states the behavior of focus, the change expected, and the time frame in which the goal is to be achieved. Role function issues in groups may have both acute and long-term phases. In setting goals, then, attention is given to both long- and short-term goals. In the case of Ms. Trotier, two goals are set in discussion with her mentor: (1) to maintain feelings of comfort in role of leader with practice group over the next 6 months and (2) to decrease the potential interrole conflict within the next month.

Nursing Intervention

According to the Roy Adaptation Model the intervention step of the nursing process focuses on the stimuli affecting the behavior identified in the goal-setting step. The management of stimuli are the interventions, and this involves altering, increasing, decreasing, removing, or maintaining them. In their discussion, Ms. Trotier and her mentor decide that she can use role negotiation to manage the level of role expectations in the new committee assignment. She will offer to be the nursing consultant to the group and specify the expertise she can offer without taking on all of the responsibilities of a committee member.

Evaluation

In the final step of the nursing process, evaluation involves judging the effectiveness of the nursing interventions. This is judged in relation to the adaptive behavior, that is, whether the behaviors stated in the goals have been achieved. Effective nursing interventions are those in which the behavior occurs as stated in the goal. However, if the goal has not been achieved, the nurse together with the person or group identifies alternative interventions or approaches by reassessing the behavior and stimuli and continuing with the other steps of the nursing process. In relation to the second goal for Ms. Trotier, to decrease the potential interrole conflict within the next month, her mentor is happy to find that when she calls back the following month, she reports no interrole conflict and continued role integration. In Ms. Trotier's role negotiations, the larger workgroup was happy to accept her more limited role of consultant for nursing. This was made more acceptable when Ms. Trotier was able to call upon her larger support system and identify a family friend who could provide occasional technical support on computerized language to the committee on the electronic medical record. The mentor agrees to keep in touch to evaluate her mentee's continued role development and satisfaction.

Summary

This chapter focused on the Roy Adaptation Model role function mode in groups. An overview of the processes of socialization for role expectation, role reciprocity, and role integration that contribute to role clarity was provided. Examples of compensatory responses related to role function in groups were described. The compromised processes highlighted included interrole conflict and caregiver role strain. Finally, guidelines for planning nursing care through assessment of behaviors and stimuli, the formulation of nursing diagnoses, goals, and interventions were explored and evaluation of nursing care was described.

Exercises for Application

1. Select a group to which you belong and identify the formal and informal roles that members play to carry out the goals of the group.
2. Think of a change related to your group that might challenge the ability to carry out your goals.
3. What is the main purpose of your educational or work institution?

Assessment of Understanding

QUESTIONS

1. Name the three processes of role function whereby role clarity is reached in groups. _____, _____, and _____.
2. Describe one compensatory process related to group role function. _____.
3. Select one situation of compromised processes of group role function and identify a way to deal with the problem. _____
4. Identify four behaviors important in assessing group role function. _____, _____, _____, and _____.
5. Identity three common stimuli that influence group role function. _____, _____, and _____.

SITUATION:

A given university has had an organization for students of minority ethnic groups for some years. Recently members of the group have begun to express a general dissatisfaction with the ineffectiveness of the group. They began to look into the history of how the group formed and to look at the challenges they face today. They have decided to redefine their goals and to look at the structure of roles that can help them meet their goals.

6. State one positive nursing diagnosis for the student organization.

   _____

7. State one goal for the nursing diagnosis identified.

   _____

8. Identify one intervention to meet the goal named above.

   _____

9. Describe how the effectiveness of the intervention can be evaluated.

   _____

FEEDBACK

1. Socialization for role expectations, reciprocating roles, and role integration.
2. Role playing or role negotiation.
3. Answers will vary. For caregiver role strain, some possible approaches are: help family to recognize the strain and the effects on the family system; help family members work through the conflicts, feelings of frustration, guilt, and anger generated by the role demands and past conflicts with parents or siblings; encourage the caregiver to maintain other roles; help to find community resources for care for elders.

4. Patterns of role performance within the group, comfort level of role adjustments, and problem-solving strategies for interrole conflict and role strain.

5. Size and complexity of role sets, the developmental stage of the group, and group stabilizer and innovator processes.

6. Answers will vary. Recognize the need for role clarity based on stage of group development.

7. Within 2 months the group will list their goals and describe role structure to meet goals.

8. Involve every member of the group in redefining goals.

9. Assess in 2 months whether the group has listed their goals and described the role structure to meet their goals.

References

Chinn, P. L. (2008). *Peace and power: Creative leadership for building community* (7th ed.). Sudbury, MA: Jones and Bartlett.

Conway, M. E. (1978). Theoretical approaches to the study of roles. In M. E. Hardy & M. E. Conway (Eds.), *Role theory: Perspectives for health professionals* (pp. 17–28). New York: Appleton-Century-Crofts.

de Carteret, N. M. (1992). The ethic of cooperation: A new approach for the decade. In U. Kirdar (Ed.), *Change: Threat or opportunity for human progress?* New York: United Nations.

Derber, C. (2003). *People before profit: The new globalisation in an age of terror, big money, and economic crisis.* London: Souvenir Press.

Fields, W. L. (1991). Mentoring in nursing: A historical approach. *Nursing Outlook, 39*(6), 257–261.

Gerrish, K. (2000). Still fumbling along? A comparative study of the newly qualified nurse's perception of the transition from student to qualified nurse. *Journal of Advanced Nursing, 32*(2), 473–480.

Global Vision Statement. (2008). Retrieved February, 19, 2008, from http://www.vbwf.org/

Goode, W. J. (1960). A theory of role strain. *American Psychological Review, 25*, 483–496.

Goshlin, D. A. (1969). *Handbook of socialization theory and research.* Chicago: Rand McNally.

Gray, J. J. (2003). Role transition. In P. S. Yoder-Wise (Ed.), *Leading and managing in nursing* (3rd ed.). St. Louis, MO: Mosby.

Gross, N., McEachern, A. W., & Mason, W. S. (1957). *Explorations in role analysis: Studies of the school superintendency role.* New York: John Wiley.

Handel, W. (1979). Normative expectations and the emergence of meaning as solutions to problems: Convergence of structural and interactionist views. *American Journal of Sociology, 84*(4), 855–881.

Hardy, M. E. (1978). Role stress and role strain. In M. E. Hardy & M. E. Conway (Eds.), *Role theory: Perspectives for health professionals* (pp. 73–110). New York: Appleton-Century-Crofts.

Homer. (1999). *The odyssey* (W. H. Rouse, Trans.). New York: Signet Classics.

Hurley, B. A. (1978). Socialization for roles. In M. E. Hardy & M. E. Conway (Eds.), *Role theory: Perspectives for health professionals* (pp. 29–72). New York: Appleton-Century-Crofts.

Kramer, M., & Schmalenberg, C. (1988). Learning from success: Autonomy and empowerment. *Nursing Management 24*(5).

Lambert, C. E., & Lambert, V. A. (2001). Preceptorial experience. In A. J. Lowenstein & M. J. Bradshaw (Eds.), *Fuszard's innovative teaching strategies in nursing* (3rd ed.). Gaithersburg, MD: Aspen Publishers, Inc.

Lowenstein, A. J. (2007). Role Play. In M. J. Bradshaw & A. J. Lowenstein (Eds.), *Innovative teaching strategies in nursing and related health professions* (4th ed.). Boston: Jones & Bartlett.

Luft, J. (1984). *Group processes: An introduction to group dynamics* (3rd ed.). Palo Alto, CA: Mayfield.

Markman, K. D., Ratcliff, J. J., Mizoguchi, N., Elizaga, R. A., & McMullen, M. N. (2007). Assimilation and contrast in counterfactual thinking and other mental simulation-based comparison processes. In J. Suls & D. A. Stapel (Eds.), *Assimilation and contrast in social psychology.* New York: Psychology Press.

Marquis, B. L., & Huston, C. J. (2006). *Leadership roles and management functions in nursing:*

Theory and application (5th ed.). Philadelphia: Lippincott Williams & Wilkins.

McMahon, E. M. (1993). *Beyond the myth of dominance: An alternative to a violent society.* Kansas City, MO: Sheed & Ward.

Merton, R. K. (1968). *Social theory and social structure.* New York: Free Press.

Murray, R. B., & Zentner, J. P. (2001). *Health promotion strategies through the life span.* (7th ed.). Upper Saddle River, NJ: Prentice-Hall.

NANDA International. (2007). *Nursing diagnoses: Definitions & classification, 2007–2008.* Philadelphia: NANDA-I.

Prestholdt, C. O. (1990). Modern mentoring: Strategies for developing contemporary nursing leadership. *Nursing Administration quarterly, 15*(1), 20–27.

Roy, C. (1997). Knowledge as universal cosmic imperative. In *Proceedings of nursing knowledge impact* conference 1996 (pp. 95–118). Chestnut Hill, MA: Boston College Press.

Roy, C., Murphy, M., & Eisenhauer, L. (2003). Mentoring: A project in process. *INDEN Newsletter, 2*(3), 3–7.

Roy, C., & Roberts, S. L. (Eds.). (1981). *Theory construction in nursing: An adaptation model.* Englewood Cliffs, NJ: Prentice Hall.

Shapiro, E., Hazeltine, F., & Rowe, M. (1978). Moving up: Role models, mentors, and the 'patron system'. *Sloan Management Review, 19*(3), 51–58.

Snelson, C. M., Martsolf, D. S., Dieckman, B. C., Anaya, E. R., Cartechine, K. A., Miller, B.,

Roche, M., & Shaffer, J. (2002). Caring as a theoretical perspective for a nursing faculty mentoring program. *Nurse Education Today, 22,* 654–660.

Turner, R. (1962). Role-taking process versus conformity. In A. Rose (Ed.), *Human behavior and social processes.* Boston: Houghton Mifflin.

United Nations Department of Public Information. (2007). Universal Declaration of Human Rights. Retrieved February 19, 2008, from http://www.unhchr.ch/udhr/index.htm

Vance, C. N. (1982). The mentor connection. *The Journal of Nursing Administration, 12*(4), 7–13.

Wedell, D. H., Hicklin, S. K., & Smarandescu, L. O. (2007). Contrasting models of assimilation and contrast. In J. Suls & D. A. Stapel (Eds.), *Assimilation and contrast in social psychology.* New York: Psychology Press.

Worchel, S. (1996). Emphasizing the social nature of groups in a developmental framework. In J. L. Nye & A. M. Brower (Eds.), *What's social about social cognition? Research on socially shared cognition in small groups* (pp. 261–281). Thousand Oaks, CA: Sage Publications.

World Health Organization. (2005). Retrieved February 2, 2008, from http://www.euro.who.int/Document/HSM/healthsys_savelives.pdf

Zohar, D., & Marshall, I. (1994). *The quantum society: Mind, physics, and a new social vision.* New York: Quill/ Morrow.

CHAPTER 20

Interdependence Mode of Relating Persons

As with the role function mode, interdependent relationships occur on an individual level and on the group level. This chapter focuses on the interdependence mode from the perspective of relating persons, that is, groups. As with the first three adaptive modes described in the Roy Adaptation Model, people in relational systems, such as families, communities, networks, organizations, and societies, increasingly are the client in nursing practice. The interdependence mode for groups involves behavior related to interdependent relationships of persons in groups. It also applies to groups relating to other groups. The interdependence mode also focuses on the social context in which groups operate.

The Roy Adaptation Model identifies the basic need of the interdependence mode for both individuals and groups as relational adequacy. The three components of the need for integrity and mastery for groups include relational adequacy, developmental adequacy, and resource adequacy. From the perspective of persons relating in groups, the components of the interdependence mode are context, infrastructure, and member capability. This chapter provides an overview of the interdependence mode of groups with a focus on three integrated life processes: relational adequacy, developmental adequacy, and resource adequacy. Illustrations of compensatory adaptive processes of relating persons are provided, and examples of compromised processes, that is, pollution and aggression, are explored. Finally, guidelines are described for planning nursing care: two levels of assessment, formulating diagnoses, establishing goals, selecting interventions, and evaluating nursing care.

OBJECTIVES

After studying this chapter, the reader will be able to do the following:

1. Describe the interdependence mode of groups according to the Roy Adaptation Model as illustrated by the three integrated life processes of group interdependence.

2. Describe compensatory processes of the interdependence mode of groups.

3. List two examples of compromised processes of relational interdependence at the group level.

4. Identify important first-level assessment behaviors for the interdependence mode of groups.

5. Identify second-level assessment stimuli that influence the interdependence mode of groups.

6. Develop a nursing diagnosis, given a relational interdependence situation.

7. Derive goals for a given situation of ineffective interdependence in a given group system.

8. Develop nursing interventions for a given situation of ineffective relational interdependence.

9. Propose approaches to determine the effectiveness of nursing interventions for adaptive group interdpendence.

KEY CONCEPTS DEFINED

Context: One of three components of the interdependence mode of groups; external includes economic, social, political, cultural, belief, and family systems and internal relates to mission, vision, values, principles, goals, and plans that influence a relational system; also viewed as stimuli.

Developmental adequacy: One of three integrated processes associated with the basic need of relational integrity of the interdependence mode of groups; learning and maturation in groups, achieved through developmental processes.

Infrastructure: The second of three components of the interdependence mode of groups; relates to the procedures, processes, and systems that exist within a group system, through which the goals of the system are accomplished.

Member capability: The third of three components of the interdependence mode of relating persons; pertains to the knowledge, skills, and commitments of individuals within the group.

Relational adequacy: One of three integrated life processes associated with the basic need of relational integrity of the interdependence mode of groups; involves receptive and contributive behaviors in interactions with significant others and support systems.

Relational integrity: The basic need of the interdependence mode; the feeling of security in relationships.

Relational interdependence: The dynamic interrelationships of systems of people.

Relational systems: Human systems, from the perspective of relating persons, participating in interdependent relationships such as families, clubs, networks, associations, and organizations; aimed at satisfying the need for relational integrity.

Resource adequacy: One of three integrated life processes of the basic need of relational integrity in the interdependence mode of groups; the need for resources such as physical space, funding, supplies, communication, and security; achieved through interdependent processes.

Significant others: For groups, other groups to whom the most meaning or importance is given.

Support systems: Persons, groups, and organizations with which a group associates in order to accomplish goals or to achieve some purpose.

PROCESSES OF INTERDEPENDENCE IN GROUPS

Much has been written about relational systems and the way goals of human adaptive systems are advanced through people working together for some purpose. According to the Roy Adaptation Model, relational interdependence is defined as the dynamic interrelationships of systems of people. Relational systems are aimed at satisfying needs for relationships, development, and resources. Satisfying these needs achieves relational integrity—the basic need of the interdependence mode of relating persons. It is through relational, developmental, and resource processes that groups continue to grow and contribute to society.

Relational systems, or groups functioning together for some purpose, may themselves be the focus of care in situations of advanced nursing practice. Nurses are familiar with the family unit as a relational system, and much has been written in this text and elsewhere about the family from a nursing perspective. Hanna and Roy (2001) addressed the use of the Roy Adaptation Model to guide practice and research with the family as the unit of care. Nurses working in a community focus on the community itself as a relational system or group. For industrial nurses, the workforce in the organization constitutes a system of focus. Even nursing as a profession can be regarded as a relational system, that is, an organizational group. Beyond the health care system, relational systems permeate society. International businesses promote their products and approaches as excelling above those of their competitors. Environmental activists band together in an effort to persuade governments and industries to curb the release of pollutants or to ban activities viewed as detrimental to survival of particular species of animal, plant, or of human beings. Groups of people act in unity to promote particular philosophies to which they are committed. They are passionate about their perspective, which they favor over other perspectives on life. All are relational systems or groups as explored in the Roy Adaptation Model.

Communities today both large and small face many demographic and societal changes, including the aging population, family breakdown, cultural integration, and transition in communities. These changes indicate that new ways of achieving relational adequacy through relational systems will be sought. Not all the outcomes produced by groups as relational systems contribute to the integrity of human systems. Some behaviors of groups may produce what the Roy Adaptation Model describes as ineffective relational interdependence adaptation. Consider the following examples. Young people, particularly boys, finding their place in society, tend to form gangs to fulfill their need for relational adequacy and security. They may be distant from their families and isolated by other cultural barriers. Such gangs become involved in illicit activities such as drug trafficking and other crimes. The notorious example of ineffective interdependence has been termed "9/11." On September 11, 2001, the world witnessed the carnage when 19 terrorists affiliated with al Qaeda hijacked four commercial passenger jet aircraft. Ineffective adaptation on the part of relations systems can result in horrific and detrimental outcomes for individuals, communities, and society as a whole. The interdependent outcome of these terrorist acts affected virtually all of humankind in one way or another.

Group relational systems can be viewed in terms of an interdependence model, adapted from Andrews and colleagues (1994). The model consists of three interrelated components: context, infrastructure, and member capability (Figure 20–1). These components

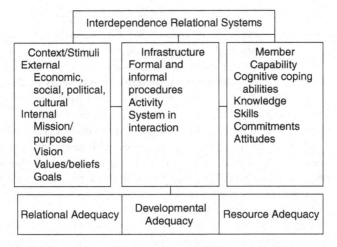

FIGURE 20–1   Interdependence Mode for groups. Theoretical basis.

provide important information for nursing assessment of behaviors and stimuli and for the other steps of the nursing process described in the Roy Adaptation Model. The *context* component is comprised of external and internal stimuli influencing the relational system. Similar to the physical mode of groups, from an interdependence perspective all groups or relational systems are influenced externally by economic, social, political, and cultural. Likewise, internally, the mission or purpose for existence of the group (its vision, that is, where it is headed), the associated values (those enduring beliefs, principles, or guidelines for action), as well as its goals (formalized or not), influence the actions and accomplishments of the group.

The *infrastructure* component relates to the processes involved in adaptation, that is, relational, developmental, and resource processes that exist within the group. These are the processes that affect adaptation levels. These processes involve formal or informal procedures, activity, and systems that are part of the interdependent interaction. For example, a funding agency may contract with several placement agencies to find homes to accommodate children in need, an activity with a related system. The placement agencies are subject to specific criteria to ensure the quality of the services they provide—a procedure. Further the placement families must undergo an evaluation process before they are accepted into the social service system, another set of procedures.

Groups and organizations proceed through developmental stages, as well. When they are forming, issues related to mission, vision, values, principles of operation, and initial plans must be addressed. A structure and its associated systems, processes, and procedures must be created and people must be in place to accomplish the objectives. As Smith and Berg (1990) described, groups struggle with ambivalence, contradiction, paralysis, and movement throughout the course of group life. A great deal is written about group effectiveness, productivity, and success. All of these processes relate to developmental adequacy. As noted in other adaptive modes, groups also are influenced by significant changes. Examples of such include mergers or separations, funding cutbacks, changes in leadership, or organizational problems in general.

The *member capability* component addresses the participants in the group and their cognitive coping abilities, such as knowledge level, skills, commitments, and attitudes. Knowledge, skills, commitments, and attitudes are important considerations in interdependent relationships of all descriptions, whether they are with significant others or support systems. Consider the example of an organization delivering primary health care to those in need in a developing country. Do the people receiving the aid have the necessary knowledge associated with cleanliness and the availability of potable water? Is there an understanding of the requirements for a balanced diet? Is access to nutritious foods a problem? Are the people welcoming of the aid or are the relief workers regarded with suspicion? Do the aid workers themselves have adequate knowledge of the local needs? Each of these questions illustrates the member capability component from the perspective of the interdependence mode of relating persons.

Another consideration when evaluating the effectiveness of these components in achieving the goals of the group and, ultimately, effective adaptation, is the congruence and alignment of these three interrelated components. Disruption occurs if any one component is not compatible with or does not complement the others. Ineffective adaptation is the outcome. For example, if a health care agency comes under scrutiny because of an outbreak of an infectious disease, the broader health care system experiences tumult and lack of integrity. If the example set by the hospital administration (member capability) differs from their instruction (context, values, and principles), the outcome will be ineffective adaptation. From the perspective of an organization, if its principles (context) advocate empowerment of staff and decentralized decision making (infrastructure), but the managers are not committed and do not demonstrate a supportive attitude (member capability), conflict will occur.

Coping processes, according to the Roy Adaptation Model, are innate or acquired ways of responding to a changing environment. The concepts of integrated, compensatory, and compromised coping processes can be applied to groups just as they are applied to persons as individuals. As previously described, the Roy Adaptation Model describes persons in groups, with coping processes acting to maintain adaptation. In all four adaptive modes, these concepts are applied to people functioning as individuals and to people in groups. Stimuli, internal and external to the group adaptive system, activate the group coping processes, the stabilizer and innovator. The responses can be either adaptive, thus promoting the integrity or wholeness of the group, or ineffective, not contributing to the goals of the group. As with adaptation level in the other modes, the Roy Adaptation Model describes three possible levels of the life processes from the interdependence perspective of groups: integrated, compensatory, and compromised.

INTEGRATED PROCESSES OF INTERDEPENDENCE IN GROUPS

At an integrated adaptation level, the structures and functions of the group processes are working as a whole to meet the needs of the system and promote adaptation. The three basic life processes of relational interdependence named in the Roy Adaptation Model are relational adequacy, developmental adequacy, and resource adequacy.

Relational Adequacy

Just as there are relational dynamics in friendships and families, relational dynamics are in all groups. Relational group dynamics are evident in communities, work settings, organizations, and other populations. On the broadest scale, relational dynamics exist in the relationship of humanity with creation as a whole. As noted in Chapter 16, interdependence needs are met through social interaction on many levels. From the individual perspective, relationships are developed with significant others and support systems. As the perspective broadens, extended families, clubs, networks, associations, organizations, corporations, and political parties, for example, occupy positions in interdependent relationships. Interdependent relationships, from the perspective of groups, are divided into two categories. Groups have significant others and support systems just as the individual in the interdependence mode. For groups, significant others are other groups to whom the most meaning or importance is given. Significant others for a group may be the government, the law enforcement agency, another gang, a God figure, a charitable organization, or the health care system, for example. These significant other groups are respected and valued, and in turn, they respect and value to a degree greater than in other relationships.

Significant others can be identified by noting the most important associations for a particular group. For most relational systems, the significant others are relatively stable for significant periods of time. For each group, there is usually at least one other group that is viewed as a significant other. For an agency that receives its funding from another organization, the funding agency is categorized as a significant other. Support systems include people, groups, and organizations with which a group associates to accomplish goals or to achieve some purpose. The meanings of relationships with support systems do not usually carry the same intensity as those of relationships with significant others. Consider the example of the nurses working in a particular specialty area confronted with a problem of infections among the patient population. The nurses may seek assistance from the infection control department and the housekeeping department in order to address the problem and develop a solution. Once the problem is resolved, the association continues to exist but, under normal circumstances, the relationship is more appropriately characterized as a support system.

Giving and receiving behavior are evident in relational group dynamics. For example, in return for time and application of knowledge, staff members receive a wage, educational benefits, opportunities to affiliate with others, and experience in their discipline of focus. From the nursing perspective, a nurse placement agency may contract with a hospital to provide replacement nursing services when additional staff is required. With respect to the placement agency, in return for a fee, that is, receiving behavior, the placement agency will locate and supply appropriately specialized nurses to meet the need, giving behavior. A group system may be associated with another relational system that assists in meeting the basic needs of relational, developmental, and resource adequacy. This assistance can take the form of family support systems, social service systems, and funding organizations, for example. Consider the system of child sponsorship in developing countries. Charitable organizations develop a network of people willing to provide financial support to enable children in developing countries to attend school, receive a nutritious meal each day, and have some health care services that they would not otherwise receive. In some situations, organizations are support systems for other organizations. The complex relationship between organized crime and legitimate business in some countries of the world is a relevant consideration. In this example, legitimate businesses contract with the criminal element for protection in return for a proportion of earnings. Without such an arrangement, the business would be unable to operate. Government subsidies for faltering businesses or service agencies could also be viewed as one organization providing for the basic needs of another organization in order to ensure continued operation.

Developmental Adequacy

Developmental adequacy refers to the processes associated with learning and maturation in groups. Groups each undergo development and transition in terms of dependence and independence throughout the life span. The appropriateness of this balance, as learning and maturation proceed, influences adaptation and the ability to achieve relational integrity. In an earlier chapter, the developmental processes associated with interdependent relationships for individuals were explored. Groups also proceed through developmental stages, as was discussed in looking at role function in groups. In the interdependence mode from the group perspective, the context, infrastructure, and member capability are important components. They are considered when defining the adaptation level of the group. The extent to which these develop as complementary and in alignment influences the effectiveness of the group in goal achievement. Within groups, isolated or as part of a larger entity, developmental stages have been described. Many are familiar with Tuckman and Jensen's (1977, p. 419) description of "forming, storming, norming, performing, and adjourning"—the stages of a relational system throughout its life span, as it becomes effective in accomplishing its goals and ultimately relinquishing its existence. Another approach to stages of group development (Worchel, 1996) was described in Chapters 18 and 19.

Several developmental perspectives have been applied to interrelationships in the workplace. Creative Nursing Management (1992) observed that employees progress developmentally in a cycle similar to that described by Erikson (1963). This suggests that leadership approaches will complement the employees' needs, requirements, and capabilities as they progress from being a novice with greater dependency to becoming more experienced, confident, and independent in their work. A well-known approach to examining development of nursing practice from novice to expert that can be helpful to nurses at all stages of their careers has been described by Benner (1984). There is much information in the literature about organizational development and group dynamics that is beyond the scope of this text. The reader is referred to sources on organizational behavior, organizational development, and group dynamics for a more in-depth understanding of the development of interrelationships and relational group systems as is needed for nursing practice.

Resource Adequacy

The third integrated life process associated with the basic need of relational integrity for groups is resource adequacy. Resource adequacy is defined as the relational system's need for resources such as physical space, funding, supplies, communication, and security. Resource adequacy is needed to achieve relational integrity. These resources are acquired through interdependent processes. A certain level of resources is necessary to support and maintain relationships and to enable groups to develop, mature, and achieve their mission. Unless resource requirements are met, a given group will struggle. It is often through interdependent relationships that these resource requirements are met. As noted in Chapter 16, in discussing the interdependence mode of individuals, Maslow (1954) outlined a hierarchy of needs—physiologic needs, safety needs, need for belongingness and love, and esteem needs. The needs are organized by the degree to which satisfaction of each is a prerequisite to the search for satisfaction of the next. This suggests that, unless the physiologic and safety requirements are met, the individual's attention is not directed toward higher order needs involving relationships with others. The application of this understanding to interdependence points to the importance of resource adequacy to support effectiveness in interdependence of groups. The implication is that physical needs of the group must be met before higher order needs can be addressed.

In groups and larger organizations there has been traditional emphasis on physical facilities, organizational structure, materials and supplies, and information processes as fundamental to effective functioning. Contemporary organizational theory is now recognizing and addressing the crucial aspect of effective relationships in the equation. Philosophic approaches such as quality management and organizational transformation are cases in point. The contemporary emphasis on the interrelationship of humanity with the environment broadens one's scope. Recognizing this complex integration and interdependence, social conscience regarding respect for and preservation of the environment has become a matter of substantial social concern. Protection of the environment, in its broadest sense, ultimately preserves and promotes resource adequacy and, in turn, the ability to satisfy basic physiologic and safety needs, so that higher order needs can be addressed.

Two factors that contribute to resource adequacy are financial resources and assisting relationships. Inadequate levels of financial resources compromise the ability of the group to continue to operate. In a family situation, if there is not an adequate income, it is difficult to provide for the family members. If an organization is not healthy financially, eventually, it will be unable to pay employees, purchase operating supplies, or, ultimately, remain in business. As noted in the physical mode for groups, capital resources are an important aspect of financial adequacy for most groups. Capital resources relate to the significant and infrequent purchases that can be required to support ongoing integrity of the relational system. In a family situation, this may be a major health care expenditure on behalf of a member or the purchase of a house for the family. For a group—a baseball team, for example—the purchase of uniforms may be the significant investment that enables the team to achieve its objectives. Organizations, communities, and societal groups often have major requirements for capital resources to support their ongoing and orderly operation. If inadequate funding persists over time, the integrity of the entire system is compromised and ineffective behaviors result. There is an abundance of literature that discusses group relationships and their effectiveness, organizational structure, problems, and keys to success. The reader is referred to sociology, psychology, and organizational literature for further information. When integrated adaptive processes of interdependence in groups are insufficient to maintain integrity and meet the needs of the relational system, compensatory adaptive processes come into play.

COMPENSATORY PROCESSES OF INTERDEPENDENCE IN GROUPS

Just as control processes are central to the functioning of individuals, control processes are inherent in the functioning of groups. With respect to relational systems, Roy and Anway (1989) categorized the control mechanisms as the stabilizer and the innovator subsystems to coincide with the regulator and cognator subsystems of the individual. At the compensatory level of adaptation, the stabilizer and innovator coping mechanisms are activated by a challenge to the integrated basic life processes. As noted, groups have two major goals, one related to stability, the other to change. Thus, the term stabilizer is used to refer to the structures and processes aimed at system maintenance. The stabilizer subsystem involves the concepts previously described as the context and infrastructure components of the relational system. The first subsystem described in the Roy Adaptation Model—the stabilizer subsystem—involves the established structures and daily activities whereby participants accomplish the primary purposes of the group and contribute to common purposes of society. For example, quality assessment processes within an organization function to ensure that the work being done and the products produced align with the standards described.

The second control process described by Roy relative to relational systems is the innovator subsystem. This subsystem involves the structures and processes for change and growth. The innovator subsystem involves cognitive and emotional strategies for change to higher levels of potential. For example, in organizations, strategic planning activities, think tanks, team-building sessions, and social functions constitute innovator strategies. Innovator compensatory processes associated with interdependence of groups may encompass involvement of significant others and support systems. For example, in 2000, three relational systems—the national health department in Canada (Health Canada, 2000, p. 7), a provincial health department, and the social planning council of a large city—gathered to establish priorities for spending of resources allocated to population health. Health Canada facilitated the discussions by commissioning a discussion paper on the topic of wellness (Andrews, 2000). This vehicle formed the basis for beginning discussions of resource allocation with a goal of innovation and interdependent involvement.

Social service programs have arisen in response to a need to provide assistance to groups to achieve relational integrity. As noted, relational integrity is comprised of relational adequacy, developmental adequacy, and resource adequacy. Agencies participating in and supporting such initiatives often include the business community, labor associations, school districts, and civic councils. There are numerous examples of business enterprises in specific communities funding a recreation center, with a goal of enhancing the level of health of those in the community. The profession of nursing, viewed as a group, provides a prime example of innovator activity. Sato and Senesac (2007) wrote on professional nursing in the year 2050. This paper was in response to Roy's (2000) challenge to nurse administrators to work toward the accomplishment of their desired futures. The authors provide examples of compensatory adaptive processes using innovator activity. When integrated and compensatory processes of relational interdependence are inadequate to promote effective or positive adaptation, an adaptation problem can result. The Roy Adaptation Model describes such situations as compromised adaptive processes.

COMPROMISED PROCESSES OF INTERDEPENDENCE IN GROUPS

Compromised processes of adaptation result from inadequate integrated and compensatory life processes, resulting in adaptation problems. Such problems become part of the nurse's consideration of the group having a compromised adaptation level. If the integrated and compensatory processes are unsuccessful in promoting adaptation, relational group problems occur. The result is isolation, inadequate development, and resource inadequacy. Not all possible adaptation problems are addressed in depth. Rather two examples of compromised processes of relational interdependence are presented, pollution and aggression.

Pollution

The adaptation problem of pollution represents a compromised process of group interdependence from the broad perspective of society as a whole. It was mentioned previously that relational integrity with the environment is vital to resource adequacy, particularly as it relates to basic physiologic and safety needs. Unfortunately, in many places of the world, pollution of the environment is causing significant resource and health concerns. Consider the following quotation related to a major nuclear plant disaster. McCullum (1996, p. 24) reported, "In addition to Chernobyl [the successor states have] ... other environmental problems to bear. Industrial areas suffer high levels of air and water pollution with resulting health-related problems. The infrastructure, such as the public water systems, is in a state of neglect, with disasters such as the breakage of the water filtration system in Kharkiv in June 1995, which resulted in sewage flowing into the city water system and the emergence of cholera." Other concerns relate to the purity of food, the conditions under which it is produced, shipped, and marketed. There are reports that bountiful crops fail to reach consumers because the mechanisms for shipment are inefficient and primitive. In many cities, water from the tap is not drinkable and water treatment systems are unreliable and rare. Speculations have been raised regarding the relationship of air quality to the incidence of respiratory disease evident in some populations. Other noncommunicable diseases are attributed to industrial hazards and contamination.

The foregoing provides examples of the interdependence adaptation problem of pollution and its impact on human groups. This situation is not unique to Eastern Europe. Pollution has become a major problem that is of concern beyond the boundaries of the countries affected. In fact, many modern industrialized countries are involved in international processes to determine how best to deal with the challenge of reversing the impact of pollution. Adaptation problems of societal proportions become issues for advanced nursing practice in collaboration with other disciplines. The Canadian Nurses Association (2005) prepared a background paper exploring the problem of pollution and its importance to nursing. Included was reference to 19 other organizations (relational systems or groups) involved in addressing the problem, as well.

Aggression—Group

Aggression has been described as the will of one person or group imposed on others, with the demand for obedience and compliance (Wheatley & Crinean, 2005). Other definitions of aggression refer to violent action, which is hostile and unprovoked; actions intended to harm the interests of others; and destructive behavior or actions. Consider the following description by Wheatley and Crinean (2005) of an aggressive society:

> These days, our senses are bombarded with aggression. We are constantly confronted with global images of unending, escalating war and violence. In our personal lives, we encounter angry people cursing into cell phones, watch TV talk shows where guests and audiences intimidate each other verbally and sometimes physically, or attend public meetings that disintegrate into shouting matches. Parents scream from the sidelines of their children's sports events: 'Get aggressive!' Employees are rewarded for aggressive timelines and plans. Dictionaries define *aggressive* action as hostile, but also positively as assertive, bold, and enterprising.
>
> Aggression destroys relationships. People believe that in order to survive, they must combat the opposition. Fear and anger destroy hope for healthy communities, workgroups, families, and organizations. Relationships fracture, distrust increases, people retreat into self-defense and isolation, paranoia becomes commonplace. (p. 2)

These authors pointed out that aggression within groups is on the rise, mirroring the societal trend. One particular example is familiar to those in the nursing profession and is termed "horizontal violence"—a concept that is introduced briefly to exemplify aggression as a compromised process of interdependence for groups. Horizontal violence is a situation where aggression, oppression, sabotage, and violence are directed at others within the same relational system or group. As Dunn (2003) noted, horizontal violence has been reported in the nursing literature for more than 20 years. Horizontal violence tends to emerge when a powerful and prestigious group controls and exploits a less powerful group. The exploited group feels powerless to confront the dominant group so the response is directed internally to the other members of the relational system.

Oppressed groups often exhibit self-hatred and dislike for members of their own group; the result is displaced and self-destructive aggression within the oppressed group. Aggression, from the perspective of groups, can be directed externally and can range from low-level group aggression such as gossiping, teasing, and swearing to mob aggression involving vigilantism, rioting, and lynching. The ultimate form of aggression is exemplified in the terrorist activities that are affecting so many parts of the world in the early twenty-first century. Having described the Roy Adaptation Model interdependence mode for groups, we now explore the nursing process as applied to group interdependence.

NURSING PROCESS RELATED TO GROUP INTERDEPENDENCE

As noted in all of Part 3 in situations of advanced nursing practice, the focus for care moves from individuals. Groups such as relational systems of families, communities, or even whole populations of people are the focus. In the delivery of nursing care to groups, the Roy Adaptation Model provides a framework for systematic nursing practice parallel to that described for the nursing care of individuals. As the six steps of the Roy Adaptation Model nursing process are presented, illustrations are provided from a variety of perspectives, one of which is population health. For purposes of this illustration, population health is described as "the interrelated conditions and factors that influence the health of populations over the life course. [It] identifies systematic variations in patterns of occurrence, and applies the resulting knowledge to develop and implement policies and actions to improve the health and well-being of those populations" (Advisory Committee on Population Health, 1999). Although it is profitable to consider all four adaptive modes in applying the nursing process to "population health," the focus in this chapter is on interdependent relationships from the perspective of group situations. Illustrations are hypothetical; they were created for descriptive purposes. They are simplistic examples that portray only small portions of very complex relational systems.

Assessment of Behavior

According to the Roy Adaptation Model, behavior is the indicator of how a human system copes or adapts in order to achieve its goals. The first step in the nursing process in the interdependence mode for groups involves gathering data about the behavior of the relational group and an initial judgment about the apparent level of adaptation. As previously presented, input, in the form of the internal and external stimuli, activates coping processes that function to maintain adaptation. The result is behavioral responses, which are identified as either adaptive or ineffective. The behavior promotes or disrupts, respectively, the goals of the group. For first-level assessment of groups in the interdependence mode, the behavior of initial concern relates to the status of the three basic life processes of relational interdependence—relationships, development state, and resources.

RELATIONSHIPS   The building blocks of interdependent relationships in groups are other groups, occupying positions of significant others or support systems. In first-level assessment, the nurse initially considers how the group fits into the bigger picture. What other groups are important in the function of the relational group of focus? Is the relational group part of a larger organization? With whom or what does the majority of interaction occur? Are other entities depending on the group for particular output? Does the group depend on other entities for particular input? Do the other groups function as significant others or support systems? Information such as this, in combination with the information associated with the second level of assessment, or stimuli, serves as a basis on which to determine the adaptation level of the relational system—be it integrated, compensatory, or compromised. In applying behavioral assessment of relationships to the example of population health, the nurse considers these questions and may identify that a number of organizations have an interest and involvement: the local government, the national health agency, the World Health Organization, for example. In addition, there may be a funding body concerned with keeping the population healthy and avoiding the costs associated with the treatment of illness.

The second consideration in the assessment of behaviors of the group is the receptive and contributive behaviors amongst the identified organization or group. What is received from each group? What is provided in return? For example, in a particular urban area, homeless people set up a "tent city." The urban area, in return, provided fencing around the compound and security personnel to enhance the level of safety in the settlement. The homeless people, in turn, agreed to work with the urban planners to address the problem of homelessness and find ways to provide more affordable housing.

DEVELOPMENTAL STATE   Of importance in the first level of assessment of the group is its current developmental state. At what stage is the family—childless, small children, teenagers, grown children? For a larger organization, a community for example, how long has it been in existence? Is it rigidly or loosely structured? Is transition occurring? Is it facing a crisis? From the perspective of the three relational system components, does the internal context reveal a shared mission, vision, and goals? Are they formal or informal? Is the infrastructure, in terms of relational, developmental, and resource processes, supportive of the developmental stage of the group? From the member capability perspective, what are the knowledge levels, skills, commitments, and attitudes of participants in the group? In the example of population health, do the groups have well-defined indicators of health? Is population health even a concern? For example, the Population Health Approach (Health Canada, 2000) noted that "the conceptualization of *determinants of health* remains problematic. Many categories overlap and the quality of evidence regarding the relationships between specific determinants and specific aspects of health is quite uneven" (p. 1111). This statement indicates that more developmental work is required with respect to determinants of health when considering the health of the population.

RESOURCES   From the perspective of resources, it is necessary for the nurse to establish the source of the resources supporting the activity of the group. Is the group self-funding? Does the government provide financial assistance? Is the group responsible for providing resources to others? Are the resources adequate to provide for the effective functioning for the relational system? From the population health perspective, the allocation of resources reflects the priorities of the relational systems involved. For example, the Government of Canada (2000) formulated the following vision statement with respect to health care resources: "Canadians will have publicly funded health services that provide quality health care and that promote the health and well-being of Canadians in a cost-effective and fair manner." From this statement, the nurse obtains an understanding of the stated priorities from the national perspective. The manner in which the funding is allocated by agencies responsible for dispensing the resources would either reflect the stated national priorities or not.

COPING PROCESS ACTIVITY   Further assessment of behavior of relational systems considers whether there is evidence of stabilizer or innovator activity. What actions are evidence of group maintenance? What are the established structures and processes? What are the activities whereby the participants accomplish the goals of the group? From the perspective of the innovator subsystem, what evidence is there of change and growth? In the population health arena, innovator activity was evident in a broad-based strategy known as the Verona Initiative (WHO/EURO, 1999). The aim of this project was to develop an understanding of how to invest to improve health at all levels in society. The project serves as an example of interdependent group innovator activity in an effort to address challenges with respect to population health. Once the behaviors are identified, a tentative judgment about whether they are adaptive or ineffective in terms of the goals of the group is made. In the second level of assessment according to the Roy Adaptation Model, the focus is on the factors that influence the behavior observed in the first level of assessment.

Assessment of Stimuli

Second level of assessment in the Roy Adaptation Model nursing process involves the identification of internal and external stimuli. Stimuli are assessed in relation to the behaviors identified in the first level of assessment. Behaviors of disrupted integrity, or the ineffective responses, are of initial concern, since the goal of nursing is to promote integrity. Adaptive behaviors also are important because they are to be maintained or enhanced. Once the stimuli are identified, the nurse classifies them as focal, contextual, or residual. As with other adaptive modes, behavior in one adaptive mode may act as a stimulus in another. In the interdependence mode of groups, there are common influencing stimuli, based on the Roy Adaptation Model description of interdependent relationships. The three components of the interdependence mode for relational systems provide a framework for the identification of the common influencing stimuli. In addition, the nurse considers the impact of other modes on integrity of interdependence for groups.

CONTEXT   In the context component, *external* stimuli stem from the economic, social, political, and cultural influences, for example, surrounding the relational system. What is the economic environment in which the relational system exists? Are there sufficient resources, monetary and otherwise, to support the purpose for which the group exists? For example, if a care center providing services for people with Alzheimer's disease does not have sufficient funding, the provision of appropriate staffing levels becomes impossible. However, if, from the social perspective, the citizens in the community are very committed to volunteerism, a shortage of staff may be mitigated for a period of time. From the interdependence perspective of population health, economic status impacts the extent to which one group can interact with others to address adaptation challenges. If funding is bare bones, there are few, if any, resources that can be directed towards addressing long-term issues with significant others and support systems.

As noted, the *internal* context encompasses the mission, vision, values, principles, goals, and plans of the group. Consider again the Alzheimer's unit. Perhaps one of the principles upon which the unit operates is family involvement. One would expect structures and processes to be in place to facilitate this involvement. Looking again at population health, each relational system that comprises or contributes to the health care system would have its own mission, vision, values, principles, goals, and plans. For initiatives to succeed in advancing population health, it is of utmost importance that each group's internal context align with, complement, and contribute to the goals and objectives directed at achievement of health for the population. If the vision of the health care system is focused on health promotion, that initiative should be reflected in the activities of the other relational systems that are part of the same system.

INFRASTRUCTURE   As described previously, the infrastructure consists of formal and informal procedures, activity, and systems. For example, if the staff members in the Alzheimer's unit were not supportive and encouraging of family members, this would serve to defeat the informal procedure of involving family members in the care and support of the unit. In the population health example, from the interdependence perspective, there would be a need for effective channels to assist in communicating the activity of health promotion and activities to involve the participating groups in determining how health promotion would be reflected in the initiatives of each organization. The developmental stage of the relational system, in addition to being a behavior of concern, also is important as a stimulus. Has the organization existed for an extended period? Are the processes and procedures entrenched? Or, is the group a newly constituted body that is just beginning to formalize its structures and processes? Is the group going through a period of change?

Developmental stage is a significant influence for interdependence, as for role function, on the effectiveness of how the group achieves its goals and promotes adaptation. Although the population health initiative has been on the agenda of the World Health Organization for many decades, for some countries, the health of the population is not a consideration. This is particularly the case where the country is ravaged by wars and internal conflicts. In these cases, survival is the primary focus and health promotion is not yet on the agenda. This is an example of how system developmental stage influences the health of a population.

System, resources, and interactions are further infrastructure considerations in second-level assessment. Within the infrastructure, there are resource processes that are important stimuli affecting groups. For example, there may be an indication that the financial resources are not being used as intended. Many organizations have experienced a problem with dishonest use of funds by an individual with access to the organization's resources. What are the resource processes in place to ensure that this does not happen? For groups where resources are tied to the national or local economy, a downturn in the economy usually means funding cutbacks. How does the organization respond to such circumstances? From the population health perspective, what impact does the adequacy of resources demonstrate? For some health care organizations, the health promotion activities associated with population health are the first to be cut if resources are limited. This is a short-sighted approach because the long-term impact of inadequate health promotion on the health care expenditures over time is not considered.

MEMBER CAPABILITY   Member capability refers to the knowledge, skills, commitments, and attitudes of the members of the group. Are people committed to the internal context, that is, mission, vision, values, principles, goals, and plans of the organization? Knowledge about relationships was presented in Chapter 16 for the interdependence mode from the perspective of the individual. From the perspective of groups, knowledge about organizational transition is an important influence within relational systems. As more is understood by the members about group dynamics and factors that influence these, development in organizations and other groups becomes more effective and efficient. From the perspective of population health, member capability can be viewed as the knowledge and understanding of those in groups about the parameters involved in population health. Are groups committed to improving the health of the population? Are the indicators of population health acknowledged and understood? Is there commitment to the priorities? Unless there is alignment of all the groups involved in contributing to population health, the progress towards the goals will be compromised.

INTEGRITY IN OTHER MODES   Just as for individual interdependence, integrity in the other modes may serve as a stimulus for interdependence in groups. If physical integrity is disrupted, for example, the group no longer has access to a facility in which to function; there is disruption in the interdependence mode, as well. If there is a problem with group identity, this may in turn cause a problem with relational integrity. For example, family members hold perceptions of how successful or dysfunctional they are. Association members feel adequate or inadequate in terms of the mission and objectives of their group. School spirit is regarded as an indicator of the group identity of the associated body of students. In some cases it is described as perceptible on entering the doors of the school. Staff in certain hospitals, and perhaps the larger community, view certain health care agencies as flagships for the industry. Each of these illustrates group identity, which in turn affects the developmental adequacy of the relating group. Related to population health, a disruption of physical integrity causes an impact on interdependent relationships. Consider the situation in 2005 when Hurricane Katrina caused its devastation along the north-central Gulf Coast of the United States. The population health concerns that ensued prompted the involvement of other groups. From an interdependence perspective, other groups such as the American Red Cross, the Canadian Armed Forces, the Salvation Army, Habitat for Humanity, and many other charitable organizations became involved, providing housing, food, and water to the hurricane victims.

Consider the following example of second-level assessment. Niska (2001) conducted an ethnographic study focused on the factors contributing to family survival, continuity, and growth in Mexican American families using the Roy Adaptation Model. She suggested that the transactional processes evident in family dynamics coincided with relational interdependence. Amongst the factors that families affirmed as essential for family survival were "having supportive parents," "having a steady job," and "having civic harmony," each of which could be characterized as illustrative of interdependence stimuli affecting adaptation within the relational system of the family.

As the various stimuli are identified, the nurse classifies them as focal, contextual, or residual. For example, if a hospital is informed by its funding agency of a budget cut, that information becomes a focal influence that requires action. A residual stimulus may be members' recollection of unpleasant situations when budget trimming was required in the past. Once the second level of assessment has been completed and the factors influencing adaptation have been identified, the nurse proceeds to the third step of the nursing process—nursing diagnosis.

Nursing Diagnoses

The third step of the nursing process as described in the Roy Adaptation Model involves the formulation of nursing diagnoses. As explained in Chapter 3, the nursing diagnosis is an interpretive statement about the individual or group. This interpretation is accomplished by considering the behaviors, as assessed in the first level of assessment, in conjunction with the stimuli affecting those behaviors, as assessed in the second level of assessment. The formulation of nursing diagnoses associated with interdependence in groups is accomplished in the same ways as in the other modes. One method involves the statement of the behaviors together with their influencing stimuli. The second approach is to use summary labels. As with each of the other modes, the Roy Adaptation Model identifies a typology of indicators of positive adaptation together with a typology of commonly recurring adaptation problems.

Consider a hypothetical situation that could have occurred in 2005 at the time of Hurricane Katrina. A particular care agency decided not to evacuate when the state order was declared. This caused a dilemma for groups focused on rescue and evacuation. An example of a nursing diagnosis formulated according to the statement of behavior and influencing stimuli is "Agency plans to not evacuate in conflict with the state-issued directive of total evacuation." The behavior is the position of the care agency, and the influencing stimulus is the order to evacuate.

The Roy Adaptation Model names three *positive indicators* of adaptation with respect to the interdependence mode of groups. These stem directly from the previously described integrated adaptation processes: relational adequacy, developmental adequacy, and resource adequacy (Table 20–1). Suppose that the hypothetical care agency mentioned above explained that they had a 2-week supply of water, food, and products with which to care for their totally bedridden patient population, that the staff was planning to remain, and that the family members all agreed that it was best not to move the patients. Perhaps a nursing diagnosis relating to this situation could be "Resource adequacy related to a 2-week inventory of supplies." The term "resource adequacy" is a summary statement that encompasses food, water, staff, and provisions. The 2-week inventory represents the infrastructure factor related to resource processes. In terms of *adaptation problems* pertaining to the interdependence mode of groups, the Roy Adaptation Model names five: isolation, ineffective development, inadequate resources, pollution, and

TABLE 20–1 Nursing Diagnostic Categories for Relational Interdependence

Positive Indicators of Adaptation	Common Adaptation Problems	NANDA Diagnostic Labels
• Relational adequacy • Developmental adequacy • Resource adequacy	• Isolation • Ineffective development • Inadequate resources • Pollution • Aggression	• Readiness for enhanced community coping • Ineffective community coping • Dysfunctional family processes: alcoholism • Interrupted family processes

aggression. The first three reflect ineffective adaptation of relational integrity, and the fourth and fifth serve to illustrate significant relational interdependence adaptation problems.

We can look again at the hypothetical example of the care agency and Hurricane Katrina. After the storm, the destruction was assessed to be far greater than anticipated. It is determined that the emergency power generators may not be sufficient in light of the damage to physical facilities and infrastructure damage to public services. Perhaps all five adaptation problems would serve as a nursing diagnosis portraying the extent of the problem. The influencing factor would be the destruction to the local infrastructure—a component of an associated relational system. In Table 20–1, the Roy Adaptation Model nursing diagnostic categories for the integrated and compromised processes of relational interdependence are shown in relation to nursing diagnosis labels approved by the North American Nursing Diagnosis Association (NANDA International, 2007). Once nursing diagnoses are formulated, the nurse proceeds to the fourth step of the nursing process—goal setting.

Goal Setting

As noted previously, each step of the Roy Adaptation Model nursing process focuses on the group's behavior, the stimuli influencing that behavior, or both. With the nursing diagnosis, the statement developed included both behavior and stimuli. With the goal-setting step, the focus is on behavior. Each goal identifies a behavior that is to be addressed. As with other group adaptive modes, many group interdependence problems have a chronic as well as an acute phase. Thus, the goal-setting process includes both long- and short-term goals, each of which states the behavior of focus, the change expected, and the time frame in which the goal is to be achieved. Considering the hypothetical example of the care agency in the wake of Hurricane Katrina, a short-term goal with respect to the previously described situation might focus on the supply of water: "Within 1 hour, 1 day's supply of bottled water will be airlifted to the agency." The behavior of focus is the supply of water, the change expected is the "1-day's supply", and the time frame is "within 1 hour." In this situation, an adaptation problem in the area of inadequate resources is addressed. A longer term goal may be "Within 1 week, a specified relief agency will provide supplies to the care agency." The behavior is the availability of supplies, the change expected is a specific source of the supplies, and the time frame is "within 1 week." This goal could be characterized as addressing the adaptation problem of "isolation."

In order to be effective in guiding the progress of providing care, goals must be established in collaboration with the groups involved. As with each step of the nursing process, system members must be active participants to ensure that accurate and relevant information is obtained, that it is interpreted appropriately into nursing diagnoses, and that achievable and relevant goals are established. This is the only way that interventions can be planned that will assist in achieving relational integrity. After formulating goals, the nurse proceeds to the identification of nursing interventions, the next step of the nursing process as described in the Roy Adaptation Model.

Intervention

The intervention step of the nursing process according to the Roy Adaptation Model focuses on the stimuli affecting the behavior identified in the goal-setting step. The intervention step is thus the management of stimuli, and this involves altering, increasing, decreasing, removing, or maintaining them. In the previously mentioned goal "Within 1 week, a specified relief agency will be providing supplies to the care agency," the factor influencing the provision of supplies is the identification of an appropriate source of what is needed. The focus of the intervention activities would be to locate an organization with the ability to provide the necessary supplies for the agency. Perhaps discussions with a particular charitable organization would be necessary. Once a source for the supplies is located, an interdependent relationship would be established to assist with the situation. The intervention would focus on ensuring the availability of the necessary supplies. This is a simplistic example of an interdependent relationship aimed at fulfilling the requirement for resource adequacy.

Returning to the example of population health, consider the situation where a problem with childhood obesity is identified for a particular population of people. Assume that assessment of the member capability component reveals that there is a lack of understanding on the part of children as to the health problems associated with unhealthy eating patterns. If the goal is focused on a change in eating habits, the intervention planned is education of children; perhaps an interdependent relationship between the health care system and the school system would serve to work toward a solution to the problem. The intervention is directed at a particular influencing factor, that is, lack of understanding. The vehicle is an interdependent relationship between two groups. The above interventions focus on stimuli (source of resources, environmental influences, and knowledge levels) that are contributing to interdependence problems for the groups involved. The next step of the Roy Adaptation Model nursing process—evaluation—returns to focus on the behaviors evident in the resulting situation.

Evaluation

Evaluation involves judging the effectiveness of the nursing interventions in relation to the group's adaptive behavior. That is, we ask whether the behaviors stated in the goals have been achieved. The nursing interventions are effective if the behavior is in accordance with the stated goal. If the goal has not been achieved, the nurse identifies alternative interventions or approaches by reassessing the behavior and stimuli and continuing with the other steps of the nursing process. In considering the previously identified goal, the lack of supplies is the behavior of concern. Once the interventions have been accomplished, the success of the plan is evident in whether the lack of supplies has been alleviated. Does the agency have an ongoing source of supplies? Is another shortage anticipated? With respect to the population health example, are children demonstrating wiser choices with respect to the types of food they select and the amount they eat? Is the average weight for specific age groups decreasing? It is important to recognize that the nursing process and the six steps are ongoing, simultaneous, and overlapping. Although they have been simplified, separated, and dealt with in an artificially linear manner for discussion purposes, often intervention is occurring at the same time that first- and second-level assessment is proceeding. Likewise, evaluation occurs on an ongoing basis, being held in mind even when nursing diagnoses are being established and as goals are being formulated.

Summary

This chapter has focused on the application of the Roy Adaptation Model to the interdependence mode of groups. An overview of the three processes, relational adequacy, developmental adequacy, and resource adequacy, associated with relational integrity, was provided. Compensatory responses related to relational interdependence were illustrated and examples of two compromised processes, pollution and aggression, were discussed. Finally, guidelines for planning nursing care through first- and second-level assessment, the formulation of nursing diagnoses, goals, and interventions were explored and evaluation of nursing care was described.

Exercises for Application

1. In relation to an organization that you are familiar with, identify the external factors (context) that influence the function and interrelations of the organization.
2. What is the mission and vision (context) associated with your educational institution?
3. Think of a nursing unit on which you have worked. Identify as many relational group systems as you can that have an impact on the activity of the unit.

Assessment of Understanding

QUESTIONS

1. The basic need of the interdependence mode for relating persons is _____ _____ which is viewed as consisting of _____, _____, and _____ adequacy.
2. Which of the following are important first-level assessment behaviors for the interdependence mode of relating persons?
   (a) _____ disease processes
   (b) _____ significant others
   (c) _____ coping process activity
   (d) _____ vital signs
   (e) _____ developmental state
   (f) _____ support systems
3. Name three stimuli that influence relational system behavior in the interdependence mode of relating persons.
   (a) _____
   (b) _____
   (c) _____
4. Name three integrated life processes of relational interdependence and provide an illustration of each from the perspective of the family.
   (a) _____
   (b) _____
   (c) _____
5. Situation:
   An industrial work site has experienced five work-related accidents in 2 days associated with the operation of all-terrain vehicles (ATVs). Provide an example of an approach to the problem by the industrial health nurse that would be illustrative of an innovator compensatory process.
   _____
6. List two compromised processes of relational interdependence.
   (a) _____
   (b) _____

SITUATION:

Ten people are now dead, and dozens remain in regional hospitals, as Smallville, USA, deals with a town water supply contaminated by *E. coli* bacteria. Hundreds of others are sick with gastrointestinal symptoms, and it could be another week before Smallville residents can drink tap water safely again. A "boil water" advisory has been issued and schools will remain closed for the rest of this week at least.

7. Formulate a nursing diagnosis for the above situation using each of the two methods described in this chapter.
   (a) _____
   (b) _____
8. Construct a short-term goal and a long-term goal with respect to the situation described above.
   (a) Short-term _____
   (a) Long-term _____
9. Since interventions are focused on stimuli, what interventions could be used to alleviate the situation described above, considering the following stimuli:
   (a) Contamination of town water supply
   _____
   (b) Supply of drinking water
   _____
   (c) Source of contamination
   _____
10. How would you evaluate achievement of one of the goals you established in item 8?

FEEDBACK

1. relational integrity, relational, developmental, resource
2. b, c, e, f

3. (a) Any three of: context, infrastructure, member capability, integrity in other modes.
4. (a) relational adequacy—family has significant others and support systems,
    (b) developmental adequacy—parents demonstrate knowledge and behavior appropriate to the ages of their children.
    (c) resource adequacy—family has sufficient resources to provide for the needs of the family.
5. The occupational health nurse could convene a meeting of the workers to generate ideas directed at increased safety when using ATVs for work.
6. Any two of isolation, ineffective development, inadequate resources, aggression, and pollution.
7. Examples of nursing diagnoses:
    (a) Multiple cases of *E. coli* infection due to contaminated water supply (behavior and relevant stimuli)
    (b) Pollution (summary label)
8. Examples of goals:
    (a) Within the next day, there will be no new reported cases of *E. coli* infection. (short-term goal)

    (b) Within 2 hours, residents will have a clean supply of water. (short-term goal)
    (c) Within 1 week, the water supply will test free of *E. coli*. (long-term goal)
9. Examples of interventions related to the stimuli identified could include:
    (a) Contaminated water supply: Communicate an alert to residents of the community to boil their water before drinking, cooking, washing, or bathing.
    (b) Supply of drinking water: Provide a supply of bottled drinking water to the residents of the community.
    (c) Source of contamination: Identify the source of the contamination in order to rectify the problem.
10. The goals would have been achieved if the following behaviors were evident:
    (a) By the next day, no new cases were reported.
    (b) Within 2 hours, affected residents were provided bottled drinking water.
    (c) Within 1 week, the water supply was approved for human consumption.

References

Advisory Committee on Population Health. (1999). *Toward a healthy future: Second report on health of Canadians.* Ottawa: Minister of Public Works and Government Services Canada.

Andrews, H. A. (2000). *Wellness: Towards a shared understanding* (pp. 1–43). A discussion paper prepared for the Consultation on Priorities Alberta section of the Population Health Fund. Health Canada Population and Public Health Branch.

Andrews, H. A., Cook, L. M., Davidson, J. M., Schurman, D. P., Taylor, E. W., & Wensel, R. H. (Eds.). (1994). *Organizational transformation in health care: A work in progress.* San Francisco: Jossey-Bass.

Benner, P. (1984). *From novice to expert: Excellence and power in clinical nursing practice.* Menlo Park, CA: Addison-Wesley.

Canadian Nurses Association. (2005). *The ecosystem, the natural environment, and health and nursing: A summary of the issues* (pp. 1–8). CAN Backgrounder. Ottawa: Canadian Nurses Association.

Creative Nursing Management. (1992). *Leaders empower staff.* Minneapolis, MN: Creative Nursing Management.

Dunn, H. (2003). Horizontal violence among nurses in the operating room. *AORN Journal, 78*(6), 977–980, 982, 984–988.

Erikson, E. H. (1963). *Childhood and society* (2nd ed.). New York: Norton.

Government of Canada. (2000). Communique on Health. Press release. Ottawa: Government of Canada, first Ministers' Meeting, September 11.

Hanna, D., & Roy, C. (2001). Roy Adaptation Model and Perspectives on the Family. *Nursing Science Quarterly, 14*(10), 9–13.

Health Canada. (2000). *Population health in Canada: A working paper. V. Definitional issues in health and social impact assessments for population health.* Health Canada: population health approach.

Maslow, A. H. (1954). *Motivation and personality.* New York: Harper & Row.

McCullum, R. (1996). Vision of a new health system for Ukraine. *Canada–Ukraine Monitor, 4*(1), 24.

NANDA International. (2007). *Nursing diagnoses: Definitions and classifications, 2007–2008.* Philadelphia: NANDA-I.

Niska, K. J. (2001). Mexican American family survival, continuity, and growth: The parental perspective. *Nursing Science Quarterly, 14*(4), 322–329.

Roy, C. (2000). A theorist envisions the future and speaks to nursing administrators. *Nursing Administration Quarterly 24*(2), 1–12.

Roy, C., & Anway, J. (1989). Roy's Adaptation Model: Theories and propositions for administration. In B. Henry, C. Arndt, M. DeVincenti, & A. Marriner-Tomey (Eds.), *Dimensions and issues of nursing administration.* St. Louis, MO: Mosby.

Sato, M. K., & Senesac, P. M. (2007). Imagining nursing practice: The Roy Adaptation Model in 2050. *Nursing Science Quarterly, 20*(47), 47–50.

Smith, K. K., & Berg, D. N. (1990). *Paradoxes of group life: Understanding conflict, paralysis, and movement in group dynamics.* San Francisco: Jossey-Bass.

Tuckman, B. W., & Jensen, M. A. (1977). Stages of small group revisited. *Group and Organization Studies, 2*(4), 419–427.

Wheatley, M. J., & Crinean, G. (2005). Transforming aggression into creative problem solving. *Leader to Leader, 36*(Spring), 19–28.

Worchel, S. (1996). Emphasizing the social nature of groups in a developmental framework. In J. L. Nye & A. M. Brower (Eds.), *What's social about social cognitions? Research on socially shared cognition in small groups* (pp. 261–281). Thousand Oaks, CA: Sage Publications.

WHO/EURO. (1999). *The Verona Benchmark I: System characteristics for implementation of investment for health approaches.* Copenhagen: World Health Organization Regional Office for Europe.

PART FOUR

Applications of the Roy Adaptation Model

The Roy Adaptation Model has been described throughout this text as a systematic framework for nursing practice. It provides the focus for knowledge relevant to nursing by taking a given approach to understanding people and their environments in ways that promote health. Part 4 focuses on the application of the model in three important areas. Chapter 21 begins with first looking at applications to nursing practice. The variety and scope of projects to apply the model in health care agencies at the unit or organizational levels are discussed. Examples of published papers that describe practice applications in a range of patient and group situations are given. The major project of the process and outcomes of implementing the Roy Adaptation Model as a basis for nursing practice at St. Joseph Regional Medical Center in Lewiston, Idaho, is described in greater detail.

Based on the dramatic impact of technology developments in health care, the second major section of the chapter focuses on the electronic healthcare record (EHR) as a significant contemporary application in nursing practice. The evolution of computers and informatics in nursing is described along with issues of nursing language. The reader's understanding will be enriched by seeing specific examples of application of the Roy Adaptation Model in the EHR based on work of colleagues in the Roy Adaptation Association of Japan.

The final section of Chapter 21 deals with research based on the Roy Adaptation Model. A perspective on model-based nursing research as involving both basic science and clinical science is presented. Then a description is provided of how 30 years of research based on the Roy Adaptation Model, that is, 218 studies published in the English language, was used to contribute to the movement of evidence-based practice. The approach was to redefine evidence-based practice and to develop strategies for cumulative knowledge. Common propositions based on the model are tested in multiple studies. This approach provides support for use of specific knowledge in practice. Examples of practice-level knowledge are provided. The closing section is a discussion of issues and future directions in the applications of the Roy Adaptation Model.

CHAPTER 21

Applications of the Roy Adaptation Model

The main purpose of any nursing model is to guide nursing practice. For the individual nurse applying the Roy Adaptation Model, this means using the knowledge of the model to assess individuals and groups, their adaptive and ineffective behaviors and the stimuli affecting them as well as their level of adaptation. In collaboration with individuals and groups, diagnoses are identified, goals set, interventions selected, and ways to evaluate effectiveness of care are determined. There are many other ways in which the model is used to improve practice. One use of the model is as the basis of the patient care services in institutions. The computerized medical record is part of practice environments. The model can guide development of computerized nursing language. Another important use of the Roy Adaptation Model is to develop the knowledge for practice in programs of research. Findings from research can be synthesized into theory-based evidence for practice. This chapter briefly describes examples of some of these applications.

Health care is experiencing unprecedented change and ever-increasing complexity, and cost issues. Expectations for high-quality, affordable, effective, and coordinated care and services are evident in both consumer and provider groups. Parker (2006) noted that, in addition to guiding practice, nursing theory "can stimulate creative thinking, facilitate communication and clarify purposes and relationships in practice" (p. 10). This creative thinking, clear purpose, and communication are even more relevant in multidisciplinary approaches to care delivery. The examples provided show how nursing based on a clear concept of the discipline can contribute to solving issues in today's health care.

OBJECTIVES

After studying this chapter, the reader will be able to:

1. Describe the potential benefits of model-based nursing practice.
2. Describe one application of the Roy Adaptation Model to a nursing practice setting.
3. Provide a rationale for nurses being involved in the development of the electronic healthcare record.

4. Identify one way that the Roy Adaptation Model can be applied to the electronic healthcare record.

5. Relate theory to research in knowledge development for nursing.

6. Classify approaches to research based on the Roy Adaptation Model.

7. Relate synthesis of research based on the Roy Adaptation Model to evidence-based practice.

KEY CONCEPTS DEFINED

Basic nursing science: Understanding of the basic life processes that promote health.

Clinical nursing science: Understanding how people as adaptive systems cope with health and illness and what can be done to promote adaptive coping.

Deductive: Using a general theory to provide a tentative hypothesis for a given situation.

Evidence-based practice: An approach to apply research in nursing practice to ensure that patients receive care that is based on the strongest possible base of knowledge.

Inductive: Identifying individual experiences that can be interpreted to provide generalizations of human experiences.

Informatics: The study of information.

Informatics competencies: Learning of both cognitive and interactive components for electronic approaches to facilitating patient care; five subject areas are suggested for developing: (1) basic concepts and applications, (2) accessing information systems, (3) utilizing data and information systems, (4) coordinating and evaluating data and information systems, and (5) integrating nursing informatics.

Model-based nursing practice: A nursing model provides structure for thinking about patient care and offers the opportunity for designing a structured, organized approach to patient care delivery, with the potential for increased efficiency and effectiveness; has benefits for both nurses and patients.

Planned change: Strategic actions toward desired objectives.

Qualitative research: Views reality as emerging and relative; approach is inductive.

Quantitative research: Views reality as discovered and measured; approach is deductive.

Standardized nursing terminologies: Include reference and interface terminologies and minimum data sets or frameworks for the inclusion in electronic healthcare records to support documentation of clinical care; ANA-listed, recognized terminologies.

Subsidiarity: Calls for vesting decision making, authority, and responsibility as close as possible to the point where the impact of the decision will be felt and at the point where individuals are most competent to make the decision.

Vision: the opportunity to turn the kaleidoscope of the past and the present to a new view of the future.

APPLICATIONS IN PRACTICE

The heritage of nursing as a profession involves a commitment to the value of providing care for people from a holistic perspective. A potential benefit of using the Roy Adaptation Model is that it provides a structure for thinking about people and their care in a holistic way. An adaptive system that is affected by a changing environment is a holistic view. Further, the model becomes the lens through which we view what is relevant to nursing. The model provides the categories for nursing assessment for both individuals and groups. The four adaptive modes and three levels of adaptation provide a focus for nursing observations. The goal to promote adaptation signifies what are the issues of concern in practice. The understanding of adaptation processes affected by three types of stimuli provides a way to organize the work of holistic and comprehensive nursing care for people. The model provides the language to describe what nurses do. Through the use of the Roy model, health care facilities can clarify the role of the nurse as a health care provider. This clarity strengthens interdisciplinary collaboration and effectiveness in the organization and delivery of health care. The use of the model assists in organizing the components of a complex health care system while centering service on each individual as a whole person. In this way enhanced outcomes associated with care delivery are possible.

According to Weiss et al. (1994), a model provides a structure for thinking about patient care and direction for organizing nursing work focused on comprehensive and holistic care for patients and families. Model-based nursing practice results in a systematic approach to organizing knowledge, so that the art and science of nursing is orderly and logical. Use of models has extended beyond nursing education and research to clinical practice settings. The clinical application of a model improves nursing practice by the integration of theory into the everyday processes of patient care and nursing administration (Allison, McLaughlin, & Walker, 1991; Rogers et al., 1991; Weiss, Hastings, Holly, & Craig, 1994). Model implementation offers the opportunity for designing a structured, organized approach to patient care delivery, with the potential for increased efficiency and effectiveness. A nursing model also assists in defining nursing roles and goals, identifying essential elements for patient databases, prescribing assessment parameters, directing nursing interventions, and providing the means for effective communication in and about nursing practice (Mayberry, 1991).

Nurses have found that model-based practice benefits both nurses and patients (Mastal, Hammond, & Roberts, 1982). The experience of Rogers et al. (1991) revealed that, although the model implementation process is complex and extensive, many beneficial outcomes are achieved. A primarily potential benefit is the clear expression in practice of nursing values, beliefs, and assumptions related to people, health, environment, and nursing.

Implementation Projects

In 2003 Senesac provided a review of published projects to implement the Roy Adaptation Model in institutional practice settings. The author identified seven distinct projects. See Table 21–1 for listing of projects by author(s), year, and focus. The projects range from ideology for a single unit to hospital-wide projects. In some cases the published project developed from a unit implementation to a full agency implementation, as in one of the early projects reported by Mastal, Hammond, and Roberts (1982). The first edition of this text included a report of implementation projects by Gray (1991). She discussed involvement in five projects, but not all completed implementation due to changes in hospital management, philosophy, or direction. Gray's initial work was at a 132-bed acute care, not-for-profit children's hospital. Others varied from a 100-bed proprietary hospital to a 248-bed nonprofit, community-owned hospital. The main focus of the implementation projects was to improve patient care through quality nursing care plans and in some cases to develop performance standards. Moreno-Ferguson (2007) reported on two implementation projects in Colombia. One was at an ambulatory rehabilitation service (Moreno-Ferguson, 2001) and the other a pediatric intensive care unit of a cardiology institute (Monroy et al., 2003).

TABLE 21–1 Implementation Projects Using the Roy Adaptation Model in Practice

Author(s) and Year of Publication	Setting	Focus
Nyqvist & Sjoden, 1993	Neonatal Intensive Care Unit	To provide ideology for nursing
Lewis, 1988	Acute Surgical Ward	To document compliance with the nursing process
Mastal, Hammond, & Roberts, 1982	An 18-bed unit in a rehabilitation facility	To integrate the professional basis of patient care
Weiss, Hastings, Holly, & Craig, 1994	Two units of a general hospital	To guide practice and as an integral part of a shared governance strategy
Rogers et al., 1991	A 125-bed orthopedic hospital	To facilitate an integrated system of nursing
Frederickson, 1991, 1993	A neurosurgical unit	To establish a professional practice environment for student training, enhance professional autonomy, and aid recruitment and retention of staff
Connerley, Ristau, Lindberg, & McFarland, 1999	A 145-bed general service hospital	To increase clarity in provider roles and strengthen interdisciplinary collaboration and effectiveness

Derived from: Senesac, P. (2003). Implementing the Roy Adaptation Model: From theory to practice. *Roy Adaptation Association Review, 4*(2), p. 7.

One of the projects Senesac identified was reported by Connerley and colleagues (1999) in the second edition of this text. The authors described the process and outcomes of implementing the Roy Adaptation Model as a basis for nursing practice at a 145-bed, nonprofit, full-service health care facility located in a rural environment. This project will be described in greater detail as reported by the authors. Services include traditional inpatient programs and diagnostic services, as well as trauma, oncology, home care, mental health, and subacute services. The hospital used a participatory leadership and management style and embraced the leadership precepts of collaboration, subsidiarity, accountability, and commitment to continuous improvement. Connerley and colleagues noted that the process of implementation of a model is a major undertaking requiring commitment and perseverance. To achieve full internalization required a period of several years.

REQUIREMENTS FOR SUCCESS Successful model implementation requires the presence of multiple positive conditions and the use of a variety of strategies and processes to support change. Paramount among these is support and recognition of the value of defining the role of nursing in the organization. Other factors include recognition of value, education, model selection, commitment and support, vision, the change process, environmental factors, and systems approach. An environment of trust needs to be pervasively present for nurses and other caregivers to make major changes in role interpretation, expression, and approach to practice. Traditional patterns of role enactment are reconstructed in the change to a model-based practice. The understanding and valuing of a model for practice is often present in nurses who have had exposure to advanced practice concepts; however, many nurses have a limited understanding of the utility of a model beyond the academic setting. A perception may be that models are disruptive, unnecessary, time-consuming, or useless. This can contribute to negativism when a nursing model is introduced. As Grahame (1987) observed, responses can include blocking implementation of the model, returning to practice as usual, or making humorous remarks about the model.

A variety of educational activities prior to the formal implementation effort is vital to ensure that nurses have opportunities to gain knowledge and form positive attitudes about models and the benefits of model application in practice. Such educational efforts require careful timing and communication of all activities to support successful implementation. It is essential that the nurses are involved in selection of the appropriate model. There must be consideration of model suitability in terms of involved areas of service and potential applications. Far more important is ensuring that the model is congruent with the mission, philosophy, values, and culture of the organization. Acceptability of the concepts and terminology by nurses and other providers will be considered, as well, in order to avoid jargon that may have little meaning to nurses or other health care disciplines.

Mayberry (1991) suggested that success or failure of implementation can be linked to the commitment and support given to the full range of implementation activities and to the clarity and sincerity of communication about the chosen model. With rapid change occurring in health care, the strong belief that a model will serve as a stabilizing environmental force will be emphasized. As this belief is shared by management and a core of care providers, the leaders of the model implementation project will be able to generate enthusiasm, participative energy, and support in the application of the model. Early demonstration that the model is an asset in designing and organizing approaches to the delivery of patient care is necessary to maintain the commitment for practice transformation.

Connerley and colleagues (1999) noted that transformation frequently occurs because of vision and visionary leadership. McFarland (1993) described vision as the opportunity to turn the kaleidoscope of the past and the present to a new view of the future. This new view helps to develop and clarify the goals and specify the means for accomplishing organizational objectives (Robbins & Duncan, 1987). The vision of the formal leader is essential for achievement of any planned change, including successful model implementation. Visionary leadership helps to actualize the vision by allowing it to drive the agenda of change including the allocation of resources (McFarland, 1993). Kouzes and Posner (1993) pointed, as well, to the importance of credibility and acceptance of the leadership—when present, they stimulate others to give more of their time, talent, and support. The nursing management team at this institution shared a vision that model-based practice would positively influence the delivery of nursing care. This vision of high-quality care, provided from a common knowledge base, served as a beacon for implementation of the Roy model.

Application of change theory augments the process of vision attainment. In a world buffeted by change and faced daily by new threats to safety, Gardner (1993) believes that the only way to conserve is by innovation. Innovation itself requires change. Thus, successful implementation of a nursing model occurs in a context of planned change. Planned change involves strategic actions toward desired objectives. As Tappen (1995) pointed out, formal leadership is instrumental in providing guidance to influence the direction of change. Planned change contrasts sharply with the unconsciousness of unplanned change that occurs to maintain system stability. Many theories and models of planned change exist. Nurses and nurse leaders will evaluate models of change and select an approach to support achievement of the desired objectives.

The degree of individual and institutional change that is required with system-wide model implementation cannot be underestimated. Change occurs on several levels, personal, professional, and organizational. Those affected by the change need to be involved in planning as early as possible in a planned change process (Marquis & Huston, 1996). Understanding and predicting people's responses to change of this magnitude is prerequisite to success. Openmindedness and sensitivity to the responses and adaptations of individuals and groups is essential for the internal changes necessary for model implementation. In regard to environmental factors, organizations serve as the center for the delivery of health care. Three premises about organizations and change are: they exist in an environment that is constantly changing; organizations should change systematically; and they must have formalized mechanisms by which environmental forces can be interpreted and new priorities determined. If this does not exist, the organization cannot change or adapt effectively and may cease to exist. If these formalized mechanisms are well established, innovation and effective adaptation can be occurring continuously (Veninga, 1982). The activity of the innovator subsystem contributes to continual growth of the organization.

At this institution, nursing leadership viewed the Roy Adaptation Model as a mechanism through which external change can be managed. The model served as the framework for the development of policies and procedures regarding practice and practitioners. All of these approaches were constantly adjusted to respond to external requirements. Successful implementation and ongoing application of a model resulted in increased stability and an orderly methodology for adaptation to a rapidly changing environment. As general systems theory contributes to the basis for the Roy Adaptation Model, so did it influence implementation of model-based practice. The model implementation project was continuously influenced by systems theory and its application to the change process. System inputs, throughputs, outputs, and feedback were identified and utilized as the basis of change activities. Input included identified goals, information, and opinions obtained from nurses and other members of the health care team; regulatory issues; and required resources. Throughput included a participatory approach, formation of an implementation committee, role clarification, and educational activities. Output included changes in procedures, documentation tools, a model-based clinical ladder, and, most importantly, an essential change in the thought process of nurses providing care. Feedback was obtained throughout the process and was used to make adjustments as implementation progressed.

DESCRIPTION OF THE PROJECT   The framework for the following description of the model implementation process is Roy's six-step nursing process, providing an illustration of application of the model to group adaptive systems. Following brief explanation of the background relating to model implementation, first- and second-level assessment of nursing is provided, diagnoses are illustrated, goals and interventions are addressed, and evaluation is explored.

The nursing management and leadership team shared a vision that collaboration, professional respect, adaptation to change, and continuity would be enhanced through implementation of a practice model used by all nurses. Preliminary activities were initiated to prepare for implementation. Through a participative approach, a formal philosophy of nursing was developed. The philosophy contained mutually owned beliefs about nursing present in the culture. A participatory approach was also utilized in selection of the model. Since the nurse manager and leadership team had varied educational backgrounds and levels of preparation, a review of theories and models was initiated to acquire a common knowledge level. The criteria for model selection were determined, and then the Roy Adaptation Model was identified as meeting the criteria. The selection criteria included the following.

- Congruence with medical center and nursing department mission and philosophy.
- Understandable process and orientation of the model, complementary to that of other health care disciplines.
- Applicability across the health care continuum.
- Consistency with regulatory requirements associated with nursing or patient assessment and care processes.
- Enough flexibility to provide a framework for practice, management, and leadership, and educational roles within the medical center.

Assessment of behavior and stimuli   Initially, the need to bring about a change in how nursing practice was carried out was recognized internally within the Medical Center. It was apparent that, to fully actualize the change, external expertise would be required. Consultation with a faculty member at the nearby college was obtained for the initial stages of model implementation. This individual had a special interest and expertise in nursing theory and its application. The assessment showed a variety of internal system forces and external events that served as catalysts and reinforcers for model implementation.
Behaviors included the following:

- Motivated, bright nursing staff, many of whom were returning to school for baccalaureate or graduate nursing degrees
- Use of multiple assessment tools and forms
- Lack of standardization in communication
- Eclectic interpretation of the role of the nurse.
- Lack of formal expression of nursing practice

Stimuli were assessed as the following.

- Recognition of the need to standardize, organize, and unify the expression of nursing practice
- A goal to prepare nurses to fulfill their role as coordinators of patient care
- A need to appropriately interpret and measure the effectiveness of nursing roles
- The need to clarify the role of the nurse for other members of the interdisciplinary health care team
- The need to demonstrate the value of nurses' knowledge base and their contribution to health care, internally and externally
- A need to create an environment where the requirements of the state Nurse Practice Act could be achieved through a holistic expression of nursing practice
- A need to operationalize the philosophy of nursing and the Institution's belief in holistic caring
- Requirements of the Joint Commission on the Accreditation of Healthcare Organizations for a written definition of nursing care
- Existing internal conditions associated with practice, documentation, and professionalism
- The shared vision of the nursing management and leadership that model-based practice would strengthen the nursing profession

Diagnoses   The diagnosis step of the Roy model nursing process calls for an interpretive statement associating the observed behaviors with their most relevant influencing stimuli. For example, one nursing diagnosis relating to the roles of the nurse is, "eclectic interpretation of the role of the nurse related to a lack of standardization, organization, and unity in the expression of nursing practice." Another diagnosis was stated as, "proliferation of unique forms and documentation systems contributing to replication of work due to lack of a standardized system of documentation." Careful analysis and interpretation of assessment data, both behaviors and stimuli, reinforced the decision to implement the model and created forward momentum. The data analysis led to stating five goals.

Goals   Outcome statements were developed to address the ineffective behaviors and their influencing factors, and to predict outcomes of implementation. These were formulated first as goals that state the purpose of a given project. In the implementation project described, these goals addressed the outcome of hospital-wide implementation of the Roy Adaptation Model. Such factors as the role of nurses, the application of their knowledge base, the perception of nursing by other disciplines, documentation, and consistency of nursing practice were the foci. A sample is goal 2: Utilizing the knowledge base to support adaptive behaviors of patients and nurses, for example, is illustrated by nurses' ongoing understanding of the value of a care delivery system guided by a defined process. Daily, nurses assess patients' progress toward expected outcomes and continue or change plans for care based on the patients' progress or lack of progress. In one instance, a registered nurse was overheard explaining the role of a registered nurse to a student. She guided the student through assessment and evaluation of patient progress. The nurse articulated the accountability registered nurses have in assuring individualized holistic patient care. It is apparent by these types of day-to-day observations that the application of the model has provided a framework while simultaneously empowering nurses to express compassionate and holistic nursing care.

A second set of goals are those that individualize how each respective unit will meet the broad set of goals. These were referred to as creative goals. In the implementation project, creative goals allowed adaptation of the model to each unique area of nursing practice (Carper, 1978; Chinn & Jacobs, 1987). For example, the first creative goal stated, "Improve communication between nursing and other health care disciplines." Creative goal 3 aimed to achieve a higher level of pride in the profession of nursing. A particular illustration of accomplishing goal 3 was noted in a community symposium held following implementation of the model with Sr. Callista Roy as a guest and participant. Nurses throughout the institution and students of local nursing programs had the opportunity to showcase their interpretations and application of the Roy model in practice. Model-based projects included a prenatal education program, clinical practice nurses' position descriptions and clinical ladder, integrated documentation system, and a framework for a nurse practice fair.

Intervention   The intervention step was actually the process of model implementation. Planning for implementation was initiated with the development of a small leadership team with representation from administration, middle management, and education. The team was committed to a dynamic planning process, recognizing that flexibility and creativity were essential. It was impossible at this stage to create an accurate blueprint for implementation, or to even accurately predict time frames, because learning needed to occur at every point. Critical components for successful implementation were identified and included management development, education, critical mass, and early application. These and other factors are described in the original report and the reader is referred to this for additional information

(Connerley, Ristau, Lindberg, & McFarland, 1999). A particular contribution of this work is the publication of a four-step clinical ladder with each step specifying growth in use of the Roy Adaptation Model and development in professional expertise.

Evaluation Implementation of a model, once undertaken, is an ongoing process. Simultaneously, this institution utilized many sources of information to evaluate model effectiveness: practicing nurses, physicians, other interdisciplinary team members, patient feedback about nursing care, quality outcome data, and surveyors. This information identified opportunities for new applications, adaptations, and refinement of earlier steps of implementation. The evaluation data provided insight into actual or potential deficits in knowledge and practice. This led to opportunities to develop educational programs consistent with the model and obtained from the evaluation data. Educational materials consistent with the Roy framework promoted ongoing synthesis of the model into approaches to thinking, caring, and problem-solving capabilities of nurses.

Model-based nursing has influenced patient care, the documentation system, and communication, while empowering nurses. Holistic nursing care is provided with patient and family participation, and patient assessments throughout the medical center consistently include all four modes as described by Roy. The daily documentation is clear and concise and allows a 24-hour view of patient assessment and responses to care. Outcomes are written with evidence of patient and family participation, and progress toward goals (or lack thereof) is easy to follow. Patient teaching guidelines that consider the four modes have been developed. Communication in both inpatient and outpatient programs is based on the four modes and the person's adaptation. In addition, interdisciplinary communication has improved as holistic care is practiced on a more consistent basis. Nurses now are able to identify and describe their practice and the influence they have on patient outcomes.

Skills fairs have become nursing practice fairs with the focus changing from tasks and procedures to nursing process—how to plan and implement patient care based on the model. Nursing orientation and ongoing nursing education are also based on the model. Throughout the implementation process, outcomes were measured and changes were made based on the findings. Outcome measurements included surveys of what nurses believed about patient care and nursing practice. Data were collected at each point of change in the implementation process to identify problems or concerns and user satisfaction. Students enrolled in nursing programs have conducted several research projects on the value and impact of model-based practice. The work completed by these students provided an external objective validation of the progress and value of the implementation of a model in a clinical setting.

Ongoing monitoring of outcomes is focused on patient adaptive responses, and this information guides practice improvements. Performance improvement is measured by continuous monitoring of the nursing process, patient education, pain, patient satisfaction, and other important indicators of the quality of care. The Roy Adaptation Model of nursing, which promotes positive adaptation to a changing environment, complements the institution's commitment to continuous improvement of service.

The implementation of the model was a transformation process that has unified the delivery of nursing care throughout the institution. The full transformation to a holistic approach to service can be achieved if there is harmony in values and philosophy of the participants and the philosophic basis and assumptions of the chosen model. Only then does it become a part of each individual's beliefs. Use of a model has been found to guide clinical, management, and educational practice. There have been many positive achievements and outcomes identified throughout this discussion. In addition, there have been many subtle but observable benefits including pride, enhanced continuity, accountability, and greater harmony in the interdisciplinary delivery of patient care. Implementation of a model is a journey. In the future, the Roy Adaptation Model will be a significant influence on the development of an interdisciplinary patient care model. The model will influence curriculum modifications and provide learning opportunities for students exploring nursing theory.

Summary of Implementation Projects

Senesac (2003) summarized what had been learned from the various projects about strategies that facilitate implementation of the Roy Adaptation Model in practice settings. The successful implementation strategies include the development of specific assessment and documentation tools emphasizing the particular areas of the model made specific for the population to be served; reformatting the principles of the model and the development of multimodal training tools for the specific learners, including just-in-time teaching and use of adult learner principles; attending to issues of authority, leadership style, and communication; establishing an implementation committee that includes early involvement of those affected by the change; and increasing the project's visibility through Roy Adaptation Model nursing care conferences, bulletin board case studies, journal clubs, and self-learning modules. The author continued her summary of implementation projects by noting that if the model is to be implemented as a practice philosophy for an entire institution, it will be reflected in the mission and vision statements of the facility, referenced in job descriptions and evaluation tools, and used as a framework for patient assessments, care plans, and related documentation.

Common challenges also were identified in the implementation projects (Senesac, 2003). The reviewer paraphrased one author noting that an issue in implementation is a lack of appreciation of the depth of the theory and practice chasm and the size of the leap required to cross it. Other advice included making the theory operational by developing concrete tools for specific practice settings; acknowledging that translating an abstract theory into practice requires hard work and determination; considering that adopting a nursing model will require changing the administrative and documentation systems around it; understanding that initially documentation will be more time consuming than whatever preceded it; developing a plan to access additional resources for implementation including people, services, material, and a budget allocation; and planning for continuing attention to varying educational needs at different stages. Finally, full implementation and internalization takes years, and is best described as a journey rather than a destination.

Reports of Roy Adaptation Model-Guided Practice

Fawcett's book on *Contemporary Nursing Knowledge* (2005) provides an in-depth presentation of the documentation of the usefulness of the Roy Adaptation Model in research, education, administration, and practice. Within this review the author provides another view of the application of the model to practice. First, she identified 64 published reports of nursing practice guided by the Roy Adaptation Model in the care of individuals from 1979 to 2002. The reports include situations such as hospitalized young children, adolescents with asthma, adults with HIV disease, women experiencing changes associated with menopause, adult cocaine abusers recovering from anesthesia for surgery, an elderly woman with rheumatoid arthritis, and community-dwelling elderly individuals. The second set of applications of the Roy Adaptation Model included 13 published reports between 1980 and 2001 of application to families, groups, and communities. Some examples include a family with a mentally retarded child, a family experiencing the terminal illness of a member, inpatient psychiatric patients in group therapy, and a county in need of a shelter for victims of domestic violence. The application of the model in practice will include how the model can inform the development and use of the electronic healthcare record. This work is ongoing and the following description includes general principles as well as some specific examples.

THE ELECTRONIC HEALTHCARE RECORD (EHR)

When identifying the health care challenges of the 21st century, Roy and Jones (2007) noted the dramatic impact of technology developments—in particular, the massive use of computerized information. Any conceptual approach to nursing will contribute to information technology being used for the good of persons and society. This section will describe some developments and applications of the Roy Adaptation Model and the EHR.

Evolution of Computers and Informatics in Nursing

Computers were first introduced into health care organizations between the 1960s and the 1970s. At that time they were used primarily for their business, financial, and reimbursement functions. The nursing literature cited that nurses' involvement with computers actually began in the 1980s when new applications emerged in various health care settings. Nurses developed computer skills and experience by attending in-services, vendor demonstrations, and on-the-job training. The subject of computer competencies and education began to be addressed in nursing in 1982. In Harrogate, England, during a workshop entitled *The Impact of Computers in Nursing,* Barry Barber and Maureen Schools recognized and coined the term *informatics* for nursing (Saba & McCormick, 1986). The concept of informatics originated from a French term, *informatique,* meaning the study of information. The specialty of Nursing Informatics was initiated as a result of this computer workshop (IFIP & IMIA, 1982), several other medical and nursing technology conferences (NIH, 1981, 1982; SCAMC, 1981), and seminal publications on computers in nursing (ANA, 1987; Grobe, 1984; NLN, 1987; Saba & McCormick, 1986; Zielstorff, 1982).

INFORMATICS COMPETENCIES IDENTIFIED IN NURSING   Early nursing informatics competency frameworks were described by Ronald and Skiba (1987) as a continuum of learning experiences. This learning included both cognitive and interactive components. The cognitive components related to specific content of basic computer concepts and applications. The interactive components related to specific skills required to operate computer systems. They further identified specific skills for three types of computer users: (1) the informed user, (2) the proficient user, and (3) the developer.

Similar work was done in 1988 by the Swedish Federation of Salaried Employees in the Health Services and the International Medical Informatics Association (IMIA) Working Group Eight Task Force on Education. They defined competencies for different types of computer users that included (1) the user, (2) the developer/modifier, and (3) the expert/innovator. The Federation and the IMIA Task Force took this one step further and defined educational content for the nursing roles of practitioner, administrator, educator, and researcher. The work was later endorsed by the National League of Nursing (NLN).

Building upon previous work, Riley and Saba introduced the Nursing Informatics Educational Model (NIEM). The model focused on three categories of curricula: Nursing Science, Information Science, and Computer Science (Riley, 1996). They suggested five subject areas for developing nursing informatics' competencies, and included (1) basic concepts and applications, (2) accessing information systems, (3) utilizing data and information systems, (4) coordinating and evaluating data and information systems, and (5) integrating nursing informatics. The nurse scholars proposed integrating informatics into undergraduate nursing curriculum, and suggested that professors consider including the following courses:

- Overview of Computer Science – Computer hardware and software
- Overview of Information Science – Data, information, and knowledge
- Overview of Nursing Applications – Patient care planning
- Overview of Evaluation of Patient Care Applications – Quality improvement

Specialty Defined and Education Endorsed by Nursing

As a result of this early work, the Council on Computer Applications in Nursing (CCAN) was created in 1986. In January 1992, nursing informatics was recognized as a new nursing specialty by the American Nurses Association Congress of Nursing Practice. A task force was formed to develop the *Scope of Practice for Nursing Informatics* (Graves & Corcoran, 1989). Competencies for an informatics nurse were defined for Beginning and Experienced Nurse Levels (i.e., requirements for a Bachelor's degree), and for Informatics Nurse Specialists and Innovator Levels (i.e., requirements for a Master's degree).

Currently, the *Scope and Standards of Nursing Informatics Practice* (ANA, 2001) has been revised several times to reflect the evolution of nursing practice in this specialty area. However, nursing informatics curricula remain elective courses in most nursing programs throughout the country. With nurses comprising 55% of the U.S. health care workforce (a number close to 3 million), in order to transform today's health care system, nursing education will be transformed in this technological area. As a result, a small group of nursing leaders and advocates met and resolved to strengthen the voice of the nursing profession to improve health care for the 21st century. In January 2005, the group held a strategy session at Johns Hopkins School of Nursing, bringing together nurses from academia, government, and industry. They confirmed the need to transform nursing education and practice, and agreed to plan for a nursing Summit focused on Technology Informatics Guiding Education Reform (TIGER).

The 2006 invitational Summit, *Evidence and Informatics Transforming Nursing*, was designed to catalyze a productive relationship between the Alliance for Nursing Informatics (ANI), which represents 22 nursing informatics professional societies, and the full range of nursing organizations. The intent of the Summit was to engage all of nursing, making informatics not just for experts in informatics anymore.

The Summit participants focused on:

- Creating a vision for the future of nursing that bridges the quality chasm with health information technology (HIT)
- Transforming the work environment for nurses; enabling them to use informatics in practice and education to provide safer, higher-quality patient care

Over 70 organizations—a diverse and comprehensive representation of nursing, informatics, and government agencies, as well as technology vendors—participated. The result was the development of the TIGER vision and action plan. The plan was aligned with the action plan of the National Health Information Technology Agenda put forth by the Office of the National Coordinator (ONC) in the Department of Health and Human Services (DHHS).

The TIGER Team released the summary report, titled *Evidence and Informatics Transforming Nursing: 3-Year Action Steps toward a 10-Year Vision*, at the 2007 Healthcare

Information and Management Systems Society (HIMSS) Annual Conference and Exhibition. The TIGER summary report (2007) provided specific action plans for each nursing stakeholder group that participated in the Summit. The Collaborative Teams that resulted from the Summit and the specific strategic action plans that are currently being developed include those listed in Box 21–1.

Nursing Language and Electronic Healthcare Records

Leaders in the field of nursing informatics practice and nurses in clinical practice both recognize the need for standard nursing terminology for use in electronic healthcare records (EHR). A series of groundbreaking reports were published (such as: *The Computer-Based Patient Record,* 1987; *To Err is Human,* 2000; *Crossing the Quality Chasm,* 2001). The Institute of Medicine (IOM) concluded that information technology held the promise for transforming health care practice to achieve foundational aims. These include safety, effectiveness, patient-family centeredness, timeliness, efficiency, and equity. Consequently, in 2004 the movement received federal standing when United States President George W. Bush issued an executive order that mandated electronic healthcare records for all Americans in 10 years. As a result, a National Coordinator for Healthcare Informatics Technology (ONC/DHHS) was appointed. The coordinator convened a National Conference on the *Cornerstones for the EHR.* EHR leaders were brought together to discuss the National Health Information Infrastructure. Only one nurse served on the panel. Recognizing the need to ensure that the nursing profession's expertise is represented in the National HIT Agenda and in EHRs, nurse informatics and executives have proliferated, advocated, and contributed to the development and use of standardized nursing languages to describe patient problems, nursing interventions, and patient outcomes (Lunney, Delaney, Duffy, Moorhead, & Welton, 2005).

To date, the American Nurses Association (ANA) has recognized standardized nursing terminologies (including reference and interface terminologies) and minimum data sets or frameworks for the inclusion in EHRs to support documentation of clinical care. The ANA recognized terminologies are listed in Box 21–2 in chronological order.

In addition to recognizing standard nursing languages, ANA has developed standard guidelines for vendors to consider when including nursing terminologies in the design of software systems. The ANA's Nursing Information & Data Set Evaluation Center (NIDSEC) is the group that develops these standard guidelines. It is imperative that nurses continue to develop common nursing terminologies that identify diagnoses, procedures, interventions, and out-

---

BOX 21–1

Specific Strategic Action Plans Developing From TIGER Summit

- National HIT Agenda and Advocacy
- Standards and Interoperability
- Informatics Competencies
- Informatics Education and Faculty Development
- Informatics Staff Development and Continuing Education
- Clinical Application Design and Usability
- Informatics Leadership Development
- Consumer-Centered Care and Personal Health Records
- Virtual Demonstration Center

BOX 21–2

ANA-Recognized Terminologies

===

- NANDA International (1992)
- Nursing Interventions Classifications (1992)
- Home Health Care Classification (1992)
- Omaha System (1992)
- Nursing Outcomes Classification (1997)
- Nursing Management Minimum Data Set (1998)
- Patient Care Data Set (1998)
- PeriOperative Nursing Data Set (1999)
- SNOMED CT (1999)
- Nursing Minimum Data Set (1999)
- International Classification of Nursing Practice (2000)
- ABC Codes (2000), and
- Logical Observation Identifiers Names and Codes (2002)

---

comes in order to predict the cost and quality of patient care in today's evidence-based practice environment. However, the real key, as described by Lunney and colleagues (2005), is that nurses must link patient-centered data with traditional medical and administrative data to accurately reflect the breadth of patient care to influence strategic decisions.

Nursing Theory Represented in EHRs

Throughout the years, nurse theorists have developed and illustrated both qualitatively and quantitatively how to represent patient-centered data with the breadth of patient care that nurses provide. However, can this breadth of patient data and nursing care be accurately captured and documented in an EHR? Much work needs to be done to answer this question positively. However, one application project is described here that has been developed using the Roy Adaptation Model.

APPLICATION OF THE ROY ADAPTATION MODEL IN THE EHR: THE JAPAN PROJECT Currently, the Roy Adaptation Nursing Theory is being used in Japan in some agencies for patients who tend to have long-term disabilities and/or care needs. These include those who need dialysis, maternity care, psychiatric care, and rehabilitation care (Hidaka & Matsuo, 2003). As a result, a team of Japanese scholars from the Roy Adaptation Association of Japan (Hidaka, Miyabayashi, Tsuhako, Ide, & Kanayama, 2007) and from St. Mary's College, Seibo College, and Seiai Rehabilitation Hospital have collaborated with vendors and have developed an application of the Roy Adaptation Model for use within their EHR system. The nurses worked with the EHR vendor to ensure accurate documentation of nursing diagnoses, appropriate patients' adaptation goals, with the related behaviors, stimuli, and interventions.[1]

Prior to the actual pilot project, the nurses advised the EHR vendor by mapping and linking the Nursing Diagnoses Screen automatically to the Behaviors, Stimuli, and Goal Assessment Screen (Screen 1). For example, when selecting the Nursing Diagnosis, *Self-Care Deficit – Bathing/Hygiene,* the EHR automatically takes the nurse to the screen to select the Patient Goal – *Ability to Brush Teeth.* Then the nurse is prompted to select (see checked items)

---

[1] The Japan Project information used with permission, lead author, Hidaka.

the Behavior (that needs improvement, adaptation) – *Inability to understand how to use tooth-brush.* Lastly, the nurse selects the description and type of Stimuli responsible for the deficit (i.e., focal, contextual, or residual) – *Apraxia Stimuli - Focal Type* (Screen 2). When this electronic Assessment Screen is completed, the nurses then assisted the EHR vendor by linking and mapping this assessment automatically to the Intervention Screen. Based on the completed assessment, the Intervention Screen is now populated with several interventions that the nurse will consider to help the patient achieve the goal of adaptation (Screen 3). In this example, the interventions such as – *If patient is able to imitate, the nurse will demonstrate brushing teeth prior to the patient performing,* or *If patient cannot use toothbrush smoothly or cannot brush teeth well, the nurse will lead the patient by the hands.* Once selected, the nurse can document the patient's progress on a daily basis, by using the Evaluation Screens.

In this EHR pilot project, the nurses wanted also to investigate the efficacy of the newly developed electronic Roy Adaptation Model at a rehabilitation hospital in Japan for patients who had central nervous system impairments. The study was conducted at Seiai Rehabilitation Hospital, a 210-bed facility. The total number of nursing-related staff was 123; 63 were registered nurses, 16 were licensed practical nurses, and 44 were nursing assistants. The therapy staff totaled 140; 53 were physical therapist, 62 were occupational

SCREEN 1 Nursing Diagnosis Screen.

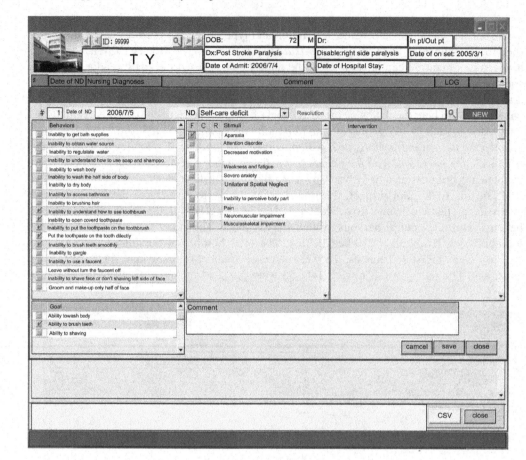

SCREEN 2   Nursing Diagnosis Screen With Stimuli Screen.

therapists, and 25 were speech therapists. At the time of this pilot project, the inpatient population that was selected comprised four medical diagnoses, as follows:

- Cerebrovascular Disorder – 46% participants
- Fracture – 24% participants
- Brain Tumor – 2% participants
- Traumatic Brain Injury – 2% participants

The top three Nursing Diagnoses recorded in the EHR for this inpatient population included:

- Self-Care Deficit
- Impaired Physical Mobility
- Risk of Falls

Self-Care Deficit was the most frequently occurring Nursing Diagnosis for this inpatient population with central nervous system impairments, so the nurses selected to investigate the causes of this particular nursing diagnosis further. They reviewed the Stimuli Database to conclude that the top causes/stimuli of Self-Care Deficit were –

- Paralysis (40%)
- Higher Brain Dysfunction (24%)

SCREEN 3   Nursing Diagnosis Screen With Stimuli Screen and Intervention Screen.

- Decline in Muscle Power (18%)
- Recognition of Functional Disorder (12%)
- Pain (4%)
- Fatigue (2%)

After reviewing this clinical information, the nurses were able to develop nursing interventions specific to the influencing stimuli and specific to the individual's patient-centered data; thereby promoting adaptation and health. The Japanese head nurses emphasized, "The Roy Model enabled stroke patients to recognize the difference between what they would like to do and what they actually can do, and it helped them affirm what they can still do. Finally, the assessment entails not only alleviating a patient's problems, but it also tries to find factors stimulating those problems. Once these factors are uncovered interventions can be put into operation to eliminate the problems" (Hidaka et al., 2007).

This study and the development of the Roy model imbedded electronically in the EHR is still in its early development. However, it provides practicing nurses and informatics nurses an exemplar for collaborating with EHR vendors to ensure the accurate capture of patient-centered data in order to provide the most appropriate and highest quality nursing care. The Japanese head nurses concluded,

At Seiai Hospital, carrying out the Roy Adaptation Model in rehabilitation for stroke patients is extremely effective in this clinical setting. The reason is that the Roy Model is an adaptation system that goes beyond physiological aspects to include aspects of self-concept, role function, and interdependence. Most of the stroke patients suffer from mobile function and high cerebral function impairment, which suddenly prevent them from doing things that they could previously do, including fulfilling their roles in family and society (Hidaka et al., 2007).

As a result of this conclusion, this group of nurses in Japan continue to collaborate with the EHR vendors, and are currently developing documentation tools and databases to collect the breadth of patient-centric data in the physiologic, self-concept, role function, and interdependence modes to develop knowledge to promote patient adaptation.

THE ROY ADAPTATION MODEL IN NURSING RESEARCH

A third major area of application of the Roy Adaptation Model is in nursing research. Nursing as both a profession and a scholarly discipline is rooted in knowledge for nursing practice. Throughout history, family members have used their cultural traditions and understanding of the other person to help increase wellness, prevent illness, assist with recovery, and comfort the suffering and dying. Today, nursing has emerged clearly as the discipline that focuses on developing an understanding of the human processes that promote health. The social concern of nursing as a profession is to contribute to health by focusing on life processes of persons integrated with their environments. Knowledge for nursing practice, then, seeks to understand how to promote interactions of persons and environment that promote health. Caring and clinical reasoning are skills used in nursing practice to fulfill the social mandate of the profession.

Application of the Roy Adaptation Model to nursing research can be described by providing a perspective for nursing research. That is, we describe what it is that nurses study and how they study it. Secondly, several reviews of model-based research are summarized. This includes analysis, critique, and synthesis of the first 30 years of English-speaking publications of research based on the Roy Adaptation Model. This analysis was used to redefine evidence-based nursing practice. In addition we acknowledge a review of Roy Model–based research from Japan (Hidaka & Matsuo, 2003) and in Latin America (Moreno-Ferguson, 2007).

Perspective of Nursing Research

Nursing is a science and an art. Science deals with understanding both how and why questions. How does something work, why does it not, and how can one help it work? Art deals with understanding and expressing the realities of life. When a child takes a small plant apart, he or she knows only the parts that make it up, not how it works. Biology looks deeper to explain how and why the plant grows. An artist such as Monet paints a water lily and both the artist and the viewer of the art know the plant in a way not known in biological science. Through science and art one knows and appreciates oneself, others, and the world.

Basic knowledge in both arts and sciences looks deeply and closely at being; such knowledge aims to understand and express the essence of what is there and how it works. Nursing has such basic knowledge just as other disciplines do. Nursing models provide a perspective from which to view the subject matter of nursing. Roy (1988) has described a general perspective for nursing knowledge as including the basic science of nursing. This basic understanding is nursing's focus on human life processes from which life patterns emerge.

Secondly, this perspective for nursing knowledge places emphasis on the related clinical science of nursing, including midrange theories of intervention and strategies related to enhancing positive life processes and patterns. According to the Roy Adaptation Model, basic knowledge is understanding people adapting within their various life situations. Basic nursing knowledge derived from this model seeks to understand and appreciate the hows and whys of persons and groups functioning as adaptive systems.

Nursing is also a practice discipline. Therefore, nursing knowledge based on a model includes a clinical art and science. Nursing has a long tradition of caring and enhancing the person's ability to handle situations of health and illness. The notes of a famous New England writer working as a nurse during the American Civil War in the nineteenth century reflect the values of this tradition. Louisa May Alcott wrote in *Hospital Sketches: An Army Nurse's True Account of Her Experience during the Civil War:*

> A few minutes later, as I came in again, with fresh rollers, I saw John sitting erect, with no one to support him, while the surgeon dressed his back. I had never hitherto seen it done; for, having simpler wounds to attend to, and knowing the fidelity of the attendant, I had left John to him, thinking it might be more agreeable and safe; for both strength and experience were needed in his case....John looked lonely and forsaken just then, as he sat with bent head, hands folded on his knee, and no outward sign of suffering, till, looking nearer, I saw great tears roll down and drop upon the floor. It was a new sight there; for, though I had seen many suffer, some swore, some groaned, most endured silently, but none wept. Yet it did not seem weak, only very touching, and straightway my fear vanished, my heart opened wide and took him in, as, gathering the bent head in my arms, as freely as if he had been a little child, I said, "Let me help you bear it, John." (1863, pp. 51–52)

The clinical art and science of nursing according to the Roy Adaptation Model uses the basic knowledge of adapting persons to understand persons in situations of health and illness. This understanding is translated to practical clinical knowledge as nurses seek to discover ways of enhancing adaptation. Understanding cognator and regulator activity for individuals and stabilizer and innovator activity for groups is basic knowledge according to the model. In addition, knowledge of human processes in situations of health and illness, and of behaviors and stimuli in each of the adaptive modes, also provides the basis for the clinical art and science of nursing. This knowledge is the basis of planning of nursing care with individual people and groups to enhance their own adaptation.

Knowledge is developed through research in many ways. Formal research can be designed to describe phenomena (what), to correlate two or more phenomena (what and how), and to experiment with the effects of one phenomenon upon another (how and why). Within each of these general types of research, there are two broad categories of research design that can answer a research question. A qualitative approach views reality as emerging and relative. The basic structure of knowledge is inductive, that is, identifying individual experiences that can be interpreted to provide generalizations of human experience. A quantitative approach sees reality as discovered and measured. Knowledge is deductive, that is, a general theory is used to provide a tentative hypothesis for a given situation. Nurses increasingly use several types of research designs and are aware of how each approach supports the other.

The broad perspective of nursing knowledge described here is basic to identifying and conducting research for nursing. The Roy Adaptation Model has a clear perspective for developing the basic and clinical art and science of nursing. Further specification of the model's focus for research is delineated by descriptions of the person and environment.

Model-Based Research to Redefine Evidence-Based Practice

The core research group of the Roy Adaptation Association conducted reviews of the first 30 years of research based on the Roy Adaptation Model in the English-speaking literature. This included 163 studies from 1970 to 1995 (BBARNS, 1999) that met selection criteria. Then 55 studies from 1995–2001 were reviewed. The 218 studies were used for secondary analysis. In one such analysis, the instruments used to measure major model concepts were evaluated and recommendations made (Barone, Roy, & Frederickson, 2008). The secondary analysis that will be described here relates to redefining evidence-based practice by using model-based research (Roy, 2007).

Nurse scholars and practitioners have for many years made efforts to bridge the gap between nursing knowledge and nursing practice. Many approaches to apply research in practice have been developed. However, there is still a lag between nursing knowledge developed and applications to practice. More recently an approach referred to as evidence-based practice (EBP) has been used as another way to ensure that patients receive care that is based on the strongest possible base of knowledge (Melnyk & Fineout-Overholt, 2005). Some have criticized the movement as being based primarily in empirical knowledge and following the approaches used to synthesize medical research.

In examining EBP, Fawcett, Watson, Neuman, Walker, and Fitzpatrick (2001) noted three key points: (1) the importance of moving from a focus on empirics to focus on diverse patterns of knowing; (2) the need for theory-guided, evidence-based holistic nursing practice; and (3) that theory, inquiry, and evidence are to be inextricably linked. Another author (Dluhy, 2007) raised the following issues about EBP:

- Standards used for evidence—nurse as medical technician for medical outcomes
- One approach for all patients—art of nursing shapes intervention for individual
- Context-based interpretation of research difficult in practice
- Use of qualitative research unclear
- Want certainty, but in nursing data are imperfect and patients do not respond predictably

In particular, the significant growth in EBP literature has not translated into the anticipated quality health care outcomes.

The research developed from the Roy Adaptation Model was used in an attempt to respond to the challenge to expand our view of evidence-based practice, to develop additional strategies for cumulative knowledge and to use approaches compatible with the heritage of nurses. It was believed that an analysis of large numbers of studies based on a given nursing model could help meet these requirements. The study purpose was to critically review theory-based research using a specific nursing model and articulate its relevance in providing evidence-based knowledge for nursing practice. The theoretical basis was the Roy Adaptation Model as described in this text. The model describes adapting persons and levels of adaptation and seeks knowledge in all ways of knowing. Figure 21–1 describes how the Roy Adaptation Model relates to EBP by showing how evidence for practice can be based on linking the model's view of persons in society, the model-based values, and integrated knowing. The 30 years of research based on the Roy Adaptation Model was used to develop a process of testing common propositions for integrating theory-based research studies.

The design used was an integrated secondary research analysis and synthesis of studies using the Roy Adaptation Model, including derivation and standardization of criteria for providing evidence of potential for implementation in practice. Standardized criteria

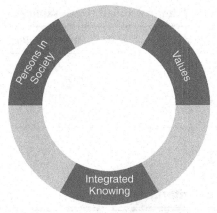

FIGURE 21–1 Roy Adaptation Model evidence-based practice.

were used for judging the quality of the research (BBARNS, 1999). The team of investigators developed criteria to evaluate links between the research and the nursing model. Propositions derived from the early work of Roy and Roberts (1981) were used to identify propositions from the model, middle-range propositions, and practice-level propositions. Figure 21–2 shows the links among the levels of propositions. Two samples were included: (1) the first 25 years of research based on the model from 1970–1994 for a total of 163 studies (BBARNS, 1999) and (2) the 5 years of Roy Adaptation Model-based research studies from 1995–2001 for a total of 59 studies (RAA, in preparation). Table 21–2 shows the results of applying the criteria to the subsamples. A total of 166 studies from the English-speaking literature were used for the analysis of knowledge as evidence for practice. Box 21–3 lists the derived criteria for EBP.

When the propositions were tested, the team found high support for the propositions (Table 21–3). In the first sample, 236 of the 275 propositions were supported. Within the sample, 60 studies met the criteria for high potential for implementation in practice. In the second sample, 95 of 118 propositions were supported and 37 studies were judged to have high potential for implementation in practice. An example of the testing of propositions is as follows. Generic Proposition 3 states: The characteristics of internal and external stimuli influence adaptive responses. This was tested a total of 156 times and supported

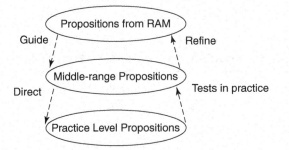

FIGURE 21–2 Linkages among levels of propositions derived from the Roy Adaptation Model.

TABLE 21–2 Data Analysis: Criteria Applied to Subsamples

	1970 to 1994	1995 to 2001
Qualitative studies met analytic criteria	n = 34/37 (92%)	n = 10/10 (100%)
Quantitative studies met analytic criteria	n = 124/138 (90%)	n = 36/38 (95%)

BOX 21–3

Derived Redefinition of Criteria for EBP

Category 1: High potential for implementation in practice

- Proposition supported by more than one study
- Unequivocal support of hypothesis
- Low risk
- High clinical need

Category 2: Need further clinical evaluation before implementation

- Proposition supported, but generalizability not clear
- Risk not clear
- High clinical need

Category 3: Need further testing before implementation

- Mixed support for proposition
- Generalizability unclear
- High risk

125 times (80%). Examples of specific knowledge relevant to nursing practice that show practice-level propositions of the broad proposition include:

- Severity of illness and adjuvant cancer treatment have the strongest association with indicators of health-related quality of life (HRQOL).
- HRQOL was strongly defined by affective status, functional status, and physical symptoms, and less by social support.

TABLE 21–3 Integrated Knowledge as Evidence for Practice Based on RAM

	1970 to 1994	1995 to 2001
	(n = 112)	(n = 50)
Propositions supported	n = 236/275 (83%)	n = 95/118 (81%)
High potential for implementation in practice	60 studies (54%)	37 studies (74%)

- HRQOL at 3 months was significantly predicted by HRQOL at baseline.

Nuamah, I, et al. (1999)

- Women with diabetes who had fewer personal resources and poorer adjustment were those with the poorest metabolic control.

Willoughby, 1995

The conclusions reached in this secondary analysis were (1) a potentially more useful description for criteria for evidence for nursing practice was proposed; (2) a process for theory-based research contributing to cumulative nursing knowledge was described; and (3) the process used provides integrated nursing knowledge based on our heritage, including theory-based research and ways of knowing that are personal, ethical, esthetic, social-political, as well as empiric.

ISSUES AND FUTURE DIRECTIONS

In reviewing some of the applications of the Roy Adaptation Model to practice, the electronic healthcare record and nursing research, one is struck by the breadth of the work over many decades. There is evidence, also recognized by others (Fawcett, 2005; Phillips, 2006), that the Roy Adaptation Model has made useful contributions to nursing. Although implementation projects in practice have been arduous efforts, and sometimes not continued to completion, many participants in the projects report positive outcomes for both patients and nurses. The wide reports of applications of the model by nurses in diverse clinical situations and cultures demonstrate how the model can guide practice in multiple settings. The initial work on the use of the model in the electronic healthcare record in Japan provides some encouragement for a potentially rich area of application. The wide body of nursing research based on the model offers many possibilities for developing integrated knowledge for practice.

Still, issues and challenges remain. Many acknowledge that the best implementation is when a nursing model becomes the basis for care throughout an institution. Still, many published projects are on given units are in small specialty hospitals. There has been a trend for health care agencies who are seeking Magnet Status certification to select a nursing model to build the philosophy and approaches to nursing care. It remains to be seen if the effects on clarifying nursing roles and improving interdisciplinary collaboration will be duplicated in some of these larger projects.

In considering the application on the individual patient level, one area for further development that has been suggested is an organized typology of interventions for use in nursing practice (Phillips, 2006). The integrated research reviews can be analyzed from this perspective. However, the caution is offered, as with nursing diagnosis, that care will always be individualized at the same time that it is derived from an established typology.

In today's information age, nursing professionals from around the world will advocate and continue to develop an electronic unifying framework for all nursing languages. This has been called a *parlance for practice,* which describes nursing practice and its quality services to society (Padovano Corliss, 1994). A unifying framework that links patient-centric data (i.e., patient's health status with the patient's ultimate health goals or outcomes) to all nursing theories, nursing diagnoses, nursing interventions, and outcomes is important to provide the depth and breadth of quality nursing care required to create *societal vitality* (Padovano & Corliss, 1994). This may seem a distant goal. However, if we look at progress in technology and in nursing knowledge over the last few decades, it is possible to believe that this will be accomplished. Such progress will take focusing on an electronic unifying framework as a priority for the future. This will require more collaboration between those known as nurse theorists and nursing informatics experts.

In regard to research issues and directions, the RAA research review team (BBARNS, 1999) had suggested that future theory development and research would focus on middle-range theories particularly related to the cognator and regulator processes and to the four adaptive modes and their relationships. Some of this work has begun. This is noted in identifying the middle-range theories related to the adaptive processes within each of the adaptive modes for both individuals and groups. Further, there is an international network of scholars working on using the Coping and Adaptation Process Scale that is based specifically on the cognator–regulator (Chayput & Roy, 2007; González, 2007; Gutiérrez, 2007). As noted earlier, and in the examples given, multiple methods are used at every stage of the work of developing knowledge based on this particular model. Scholars are encouraged to develop philosophic and empiric inquiry. Dialogue among scholars about methods related to multiple ways of knowing will enrich the work of all.

Specific recommendations for developing research instruments have been made (Barone, Roy, & Fredrickson, 2008). Limitations were noted in the review of instruments used over the past 30 years. Some of the high-priority areas for locating or developing tools included physiologic adaptation and regulator activity; body image, self-ideal, and the moral-ethical-spiritual self; role-taking processes, role transition, and social integrity; affectional adequacy and relational integrity; as well as further work on cognator effectiveness and adaptation in multiple modes or integrated adaptation. The authors also noted that much of the research to date focused on the individual and the family or a dyad. Thus we see that the future of measurement using the Roy Adaptation Model also will focus on adaptation of groups such as group integrity and infrastructure relations.

Further, this model and other approaches to understanding nursing knowledge profess a belief in holism. The notion of individual patterns is strongly represented, but this presents difficulties in describing the commonalities that make for understanding beyond an experience that is too unique to communicate. Thus clinical investigators seek ways to understand infinite variety, holism, and control of variables. This is particularly true with outcome measures. For example, the definition of health within the model includes a process of being and becoming whole and integrated. The methodology then will be designed to tap the manifestation of the experience of being whole and integrated. The need for longitudinal studies, for refinement and replication, and for programs of research has been identified by a number of reviewers, including the RAA core research team. Research in nursing and research based on the Roy model's perspective of knowledge are beyond simply accumulating more facts. The opportunity to seek meaning and understanding is provided. The philosophic, scientific, and cultural assumptions, the essential elements of the model, and ongoing research efforts can guide further programs of research. The work to be done in the future likely will make more contributions to nursing and to nursing practice than are noted in the applications reviewed in this chapter.

Exercises for Application

1. Select a classmate or another nurse you know and discuss your first experience of using a nursing model as the basis of your practice—your feelings, reactions, successes, and difficulties.

2. Evaluate the electronic healthcare data systems in an institution you know for how helpful they are in communicating nursing practice.

3. Identify one research topic based on your understanding of the Roy Adaptation Model that you think would be useful to explore.

Assessment of Understanding

QUESTIONS

1. Describe two potential benefits of model-based nursing practice. _____ , _____

2. Describe one important condition or strategy in applying the Roy Adaptation Model to a nursing practice setting. _____

3. Give one reason why nurses are involved in the development of the electronic healthcare record. _____

4. Describe one way that a nursing model can be used to guide research for knowledge development for nursing. _____

_____

5. Classify the following statements as qualitative (QL) or quantitative (QN) in their approach to knowledge development.
   (a) _____ reality as emerging and relative
   (b) _____ deductive reasoning
   (c) _____ generalizes from individual experiences
   (d) _____ inductive approach
   (e) _____ measurement of reality
   (f) _____ provides tentative hypothesis

6. What is one possible advantage of using a nursing model to redefine evidence-based practice?

_____

FEEDBACK

1. Answers will vary. Can include: provides direction for data gathering, is a systematic approach to organizing knowledge, provides a means of effective communication, assists in role definition.

2. Answers will vary. Can include: administrative support, education, model selection, supportive communication, early success, vision.

3. Answers will vary. Can include: reality of massive use of computerized information; the need to transform nursing education and practice in keeping with the current and future use of electronic healthcare records; as a way to make health care informatics relevant to patient care nurses provide.

4. Answers will vary. Can include: provide a perspective for research, provide the basis for the phenomena to be studied and the research question to be asked, direct education.

5. (a) QL (b) QN (c) QL (d) QL (e) QN (f) QN

6. Answers will vary. Can include: recognizes the importance of moving from a focus on empirics to focus on diverse patterns of knowing; addresses the need for theory-guided, evidence-based holistic nursing practice; links theory, inquiry, and evidence; provides integrated nursing knowledge based on our heritage, including theory-based research and ways of knowing that are personal, ethical, esthetic, social-political, as well as empiric.

References

Alcott, L. M. (1963). *Hospital sketches: An army nurse's true account of her experience during the Civil War.* Concord, MA (Edition Cambridge, MA: Applewood Books, 1986).

Allison, S. E., McLaughlin, K., & Walker, D. (1991). Nursing theory: A tool to put nursing back into nursing administration. *Nursing Administration Quarterly, 15*(3), 72–75.

American Nurses Association. (1987). *Computers in nursing education.* Washington, DC: American Nurses Publishing.

American Nurses Association. (2001). *Scope and standards of nursing informatics practice.* Washington, DC: American Nurses Publishing.

ANA Council on Computer Applications for Nursing. (1992). *Report on the designation of nursing informatics as a nursing specialty.* Washington, DC: CCAN, Congress of Nursing Practice, ANA.

Barone, S., Roy, C., & Frederickson, K. Instruments for RAM research: Critique, examples, and future directions. *Nursing Science Quarterly, 21(4),* 270–276.

Boston Based Adaptation Research in Nursing Society. (1999). *Roy Adaptation Model-based research: 25 years of contributions on nursing science.* Indianapolis, IN: Sigma Theta Tau International Center Nursing Press.

Carper, B. A. (1978). Fundamental patterns of knowing in nursing. *Advances in Nursing Science, 1*(1), 13–23.

Chayput, P., & Roy, C. (2007). Psychometric testing of the Thai version of coping and adaption processing scale—short form (TCAPS-SF). *Thai Journal of Nursing Council, 22*(3), 29–39.

Chinn, P., & Jacobs, M. (1987). *Theory and nursing* (2nd ed.). St. Louis, MO: Mosby.

Connerley, K., Ristau, S., Lindberg, C., & McFarland, M. (1999). The Roy model in nursing practice. In C. Roy & H. Andrews (Eds.), *The Roy Adaptation Model* (2nd ed.). Stamford, CT: Appleton & Lange.

Detmer, D. E., Dick, R. S., & Steen, E. B. (Eds.). (1997). CPRI. *The computer-based patient record: An essential technology for health care.* Washington, DC: National Academy Press.

Dluhy, N. (2007). *Uncertainty, transparency, control: The allure of EBP.* Presentation at Theory Research Interest Group Pre Conference Workshop, Eastern Nursing Research Society, Providence, RI.

Fawcett, J. (2005). *Contemporary nursing knowledge analysis and evaluation of nursing models and theories* (2nd ed.). Philadelphia: F.A. Davis Company.

Fawcett, J., Watson, J., Neuman, B., Walker, P., & Fitzpatrick, J. (2001). On nursing theories and evidence. *Journal of Nursing Scholarship, 33*, 115–119.

Gardner, J. (1993). *Self renewal.* New York: Harper & Row.

González, Y. M. (2007). Efficacy of two interventions based on the theory of coping and adaptation processing. *Roy Adaptation Association Review, 11*(1), 4.

Grahame, C. (1987). Frontline revolt. *Nursing Times, 83*(16), 60.

Graves, J. R., & Corcoran, S. (1989). The study of nursing informatics. *Image: Journal of Nursing Scholarship, 21*(4), 227–231.

Gray, J. (1991). The Roy Adaptation Model in nursing practice. In C. Roy & H. A. Andrews (Eds.), *The Roy Adaptation Model: The definitive statement* (pp. 429–443). Norwalk, CT: Appleton & Lange.

Grobe, S. J. (1984). *Computer primer and resource guide for nurses.* Philadelphia: Lippincott.

Guitierrez, M. dC. (Ed.). (2007). *Adaptacion y cuidadao en el ser humano: Una vision de enfermeria* (pp. 1–12). Bogota: Editorial El Manual Moderno, Universidad de la Sabana.

Hidaka, T., & Matsuo, M. (2003). Trends and perspectives of nursing research based on the Roy Adaptation Model in Japan. *The Japanese Journal of Nursing Research, 36*(1), 31–40.

Hidaka, T., Miyabayashi, I., Tsuhako, S., Ide, N., & Kanayama, M. (2007). *The application of the Roy Adaptation Model in Japanese stroke patients.* Los Angeles: Mount St. Mary's College.

Institute of Medicine. (2000). *To err is human.* Washington, DC: National Academy Press.

Institute of Medicine. (2001). *Crossing the quality chasm: A new health system for the 21st century.* Washington, DC: National Academy Press.

Kouzes, J., & Posner, B. (1993). *Credibility.* San Francisco: Jossey-Bass.

Lunney, M., Delaney, C. W., Duffy, M., Moorhead, S., & Welton, J. (2005). Advocating for standardized nursing languages in electronic health records. *JONA: The Journal of Nursing Administration, 351*, 1–3.

Marquis, B., & Huston, C. (1996). *Leadership roles and management functions in nursing.* Philadelphia: Lippincott.

Mastal, M. F., Hammond, H., & Roberts, M. P. (1982). Theory into hospital practice: A pilot implementation. *The Journal of Nursing Administration, 12*, 9–15.

Mayberry, A. (1991). Merging nursing theories, models and nursing practice: More than an administrative challenge. *Nursing Administration Quarterly, 15*(3), 44–53.

McFarland, M. R. (1993). The process of vision development described by six college and university presidents (Doctoral dissertation, Gonzaga University, 1993). *Dissertation Abstracts International, DAI-A 54/04,* 1256–1386.

Melnyk, B., & Fineout-Overholt, E. (2005). *Evidence-based practice in nursing and health care: A guide to best practice.* Philadelphia: Lippincott Williams & Wilkins.

Moreno-Ferguson, M. E. (2001). Rehabilitation ambulatory service in Clínica Puente del Común-Teletón, Chía, Colombia. From Moreno-Ferguson, M. E. (2007). *Application of the Roy Adaptation Model in Latin America: Literature review.* Roy Adaptation Association Conference 2007, Los Angeles, CA.

Moreno-Ferguson, M. E. (2007). *Application of the Roy Adaptation Model in Latin America: Literature review.* Roy Adaptation Association Conference 2007, Los Angeles, CA.

Monroy, et al. (2003). Pediatric Intensive Care Unit at Fundación Cardio Infantil–Cardiology Institute, Bogotá, Colombia. From Moreno-Ferguson, M. E. (2007). *Application of the Roy Adaptation Model in Latin America: Literature review.* Roy Adaptation Association Conference 2007, Los Angeles, CA.

National League for Nursing. (1987). *A guideline for basic education in nursing.* New York: National League for Nursing.

Nuamah, I. F., Cooley, M. E., Fawcett, J., & McCorkle, R. (1999). Testing a theory for health related quality of life in cancer patients: A structural equation approach. *Research in Nursing and Health, 22*(3), 231–242.

Padovano, C., & Corliss, C. (1994). *Universals of nursing: Consensus and action.* University Microfilms International. Ann Arbor: MI. University of Michigan.

Parker, M. (2006). *Nursing theories and nursing practice* (2nd ed.). Philadelphia: F.A. Davis Company.

Phillips, K. D. (2006). Sister Callista Roy: Adaptation model. In A. M. Tomey & M. R. Alligood (Eds.), *Nursing theorists and their work* (6th ed., pp. 355–385). St. Louis, MO: Mosby.

Riley, J. B. (1996). Educational applications. In V. K. Saba & K. A. McCormick (Eds.), *Essentials of computers for nurses* (2nd ed., pp. 527–573). New York: JB Lippincott Company.

Robbins, S. R., & Duncan, R. B. (1988). The role of the CEO and top management in the creation and implementation of strategic vision. In D. Hambrick (Ed.), *The executive effect: Concepts and methods for the study of top managers.* Greenwich, CT: JAI Press.

Rogers, M., Paul Jones, L., Clarke, J., Mackay, C., Potter, M., & Ward, W. (1991). The use of the Roy Adaptation Model in nursing administration. *Canadian Journal of Nursing Administration,* June, 21–26.

Ronald, J. S., & Skiba, D. J. (1987). *Guidelines for basic computer education in nursing.* New York: National League for Nursing.

Roy, C. (1988). An explication of the philosophical assumptions of the Roy Adaptation Model. *Nursing Science Quarterly, 1*(1), 26–34.

Roy, C. (2007). *Nursing theory-guided practice: Focusing on evidence-based care.* Poster presented at American Academy of Nursing Annual Conference, Washington, DC, November, 2008.

Roy, C., & Jones, D. (Eds.). (2007). *Nursing knowledge development and clinical practice.* New York: Springer.

Roy, C., & Roberts, S. (Eds.). (1981). *Theory construction in nursing: An adaptation model.* Englewood Cliffs, NJ: Prentice Hall.

Saba, V. K., & McCormick, K. A. (1986). *Essentials of computers for nurses.* Philadelphia: JB Lippincott Company.

Senesac, P. (2003). Implementing the Roy Adaptation Model: From theory to practice. *Roy Adaptation Association Review, 4*(2), 5.

Tappen, R. M. (1995). *Nursing leadership and management* (3rd ed.). Philadelphia: Davis.

The TIGER Initiative (2007). Evidence and informatics transforming nursing: 3-Year action steps toward a 10-year vision. Retrieved from http://www.amia.org/inside/releases/2007/tigerinitiative_report2007_color.pdf

Veninga, R. L. (1982). *The human side of health administration.* Englewood Cliffs, NJ: Prentice Hall.

Weiss, M. E., Hastings, W. J., Holly, D. C., & Craig, D. I. (1994). Using Roy's Adaptation Model in practice: Nursing perspectives. *Nursing Science Quarterly, 7*(2), 80–86.

Willoughby, D. (1995). The influence of psychosocial factors on women's adjustment to diabetes. (Doctoral dissertation, Georgia State University, 1995). *Dissertation Abstracts International,* 56(08B), 4247.

Zielstorff, R. D. (Ed.). (1982). *Computers in nursing.* Rockville, MD: Aspen Systems Corp.

Conferences

Fifth Annual Symposium at Computer Applications in Medical Care (SCAMC). (1981).

Healthcare Information and Management Systems Society (HIMSS) Annual Conference and Exhibition. (2007). *Evidence and Informatics Transforming Nursing: 3-Year Action Steps Toward a 10-Year Vision,* New Orleans, LA.

International Federation for Information Processing (IFIP), and the International Medical Informatics Association (IMIA). (1982). *The Impact of Computers in Nursing,* Harrogate, England.

National Institutes of Health (NIH). (1981). *First National Conference on Computer Technology and Nursing.*

National Institutes of Health (NIH). (1982). *Second National Conference on Computer Technology and Nursing.*

Technology Informatics Guiding Education Reform (TIGER) Summit. (2006). *Evidence and Informatics Transforming Nursing,* Bethesda, Maryland.

Relevant Web Sites for Nursing Languages

NANDA International, http://www.nanda.org/

Nursing Interventions Classifications, www.nursing.uiowa.edu/centers/cncce/

Home Health Care Classification, http://www.health.wa.gov.au/hacc/quality/docs/isd_nsig.pdf

Omaha System, http://www.omahasystem.org/systemo.htm

Nursing Outcomes Classification, www.nursing.uiowa.edu/centers/cncce/

PeriOperative Nursing Data Set, www.aorn.org

SNOMED CT, http://www.snomed.org/

International Classification of Nursing Practice, www.icn.ch/icnp.htm

ABC Codes, www.abccodes.com

Logical Observation Identifiers Names and Codes, www.loinc.org

Relevant Publications

Institute of Medicine. (2003). *Health professions education: A bridge to quality.* Washington, DC: National Academy Press.

Institute of Medicine. (2004). *Keeping patients safe: Transforming the work environment of nurses.* Washington, DC: National Academy Press.

Peterson, H. E., & Gerdin-Jelger, U. (1988). *Preparing nurses for using information*

systems: Recommended informatics competencies. New York: National League for Nursing.

Pravikoff, D., Pierce, S., & Tanner, A. (2003). Are nurses ready for evidence-based practice? *American Journal of Nursing, 103*(5), 95–96.

Pravikoff, D., Pierce, S., & Tanner, A. (2005). Readiness of U.S. nurses for evidence-based practice. *American Journal of Nursing, 105*(9), 40–52.

INDEX

Pages numbers followed by f indicate figure. Page numbers followed by t indicate table.

A